Advanced Concepts of Personal Training

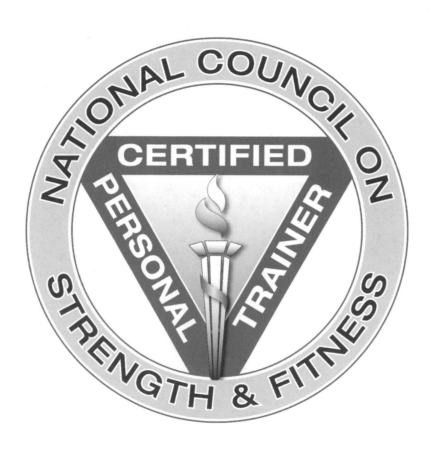

Brian D. Biagioli, EdD
Florida International University

Editorial Staff
Matthew Biagioli, MD
Wesley Smith, PhD
Sean Grieve, MS
Anthony Wyrwas, DC
Steven Wermus, MS

Book Development Staff
Paul Garbarino, MS
Tyler Poynton
B Glass Typography

© 2007 National Council on Strength & Fitness

Printed in the United States of America

Library of Congress Control Number: 2007925963

ISBN 978-0-9791696-0-1

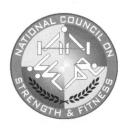

Table of Contents

Chapter 1

Functional Anatomy

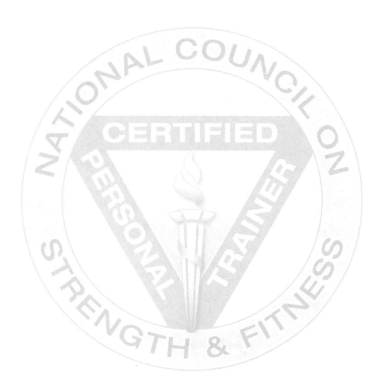

Knowledge of functional anatomy is critical to the success of the personal trainer. Because voluntary movement stems from the application of force produced by the muscle on the attached bone, having clear comprehension of the musculoskeletal structures and their function is fundamental to understanding human movement. Employing knowledge of the body's structures and how they work in a coordinated manner allows personal trainers to use appropriate decision-making criteria for individual exercise prescription.

Composition of Bones

The human skeletal system is uniquely designed to resist stress, providing shape and support to the body. The skeleton has a mineral component which provides rigidity, and a protein component that makes bone resistant to tension. The organic compounds or protein, mainly in the form of collagen fiber, represent 33% of bone, while the mineral component represents the other 67% (1). The resilience of the bony tissue makes the body capable of managing force, while the connective tissues provide for the application of force. Together, the tissues function to systematically produce and control motor function.

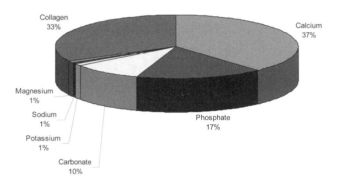

Bone tissue is hardened by calcium salts which represent approximately 98% of the calcium storage in the body. Although it is the most significant location of calcium in the body, bone is not simply mineral composite; it is actually very dynamic, with a fairly complex vascular system, which acts as a reservoir of calcium usable in the maintenance of extracellular calcium concentrations. When extracellular calcium levels fall too low, calcium is recruited from bone storage and mobilized to alternate physiological destinations based on the need of the internal environment. This process is a normal interchange by the body to maintain homeostasis. When daily calcium intake is insufficient for prolonged periods of time, bone stores of calcium become compromised as the mineral density declines. A significant reduction in bone mineral density causes a predisease condition called **osteopenia**, before progressing to the disease state called **osteoporosis**.

Sagittal Cross-Section of Bone

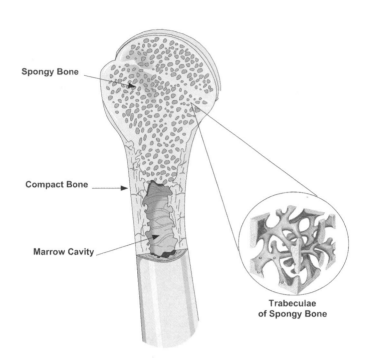

Trabeculae
of Spongy Bone

The skeleton is actually a system of levers, support structures, and struts which allow the body to maintain erect postural equilibrium, perform movement, and protectively house vital organs. The skeleton consists of two segments: 1) the axial skeleton which consists of the skull, hyoid bone, vertebral column, and rib cage; and 2) appendicular skeleton consisting of the limbs and their respective girdles. For the most part, the axial skeleton serves a protective role for the central nervous system, heart and lungs, and is the structural segment for erect posture, while the appendicular skeleton supports locomotion and everyday movements. Each segment is comprised of various bones to support its respective role and function.

The shape of a bone is specific to its purpose. Bones come in several shapes and sizes, which also define how they are classified. The bones of the arms and legs are long bones; in the hands and feet they are called short bones; the unique shape of the vertebra are called

~Key Terms~

Osteopenia- Refers to bone mineral density (BMD) that is lower than normal peak BMD but not low enough to be classified as osteoporosis.

Osteoporosis- Irreversible decrease in mineralized bony tissue.

irregular bones, while bones with a broad connective surface, like that of the scapulae, are called flat bones. As stated, each bone's shape has distinctions which support its function. Long bones, for instance, serve as levers that allow for bipedal movement and include an elongated diaphysis (shaft) which contains a significant marrow cavity where 2.5 million red blood cells are formed every second. Short bones make up the intricate formations of the hands (providing for dexterity) and feet (serving as a platform for postural balance). The flat bones allow for broad muscular attachments, which are often used to support significant force requirements, as seen with the insertion sites of the rhomboids on the scapula and pectoralis major on the sternum. Irregular bones are intended to manage uniquely designed muscle arrangements, as seen with the spiny process of the vertebrae. These bones support the numerous muscular attachments to the spine and function to accommodate the specific action capabilities of the trunk.

Bone Growth

The skeleton begins as a cartilaginous structure and is replaced by bone through a maturation process called ossification. Increases in bone mass (width or diameter) occur from the formation of new bone on the surface of existing bone tissue called **appositional growth**. During normal maturation, the bone increases in size and is remodeled by the removal and replacement of bone. Bone length is attributed to **endochondral growth,** where cartilage is ossified in the **epiphyseal plates** of long bones. As humans age, new cartilage is formed to promote growth that eventually turns to bone. Vertical growth ceases when no further cartilage is formed and the present cartilage becomes ossified. In most humans, 90% of bone mass is reached by age 18 (2). The integrity of bone is often measured by mass and density. **Bone mass** represents the surface area of bone, while **bone mineral density** reflects the concentration of minerals within bone.

To promote bone development, it is critical that children consume adequate vitamin D and calcium and participate in regular physical activities. Once bone mass has reached maturity, the mineral density is still subject to variations based upon diet and activity. Improvements in bone mineral density can be attained until approximately age thirty, at which time, genetics, behavior, and lifestyle become the primary factors dictating the rate of decline (2). One key factor in maintaining healthy bones is the application of resisted movement activities. There is a correlation between bone mineral density and the strength of the attached musculature, which suggests that resistance training can be an important activity used to maintain bone health (3). This holds true for all populations and age ranges. It is believed that skeletal benefits can be attained by even older adults and children via routine age-appropriate strengthening activities (2).

~Quick Insight~

Calcium ion concentration requires close management by the body to prevent dysfunction. Even small variations in calcium concentration can disrupt physiological function. For example, hypocalcemia (low blood calcium) can lead to neuromuscular excitability, muscle spasms and tetany, while hypercalcemia (high blood calcium) can cause abnormally high deposits of calcium phosphate in tissues leading to organ dysfunction and failure. Due to the key role calcium plays in motor neuron activities, calcium deficiency within the body can cause muscles to lose normal function, becoming unresponsive. This can be life threatening when cardiac muscle activity is altered. Fortunately, the calcium levels of the extracellular fluid are closely regulated by the endocrine system. During hypocalcemia, parathyroid hormone will cause increased intestinal absorption of calcium via activation of Vitamin D, tubular reabsorption of calcium from the kidneys, and release of calcium and phosphate from bone tissue. In contrast, hypercalcemia suppresses parathyroid hormone activity and leads to the secretion of calcitonin, which reduces urinary excretion of calcium and inhibits calcium loss from the bone. Therefore, prolonged dietary deficiency causes the calcium needs of the body to be met by the bone calcium stores, which reduces bone mineral density. When this activity parallels the natural loss of bone mass that occurs after age 30, the risk for bone disease is dramatically increased. Women will lose approximately 8% of bone mass (men 3%) naturally per decade from the aging process (2). Sex hormones are key endocrine factors in the maintenance of bone mineral density. Lower levels of circulatory estrogen increase the risk for developing osteoporosis, which is of particular concern for menopausal females. Males lose far less bone because of the relatively high amounts of androgens produced later in life (2). The bone disease *osteoporosis* occurs when bone function is compromised due to excessive bone loss. Commonly, the epiphyses (ends) of long bones, the vertebral column, hip, and jaw experience the greatest decline, placing these areas at high risk for fracture. Osteoporosis is linked to premature death due to functional decline. One out of two women and one out of four men will suffer from an osteoporotic fracture after age 50 (4). Approximately one out of four hip fracture patients die within one year after the hip fracture, commonly from pulmonary thrombosis due to the significant reduction in movement. It is estimated that the public health cost attributed to osteoporotic fractures is in excess of $17 billion annually, and approximately 90% of women and 50% of men will have osteoporosis before they die (5).

Resistance training activities performed by children and adolescents have raised concerns due to the potential risk of damage or premature ossification of the epiphyseal (growth) plates of long bones (6). The risk of epiphyseal fracture in children performing resistance exercise is equivocal as no clinical trials have demonstrated an adverse effect. However, due to the developmental stage of the bone and the stress associated with resisted movement it is believed there may be some increased vulnerability. Premature cessation of bone growth may be another potential adverse event associated with intense resistance training in children. The epiphyseal plates close naturally in response to high levels of sex hormones that exist during post-pubescence. Some theorize that the increased androgenic hormones produced in response to intense resistance training may promote a premature ossification of the epiphyseal plates, attenuating natural bone growth. Nevertheless, there is no clear evidence to support this notion. In fact, most physicians will encourage age-appropriate resistance activity when performed under supervision of a prudent professional. No clinical trial to date has indicated that appropriately applied resisted movement damages the epiphyseal plates of long bones. Analysis of bone stress during play, where jumping and landing activities are engaged in, shows that stress from daily activity supercedes that of controlled resisted activities such as squatting and pressing when performed with 10 RM resistance (7). Children and adolescents have greater risks to bone health from malnutrition, disease, and trauma.

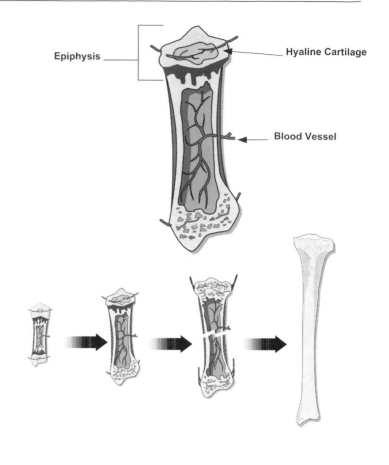

Illustration of Bone Growth

~Quick Insight~

Contrary to popular belief, bone is not static or inert. In fact, bone is extremely active, continually recycling and renewing the organic and mineral components in the process of remodeling. To remodel the bone matrix without weakening the bone, an interplay of supporting activities must occur between the bone cells: osteocytes, osteoblasts, and osteoclasts. In adult bones, the osteocytes are constantly removing and replacing the calcium salts, while the osteoblasts and osteoclasts manage the balance of forming new bone, while destroying old bone. In young adults, the annual turnover rate is about 20% of the skeleton (1). The bone remodeling occurs at selected areas within the bone, identifying areas for greater formation activity and areas where bone turnover is more suppressed.

This ability to turn over bone and manage the component salts allows the body to adapt to new stress. The theory supporting bone's ability to identify stress suggests osteoblasts are sensitive to electrical variations. When the bone is stressed, the electrical fields communicate to the osteoblasts to form more bone. This explains why a person performing weight training experiences bone enlargement at the site of the attachment to accommodate tissue hypertrophy and strength. Bones that experience heavy stress become thicker and stronger, whereas bones that do not experience stress weaken and become brittle. Recent evidence has demonstrated significant increases in bone stiffness and strength, as well as increased quantity and quality of trabecular bone in response to low-level, high frequency skeletal vibration (9,10). This experimental evidence supports the association between physical activity and bone cell activity. Moreover, vibratory stimulus may be a useful intervention in the future to treat osteoporosis or ameliorate bone loss in post-menopausal women (10).

Notable amounts of degenerative changes occur in a relatively short period of time when the body is inactive. In fact, an individual loses approximately a year of bone mass in one week of bed confinement (11). This explains why astronauts have a high risk for osteoporosis. Fortunately, bones regenerate about as quickly as they degenerate in response to acute changes in physical activity and weight-bearing or resisted movements. This again reinforces the need for daily physical activity and strength training exercise.

~Key Terms~

Appositional growth- Growth by the addition of new layers on those previously formed. Characteristic of tissue formed of rigid materials.

Endochondral growth- Process of bone formation whereby a cartilage model is replaced by bone.

Epiphyseal plates- Transverse cartilage plate near the end of a child's bone responsible for growth in length of the bone.

Bone mass- The volume of bone in the body measured by mineral content.

Bone mineral density- The mineral content in a given volume of bone, used as a measure of bony health and in the diagnosis of osteoporosis.

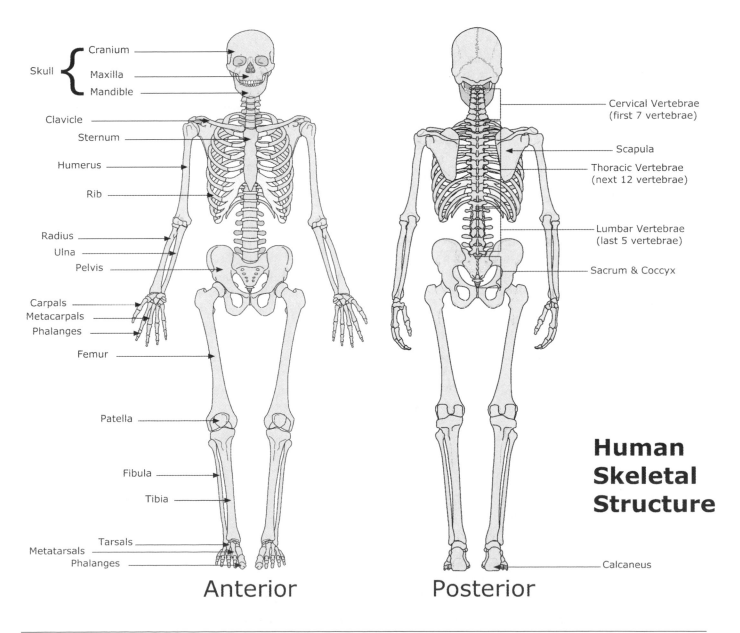

Human Skeletal Structure

Anterior

Posterior

Joint Classifications

The intersection of two bones is called an articulation or a **joint**. Depending on the role of the joint, its movement may have a broad range, such as the shoulder's glenohumeral joint, or it may be limited for structural purposes, such as the acromioclavicular joint. The structure of a joint relates to its movement capabilities. The more movement that is afforded to a joint, the more it is able to reduce friction.

The three major classifications of joints are **fibrous, cartilaginous**, and **synovial**. The connective tissue characteristics determine how they are classified. Fibrous joints are not intended to move, or exhibit very little movement, so they are tightly connected by fibrous tissue and do not possess a joint cavity. Cartilaginous joints unite articular surfaces with **hyaline cartilage** which allows for very slight movement, or **fibrocartilage** which has slightly greater movement capabilities due to the tissue's flexible nature. The primary role of the aforementioned joints is to support the structural integrity of the skeletal system or serve as connectors for growth. In contrast, synovial joints are designed to manage movement. To allow for the considerable movement range between articulating joints, synovial joints are more complex anatomically than fibrous and cartilaginous joints.

Synovial Joints

The joints of the appendicular skeleton are predominantly synovial to accommodate the movements required for locomotion and daily activity. Synovial joints rely on several mechanisms to reduce friction and maintain the joints' integrity when forces are applied. The articular surfaces are covered with hyaline cartilage which provides for a smooth surface at the site where the bones meet. In areas where compressive or shock forces are often applied, the surfaces are additionally supported by fibrocartilage and fat pads. The fibrocartilage forms **articular discs** which provide added strength and support to the joint, as for example the meniscus in the knee. The fat pads are often found around the edges of joints to provide protection for the cartilage. Each joint is enclosed by a dual layer **joint capsule**. The articular capsule is made up of fibrous tissue extending from the **periosteum** that covers the bone. The fibrous capsule may have thickened regions which provide ligamentous support to the joint. **Ligaments** and **tendons** may further add structural support to strengthen the joint. Lining the joint capsule is a **synovial membrane**. This inner lining secretes synovial fluid to form a thin lubricating film which covers the articular surfaces to further reduce the frictional coefficiency created by movement. In some synovial joints the lining extends to form a pocket or

sac called a **bursa**, which serves as a fluid filled cushion between surfaces to prevent contact or the rubbing of connective tissues during movement.

Synovial Joint

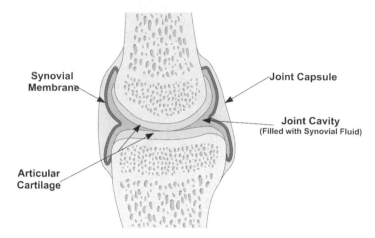

~Key Terms~

Joint- A point of articulation between two or more bones, especially such a connection that allows motion.

Fibrous joints- Consist of two bones that are united by fibrous tissue and exhibit little or no movement.

Cartilaginous joint- Unites two bones by means of either hyaline cartilage or fibrocartilage.

Synovial joints- Contain synovial fluid and allow for considerable movement between articulating bones.

Hyaline cartilage- A tough, elastic, fibrous connective tissue found in various parts of the body, such as the joints, outer ear, and larynx.

Fibrocartilage- Cartilage that allows for greater movement capabilities due to its flexible nature.

Articular discs- A plate or ring of fibrocartilage attached to the joint capsule and separating the articular surfaces of the bones.

Joint capsule- A sac enclosing a joint, formed by an outer fibrous membrane and an inner synovial membrane.

Periosteum- The dense fibrous membrane covering the surface of bones except at the joints and serving as an attachment for muscles and tendons.

Types of Synovial Joints

There are several types of synovial joints which are classified according to the shape of the adjoining articular surfaces. The six types of synovial joints include: Ball and Socket joints, which consist of a rounded articular surface of one bone that fits into the socket (cup shaped depression) of the corresponding bone, allowing for complementary movements (shoulder and hip); Plane or Gliding joints, consisting of two opposed flat surfaces that are relatively equal in size and may glide across or twist slightly over each other (spinal vertebrae); Hinge joints, which work by fitting a convex cylinder inside a concave articular surface, allowing for movement in a single plane (elbow and knee); Pivot joints, which restrict movement to rotation around a single axis (radius/ulna); Saddle joints, which have similarly shaped (saddle) articular surfaces which fit into one another, allowing for two planes of movement (thumb); and condyloid joints which are uniquely structured shallow ball and sockets with limited movement range similarly to a hinge (wrist).

The ability of the joint to move depends upon the muscular attachment location called the insertion site, the type of joint, and the shape of the articular surface. The joints that have the greatest mobility have the least stability and are often considered to be weak when compared to limited moving synovial or non-moving fibrous and cartilaginous joints. The shoulder or glenohumeral joint is a good example. Although freely moving, the shoulder joint loses stability when fully abducted, flexed, or externally rotated. The body has put defense mechanisms in place to help manage the risk for injury in highly moveable joints by attempting to limit movement range. This is accomplished by the location of fibrous connective fibers in and around the joint capsule, the particular shape of the articulating surface in relation to the muscle attachment sites, the presence of other structures including disks and fat pads, and the activity of proprioceptors that manage muscle and tendon tension. When these mechanisms can not manage an external force, a joint may dislocate, causing the articular surfaces to come apart. This may damage the joint capsule, articular cartilage, and ligaments. Individuals with extremely flexible joints are often referred to as having **joint laxity** or **hypermobility** and should strengthen the surrounding

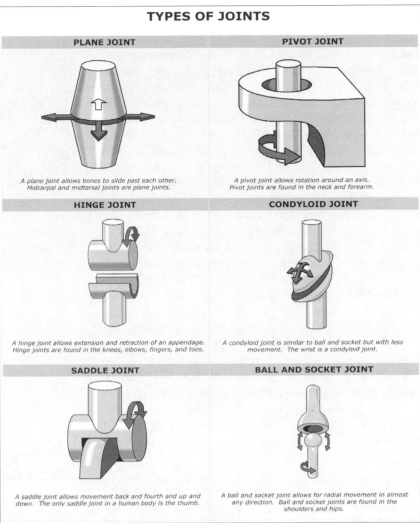

TYPES OF JOINTS

PLANE JOINT

A plane joint allows bones to slide past each other. Midcarpal and midtarsal joints are plane joints.

PIVOT JOINT

A pivot joint allows rotation around an axis. Pivot joints are found in the neck and forearm.

HINGE JOINT

A hinge joint allows extension and retraction of an appendage. Hinge joints are found in the knees, elbows, fingers, and toes.

CONDYLOID JOINT

A condyloid joint is similar to ball and socket but with less movement. The wrist is a condyloid joint.

SADDLE JOINT

A saddle joint allows movement back and fourth and up and down. The only saddle joint in a human body is the thumb.

BALL AND SOCKET JOINT

A ball and socket joint allows for radial movement in almost any direction. Ball and socket joints are found in the shoulders and hips.

tissues to encourage stability and be cautious during high force activities (8).

~Key Terms~

Ligaments- Tough fibrous band of connective tissue that supports internal organs and holds bones together properly in joints.

Tendons- A tough band of fibrous connective tissue that connects muscles to bones.

Synovial membrane- A layer of connective tissue which lines the joint and produces synovial fluid.

Bursa- A bursa is a tiny fluid-filled sac that functions as a gliding surface to reduce friction between tissues of the body.

Hypermobility- Describes joints that stretch further than is normal.

How Joints Work

Joints move when internal forces or external forces are applied to the skeleton. Voluntary movements require muscles to contract in a coordinated manner to produce internal forces which act on the bone. Muscle connects to bone by tendons which extend from the musculotendinous junction at the muscles end to the periosteum, a fibrous connective tissue which makes up the outer surface of the bone. The periosteum isolates the bone from surrounding tissues and encases a network of nerves and vessels which provides nutrients and participates in bone remodeling. Near joints, the periosteum becomes continuous with connective tissue to hold bones together and form the joint capsule. The fibers of the periosteum are also interwoven with the tendons that attach to the bone. The connective tissues are further secured to the bone by collagen fibers, which provide for an extremely strong attachment. So strong that an exertion of force beyond the tissue's strength will most often break a bone before snapping the collagen fibers at the bone's surface. This tension is monitored by special neuronal cells (golgi tendon organs) which send reflexive signals back to the spinal cord. These signals are part of a protective mechanism involving inhibitory signals to the contracting muscle when the tension on the bone reaches a critical threshold prior to damage (see Chapter 4 for more detail).

On the other end of the tendon, connective tissue is structured in a way that produces and manages efficient force development. The muscle anatomy that causes movement is arranged to serve several purposes. The obvious first role of skeletal muscle is to pull on the tendons attached to the skeleton for movement. The skeletal muscles also must produce tension to maintain posture and sustain body positions. In addition, skeletal muscles serve to support soft tissues, such as the visceral organs, guard entrances and exits, including the digestive and urinary tracts for swallowing, defecation, and urination, as well as assist the maintenance of body temperature by releasing heat.

Skeletal Muscle Architecture

Skeletal muscles are organized into several layers. The outer layer is the **muscle fascia,** which is a fibrous connective tissue that separates individual muscles, and in some cases muscle groups, providing shape to the arranged fibers it contains and maintaining intramuscular tension. Just beneath the fascia is the epimysium, which is a dense collection of collagen fibers covering the entire surface of the muscle. Inside the epimysium lie bundles of fibers enclosed by the perimysium. Each bundle is called a fasciculus, which contains packages of muscle fibers called myofibrils.

Muscle Fiber Anatomy

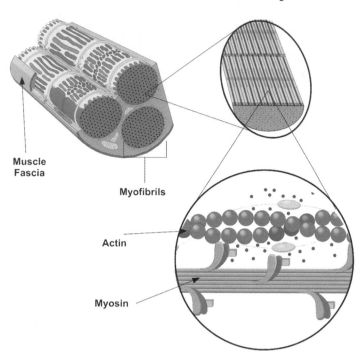

Muscle Fascia

Myofibrils

Actin

Myosin

Myofibrils are made up of long cylinder-like muscle fibers (muscle cells). The individual muscle fibers are encompassed by the endomysium. The muscle fibers are further encased by sarcolemma, a delicate external lamina of reticular fibers which serves as an extension of the muscle fiber for connective purposes. The individual muscle fibers themselves can be further broken down to their constituent parts, called **myofibrils**. The myofibrils are comprised of proteins called **myofilaments**, which set the actions of the muscle into motion. The thick myofilaments are **myosin,** and the thin filaments are **actin**. Together, actin and myosin are arranged in functional sequence along the myofibril and are used to create tension inside the muscle tissue.

Each subsequent layer of muscle tissue maintains an intricate network of nerve and circulatory branches to fuel and run the muscle cell operations. This enables the muscle tissue to efficiently manage neural information while satisfying energy and oxygen requirements of the working tissue. When tissue is trained, it responds with cellular enhancements to allow the body to adapt to the demands of the stress. By now, it should be fairly clear that there is a close-knit relationship between the tissues within a system.

~Key Terms~

Muscle fascia- Thickened connective tissue that envelops a muscle or a group of muscles.

Myofibrils- Thread-like fibrils that make up the contractile part of a striated muscle fiber.

Myofilaments- Filaments, made up of actin and myosin, that are the structural units of a myofibril.

Myosin- A contractile protein in muscle cells, responsible for the elastic and contractile properties of muscle. It is commonly referred to as the thick contractile protein.

Actin- A protein found in muscle that together with myosin functions in muscle contraction. It is commonly referred to as the thin contractile protein.

Spatial and Directional Terminology

When the musculoskeletal system is put into action, the outcome is often dynamic. Contractile forces extending from the myofilaments make their way through the muscle fibers to the muscle's epimysium and fascia, pulling on the tendon. This in turn, pulls on the bone to put action into a joint. When voluntary movement occurs at a given joint, the movement will be specific to the location of the contractile force, the shape of the joint, and the structures that act on the joint. In most cases, anatomical movement either occurs to move a body segment away from the body or back to the body. Although this is well illustrated when viewed with regard to basic anatomical positions, there are occasional exceptions.

Describing the actions or motions of synovial joints requires anatomical terminology. For instance, lifting the arm could apply to abduction, flexion, extension, and even rotation depending on the start position and the plane of movement where the action occurs. These directional terms are applied to anatomical structures and function.

Describing movement anatomically requires both the starting position, axis of joint rotation and the plane in which the movement occurs. **Anatomical position** is the standard reference position for the body when describing locations, positions, and movements of limbs or other anatomical structures. Anatomical position is assumed when the body is standing with erect posture, facing forward with both feet aligned parallel and the toes forward, the arms and hands hanging below the shoulders at the side with the elbows and fingers extended, palms facing forward. From this reference position, spatial and direction terms can be easily applied.

Positional Lines and Movement Planes

Spatial term comprehension and accuracy can be further enhanced by the defined lines of origin along the anatomical position. These lines correspond with the planes of movement. The line that dissects the body down the center, splitting it into side by side halves, is called the **Midline,** which lies along the **Sagittal Plane**. When that line is shifted over to align with the crease of the arm it is referred to as the **Anterior Axillary Line**. If the line dissected the body into front and back halves, it would be called the **Midaxillary Line,** which runs along the **Frontal Plane**. The last plane is called the **Transverse Plane.** It runs side to side and anterior to posterior, dissecting the body into superior (top) and inferior (bottom) parts. Sometimes the word cardinal, or cross, is attached to planes to identify the center of gravity of the body. Planes will be further reviewed under movement terminology.

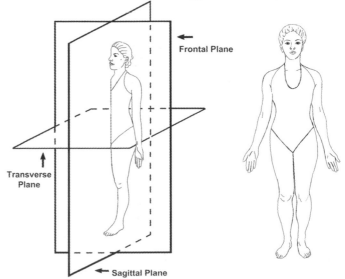

Movement Planes   **Anatomical Position**

Spatial Terms

When spatial terms are used they may be referencing location or direction. They describe the area of space relative to the body's anatomical position. For instance, if something is in front of the body or the body segment moves forward, the space descriptor for the movement or location would be **anterior**. If the location of space is behind the body or a segment of the body is moved backward, the space location would be **posterior**. In some cases, other words can be used to describe the same area of space. For instance, anterior is synonymous with **ventral** and posterior is synonymous with **dorsal**. This may also occur when spatial terms are used as directional movement terms, as is the case with **medial**, **internal**, and **inward rotation**, or **lateral, external**, and **outward rotation**. When applied to rotation, these terms have a synonymous relationship. **Medial** refers to the direction or location toward, or closer to, the midline, while **lateral** refers to a position or movement away from, or farther from, the midline of the body.

When locating a point or direction along a limb, the terms **proximal** and **distal** are used. Proximal refers to the direction or location close to where the limb attaches to the body. Distal refers to the point toward the end of the limb or location farthest away from the limb's attachment site. When the limbs are viewed from a particular side, they are often referenced by the terms **ipsilateral** (same side) and **contralateral** (opposite side) rather than left or right side. The terms **superficial** and **deep** also refer to locations on (or within) the body. The location descriptors refer to positions relative to the exterior surface of the body. The superficial layers of tissue, for instance, lie just below the skin, while deep tissues are more internally located in reference to the skin layer. So, one might refer to the deep muscles of the spine or identify the trapezius as superficial to the rhomboids. Another way to view it is a superficial or surface wound, compared to a deep wound.

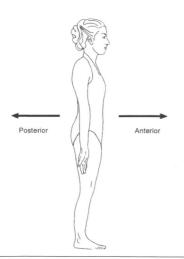

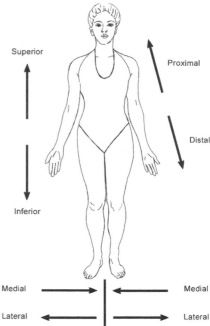

When the terms are applied to movement, the planes and axes of motion are applied to the anatomical positions and often reference spatial descriptors to add conciseness to the movement description. The three movement planes dissect the body, each with a corresponding axis that passes perpendicularly through the plane. The sagittal plane is probably the most referenced due to the number of activities and movements the body performs in the plane. The two dimensional surface connects anterior to posterior and superior to inferior, in layman's terms it runs front to back and top to bottom. The axis that corresponds with the sagittal plane is the **transverse axis**. The frontal, or coronal, plane dissects the body into front and back. It runs side to side and superior to inferior (top to bottom). The respective plane of movement is the **anteroposterior axis**. The transverse plane runs perpendicular to the sagittal plane, splitting the body into top and bottom. The axis of rotation for the transverse plane is called the **longitudinal axis**.

With the planes and axes of rotation defined, the application of movements can be described accurately. The movements can be categorized by the plane that they occur in. Movements around the transverse axis (sagittal plane) include **flexion, extension, hyperextension, plantar flexion,** and **dorsi flexion**. The joint movements that occur around the anteroposterior axis (frontal plane) include **abduction, adduction, lateral flexion** (right and left), **inversion, eversion, radial deviation,** and **ulnar deviation**. The longitudinal axis (transverse plane) perpetuates different types of rotational movements. These include **internal** and **external rotation, supination, pronation, horizontal abduction,** and **horizontal adduction**.

Positional Terms

Anatomical Position- A reference posture used in anatomical description in which the subject stands erect with feet parallel and arms adducted and supinated, with palms facing forward.

Midline- The median plane of the body.

Anterior Axillary Line - Crease of the axilla (underarm).

Midaxillary line- A perpendicular line drawn downward from the apex of the axilla.

Anterior- Placed before or in front.

Posterior- Located behind a part or toward the rear of a structure.

Proximal- Situated nearest to point of attachment or origin.

Distal- Situated farthest from point of attachment or origin, as of a limb or bone.

Medial- At, in, near, or being the center; dividing a person into right and left halves.

Lateral- Situated or extending away from the medial plane of the body.

Ipsilateral- On, or relating to, the same side of the body.

Contralateral- On, or relating to, the opposite side of the body.

Superficial- Shallow proximity in relation to a surface.

Deep- Extending inward in relation to a surface layer.

Movement Definitions

Flexion - To bend; in hinge joints, the articulating bones move closer together; in ball and socket joints, the limb moves anterior to the midaxillary line.

Extension - To straighten or extend; in hinge joints the articulating bones move away from each other; in ball and socket joints, the limb moves posterior to the midaxillary line.

Lateral Flexion - Spinal movement to the left or right occurs at the neck and trunk.

Protraction - Movement of a structure toward the anterior surface in a straight horizontal line.

Retraction - Movement back to the anatomical position or additionally, posterior to functional range of motion.

Dorsi Flexion - Movement of the ball of the foot towards the shin.

Plantar Flexion - Foot movement towards the plantar surface.

Pronation - Unique rotation of the forearm which crosses the radius and ulna. The palm faces posterior. (Prone means lying face down.)

Supination - Unique rotation of the forearm where the radius and ulna uncross. The palms face anteriorly. (Supine means lying face up.)

Inversion - Confined to the ankle; consists of turning the ankle so the plantar surface of the foot faces medially

Eversion - Confined to the ankle; consists of turning the ankle so the plantar surface of the foot faces laterally.

Abduction - Movement away from the midline.

Adduction - Movement toward the midline.

Anatomical Movements

Trunk & Neck

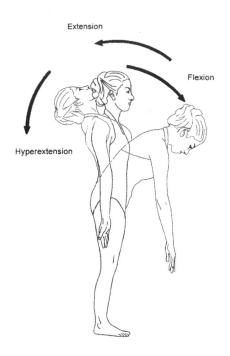

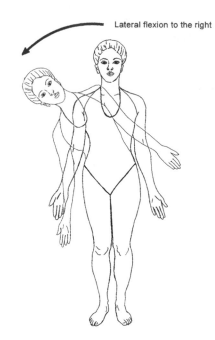

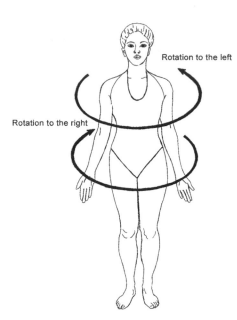

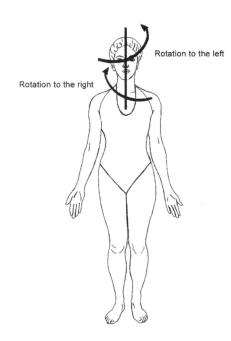

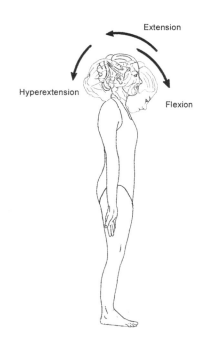

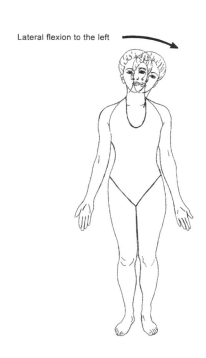

Shoulder

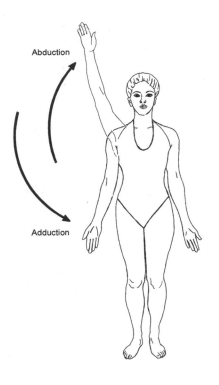

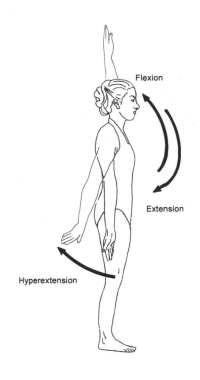

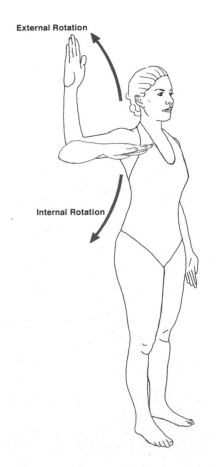

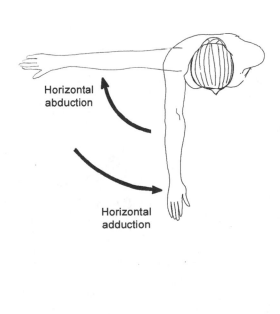

<u>Elbow & Wrist</u>

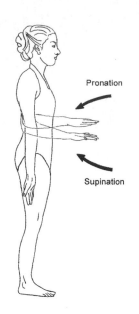
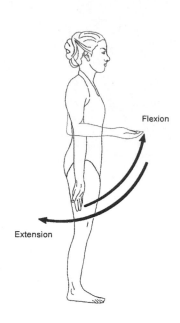
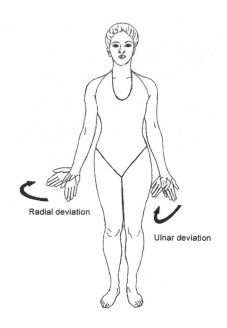

<u>Hip</u>

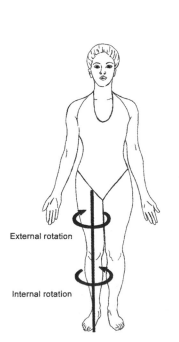
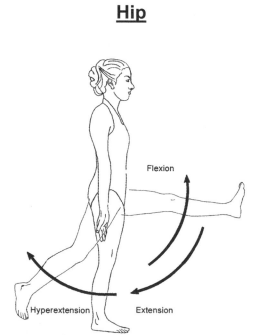
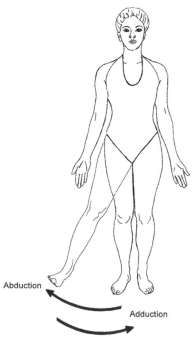

Knee & Ankle

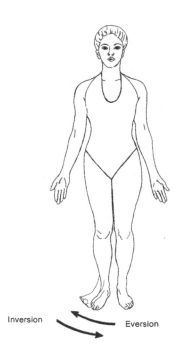

Inversion   Eversion

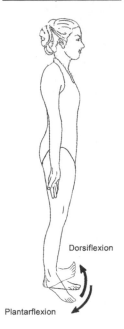

Dorsiflexion

Plantarflexion

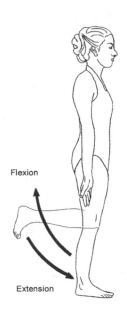

Flexion

Extension

~Movement Definitions~

As previously stated, joint function is dictated by its architecture and the surrounding connective tissue. The joint's actions are largely determined, both in direction and range, by the articulating surfaces of the intersecting bone. The ball and socket joints, for instance, allow for significant movement, whereas a hinge joint has restrictions in both direction and range to prevent injury to the connective tissue. Bone impingement, ligament attachment sites, and elasticity are the primary contributors to joint range of motion. Muscle and tendon tissue are secondary contributors. The extent and frequency of joint use will determine the motion range of these structures. The muscle and fascia are considered to have a visco-elastic property (12). That is, the tissue can be stretched and lengthened and then can return to its original length again. But instead of being simply elastic with rapid changes in length, it is a more gradual viscous process; like a thick fluid (ketchup) changing length gradually and slowly.

The appendicular skeletal muscles are the most commonly targeted in resistance exercise prescriptions. For example, muscles of the shoulder joint, shoulder girdle, the elbow, and wrist as well as the pelvis, hip, knee, and ankle are commonly the only muscles included in a selectorized weight training circuit. In contrast, the axial skeletal joint movements predominantly come from the spine. Since spinal position will affect the movement capabilities of the appendicular joints, it will be discussed first.

Ulnar deviation– Joint action at the wrist that causes the hand to move medially toward the little finger in the frontal plane.

External rotation– Action at the shoulder and hip joint where the articulating bone is rotated away from the body from anatomical position.

Internal rotation- Action at the shoulder and hip joint where the articulating bone is rotated toward the body from anatomical position.

Circumduction– Multiple-axis joint action where flexion is combined with abduction, and then adduction or extension and hyperextension are combined with abduction and then adduction.

Elevation– Superior movement of the bone.

Depression– Inferior movement of the bone.

Horizontal abduction– Movement away from the midline in the transverse plane.

Horizontal adduction– Movement toward the midline in the transverse plane.

Rotation– The turning of a structure around its long axis.

Radial deviation– Joint action at the wrist that causes the hand to move laterally toward the thumb in the frontal plane.

Spine and Neck

The vertebral column is composed of five regions serving a variety of functions, including support and movement of the head and trunk, protection for the spinal cord, allowing nerve outlets from the spinal cord, and providing sites for muscle attachment. The five segments include seven (7) cervical vertebrae, twelve (12) thoracic vertebrae, five (5) lumbar vertebrae, one (1) sacral bone (5 fused vertebrae) and one (1) coccygeal bone (4 or 5 fused vertebrae). In addition to the regions, the vertebral column has four major curvatures that assist in shock absorption and movement. The cervical and lumbar regions have lordotic curvature, represented by a natural concavity. If the forward curvature is exaggerated in an undesirable manner, it is termed **lordosis**. The curvature of the thoracic and sacral spine is convex or kyphotic. When the thoracic spine experiences an exaggerated curvature, it is referred to as being in a state of **kyphosis,** as is commonly seen in elderly populations. The exaggerated curves are detrimental to the function of the articulations within the area as well as those joints that depend on spinal position for proper function. For instance, a person with a structural kyphosis will lose range of motion in the shoulder complex and shoulder joint. Try rounding your back and externally rotating your arm. Range of motion capabilities of the shoulder will significantly decline. When the term **neutral spine** is applied, it refers to the state of functional curvature seen in an erect posture.

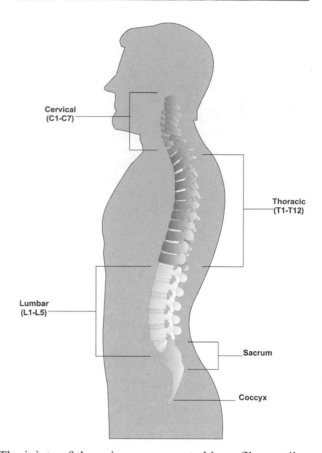

Spinal Curves

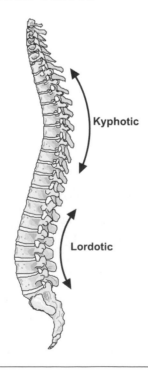

The joints of the spine are separated by a fibrocartilage **intervertebral disc** which provides support and prevents the bone surfaces from making contact. The discs are comprised of an outer annulus, which encases the gelatinous disc nucleus-pulposus, looking much like a fried egg. With age, the discs become more compressed and gradually lose water, which decreases the cushioning capabilities and explains the shortening phenomenon that occurs as a person gets older (13). If the disc is compressed from repetitive microtrauma or blunt trauma it may bulge or herniate. This often causes a partial or complete release of the nucleus pulposus. The bulging or herniated portion may impinge upon the spinal nerves compromising their function and causing pain. The design of the motion segments of the spine allows the spine to perform several movements. The spine is capable of flexion and extension (hyperextension) of the trunk, lateral flexion of the neck and trunk, as well as rotation of the trunk and head. In many cases, the spinal movements are enjoined with movements of the appendicular skeleton to allow for the completion of everyday movements, as well as those engaged in during sports and other physical activities. Limitations in the movement of these articulations often lead to premature functional decline (13). With age, the ability to extend and rotate the spine is often reduced due to lack of use.

Motion Segment

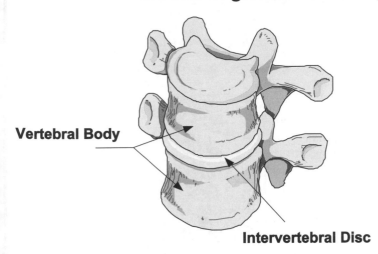

Vertebral Body

Intervertebral Disc

~Key Terms~

Lordosis- Anterior curvature of the spine, creating a swayback appearance.

Kyphosis- An abnormal convex (outward) curvature of the upper portion of the spinal column, sometimes called a humpback or hunchback.

Neutral spine- A spinal position that retains the three natural curves: a small lordotic curve at the base of the neck, a small kyphotic curve at the middle back, and a small lordotic curve in the low back.

Intervertebral disc- A fibrocartilaginous disc serving as a cushion between the vertebrae of the spinal column.

~Quick Insight~

Disc damage and injury can lead to physical debilitation. A disc does not always become damaged from a single dose of excessive force. In fact, most disc related injuries occur from repetitive microtrauma (13, 14). If a heavy object is suspended in the air from a thick rope, and the rope is hit by something as blunt as a butter knife, the thickness of the rope will prevent the object from falling. But if the rope is struck with the object in the same place everyday for a year, its integrity will eventually become compromised to the point that it can no longer hold the weight of the object, and it will break. This is analogous to what happens with people who experience back pain and disc problems. The daily stress from poor movement biomechanics, poor posture, muscle weakness and tightness, and poor lifting techniques eventually wear down the ligaments and supporting structures so that when a single high force event occurs, the disc is damaged.

In most cases, the discs at the greatest risk are in the lordotic curvatures of the spine, specifically between C5-C6, L4-L5, and most commonly L5-S1. The reason for the frequent occurrence of injury in these areas is that these are the vertebral segments with the greatest movement capabilities (2, 14). They often experience anterior, posterior, and/or lateral compressive forces from the aforementioned contributing factors. When the disc is damaged and the nucleus pulposus breaks through the annulus fibrosus, it penetrates the vertebral canal distorting sensory nerves and effecting sensory function. Additionally, the protruding section compresses the nerve roots, causing severe pain often leading to abnormal posture and radiating sensation through the lower back and limbs. In some cases, the compressed nerve loses its ability to properly innervate muscle tissue, and a partial loss of muscle control is experienced (15).

The radiating sensations often identify the area of injury. A herniation between L5-S1 is most often felt in the posterior aspects of the buttocks, upper leg, calf, and the bottom of the foot (15). A herniation between L4-L5 tends to cause more laterally experienced discomfort, including the lateral hip and lateral posterior portion of the leg, lateral surface of the calf, and top of the foot. Most therapies for lumbar disc herniation include pain medication, rest, braces, and physical therapy. Only about 10% of the disc herniations are treated with surgery to repair the damaged area (15).

Spinal & Trunk Musculature

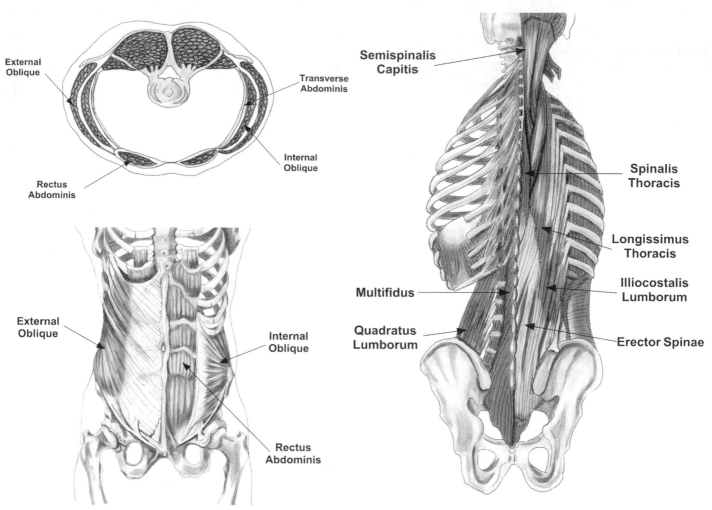

Cross Sectional View

External Oblique

Transverse Abdominis

Internal Oblique

Rectus Abdominis

Anterior View

External Oblique

Internal Oblique

Rectus Abdominis

Semispinalis Capitis

Spinalis Thoracis

Longissimus Thoracis

Illiocostalis Lumborum

Multifidus

Erector Spinae

Quadratus Lumborum

Posterior View

Trunk Muscles	Movement Function	Example Exercise
Rectus Abdominis	Trunk Flexion	Ab curl-up
External Oblique	Flexes and rotates vertebral column	Diagonal chop
Internal Oblique	Flexes and rotates vertebral column	Cable torso twist
Transverse Abdominis	Compresses abdomen	Draw in
Erector Spinae Group	Extends vertebral column	Good morning
Quadratus Lumborum	Abducts vertebral column	Lateral flexion

Pelvic Positioning

The pelvis has a relationship with the spine, based on the movements that occur, mainly at the lumbosacral joint, which is formed by the pelvis and lowest lumbar vertebrae. When the spine of the ilium is rotated forward, the movement is termed an **anterior pelvic tilt**. When the same anatomy is rotated backward, the pelvis is considered to be in a **posterior pelvic tilt**. When these movements are performed, they change the curvature of the spine. An anterior pelvic tilt increases the convexity (lordosis) of the lumbar spine which, consequently, may place excessive stress on the posterior aspect of the discs in the region. A posterior pelvic tilt reduces the convexity, flattening the lumbar spine. This interaction of the pelvis and spine points to the need to properly control the pelvis when lifting resistance or maintaining posture for prolonged periods of time. Weakness or tightness in the muscles that attach to the pelvis and spine can lead to pelvic instability, often manifesting into low back pain.

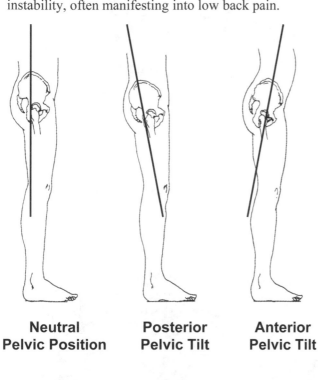

| Neutral | Posterior | Anterior |
| Pelvic Position | Pelvic Tilt | Pelvic Tilt |

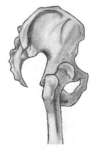 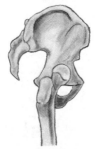 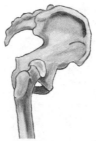

| Posterior | Neutral | Anterior |
| Pelvic Tilt | Pelvic Position | Pelvic Tilt |

~Quick Insight~

Due to the importance of pelvic control, it is important to maintain a healthy balance in the muscles that act on the articulating bones. Tightness in the hip flexors (iliopsoas muscle group) often pulls the pelvis forward and increases lumbar convexity due to the insertions of the psoas major and iliacus. The gluteus maximus muscle, if tight, may pull the pelvis into a posterior tilt particularly in conjunction with hip flexion. If this muscle is weak, the pelvis may gravitate forward, contributing to anterior tilt. Likewise, the quadratus lumborum, which attaches the pelvis and lumbar vertebrae laterally, may pull on the pelvis, reducing the stability in the frontal plane.

Shoulder

The glenohumeral joint is a ball and socket joint which allows for the most movement of any joint. As previously mentioned, the shallow glenoid fossa allows for substantial movement capabilities by the humerus. In the hip, these same movements are more closely limited by the articulating surfaces of the joint, causing it to be more stable. For instance, abduction at the shoulder joint far surpasses the 45 degrees attainable at the hip. In humeral or shoulder flexion, the arm can be raised far above the shoulder when the hand is held in neutral position. Additionally, the joint allows for movement in all planes including flexion, extension, hyperextension, abduction, adduction, horizontal adduction, horizontal abduction, internal and external rotation, and **circumduction**. The vast movement capabilities decrease the stability due to a reduced contact area. To counteract the lack of stability, the body uses three sets of ligaments and four muscles, which collectively make up the rotator cuff. The rotator cuff, which is comprised of the supraspinatus, infraspinatus, teres minor, and subscapularis, also serve to assist movement at the shoulder. The teres minor and infraspinatus extend and externally rotate the humerus, the supraspinatus abducts the humerus to 30 degrees, while the subscapularis extends and medially rotates the humerus.

~Key Terms~

Anterior pelvic tilt- Anterior pelvic movement, originating from the lumboscacral joint and affecting the curvature of the spine.

Posterior pelvic tilt- A posterior pelvic movement, originating from the lumboscacral joint and affecting the curvature of the spine.

Shoulder Musculature

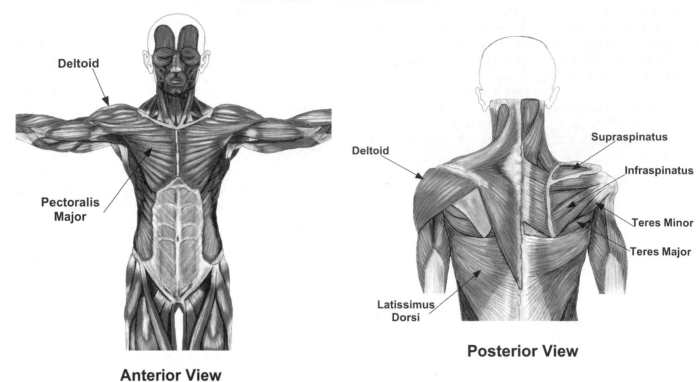

Anterior View

Posterior View

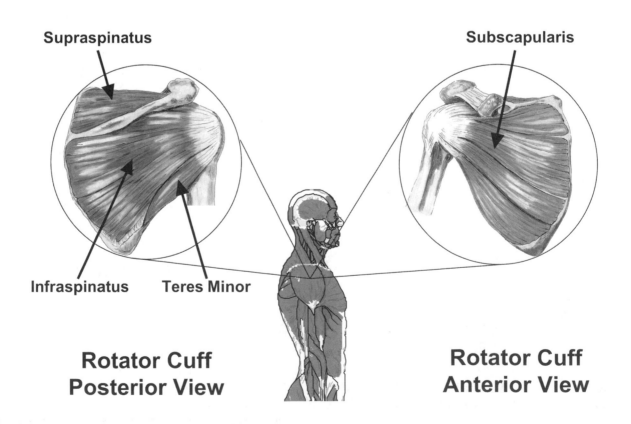

**Rotator Cuff
Posterior View**

**Rotator Cuff
Anterior View**

Shoulder Muscles	Movement Function	Example Exercise
Deltoids	Horizontally abduct, flex, extend, and rotate humerus	Side raise
Latissimus dorsi	Adduct, medially rotate, and extend humerus	Pull up
Pectoralis major	Horizontally adduct, flex, extend, and medially rotate humerus	Bench press
Teres major	Adduct, extend, and medially rotate humerus	Single arm row
Coracobrachialis	Adduct and flex humerus	Front raise
Infraspinatus	Extend and externally rotate humerus	External band rotation
Subscapularis	Extend and internally rotate humerus	Internal band rotation
Supraspinatus	Abduct humerus	Empty can raise
Teres minor	Adduct and externally rotate humerus	External band rotation

~Quick Insight~

The rotator cuff muscle group is very important to the health and integrity of the shoulder joint. Injuries to the rotator cuff are common in both the sedentary population and active population, which suggest the tissue often has deficiencies. Additional concerns arise when the external accelerators and decelerators are imbalanced or are considerably stronger than the appropriate strength balance between the stabilizers and prime movers of a joint. Rotator exercises should be included in any comprehensive exercise program to prevent these imbalances and associated pain, instability, and injury.

Shoulder Girdle

The movements of the shoulder girdle complement the actions of the glenohumeral joint. Rather than a single joint, the shoulder girdle is a joint complex that includes the articulations between the sternum and clavicle and the clavicle and the scapula. The movements, defined by scapular action, can be performed without shoulder joint movement but most often are employed to enhance the movements of the shoulder. Although gliding movements occur at the respective articulations of the sternoclavicular (sternum and clavicle) and acromioclavicular (scapula and clavicle) joints, the actual movement terms are applied to actions of the scapula. The scapula can be elevated and depressed, abducted (protracted) and adducted (retracted), and rotated upward and downward. As mentioned, these movements are often combined with shoulder movements. For instance, the scapula may be adducted while the humerus is hyperextended to allow for the action of a seated row, or the scapula may be depressed and rotated downward while the arm is adducted to allow for the movements of the lat pulldown. These movements should be taught for correct exercise performance.

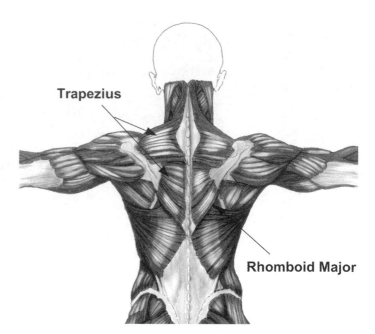

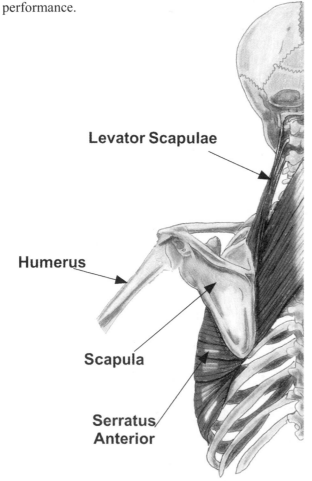

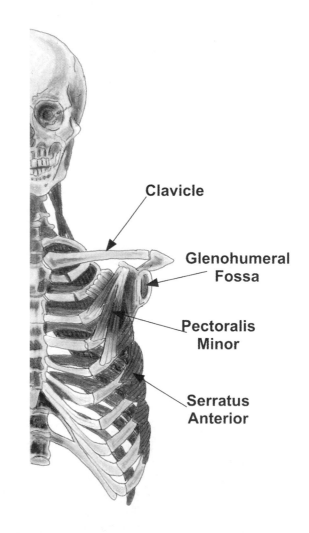

Posterior View   **Anterior View**

Shoulder Girdle Muscles	Movement Function	Exercise
Trapezius	Elevates, depresses, rotates, and fixes scapula; extends neck	Shoulder shrug
Rhomboid major	Retracts, rotates, and fixes scapula	Seated row
Pectoralis minor	Depresses scapula	Chest flyes
Levator scapulae	Elevates and retracts scapula; abducts neck	High row

Elbow

The elbow joint, like the knee, is a hinge joint which allows for flexion and extension of the arm. The bicep muscle crosses the elbow and attaches to the radius to allow for arm flexion. The triceps muscle crosses the elbow and attaches to the ulna to straighten or extend the arm. The elbow is very stable because the surface of the humerus and ulna interlock; if a person can hyperextend their arm it is due to the irregular shape of their articulating surfaces. The elbow is most at risk when a person falls and uses the arm to brace the impact.

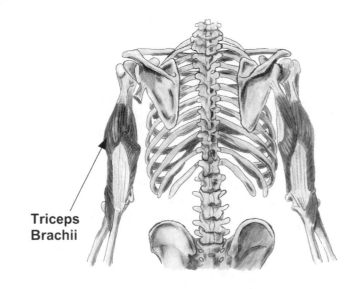

Triceps Brachii

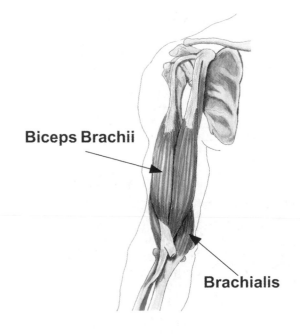

Biceps Brachii

Brachialis

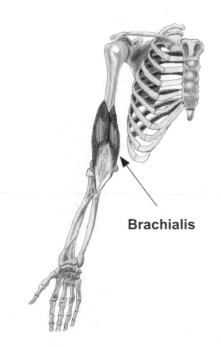

Brachialis

Radioulnar Joint

The radius and ulna of the forearm come together to form a pivot joint which allows the bone to cross and uncross so the hand is supinated (facing forward) or pronated (facing backward). When supinated, the radius and ulna are parallel; when pronated, the radius lies across the top of the ulna. Hand position variations when lifting will change the resistive load application to different structures. For instance, if the arm is flexed and hand pronated, the brachioradialis performs more work. If the hand is supinated during arm flexion (bicep curl) the bicep brachii experiences greater resistive force.

Wrist

The movements of the wrist generally occur in two planes, which allow for radial and ulnar deviation, also called abduction and adduction, in the frontal plane, and flexion and extension in the sagittal plane from the anatomical position. The wrist has the ability to hyperextend, which occurs as the back of the hand moves closer to the top of the forearm from a neutral wrist position. Forceful extension of the wrist over time can result in wrist extensor inflammation called tennis elbow (16).

Elbow Joint Muscles	Movement Function	Exercise
Biceps brachii	Flexes arm	Bicep curl
Brachialis	Flexes arm	Reverse grip curl
Brachioradialis	Flexes arm	Hammer curl
Triceps brachii	Extends arm	Cable pushdown

Wrist Muscles	Movement Function	Exercise
Flexor carpi radialis	Flexes and abducts wrist	Wrist curls
Flexor carpi ulnaris	Flexes and adducts wrist	Wrist curls
Extensor carpi radialis	Exends and abducts wrist	Rev. wrist curls
Extensor carpi ulnaris	Extends and adducts wrist	Rev. wrist curls

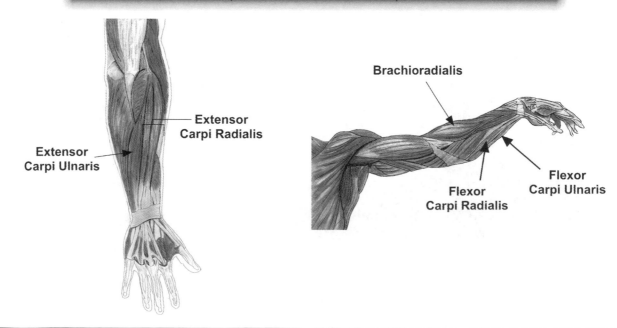

Hip

Movements of the hip occur at the articular surface of the acetabulum and femoral head. Due to its connective make-up, the joint capsule of the hip is very dense, providing for strength and stability. The shape of the joint, organization of the articular capsule, and four broad ligament attachments supporting the ball and socket joint ensure the femoral head stays securely inside the acetabulum. The hip joint allows for similar movements as the shoulder joint. The hip can flex, extend, hyperextend, abduct, adduct, and internally and externally rotate. It has greater limitations to its specific range of motion in some movements due to the deeper socket and supportive connective structures. For instance, bone impingement limits true hip abduction to about 45 degrees and hyperextension of the hip is limited in range compared to that of the shoulder. In young adults, the hip is injured less frequently than the shoulder because the comparable decrease in mobility encourages greater stability (16).

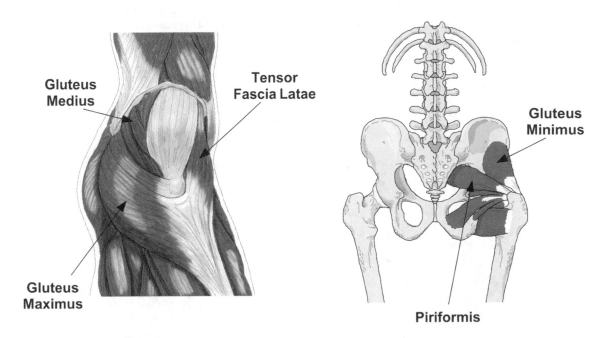

Hip Muscles	Movement Function	Example Exercise
Psoas major	Flexes thigh (hip)	Knee raise
Iliacus	Flexes and medially rotates thigh (hip)	Diagonal knee raise
Gluteus maximus	Extends, adducts, and laterally rotates thigh	Squat
Gluteus medius	Abducts and medially rotates thigh	Lateral squat
Gluteus minimus	Abducts and medially rotates thigh	Lateral squat
Tensor fascia latae	Abducts and medially rotates thigh	Supine leg abduction
Piriformis	Laterally rotates and abducts thigh	Rotational step outs
Quadratus femoris	Laterally rotates and abducts thigh	Rotational step outs

Knee

The relationship between the shoulder and hip is similar to that of the knee and the elbow. The elbow and knee are both hinge joints and perform flexion and extension, but the knee is far more complex than the elbow joint. The femoral condyles actually allow for variations in contact with the tibia, which change during movement, and the patella-femur relationship adds to the differences seen between the joints. Additionally, the knee does not have a unified capsule or common synovial cavity. The knee uses fibrocartilage discs called menisci for cushioning, shape, and lateral stability, as well as fat pads to reduce friction. In addition, a fairly complex organization of ligaments aids in stability. Due to the nature of movements encouraged by physical activity these ligaments and menisci are subject to injury. In activities that use resistance, the risk of ligament injury is decreased compared to sport participation because the movements

are slower and more controlled. Risk still exists however, when the knee does not follow proper biomechanics of movement. When the knee passes the plane of the toe during flexion, the action forces undesirable movement of the tibia called tibial translation, which disrupts the patella tracking. When this occurs frequently the patellar ligament is subject to inflammation termed chondromalacia patellae, often referred to as "jumper's knee," or "runner's knee." The knee joint also has the ability to lock in place to allow for prolonged periods of standing without contracting the knee extensors. This action is undesirable during lifting activities because the mechanism requires the meniscus to be compressed between the tibia and femur to maintain the position. Under load, the risk for damage is dramatically increased compared to unloaded standing with the knee in the same position (16).

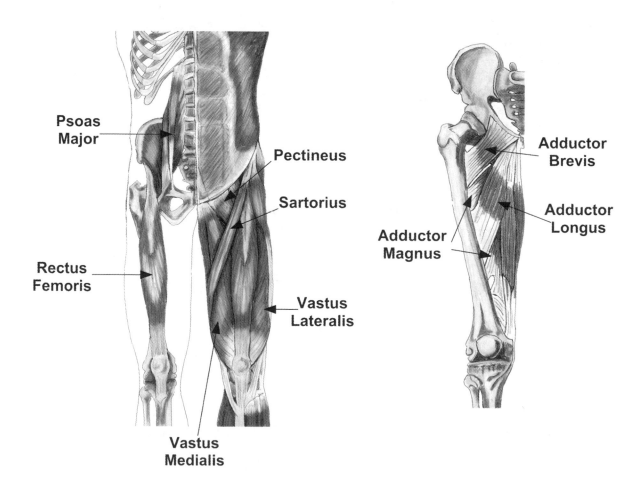

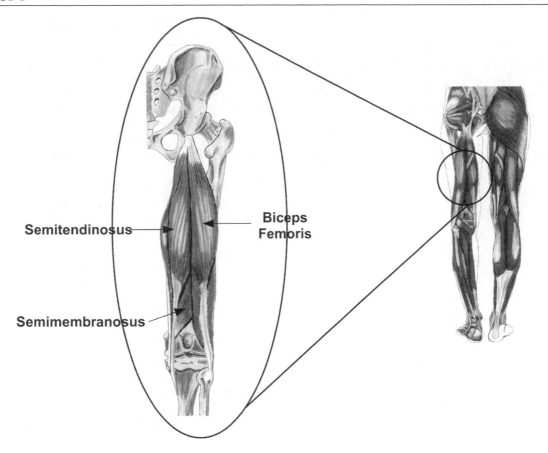

Knee Muscles	Movement Function	Example Exercise
Rectus Femoris	Extends leg, flexes thigh (hip)	Front squat
Vastus Lateralis	Extends leg	Lunge
Vastus Intermedius	Extends leg	Leg press
Vastus Medialis	Extends leg	Leg extension
Sartorius	Flexes hip and leg, rotates leg medially and thigh laterally	Lateral step up
Biceps Femoris	Extends thigh (hip);Flexes and laterally rotates leg	Romanian deadlift
Semitendinosus	Extends thigh (hip);Flexes and medially rotates leg	Supine leg curl
Semimembranosus	Extends thigh (hip);Flexes and medially rotates leg	Standing leg curl
Adductor Brevis	Adducts, flexes, and laterally rotates thigh	Lateral lunge
Adductor Longus	Adducts, flexes, and laterally rotates thigh	Side step ups
Adductor Magnus	Adducts, extends, and laterally rotates thigh	Seated adduction
Pectineus	Adducts and flexes thigh	Cable adduction

Ankle

The ankle joint is also a hinge joint which allows for two primary movements: plantar flexion (extended ankle) and dorsi flexion (flexed ankle). The foot can also be inverted and everted through a limited range at the intertarsal joints (gliding joints). Injuries can occur when the foot is inverted or everted under load. This commonly occurs during jumping or running activities when body weight is applied to an uneven surface, such as landing on a person's foot during a rebound in a basketball game or stepping in a divot when running.

~Quick Insight~

A common injury experienced by runners is shin splints. The term could apply to any of four injuries associated with anterior pain of the lower leg. In most cases, the injuries are caused by muscle imbalance, limited acclimation to the exercise stress, overuse, uneven running surfaces, the wrong foot wear, or improper technique. Shin splints are commonly attributed to overstressing the posterior tibialis, inflammation of the tibial periosteum (tibialis periosteum), anterior compartment syndrome where compressed nerves and vessels cause pain due to excessive blood flow to the anterior compartment muscles with concurrent tightness in the overlying fascia, and stress fractures of the tibia. Rest and ice often help to treat these ailments along with changing footwear and running surface (16).

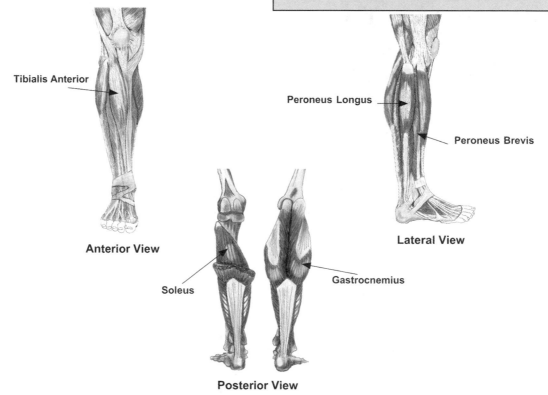

Tibialis Anterior

Peroneus Longus

Peroneus Brevis

Anterior View

Lateral View

Soleus

Gastrocnemius

Posterior View

Ankle Muscles	Movement Function	Example Exercise
Gastrocnemius	Plantar flexes foot; flexes leg	Standing calf raise
Soleus	Plantar flexes foot	Seated calf raise
Tibialis Anterior	Dorsi flexes and inverts foot	Toe raise
Peroneus Tertius	Dorsi flexes and everts foot	Toe raise
Peroneus Brevis	Plantar flexes and everts foot	Calf raise
Peroneus Longus	Plantar flexes and everts foot	Calf raise

CHAPTER ONE REFERENCES

1. Seeley RR, Stephens TD, Tate, P. *Anatomy and Physiology*. St. Louis, Mo: Times Mirror/Mosby College Publishing; 1989.

2. Beck BR, Snow CM. Bone health across the lifespan--exercising our options. *Exerc Sport Sci Rev* 2003; 31(3):117-22.

3. Suominen H. Muscle training for bone strength. *Aging Clin Exp Res*. 2006;18(2):85-93.

4. Lane NE. Epidemiology, etiology, and diagnosis of osteoporosis. *Am J Obstet Gynecol*. 2006; 194(2):S3-11.

5. Siris ES, Miller PD, Barrett-Connor E, Faulkner KG, Wehren LE, Abbott TA, Berger ML, Santora AC, Sherwood LM. Identification and fracture outcomes of undiagnosed low bone mineral density in postmenopausal women: results from the National Osteoporosis Risk Assessment. *JAMA*. 2001; 286(22):2815-22.

6. Maffulli N, Bruns W. Injuries in young athletes. *Eur J Pediatr*. 2000; 159(1-2):59-63.

7. Micheli LJ. Sports injuries in children and adolescents. Questions and controversies. *Clin Sports Med*. 1995l;14(3):727-45.

8. Engelbert RH, van Bergen M, Henneken T, Helders PJ, Takken T. Exercise tolerance in children and adolescents with musculoskeletal pain in joint hypermobility and joint hypomobility syndrome. *Pediatrics*. 2006; 118(3):e690-6.

9. Rubin C, Turner AS, Bain S, Mallinckrodt C, McLeod K. Anabolism. Low mechanical signals strengthen long bones. *Nature*. 2001; 412(6847):603-4.

10. Rubin C, Turner AS, Mallinckrodt C, Jerome C, McLeod K, Bain S. Mechanical strain, induced noninvasively in the high-frequency domain, is anabolic to cancellous bone, but not cortical bone. *Bone*. 2002 Mar;30(3):445-52.

11. Ziambaras K, Civitelli R, Papavasiliou SS. Weightlessness and skeleton homeostasis. *Hormones*. 2005;4(1):18-27.

12. Wang K, McCarter R, Wright J, Beverly J, Ramirez-Mitchell R. Viscoelasticity of the sarcomere matrix of skeletal muscles. The titin-myosin composite filament is a dual-stage molecular spring. *Biophys J*. 1993; 64(4):1161-77.

13. Pfirrmann CW, Metzdorf A, Elfering A, Hodler J, Boos N. Effect of aging and degeneration on disc volume and shape: A quantitative study in asymptomatic volunteers. *J Orthop Res*. 2006; 24(5):1086-94.

14. Harris JH Jr. Apophyseal joint and intervertebral disk injuries caused by hyperflexion and hyperextension. *Radiology*. 2002; 224(3):932

15. McCall IW. Lumbar herniated disks. *Radiol Clin North Am*. 2000; 38(6):1293-309

16. Neviaser TJ. Weight lifting. Risks and injuries to the shoulder. *Clin Sports Med*. 1991;10(3):615-21.

Chapter 2

Biomechanics

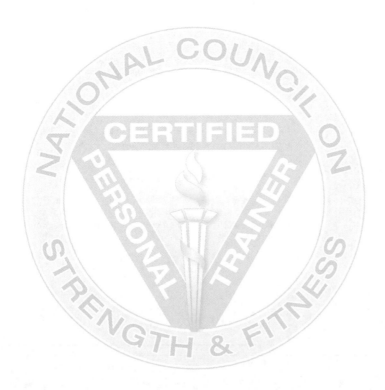

Introduction

Biomechanics is an encompassing term that joins human anatomy and physiology with movement physics and mathematics to identify how both internal and external forces affect the body. Dynamic mechanics, or objects in accelerated motion, is sectioned into kinematics and kinetics. Kinematics describes the occurring motion, whereas kinetics describes the forces that cause or have a tendency to change the motion. As with movement descriptors, force applications also have descriptors that allow for precise identification of what occurs with the body or the objects that interact and consequently, affect the body in some fashion.

Laws of Motion

Common terms used to describe motion include momentum, power, force, inertia, mass, and weight. Length and time are also considered with movement or motion and aid in determining the force considerations. All of these terms will be practically applied and used to develop a better understanding of biomechanics as it relates to motion and physical activity. Sir Isaac Newton's Laws of Motion assist in understanding motion through three basic laws. The first law suggests that if an object is static or motionless, it will remain that way unless a force acts upon it. Likewise, if an object is in motion, it will stay in motion unless something acts to change the motion. This concept is more easily understood when looked at from an outer space perspective where there is negligible gravity. If no force is applied, nothing exists to affect motion. Therefore, an object moving has nothing to slow it down or cause it to change its course. The same is true of a static object.

Newton's second law states that if an external force is applied to an object, the object will accelerate directly proportionate to the net external force and inversely proportionate to its mass. A bulldozer exemplifies this law. If a bulldozer pushes dirt, the dirt will move in the same direction the bulldozer is moving and will accelerate at the speed it is being pushed. The same can be said with a baseball throw or a weight being lifted. The resistance will accelerate in the direction of the force, at a speed determined by the weight of the object and the force applied.

The third law states that if an object exerts a force on another object, the reacting force from the other object will be equal and opposite. This case might lead one to believe that, given equivalent forces acting upon them, both objects will respond to these forces in the same manner; however, each object's mass determines it acceleration potential. For instance, if a car moving at thirty miles an hour hits a trash can, the trash can will be pushed in the direction the car is moving (2nd law), but the force the car and trash can both experience will be the same. Obviously the outcome, from a movement standpoint, will be different. The car's mass enables it to continue in motion; whereas the trash can's disproportionate mass causes it to move in the direction of the force.

Forces

Forces, including gravity, act on the body everyday. Manipulating these forces allows for voluntary movement and the maintenance of a desired static position. If the body could not control force, it would not be able to move efficiently, or even stand or sit in an upright position. In general, forces are often defined as a push or a pull, with the ability to start, speed up, slow down, stop or change the direction of an object. Force is

Newton's Three Laws of Motion

1. Law of Inertia: An object at rest tends to stay at rest and an object in motion tends to stay in motion with the same speed and in the same direction unless acted upon by an unbalanced force.

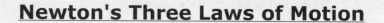

Constant speed
x

Unbalanced force

2. The force exerted on a body equals the resulting change in the body's momentum divided by the time elapsed in the process.

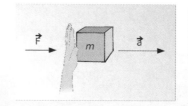

F = Force
m= Mass
a = Acceleration

3. To every action there is always an equal and opposite reaction.

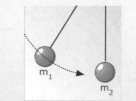
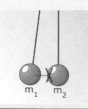
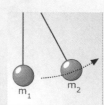

universally measured using the **Newton**, but a more common expression is the pound. By identifying or quantifying the force, it is possible to manipulate the event using other forces.

Forces are often classified as **internal forces** and **external forces**. Internal forces act within the object or system, while external forces are those that act on an object through some interaction. Internal forces in the body are produced by the actions of tissues, which exert forces upon each other. Inside the body, the forces are categorized as **tensile forces**, those in which tension results in a pulling force, and **compressive forces**, those that exert a pushing force. The two types of forces interact everyday for human function.

Even though the body can produce internal forces, it cannot change the motion of the center of mass without external forces, such as the ground. The tension created from muscle contractions can move the limbs of the body, but the body's center mass will remain the same unless the body can push or pull against another object in a force/counter-force relationship. Picture yourself floating in outer space and trying to run somewhere. Your legs may perform the actions used to propel the body on earth, but without the ground reaction forces to push against, you would not be able to go anywhere. Thus, external forces are required to change the body's center of mass, allowing for locomotion and enabling living things to run, swim, and jump. External forces do not have to contact the body to apply force to it. Gravity is a non-contact force that in many cases, determines the acceleration requirements of the body to perform tasks, as gravity determines terrestrial weight. **Contact forces,** on the other hand, occur when two objects contact one another. These objects include wind, water, the ground, or anything else that contacts the body. Contact in this sense means an interaction between "forces" not only solid objects.

Contact forces are further described as normal contact force, which acts equally and opposite to the interacting objects, and **frictional force**, which runs parallel to the two surfaces of the object. A runner will be able to accelerate using ground reaction forces by 1) the normal contact pushing down against the ground, and 2) the forward frictional force between the shoe's surface and the ground surface. The normal force applies the vertical component so the foot leaves the ground, and the frictional force applies the horizontal component, which allows the runner to move forward. When internal and external forces work synergistically, they allow for stability, while also producing movement.

~Key Terms~

Newton - The unit of force required to accelerate a mass of one kilogram one meter per second squared.

Internal forces – A force exerted by one part of a system on another part within the same system.

External forces- A force exerted on a system or on some of its components by a source outside the system.

Tensile forces- A stretching force (tension) pulling at both ends of a component or structure along its length.

Compressive force- A pushing force whose direction and point of application would tend to shorten or squeeze an object along the dimension coinciding with the line of action of the force.

Contact force- a force between two objects (or an object and a surface) that are in contact with each other.

Frictional force- the force acting on a body when the body is not in motion, but when a force is acting on it.

Stabilizer- A muscle whose torque prevents movement at a joint.

Neutralizer- Role of a muscle whose torque cancels or eliminates the undesired effect of the torque produced by another muscle at that joint to allow a desired movement only.

Prime mover- The muscle that causes an action.

Asymmetrical load- A single sided or unbalanced load or weight distribution.

Action and Reaction Forces

Newton's third law identified that forces come in pairs or couples, illustrating the concept of action and reaction forces, which act on different parts of the body. This explains why the more complex an activity becomes, the more difficult it is to perform. Chest pressing 50 lbs. using a machine is relatively easy because of the stable environment. The body contributes external force beyond the quantity of the resistance, but has limited other responsibilities to manage the environment. Essentially, forces contribute to the acceleration of the resistance in a single plane. When the same person performs a 50 lb. bench press, additional force requirements are added to stabilize the bar and prevent undesirable actions while exerting the forces to accelerate the weight against gravity. In this case, the **stabilizer** and **neutralizer** forces used to control the bar are added to the **prime mover** force, identifying an increase in total force requirements. Performing the same lifting movement on a physioball using a pair of 25 lb. dumbbells further adds difficulty due to the addition of greater force requirements to stabilize the body on the ball, while stabilizing the resistance, and concurrently producing the necessary force to move the weight. Making the resistance **asymmetrically loaded** increases the force requirements even more dramatically (5).

Balance

When the body is able to manage the sum of all external forces so that the net forces acting on the body equal zero, the body will be in **static equilibrium**. Static equilibrium determines a person's ability to **balance**. The ability of the body to manage force determines its voluntary capabilities and consequently, the efficiency of the movement or non-movement depending on the desired effect.

Measuring Motion

When the body is in motion, it is measured using space and time. The body will move through a quantifiable space in a period of time. The motion that is accomplished will either be linear, angular, or both. **Linear motion**, or translation, occurs when the body or body segment moves the same distance, in the same direction, and at the same time. **Angular,** or rotary motion, occurs when all points on a body move in circles around a fixed axis. Together, the two classifications of motion combine to produce **general motion**. General motion is the most common motion used in physical activities because angular motion of the joints move the distal portion of the limb linearly. If the starting position is known, the motion can be quantified into **speed** and **velocity** at defined points. The rate of change in velocity is defined as **acceleration**. Acceleration explains why things move.

Gravity and Motion

Remember Newton's second law of motion? The change of motion of an object is proportional to the external force applied to it. If the internal and external forces do not balance, then an object will be accelerated in the direction defined by the greater of the two forces. This explains why a person can lift a resistance. When a person rises up from a chair the internal forces apply adequate force to the ground to lift the body upward. When the same person performs a squat with resistance, the same rules apply. The force produced must be greater than the gravitational pull on the mass. If the internal and external acceleration forces are not greater than the external force of gravity, the person will not be able to rise from the chair or lift the weight upward.

What if the mass of the object is greater than the mass of the body? The reason a person can lift more than his or her body weight is due to contact reaction forces. When a 200 lb. man bench presses 250 lbs., the body's internal forces exert enough force to lift the weight because the internal forces combine with the external forces that the bench and ground supply. Together, the forces combine to produce an acceleration force greater than the mass of the man and the resistive force of the object; in this case, the weight. In space this scenario would not be possible. Based on Newton's third law, the body could only push things away from it if the mass of the object were less than the body's mass. If the mass was the 250 lb. weight, the man could not push the weight off the body, but the weight would push the man away from it due to its greater mass. So, in effect, the body would move in the direction of the force produced by the weight.

In some cases, the acceleration of a mass is greater than the acceleration forces produced by the body. When this occurs, the object may be decelerated but not accelerated.

~Key Terms~

Static equilibrium- Sum of all forces and torque acting on a body are equal.

Balance- A stable state characterized by the cancellation of all forces by equal opposing forces.

Linear motion- Change in position that occurs when all points on an object move the same distance, in the same direction, and at the same time.

Angular motion- occurs when all points on a body move in circles around a fixed axis.

General motion- When an object displays a combination of both rotary and translatory movement.

Speed- The time rate of change of position of a body without regard to direction.

Velocity- Rate of motion or performance.

Acceleration- A change in the velocity of an object.

Linear momentum- Mass of an object times the linear velocity of the object.

For example, if a person with a maximum bench press of 200 lbs. performed a bench press with 210 lbs. of resistance, he would be able to lower the bar to the chest in a controlled manner but would not be able to return the bar in the opposite direction because the downward acceleration force is greater than the upward acceleration force. The deceleration concept must also be considered when objects are thrown. For instance, if a 20 lb. medicine ball was thrown to a 150 lb. person seated on a bench at 10 mph, the force required to decelerate and stop the ball when caught would be substantially more than the 20 lb. mass itself due to the medicine ball's **linear momentum**. Linear momentum is the product of the mass and its linear velocity. If the sum of forces created by the body were not enough to attenuate the forces acting on the medicine ball, the 150 lb. person could be knocked off of the bench. But because humans can produce internal force and apply external forces to achieve force sums greater than their mass, projectile objects with a sum of force that would normally disrupt equilibrium can be managed. This case illustrates the importance of understanding forces and motion when prescribing or performing activity.

Energy and Work

The body produces forces for all types of purposes. To do so requires **energy**. Before we can explain mechanical energy however, we must first define **work**, since this term is used in the description of energy. Work, in mathematical terms, and as defined by Webster's dictionary, is the product of force and the amount of displacement in the direction of that force (W= F x d). Work can be either positive or negative as long as there is movement. If a weight is pressed overhead this action is positive work; when the weight is lowered back down, the work is considered negative. Positive work suggests the displacement is in the direction of the force, whereas negative work occurs when the displacement is opposite the direction of the force: think concentric vs. eccentric contractions. The body can actually produce more force negatively than it can positively. Going back to the bench press example, the weight lifter was able to decelerate the 210 lbs. down to the chest by performing negative work but did not have the force capabilities to move the resistance in the direction of the force to produce the positive work required to raise it back to its starting point. Both negative and positive work contribute to improvements in strength.

Work
W = F(d)
W = work
F = force applied to an object
d = distance traveled

Kinetic and Potential Energy

To perform work, the body uses energy. Although energy has many meanings, in the mechanical sense, energy is defined as the capacity to do work. Although the body uses heat, electric, chemical, and mechanical energy, for the purposes of this chapter we will focus on mechanical energy. Mechanical energy has two forms, **kinetic** and **potential**. Kinetic energy implies motion, whereas potential energy suggests no movement, but does imply energy due to position, such as with a stretched rubber band or muscle. Kinetic energy or energy in motion is easily illustrated by the dynamics of a wrecking ball. When the heavy ball is swung from a crane, its energy is obvious when it hits a building. The ball displaces the building, knocking it apart. The kinetic energy of the object is affected by its mass and velocity. In this case, the bigger the wrecking ball and greater the velocity in which it is swung, the more energy it maintains and exerts on objects it contacts.

When energy is in a potential state, it is able to do work due to its position. For instance, a weight held off the roof of a building has potential energy. If it is released, it will accelerate at the rate of gravity. With gravity, the object's location in relationship to the earth determines its potential energy. If the object is high enough to reach terminal velocity it will maximize its potential energy. On the other hand, if it is only four feet off the ground its potential energy will be less. As kinetic energy increases, potential energy proportionately decreases. The rubber band example also demonstrates the role of position in potential energy. The further the rubber band is stretched, the more energy it possesses upon release. Again, as the stretch in the band decreases, so does the potential energy, but as the band stretch decreases, the potential energy is turned into kinetic energy in equal and opposite proportion. The human body has systems in place that work very similarly to the rubber band. One mechanism we will visit later in this text is called the stretch-shortening cycle, which uses kinetic energy transferred into potential energy and back into kinetic energy for increased force output. A difference in living tissue is that potential energy may be gained or lost depending on certain neural factors.

Since work is always done when kinetic energy is produced, it is obvious a relationship exists between the two (energy ~ work). When potential energy is employed, there is no work, but forces are still being applied to maintain the potentiality of the energy. Remember, energy was defined as the capacity to do work. This explains why the human body burns calories to remain in a static position. Without movement, technically no work is being done. But to produce the tensile and compression forces necessary to hold the body upright, in the static position, energy is required.

Mechanically speaking, energy can be increased or decreased by the performance of work. For instance, if a bow is drawn halfway back, the arrow will have less kinetic energy when released than if it were pulled back the full distance. In this case, the more work performed, the more energy produced. On the other hand, work can be done to decrease energy. When a medicine ball is thrown, the person throwing it creates kinetic energy through positive work. The person catching the medicine ball reduces the ball's energy by performing negative work in the process of decelerating it. In both cases, the energy referred to is the energy of the moving object, not the energy of the accelerating object. When the body does work to manage energy, it increases its own energy usage. So energy can be viewed as external or internal depending on what is being analyzed. Internal energy will be covered under the section on bioenergetics (Chapter 5).

Power

Since work is the product of force and displacement, it can be accomplished in any variable of time. For instance, a 25 lb. object moved four feet requires the same amount of work no matter how long it takes to move it the full distance. The faster the rate of work is performed, the more **power** produced by the movement. Power is work divided by time ($P = F \times d/t$). This is illustrated by a race between two cars that have the same mass. If both cars weigh the same and drive the same distance in the race, they produced the same amount of work. The car that wins the race though, is the more powerful of the two vehicles. Power is an extremely important component of performance-related fitness, as it contributes to momentum, which assists in enabling the body to perform certain tasks, such as getting up from a chair. Power is expressed in **watts,** much like the power in a light bulb, which is why the electrical company is synonymous with the power company. Human power is also measured in watts. This can be seen on many pieces of aerobic equipment. The machines display the power output in watts and energy output in kilocalories.

> ## Power
>
> ## P = W/T
>
> P = power
> W = work
> T = time taken to do the work

Power production characteristics of muscle can provide further insight as to how to maximize the performance of the human body. Power output depends upon the muscle's contractile velocity. Interestingly, as a muscle's contraction velocity increases, its maximal force output decreases. When velocity of a contraction is multiplied by the maximal force at that respective velocity, maximal power can be calculated for each contraction velocity. In general, a muscle's maximal power occurs at a velocity that is approximately 50% of the muscle's maximal contractile velocity. Using this information, the optimal method to perform tasks to maximize power can be calculated. Advanced training environments, such as those found in preparation for the Tour de France use this information to find the ideal gears, seat heights, and cranking speeds for the cyclist to optimize performance.

As stated earlier, power is a valuable tool for human performance, but the metabolic systems that generate the power fail to provide for the ability to sustain its output over a prolonged period of time. Power output is dependent upon the quantity of power and the time it is sustained. For instance, a sprinter uses high power outputs to generate great speeds in a short period of time, often referred to as burst power. Unfortunately, this power cannot be sustained. Therefore, beyond the point of peak power output, the sprinter's speed will no longer increase, but rather begin to slow down. When power requirements are prolonged, the outputs are inversely related, meaning the longer the power is required the less power will be provided. This limitation is an inherent flaw in the metabolic systems of the body. Even when all systems are optimal, this limiting relationship still exists.

Torques

The body is constantly managing different types and applications of force. One of the most common applications within the body is the moment of force, or **torque** that causes change in angular motion. Simply put, torques cause rotation. The forces muscles produce move the limbs around their respective axis of rotation, as defined by the joint. But torques can also be applied without movement. Equilibrium, stability, and balance are attainable with the help of torques.

Since torque causes rotation, it changes the linear and angular motions of an object to cause general motion. If the external force is **centric**, meaning the force is directed through the center of gravity, it will not cause rotation, and therefore, remain linear. If the external force is directed against an object at a line other than the center of gravity, referred to as **eccentric** force (not to be confused with an eccentric contraction), some level of rotation will occur, thereby creating torque. This force can be easily demonstrated by placing a

Torque

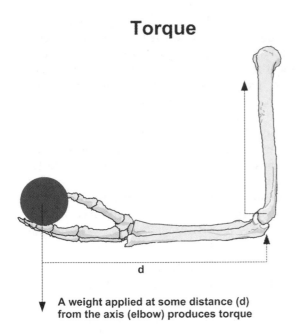

A weight applied at some distance (d) from the axis (elbow) produces torque

similar force acts on the bottom of the pencil in the opposite direction, the pencil will experience the coupled torques and therefore rotate more easily. A sea-saw works under the same premise. If two children of equal weight are on a sea-saw, they can easily perform the up-down motion across the fulcrum of the board. One child applies upward force, while the gravitational force applied to the other child from the earth pulls downward to create the force couple. The force couple increases the torque to cause playful rotation. This can be accomplished even if the children have different weights due to the coupling effect of the forces. If one child tries to play on the sea-saw alone, however, the same phenomenon will not be duplicated. The single child would produce some torque but not have the force capabilities to cause the torque in the way the two children's force couple did. The child may get the see-saw to rise to a limited degree, but the low level of torque would limit the attainable motion.

pencil flat on a table. If the pencil is pushed in its center it will slide, or translate, across the table in the direction of the force without change in its orientation. However, if the pencil is pushed from the top or bottom, it will rotate away from the line of force. The closer the force is to the middle of the pencil, the less it will rotate; therefore, the closer a force is applied to the center of gravity, the less torque it will experience. On the contrary, the further the line of force is from the center of gravity the greater the torque created. When this occurs in the body, the more torque that is applied, the greater the internal force will need to be to manage the eccentric force. For instance, if a person performs an abdominal curl-up while holding a medicine ball on their chest they will experience an increase in torque and noticeable difficulty added to the movement when compared to performing the exercise without the resistance. When that same resistance is held with arms extended overhead, the torques increase by the magnitude of the distance the weight is located from the center of gravity. The same can be said for the side raise exercise. The further the resistance is held from the body, the longer the **resistance arm**, and consequently the greater the magnitude of torque applied. The more torque experienced during exercise, the greater the difficulty of the movement, even when the weight remains constant.

Torque is increased to an even greater degree when **force couples** act upon an object. Back to the pencil example, if a linear force is applied to the top of the pencil in one direction, while at the same time a

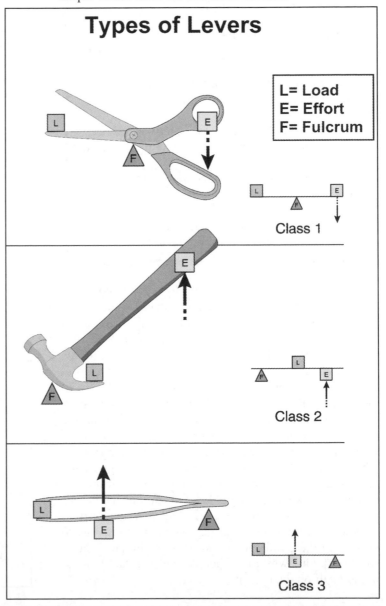

Types of Levers

L= Load
E= Effort
F= Fulcrum

Class 1

Class 2

Class 3

~Key Terms~

Energy- The capacity to do work.

Work- Transfer of energy by a force acting to displace a body. Work is equal to the product of the force and the distance through which it produces movement.

Kinetic energy- The energy possessed by a body because of its motion.

Potential energy- Energy stored by an object by virtue of its position.

Power- Time rate of doing work.

Watt- A unit of power in the International System of Units equal to one joule per second.

Torque- The turning effect created by a force about an axis.

Centric force- Force whose line of action passes through the center of gravity of an object.

Eccentric force- Force whose line of action does not pass through the center of gravity of an object.

Resistance arm- The distance between the fulcrum and the resistance point.

Force couples- Torque created by a pair of oppositely directed forces about an axis.

The torques created by the muscles of the body are dependent upon the force and attachment location. This is called the **line of action,** or line of pull. The line of action is most often in the direction of the tendons. Tendon attachment locations cross joints to pull the limbs in the desired direction. Generally, the more distal the attachment, the more rotation or torque created. In most cases, the muscles work in pairs, so as rotation occurs from one muscle, other muscles aid in the production of torque or counter torque. For instance, when the elbow flexes, the bicep brachii crosses the elbow and pulls on the proximal radius, whereas the brachioradialis which crosses the elbow from the humerus and attaches to the distal portion of the radius, pulls from a different location. Together they act to enhance arm flexion capabilities. The hamstring muscle group and the gastrocnemius work in a similar fashion, which explains why many people feel contractile force in their calf on the leg curl.

With this in mind, the design concept behind weight training equipment and resisted movements becomes apparent. For instance, a leg extension or curl machine is designed to place the resistance at the distal end of the limb to create higher levels of torque. If the same machines had shorter swing arms, or if they were not properly adjusted to match a person's limb length, the exercise would become easier. Likewise, the exercise machines with longer lever arms make it mechanically easier to move a respective resistance due to the lever advantage compared to the machines that have shorter levers like those that more closely resemble the free weight movement. The more cables and levers, the less resistance that is actually lifted.

Determining Torque

To determine the actual resistance, or torque, a muscle must overcome, some basic facts must be known. Algebraically, torque that produces movement is expressed as T= F x FA, or torque equals applied force, multiplied by the length of the force arm. Torque that resists movement is expressed as T = R x RA, or torque equals the resistance multiplied by the length of the resistance arm. The heavier the resistance or longer the resistance arm, the more difficult it is for the body to move the resistance. Holding a dumbbell close to the body is much easier than holding the dumbbell away from the body. The resistive torques increase as the

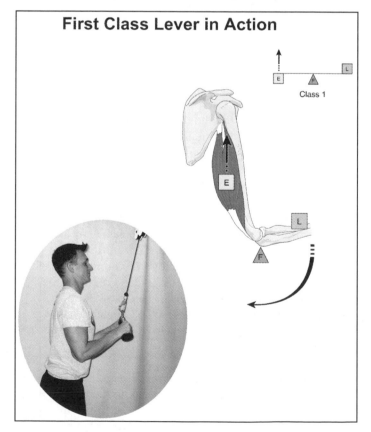

First Class Lever in Action

resistance arm lengthens. This is why a person can perform a lift with more weight on the bench press compared to the chest fly, or on the upright row compared to the side raise. The shortened resistance arm provides for mechanical advantage, particularly when the force arm is long.

From this, it follows that exercise difficulty can be manipulated by adjusting the factors that contribute to resistive torques or by changing the mechanical advantage of the lever system. If a person has difficulty with a movement, they can simply reduce the resistance, shorten the resistance arm, or lengthen the force arm to better perform the movement. In many cases with body weight exercises, shortening the resistance arm is the easiest variable to adjust. If a new exerciser has difficulty performing abdominal curl-ups from the ground, have them perform the exercise from an inclined bench with their feet on the ground. The muscle action and movement are the same, but the shortened resistant arm will make the movement easier. If they cannot do a push-up from the floor, have them perform the exercise from an elevated surface. Mild adjustments can make the difference between correct and successful performance and failure or poor movement technique and possible injury.

Second Class Lever in Action

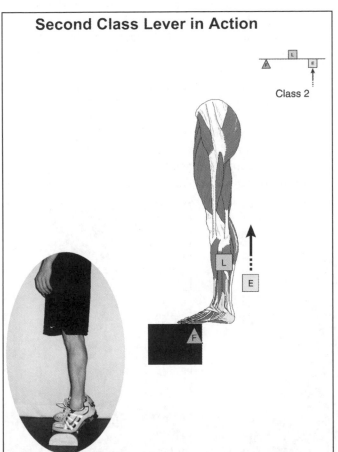

Class 2

Stability

When the body is in general motion, torques are contributing to the angular motion while other forces are creating linear motion. As stated earlier, when all external forces and torques are accounted for so that the net sum of all forces and torques is equal, static equilibrium is attained. Static equilibrium means non-movement balance, but in exercise and physical activity non-movement would be contrary to the exercise's purpose. So, with dynamic activities, balance and stability are more appropriate considerations for managing external forces and torques.

To understand balance and stability, it is important to first identify the major contributing factor that works against it: gravity. The constant 9.81 m/sec^2 applied to the body requires it to constantly manage the external force created by the gravitational pull. Gravity pulls on the center of mass of an object, commonly referred to as the **center of gravity**. The center of gravity, as defined by Webster's dictionary is "that point in a body or system around which its mass or weight is evenly distributed or balanced, and through which the force of gravity acts." With regard to Newton's laws of motion, the center of gravity is the site by which the laws apply. The body rotates around its center of gravity.

The human body is slightly more complicated than a rigid mass when it comes to identifying the center of gravity. This is due to the fact that the body can be in different positions, which causes the center of gravity to migrate to the movement of the greatest mass. A shot put, for instance, always has the same center of gravity because it has no limbs. But humans have many joints which can move the center of gravity in all directions. When standing in anatomical position, the center of gravity is centrally located since most people are symmetrical from side to side. The same symmetry does not exist from front to back. A view of any person from the side will illustrate this fact. This is particularly true for individuals carrying excessive mass. The changes related to lean mass build up or fat storage may raise, lower, or shift the center of gravity forward or backward. Changes in the center of gravity may cause the body to work harder to establish static equilibrium, balance, or stability (4; 29). A pendulous belly for example, causes the center of gravity to shift anteriorly, increasing strain on lumbar joints as the soft tissues work to counteract the force. This identifies why added fat mass makes activity more difficult to perform, which can contribute to a decline in activity status.

Since stability is a key factor in the application of human force and the subsequent movement created by the force produced, its relationship with gravity must be

Third Class Lever in Action

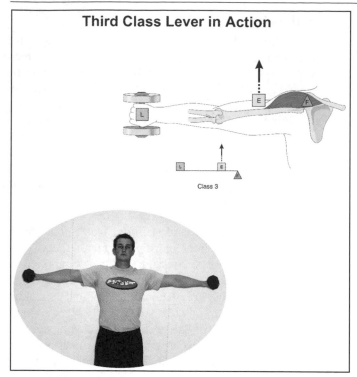

Class 3

well understood. Webster's dictionary says that an object is stable when it is not easily moved or thrown off balance. The ability of the body to stabilize its segments ultimately determines performance. This is true of lifting weights, running on a treadmill, or standing still. External force energy must be transferred through the body's **kinetic chain** to effectively join it with internal force (11). It is very important that the force remains as close to its starting magnitude as possible. If any of the energy leaks out to unstable segments on the chain, the application of the internal force will be limited by the loss of the external force. This suggests a person completing a military press may not be able to reach their potential because part of the ground reaction force is lost due to instability in the

trunk. The more stable the body becomes, the more efficiently external force can be applied.

Components of Stability

The body achieves stability by manipulating several variables. The mass of the object, height of the center of gravity, line of gravitational pull, and the base of support all affect the stability of the object (4; 13). Since the mass is constant, the three variables which can be managed are the base of support, the height of the center of gravity, and line of gravitational pull(14; 24). By manipulating these variables effectively, less internal and external force is required for stability.

The more central the line of gravity falls within the base of support, the more stable the object becomes. If the line of gravity migrates to the outer regions of the base, the object becomes less stable. If the line of gravitational pull exceeds the outer limits of the base of support, the object will no longer be able to maintain stability (13). This being said, the wider the base of support, the more stable an object will be as long as the line of gravitational pull is centered within the base. Again, moving the line of gravity toward the outer limits of the base of support will proportionally disrupt the object's stability consistent with the distance from the center line of gravity (14). This is also true when the center of gravity is elevated. The degree of stability is indirectly proportional to the height of the center of gravity. If a person lies on the ground, they are difficult to move and therefore stable. A large pushing force would be required to disrupt their stability. When the same person stands up, the center of gravity is elevated with their elevated position. The pushing force required to disrupt an individual when they are standing is much less than the force needed to disrupt their stability when they are lying on the ground. If that same person stands

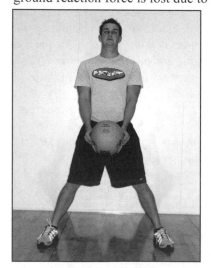

Gravitational pull is centered

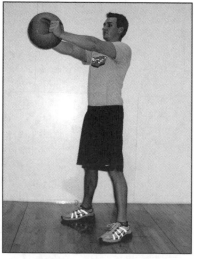

Line of gravity moved toward the outer limit of the base of support

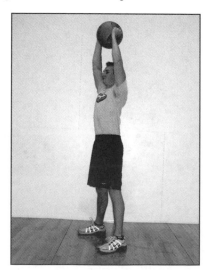

Elevated center of gravity

on one foot, even less external force would be needed to disrupt their stability because the base of support has been reduced.

Another key to stability is the width of the base of support as it applies to the direction of the external or disruptive force. For instance, in a tug-of-war, a wide stance in the direction of the pull would be more stable than a wide stance perpendicular to the line of pull. To enhance stability, the base of support width must be widest in the direction of the resistance. When objects are lifted overhead, the direction of the force is directly down, so a wide natural stance or wide split stance would each enhance stability.

In physical activities such as running, the base of support must constantly be changed to account for the movement of the centerline of gravitational pull (17). As the line of gravity moves outside the base of support, the person loses stability in the process to create mobility. This explains why a person will fall if one leg gets held up when running. Since the line of gravity is moving forward, the trip leg cannot swing through to re-establish a base of support outside of the line of gravity, stability is lost and the runner falls. If he or she trips, but can re-adjust and get the limb past the line of gravity in time, a stumble occurs but not a fall, since stability was lost and re-attained. Essentially, for activities where locomotion occurs, the body moves by constantly losing and regaining stability. The ability to regain stability helps define the efficiency by which the movement is performed.

This also explains why we may be able to accomplish a movement pattern with limited success but not in an efficient manner. If stability is disrupted or difficult to attain, or attained to a limited degree, the movement will suffer proportionate to the level of stability. If stability is lost, the movement will fail. But when complete stability is attained, the movement will become fluid. This supports the trend toward the inclusion of stability training in exercise programs. The more efficiently the body can attain stability and the more stable it can become, the better it will perform.

Practical Application
The Body's Stabilizing Units

The ability to stabilize its segments determines how effectively the body can manage forces to perform tasks. An inability to stabilize the body segments leads to dysfunction. Static and dynamic stability is achieved when passive, active, and control systems work together to manage forces and transfer load (5; 7). The ability to transfer force through a joint is dependent upon 1) the integrity, mechanics, and function of the tissue of the joint, often referred to as form closure, 2) the coordinated tensile and compression force produced by tissues to manage the other forces acting on the joint called force closure, and 3) the appropriate neural activity to orchestrate the pattern of motor control often referred to as kinesthetic awareness. Stability depends more upon accelerating force "harmony" than the independent factors such as the joint structure or strength of the attached tissue. This suggests that to become more stable, the objective should be to control motion as a whole, rather than addressing the independent parts, since it is the coordination of the parts that ultimately enhances stability.

Due to the fact that the stable segments of the body allow it to transfer external energy from the ground and other objects, the ability to recognize the areas of inefficiency is necessary to improve force transference through the kinetic chain (11). The multiple segments of the spine and pelvis need to transfer energy to and from the upper limb and lower limb segments. This suggests that the trunk is a key point of stability (5; 9). This is further demonstrated when increased limb velocities require the transfer of angular momentum. A motion segment must become stable to pass its angular momentum to another segment. If the trunk cannot attain an adequate level of stability, the force cannot be effectively transferred from the bottom to the top or from top down. Throwing, running, and jumping, as with most dynamic movements, require force transfer from the limbs through the trunk or the trunk through the limbs.

The body has two primary systems of stability for energy transfer at, and around, the lumbo-pelvic region. The inner unit, or local stabilizers, describes the tissues that stabilize the joints from deep within the body, while the outer unit, or global stabilizers, stabilizes and moves body segments using the more superficial prime mover musculature. The inner unit is comprised of the transverse abdominis, pelvic floor, multifidus, and the diaphragm. These muscles work together to create internal forces that support the spine (5; 8; 9). The outer unit is composed of groups of tissues that make up four independent systems, sometimes called sling systems, which work via the continuity of fascial attachment. They include the posterior oblique, the deep longitudinal, the anterior oblique, and the lateral oblique systems. Historians suggest that the ancient Egyptian theorists had an understanding of these relationships in the development of human stability and movement.

The Inner Unit

The inner unit features the hoop tension created by the transverse abdominis (TVA) and the multifidus muscles, which represent the primary stabilizers for the lumbo-pelvic region (5; 8; 9). It has a large attachment to the middle layer and the deep lamina of the posterior layer of the thoraco-dorsal fascia and is recruited prior to any upper or lower extremity movements (31). When the TVA contracts, tension increases in the thoraco-dorsal fascia called thoraco-lumbar fascia gain, and intra-abdominal pressure increases as the relatively non-compressible viscera pushes against the supportive structures of the diaphragm and pelvic floor. The collective effect of the thoracolumbar fascia gain, increased intra-abdominal pressure, and hydraulic amplifier effect caused by the spinal musculature, enhance stability in the lumbopelvic and upper spinal regions (9).

In upper body movements, TVA contractions should occur at least 30 milliseconds prior to the movement and 110 milliseconds before the initiation of a lower body movement for sufficient stability (9). TVA activation requirements seem to be consistent, regardless of the movement pattern or the plane in which the movement is performed (21). According to studies, individuals with a timing delay of TVA activation beyond the aforementioned requirements are more likely to suffer chronic low back pain (23). It is suggested that significant motor control deficit is present in people with chronic low back pain which is primarily associated with the control of the contraction of the transverse abdominis" and is worsened by atrophy of the multifidus (6; 28).

The Outer Unit

The outer unit works in conjunction with the stability created by the inner unit. Each sling system is comprised of connective tissues, which act to stabilize or move body segments. The posterior oblique system is comprised of the latissimus dorsi, gluteus maximus, and intervening thoraco-dorsal fascia. When added to the superficial layer of the trapezius, transverse abdominis, and deep layer of the internal oblique, in conjunction with the hydraulic pump of the multifidus and erector spinae muscles, a structural force bridge is created. This bridge between the lumbar spine and pelvic girdle created by these active tissues is fundamental to safe exercise performance because these muscles are significant contributors to the transference of load through the pelvic girdle (31). The deep longitudinal system includes the deep lamina of the thoraco-dorsal fascia, the sacrotuberous ligament, and the biceps femoris muscle. This system serves as an extension of the inner unit by contributing to tension in the thoraco-dorsal fascia and facilitating compression through the sacroiliac joint. This support mechanism adds to dorsal and inferior lumbo-pelvic stabilization.

On the other side of the body, the anterior oblique system combines the abdominal obliques, the adductor muscles of the thigh and the intervening abdominal fascia. This system is considered important for phasic actions such as the initiation of movement and high load control activities (2). The oblique muscles are active whenever actions of the trunk, upper, and lower extremities occur (1; 22).

The final system to make up the outer unit is called the lateral system and includes the gluteus medius and minimis, the tensor fascia lata, and the adductors of the thigh. These muscles are important to bipedular motion and standing, providing frontal plane stability. As with all systems of the outer unit, the phasic actions of this system depend upon internal stabilizing force. If the inner unit cannot manage the forces produced by the outer unit, injury is a likely occurrence.

The relationship between the inner and outer unit is probably the best supporting evidence for the inclusion of functional-based activities for performance enhancement. The concept of harmonized movement suggests that stability is efficiently attained and forces are transferred effectively through body segments for desired outcomes. Training to emphasize improvements to inner unit stability, while utilizing resisted movements consistent with the natural functional systems of the outer unit, is well justified in an exercise program for optimal stability and function of the body (31).

Rotational Inertia

The necessity for harmonious interaction between the inner and outer units is even more evident when the body must manage dynamic forces at high velocities. Since the body has limb segments, forces and torques that cause rotation contribute to the disruption of stability as seen by the running example (18). People most often fall down when they move, not when they are standing still. The faster the rate of movement, the harder it is to manage the movement. Therefore, the faster a body segment moves, the greater the stability requirements assumed by the body. In the case of ballistic movements where the body segments are accelerated for power, such as throwing, running, or swimming, it is important to recognize the additional contributing factors that affect stability. **Rotational inertia** and its product, **angular momentum** are created when the segments of the body move. The faster the movement, or the larger the segment, the more rotational inertia and subsequent angular momentum produced.

Rotational inertia, as it pertains to the body, is defined as the reluctance of the body segment to move around its axis. The distribution of mass and length of the swing arm dictate the amount of rotational inertia. A baseball bat has its proportionate mass toward the distal end when held correctly. In this position, it has less rotational inertia than if the bat were flipped around so the thin end is distal. This explains why the leg has greater rotational inertia around its joint than the arm. The longer length and greater mass proximal to the body makes it more reluctant to rotate. This is exemplified when running. The recovery leg is bent when it passes the hip. This way, it more efficiently re-establishes stability. The bent knee has less rotational inertia to overcome than a straight leg. This also explains why an overhand pitch used in baseball has greater velocity than the underhand pitch used in softball. The arm flexes during the overhand throw creating less rotational inertia than the straightened arm wind up of the softball throw.

Angular Momentum

The amount of rotational inertia produced depends upon the total mass, distribution of the mass, and the angular velocity. Collectively, this product is the angular momentum. The force required to change angular momentum is proportionate to the quantity of momentum. Momentum is either desirable or completely undesirable, depending on the purpose of the movement. Desirable momentum would be that created in the hammer throw. In this case, the momentum can be built upon as the thrower rotates to throw the object further. In cases of resistance training, momentum may be less desirable because it applies less resistive force to the tissue being trained. Swinging the bar may allow for greater weight to be moved, but will likely place less stress on the targeted contractile tissues. This is commonly seen in many exercises when too much resistance is used. The lifter applies angular momentum, most often generated from hip extension or flexion to move greater resistance. Adaptations to the muscle are based on the force generated by the tissue and the duration those forces are applied for, not just the load moved. When using the hips to lift weight the prime movers perform less work and experience minimal training stress compared to the employment of proper lifting technique.

In other cases, it is desirable to use momentum to perform a lift or task. When momentum is employed to perform a task, it is usually transferred from one body segment to another. This is accomplished by stabilizing the initial moving part so the momentum transfers to the next segment. When Olympic weightlifters perform the clean and jerk exercise, they take advantage of the momentum forces to perform the lift. The lifter generates a powerful movement using hip extension, which causes the bar to accelerate upward. During the period of acceleration (caused by angular momentum) that is greater than gravity, the lifter has time to drop under the bar to catch it before it reaches neutral gravity. If the lifter does not get under the weight by the time it reaches neutral gravity, the lifter will have increasing difficulties successfully completing the lift because the bar will begin accelerating back to the ground at the rate of gravitational pull. Another example of the body's ability to transfer momentum occurs when we run or jump. Humans can both run and jump without the use of arm movements, but the performance of the tasks will be compromised compared to when the arms are employed during the movements. When we swing our arms during a forward or upward jumping motion, the angular momentum from the rotational inertia of the arm swing is transferred to the trunk to help propel the body in the direction the center of mass is moving (10; 30). Running works the same way. The alternating arm swing occurs contralaterally to the alternating leg movement for the purposes of balance and the generation of angular momentum. The arms are bent to accelerate more efficiently so as to mirror the speed of the recovery leg. The recovery leg is also flexed so the hip flexors can move it forward rapidly to regain stability.

Agonist and Antagonists

Managing angular momentum is as important as generating it. Whenever the body produces angular momentum from rotational inertia, a force proportionate to the angular momentum is required to stop the movement. This is an important concept to apply in physical activity in order to prevent undesirable outcomes and injuries. The throwing example illustrates this concern. When a pitcher winds up during a pitch, additional angular momentum is supplied to further accelerate the baseball beyond the arm's relative rotational force capabilities. The forward acceleration of the limb allows the ball to travel at a high velocity, but the limb must be decelerated using forces proportionate to the forces that caused the acceleration. If the deceleration muscles, or **antagonists**, are not comparable in force production capabilities (relative to their role) to the acceleration producing muscles, or **agonist**, the joint and tissues of the movement segment they serve are at risk. In fact, other muscles may strain in support of deceleration, as they are not serving as antagonists to the prime movers but acting as assistive decelerators.

A pitcher who strains the muscles of the low back or rotator cuff during the follow-thru of a pitch will do so because the acceleration was beyond the magnitude of the tissue's eccentric deceleration capacity (25). When the prime antagonists cannot manage the deceleration requirements, they employ assistive musculature all the way down the kinetic chain to help slow the movement. This would explain a back strain that occurs when decelerating the throwing motion (20). If the sum of the deceleration forces does not equal acceleration, something has to give. Either a tissue will be compromised or stability will be lost. Individuals engaged in sports or activities where momentum forces are common should strengthen the muscles that aid in deceleration. In many cases, athletes and exercisers routinely focus on strengthening the muscles that accelerate movement without addressing the muscles that must slow the movement down. When the agonist muscle group surpasses the antagonist muscle group's **strength balance** requirements, injuries will occur (12; 19; 26). This is actually the most common reason individuals suffer soft tissue strains.

A common example is seen in the frequency athletes "pull" or strain their hamstrings. This occurs because the hip flexors and knee extensors become disproportionately stronger than the hamstrings. In this relationship, the minimum strength balance is 2:1, or the hamstrings must have at least 50% of the strength of the quadriceps (12; 16). A better balance would be a 25% difference, also stated as a quadriceps/hamstring ratio of 4:3 (15).

Each agonist/antagonist relationship has a specific muscle balance requirement depending on the relative factors of the joint where the movement occurs. In most cases, injury will occur when the weaker antagonist takes on agonist responsibilities. Analysis of a hamstring pull illustrates this phenomenon. The hamstring is the antagonist muscle to the quadriceps during a leg extension but switches roles to become the agonist in the leg curl. In this scenario the majority of force is produced solely by a single muscle group; either the quadriceps is producing the force or the hamstrings are producing the force. In this environment, the imbalance is not as much a concern. The problem occurs when they produce force together. The hamstring pull occurs during activities such as running where hip extensors and knee flexors combine with the hip flexors and leg extensors to produce high-speed locomotion. The stress from the contraction, in addition to the stress of the active imbalance, produces the double stress phenomenon that causes the strain.

In weight training and physical activity, muscle imbalances are very easy to develop. Every sport or activity has the potential to cause imbalances because, more often than not, particular movements and muscles are employed repeatedly and chronically. A notable example occurs in swimmers and wrestlers, who often develop upper cross syndrome, identified by the rounded, internally rotated shoulders and kyphotic spine postures (3; 27). Due to the frequency of the strokes and the muscles used to generate the force in swimming or the constant squeezing which occurs in wrestling, viewable structural shifts can be observed during postural analysis. If imbalances are identified, they should receive priority within the exercise program matrix. With imbalance comes injury, and with injury comes limitation to movement or activity attrition.

~Key Terms~

Line of action- The relation of a muscle's pull to the joint.

Center of gravity- The point where the mass of the object is equally balanced. The center of gravity is also called the center of mass.

Kinetic chain- A group of body segments that are connected by joints so that the segments operate together to provide a wide range of motion for a limb.

Rotational inertia- As a rotating body spins about an external or internal axis (either fixed or unfixed), it opposes any change in the body's speed of rotation that may be caused by a torque.

Angular momentum- The product of the momentum of a rotating body and its distance from the axis of rotation. In lay terms, angular momentum can be thought as the "amount of rotation" of the body.

Antagonist- Role of a muscle whose torque opposes the action referred to or muscle referred to.

Agonist- Role of a muscle whose torque aids the action, referred to as the prime mover.

Strength balance- The force production relationship between an agonist and antagonist muscle or group of muscles.

Common Errors in Movement and Exercise

Biomechanical limitations to performance can also occur when the muscle or connective tissue is inflexible or weak along the kinetic chain. In some cases, movement execution is poor due to improper technique. In other cases, the improper movement is caused by limitations in the functioning tissue. Common errors in movement and exercises can provide information about kinetic chain deficiencies. The following identifies some of these common errors.

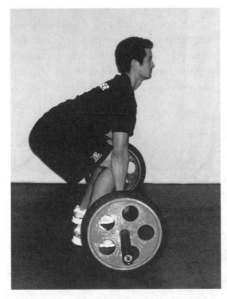

Correct Starting Position

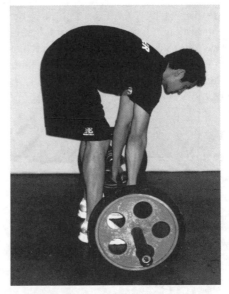

Incorrect Starting Position

Deadlift

The traditional deadlift exercise uses a flexed knee and hip position with the feet in relative close proximity, or about hip width apart. The bar is grasped using an alternate grip outside the knees, with chest elevated to maintain a flat back position with a slight lumbar curve. The common error in this movement occurs when the legs are extended, but weakness in the trunk causes a forward and downward pull leading to a rounded back position during the ascent. Likewise, if the glutes are inflexible, the start position may cause a posterior shift in the pelvis, leading to a decreased convexity of the lumbar spine. In either case the round back position caused by the lift will place stress on the spinal ligaments and may cause excessive disc compression. To correct the error, more attention should be placed on the back position during the lift. This may require better cueing during the instruction of the exercise, a decrease in weight, or a modification to the position to allow the hips to extend sooner. A common modification is a wider stance with an inside the knee grip on the bar. This leads to greater hip extension ability earlier in the lift and increases adductor contribution. However, the change does reduce the leg extension requirements proportionally to the added hip and adductor contributions.

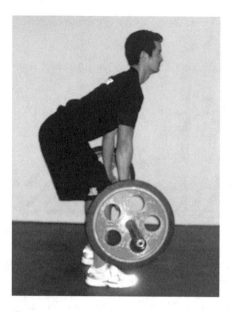

Correct

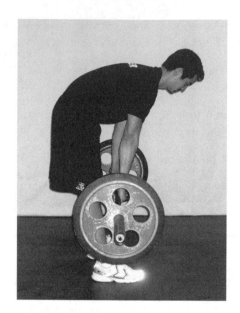

Incorrect

Romanian Deadlift

The Romanian deadlift (RDL) requires a slightly flexed knee position and maintenance of a neutral spine throughout the movement. The maintenance of proper spinal alignment is where errors frequently occur. Rounding the back either suggests weakness relative to the weight or incorrect instruction. Cueing an exerciser to elevate the chest causes the back extensors to better control a straight spine position. If the exerciser continues flexing the knees as they lower the resistance, it suggests tightness in the hamstrings. Performing the exercise using a staggered stance with less weight can enhance range of motion through dynamic flexibility.

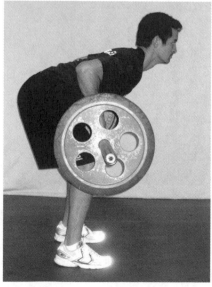

Correct

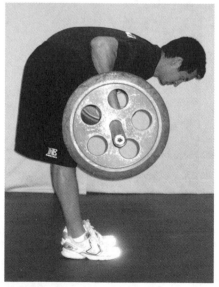

Incorrect

Bent-Over Rows

Similar to the lower body position of the Romanian deadlift, the bent-over row exercise requires the maintenance of a flat back position. Ideally, the lift is performed with mild knee flexion with hips flexed so the line of the spine approximately parallels the floor. Rounding of the back stresses spinal ligaments and places compressive force on the intervertebral discs. Similar to the RDL, inability to maintain the position often suggests too much resistance, stabilizer weakness in the trunk, and/or lack of flexibility in the hip extensors. If the exerciser extends the hip during the row phase of the movement, it again suggests too much resistance.

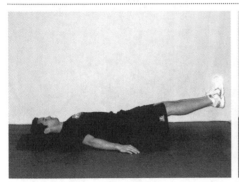 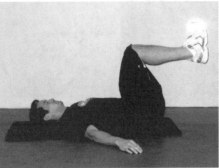 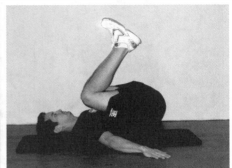

Incorrect   **Correct Starting Position**   **Correct Ending Position**

Leg Lifts

Supine leg lifts have classically been used to train the abdominals. The blatant error common in the employment of this movement is the abdominals do not attach to the femur, so the exercise is actually controlled by the hip flexors. The insertion of the hip flexors place excessive stress on the lumbar spine and pull the pelvis into an anterior pelvic tilt, increasing lumbar convexity and disc compression forces. For this reason, the movement is contraindicated. Modifying the movement by beginning the exercise with a flexed hip and contracting the abdominals to pull the pelvis posteriorly reduces spinal stress and increases abdominal activation.

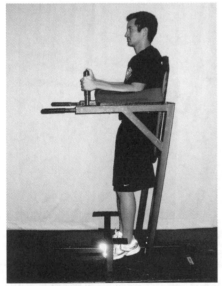 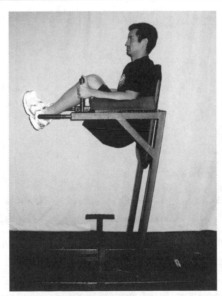 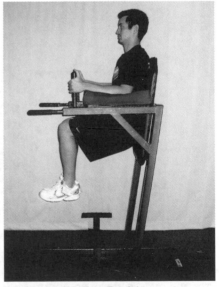

Correct Start   **Correct Ending Position**   **Incorrect Ending Position**

Knee Raise

The hanging leg or knee raise is subject to the same concerns as the supine leg lift, but disc compression occurs at a lesser degree. The common error is to raise the thigh to a ninety degree flexed hip position with an anterior pelvic tilt. This movement is caused by contraction of the iliopsoas muscle group, whereas the abdominals serve as a stabilizer to the trunk. To correctly perform the exercise so the abdominals serve as the prime mover, a posterior pelvic tilt must be attained. For many exercisers performing the movement from an inclined body position is more desirable for proper movement execution.

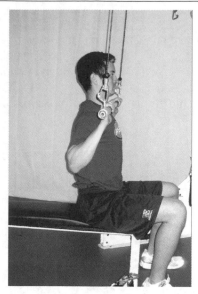
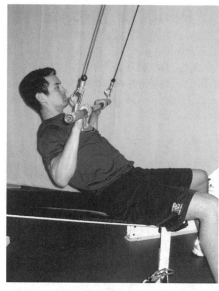
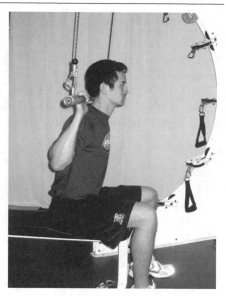

Correct Ending Position   **Incorrect Ending Position**   **Incorrect Ending Position**

Lat Pulldown

Two common errors exist in the lat pulldown exercise. The first is incorrectly pulling the resistance to the back of the neck. This technique causes excessive external rotation in the shoulders, which may damage the shoulder capsule and increases risk of injury to the cervical spine, making the exercise contraindicated. To correct this error, the bar should be pulled to the chest. The second error is common in many back exercises, where hip extension serves to create angular momentum to move more resistance. This action reduces the tension in the desired musculature. To correct this error, the hip and spine relationship should remain virtually unchanged throughout the movement performance.

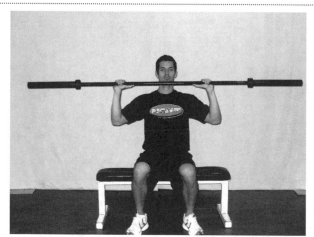
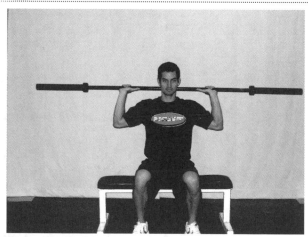

Correct Position   **Incorrect Position**

Overhead Press

Pressing overhead can compromise the shoulder, as excessive force is placed on an open joint. To reduce the stress in the shoulder and prevent humeral head translation, the exercise should not be performed behind the head. Instead, the bar should be lowered in front of the head to the chest, or dumbbells should be used to resist the overhead shoulder abduction movements. During the overhead press, particularly during the standing military press, it is also important to pay attention to the hip and low back position. A common error when too much resistance is used is to lean backward to employ the pectoralis major and gain some mechanical advantage. The backward lean extends the hips and low back, increasing spinal compression forces. The hip and spinal positions should not change from the starting posture during the movement.

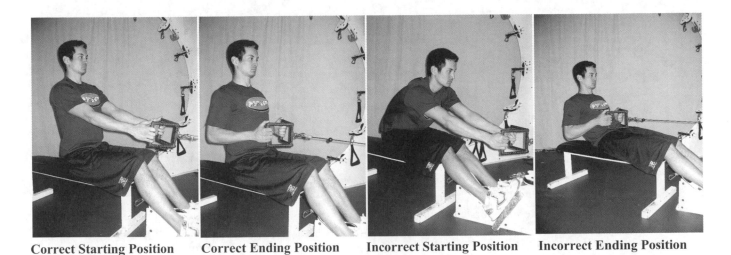

Correct Starting Position   **Correct Ending Position**   **Incorrect Starting Position**   **Incorrect Ending Position**

Seated Row

As alluded to during the discussion of other pulling exercises, the employment of hip extension is a common error used to generate angular momentum to move the resistance. Correctly performing the seated row, as with the bent-over row, requires a stable trunk and spinal position. Flexing and extending the hip are undesirable during the movement. Additionally, the back musculature acting on the scapula should initiate the movement via scapular retraction. Arm flexion with limited scapular retraction is another common error seen during the performance of row exercises. Due to the fact that the rhomboids do not attach to the humerus, the shoulder complex movements should precede flexion of the arm to increase the effectiveness of the exercises.

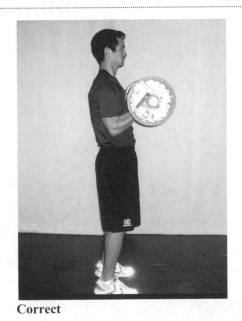
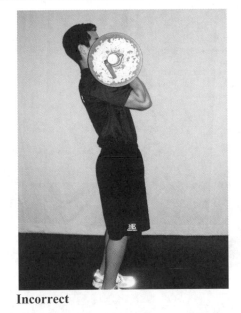

Correct   **Incorrect**

Bicep Curl

When too much resistance is used in arm flexion exercises, such as the standing bicep curl, the tendency is to use swing to generate angular momentum. The two most common errors in bicep curling exercises are to flex the shoulder and, or extend the hips during the concentric movement. The humerus should remain fixed against the midaxillary line during the entire movement, and movement at the hip should be minimal.

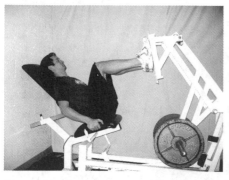 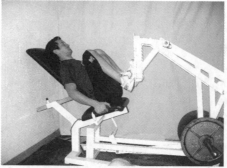 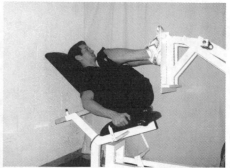

Correct   **Incorrect**   **Incorrect**

Leg Press

The leg press is a popular exercise for leg training because very little skill is required to perform the movement. The most common errors exist when placing the feet on the foot plate. Low foot position causes the ankle to dorsi flex and the knees migrate past the toes during the descent. This will cause the resistive forces to be directed into the balls of the feet rather than the heels and often leads to tibial translation and knee ligament stress. To correct the problem, the feet should be placed higher on the foot plate, so the ankle position remains fairly neutral throughout the movement. The second error usually relates to tightness in the hip extensors. During the descent, tight musculature pulls on the pelvis, causing it to migrate posteriorly, reducing the lumbar curvature. This causes low back stress and can lead to injury. To correct this problem requires either improvement in range of motion or performing the exercise within functional range. The third error seen in the movement occurs when too much resistance is used. Frequently, exercisers will allow the resistance to accelerate downward to take advantage of the pre-stretch recoil response. This lack of controlled deceleration often pushes the body into a posterior pelvic tilt, again leading to increased risk for injury.

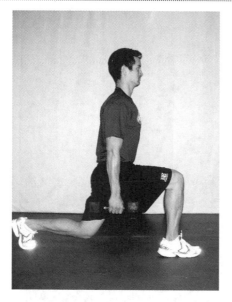 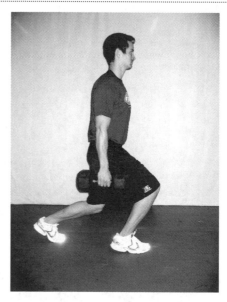

Correct   **Incorrect**

Lunge

One of the most common errors in lower body exercise is to allow the knee to cross the plane of the toe. This occurs due to an incorrect hip flexion-knee flexion relationship during the descent of the squat, lunge, or step-up. During the step-up and lunge, anterior movement of the hip, combined with a shallow lead step pushes the femur over the heel and consequently, forces the tibia to translate. During the squat, a similar action occurs when knee flexion supercedes appropriate hip flexion. The hips stay forward rather than driving backward, causing the femur to slide over the heel. Pushing the glutes backward to initiate the movement and sitting back into the squat will help prevent anterior knee movement during its performance. Taking a broad step and flexing the back knee early in the movement can correct the lunge technique. To correct the step-up errors, the lead foot should be placed into the center of the step with the weight directed into the heel, and upon the descent, the initial back step should be broad to pull the forward knee back behind the heel.

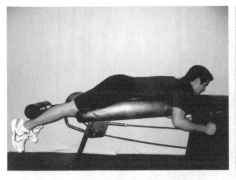 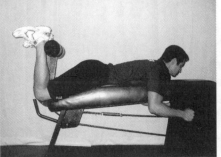 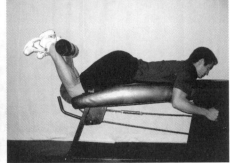

Correct Starting Position   **Correct Ending Position**   **Incorrect Ending Position**

Prone Leg Curl

The most common error in the prone leg curl exercise is the use of hip flexion to aid in the movement. The tendency for the body to assume a position of mechanical advantage explains the reason the hips flex and the pelvis moves anteriorly during performances when too much resistance is used. If cueing does not correct the error the exerciser can reduce the resistance or switch to performing the movement one leg at a time, which will often correct the problem.

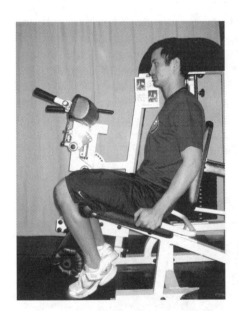 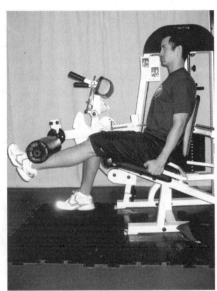 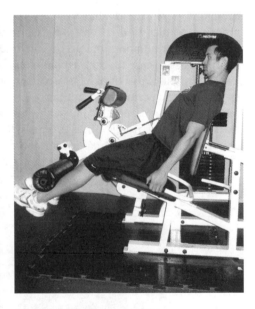

Correct Starting Position   **Correct Ending Position**   **Incorrect Ending Position**

Leg Extension

Similar to the leg curl, the common error with the leg extension most often occurs with too much resistance, as the body compensates by extending the hips. The extended hips provide greater mechanical advantage for the rectus femoris and shorten the resistance arm. To combat this error, the resistance can be reduced or single leg extension can be substituted.

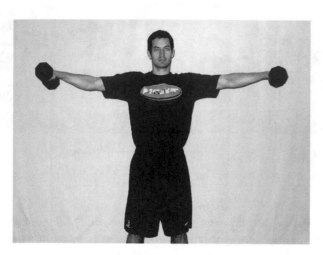

Correct Ending Position

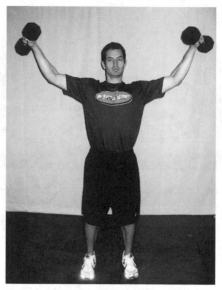

Incorrect Ending Position

Side Raise

Shoulder flexion and abduction exercises are prone to the same common performance errors. Consistent with the mistakes of many other exercises, incorrect resistance selection is often the cause. The three major errors in the lift are incorrect starting point, the use of hip extension to create angular momentum, and too high an ending position during the ascent phase. Since the supraspinatus is the prime mover in initial humeral abduction and the first twenty degrees of the movement basically transfers resistance across gravity, the ideal starting position would be 20-30 degrees off of the hip to increase the deltoid contractile requirements. Many exercisers start and end the movements by swinging the weights so momentum forces contribute to the ascent phase of the lifts. When this occurs along with the added force from hip extension, the deltoids contribute less to the exercise's performance. Too high an ascent can also be problematic, as acromion impingement may occur. To reduce the risk, the side and front raise should end at approximately 90 degrees. Additionally, the hand grip for the front raise should be neutral.

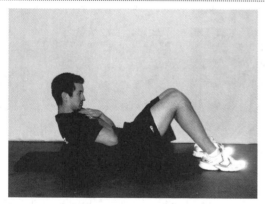

Correct

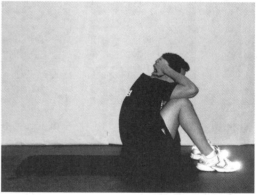

Incorrect

Sit-up

The full sit-up is a contraindicated exercise because the hip flexors take over as the prime mover at about 40 degrees of the movement, placing excessive stress on the intervertebral discs and spinal ligaments. The employment of the hip flexors is further enhanced when the feet or ankles are secured by an external object or person, or when the movement is performed on an inverted incline bench. To correctly perform the exercise for the abdominals, the abdominal curl-up movement should be executed with a draw-in of the umbilicus to stabilize the spine using the transverse abdominis, accompanied by a posterior pelvic tilt to reduce hip activity and trunk flexion to 30 degrees. Additionally, the exerciser should avoid pulling the cervical spine into flexion and perform the movement at a controlled rate of speed, maintaining contractile stress on the abdominals at all times during the execution.

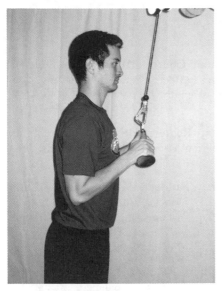
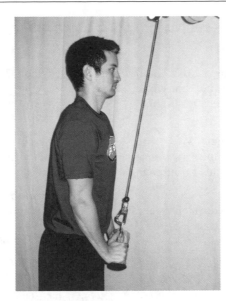
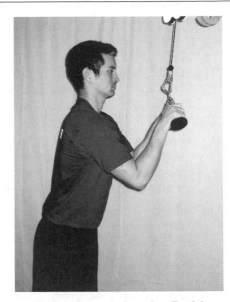

Correct Starting Position   **Correct Ending Position**   **Incorrect Starting Position**

Triceps Extension/Pushdowns

The most common error in triceps exercises involves movement of the humeral position during the execution of the movement. In many cases, shoulder movements are used to increase angular momentum. The incorrect momentum forces in the triceps extension and pushdown exercises are generated by a starting position in shoulder flexion and use of latissimus contractions to cause shoulder extension prior to arm extension. Momentum may also be caused by hip flexion when the resistance is incorrectly applied. Another error is the use of humeral horizontal abduction and adduction to increase pectoralis major contribution by making it more of a press down. To correct these errors requires a static humeral, spinal, and hip position during the movement and often an appropriate reduction in resistance.

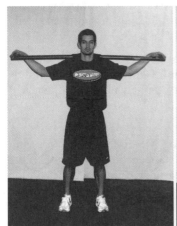
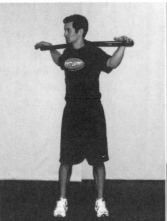
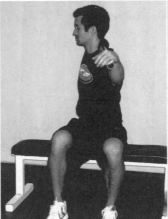
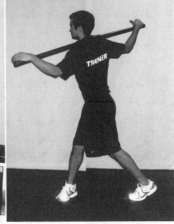

Correct Starting Position   **Correct Ending Position**   **Correct Ending Position**   **Incorrect Ending Position**

Trunk Rotation

Errors in the performance of trunk rotation usually occur due to a lack of flexibility or inefficiency because the movement is more often combined with hip rotation than isolated. Many people have limited range in true trunk rotation, so they compensate by movement at the hip. To correct these problems, exercisers should be cued to stabilize the hip during rotational movements of the trunk. Stability can also be assisted by having the exerciser perform the movements in the seated position. When the arms are employed to move resistance, it is important to make sure the shoulder position does not change horizontally, so the action occurs at the spine.

CHAPTER TWO REFERENCES

1. **Ainscough-Potts AM, Morrissey MC and Critchley D**. The response of the transverse abdominis and internal oblique muscles to different postures. *Man Ther* 11: 54-60, 2006.

2. **Ainscough-Potts AM, Morrissey MC and Critchley D**. The response of the transverse abdominis and internal oblique muscles to different postures. *Man Ther* 11: 54-60, 2006.

3. **Bak K**. Nontraumatic glenohumeral instability and coracoacromial impingement in swimmers. *Scand J Med Sci Sports* 6: 132-144, 1996.

4. **Clark S and Rose DJ**. Evaluation of dynamic balance among community-dwelling older adult fallers: a generalizability study of the limits of stability test. *Arch Phys Med Rehabil* 82: 468-474, 2001.

5. **Danneels LA, Vanderstraeten GG, Cambier DC, Witvrouw EE, Stevens VK and De Cuyper HJ**. A functional subdivision of hip, abdominal, and back muscles during asymmetric lifting. *Spine* 26: E114-E121, 2001.

6. **Davis JR and Mirka GA**. Transverse-contour modeling of trunk muscle-distributed forces and spinal loads during lifting and twisting. *Spine* 25: 180-189, 2000.

7. **Diener HC, Dichgans J, Guschlbauer B and Mau H**. The significance of proprioception on postural stabilization as assessed by ischemia. *Brain Res* 296: 103-109, 1984.

8. **Granata KP and England SA**. Stability of dynamic trunk movement. *Spine* 31: E271-E276, 2006.

9. **Granata KP, Orishimo KF and Sanford AH**. Trunk muscle coactivation in preparation for sudden load. *J Electromyogr Kinesiol* 11: 247-254, 2001.

10. **Hara M, Shibayama A, Takeshita D and Fukashiro S**. The effect of arm swing on lower extremities in vertical jumping. *J Biomech* 39: 2503-2511, 2006.

11. **Heiss DG and Pagnacco G**. Effect of center of pressure and trunk center of mass optimization methods on the analysis of whole body lifting mechanics. *Clin Biomech (Bristol , Avon)* 17: 106-115, 2002.

12. **Hiemstra LA, Webber S, MacDonald PB and Kriellaars DJ**. Hamstring and quadriceps strength balance in normal and hamstring anterior cruciate ligament-reconstructed subjects. *Clin J Sport Med* 14: 274-280, 2004.

13. **Holbein MA and Chaffin DB**. Stability limits in extreme postures: effects of load positioning, foot placement, and strength. *Hum Factors* 39: 456-468, 1997.

14. **Holbein MA and Redfern MS**. Functional stability limits while holding loads in various positions. *Int J Ind Ergon* 19: 387-395, 1997.

15. **Holcomb WR, Rubley MD, Lee HJ and Guadagnoli MA**. Effect of hamstring-emphasized resistance training on hamstring:quadriceps strength ratios. *J Strength Cond Res* 21: 41-47, 2007.

16. **Hortobagyi T, Westerkamp L, Beam S, Moody J, Garry J, Holbert D and DeVita P**. Altered hamstring-quadriceps muscle balance in patients with knee osteoarthritis. *Clin Biomech (Bristol , Avon)* 20: 97-104, 2005.

17. **Iida H and Yamamuro T**. Kinetic analysis of the center of gravity of the human body in normal and pathological gaits. *J Biomech* 20: 987-995, 1987.

18. **Lee DV, Walter RM, Deban SM and Carrier DR**. Influence of increased rotational inertia on the turning performance of humans. *J Exp Biol* 204: 3927-3934, 2001.

19. **Mayer F, Axmann D, Horstmann T, Martini F, Fritz J and Dickhuth HH**. Reciprocal strength ratio in shoulder abduction/adduction in sports and daily living. *Med Sci Sports Exerc* 33: 1765-1769, 2001.

20. **Nadler SF, Malanga GA, Bartoli LA, Feinberg JH, Prybicien M and Deprince M**. Hip muscle imbalance and low back pain in athletes: influence of core strengthening. *Med Sci Sports Exerc* 34: 9-16, 2002.

21. **Ng JK, Parnianpour M, Richardson CA and Kippers V**. Effect of fatigue on torque output and electromyographic measures of trunk muscles during isometric axial rotation. *Arch Phys Med Rehabil* 84: 374-381, 2003.

22. **Ng JK, Richardson CA, Parnianpour M and Kippers V**. EMG activity of trunk muscles and torque output during isometric axial rotation exertion: a comparison between back pain patients and matched controls. *J Orthop Res* 20: 112-121, 2002.

23. **Ng JK, Richardson CA, Parnianpour M and Kippers V**. EMG activity of trunk muscles and torque output during isometric axial rotation exertion: a comparison between back pain patients and matched controls. *J Orthop Res* 20: 112-121, 2002.

24. **Nichols DS, Glenn TM and Hutchinson KJ**. Changes in the mean center of balance during balance testing in young adults. *Phys Ther* 75: 699-706, 1995.

25. **Noffal GJ**. Isokinetic eccentric-to-concentric strength ratios of the shoulder rotator muscles in throwers and nonthrowers. *Am J Sports Med* 31: 537-541, 2003.

26. **Noffal GJ**. Isokinetic eccentric-to-concentric strength ratios of the shoulder rotator muscles in throwers and nonthrowers. *Am J Sports Med* 31: 537-541, 2003.

27. **Pasque CB and Hewett TE**. A prospective study of high school wrestling injuries. *Am J Sports Med* 28: 509-515, 2000.

28. **Teyhen DS, Miltenberger CE, Deiters HM, Del Toro YM, Pulliam JN, Childs JD, Boyles RE and Flynn TW**. The use of ultrasound imaging of the abdominal drawing-in maneuver in subjects with low back pain. *J Orthop Sports Phys Ther* 35: 346-355, 2005.

29. **Tucker CA, Ramirez J, Krebs DE and Riley PO**. Center of gravity dynamic stability in normal and vestibulopathic gait. *Gait Posture* 8: 117-123, 1998.

30. **Vanezis A and Lees A**. A biomechanical analysis of good and poor performers of the vertical jump. *Ergonomics* 48: 1594-1603, 2005.

31. **Willson JD, Dougherty CP, Ireland ML and Davis IM**. Core stability and its relationship to lower extremity function and injury. *J Am Acad Orthop Surg* 13: 316-325, 2005.

Chapter 3

Muscle Physiology

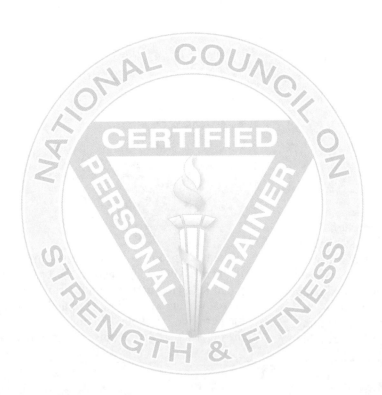

Types of Muscle Tissue

The muscular system is comprised of three types of muscle tissue: **skeletal**, **cardiac** and **smooth**. Each performs specialized functions within the body. Skeletal muscle acts on the skeleton to maintain posture, create voluntary movement, manage force transfer, and prevent undesirable body actions. The cardiac muscle tissue, located only in the heart, pushes blood through the circulatory system. Smooth muscle comprises the muscular walls of blood vessels as well as the gastrointestinal tract, which includes the esophagus, stomach, small intestine, large intestine, and rectum. Smooth muscle moves fluids and solids, dilates and constricts small arteries, and performs a variety of other functions to help keep the body in a state of balance. For the purposes of personal training, this chapter will focus on the functions and adaptations of skeletal muscle.

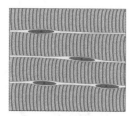

Skeletal

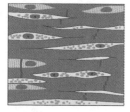

Cardiac

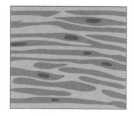

Smooth

How Muscles Contract

To produce the internal tensile and compression forces described in Chapter 2, skeletal muscle must contract. To do so, the body requires multiple systems to work concurrently and synergistically. Using signals primarily initiated in the brain, the nervous system stimulates the muscle, causing it to contract and produce tension. If the force requirements are ongoing, the muscle needs a continuous supply of energy and

blood. In Chapter 1, we learned that the epimysium and perimysium (interwoven muscle layers) contain the nerves and blood vessels that support muscular contraction and the production of force. These networks are extremely important, as they carry the motor information via **action potentials** from the **central nervous system** and allow the vascular system to deliver energy and oxygen and remove by-product waste produced from the metabolic production of energy. The peripheral nervous system and vascular system run together through the muscle tissue, branching into smaller units all the way down to the muscle fiber, where **capillaries** and nerve fibers interact with the contractile proteins.

The muscle fiber is arranged like a small factory, with each structure serving a particular function to create contractile tension. Working from the inside out, the myofibrils are cylindrical structures that contain the myofilaments actin (thin filament) and myosin (thick filaments). These protein filaments are where the contractile action of the sliding filament theory takes place. This process will be explained in the next paragraph. Surrounding the myofibrils are a calcium housing network called the **sarcoplasmic reticulum** (SR), tube-like structures called **T-tubules** used to transfer nerve signals, and **mitochondria,** which will eventually be used to produce energy. The whole package is encased by the muscle fiber's cell membrane called the **sarcolemma**. The muscle fibers are encased by the **endomysium** which is where the capillaries and nerve endings are located.

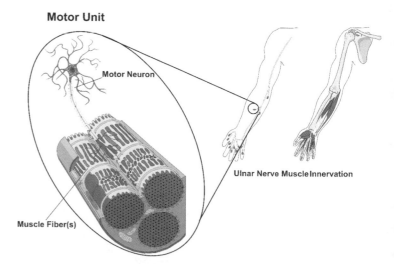

Motor Unit

Motor Neuron

Ulnar Nerve Muscle Innervation

Muscle Fiber(s)

If the body needs to create tension in a group of muscle fibers, a signal is initiated in the brain called an action potential. The action potential travels via electrical current through the spinal cord and is then transferred to the peripheral nervous system. The current runs through the outer levels of the muscle tissue to very small nerve fibers, which connect to the particular fibers to be contracted. These small nerve fibers are called **motor neurons**. Together, the motor neuron and all the muscle fibers it innervates are called the **motor unit**. Within the motor unit, the motor neuron extends branches of individual nerve fibers to individual muscle fibers. The action potential enters the individual muscle fibers at the neuromuscular junction, formed by the end of the nerve fiber and sarcolemma. Here, it stimulates the sarcolemma via an electrically-gated channel. This connection between the nerve and the muscle fiber is called an excitation-couple. The excitation-couple acts as a bridge between the nerve and the muscle, allowing the electrical impulse to jump from the nerve fiber to the muscle fiber.

Inside the muscle fiber, the action potential travels down the T-tubules and stimulates the sarcoplasmic reticulum. This initiates the contraction cycle by releasing calcium from the SR. In a relaxed state, the muscle fiber protein filaments inside the **sarcomere** are blocked from interacting with each other by a protein complex consisting of troponin and tropomyosin. Calcium released from the SR acts like a key to unlock the bond between the thin actin contractile filament and troponin via a conformation change of the troponin molecule. When the calcium unlocks the bond, the **troponin** molecule moves, rotating the **tropomyosin** molecule out of the way of the binding site just like opening a door. When this occurs myosin is free to attach to actin by what is referred to as a cross bridge attachment. At the myosin/actin attachment site, **adenosine triphosphate (ATP)** is split, and the energy released allows the muscle fiber to contract and produce force. This complex chain of interactions, allowing the

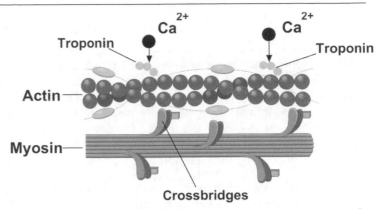

actin and myosin filament proteins to slide over each other, is known as the **sliding filament theory.**

The movement of the myosin head resembles the movement of an oar when rowing a boat. In the same way the oar enters the water, gets pulled across the surface of the water, and is pulled out before being repositioned for the next rowing cycle, the myosin head attaches, pulls, detaches, re-cocks, and starts the process again. If the excitation is maintained and adequate ATP exists, this process can be repeated up to five times per second. The amount of tension produced is proportionate to the number of active **cross bridges** along a myofibril's length.

Force Production

A muscle fiber is either in a state of producing maximum tension or not producing any tension at all. This is often referred to as the "all or none" principle. This suggests that the tension produced by a muscle is dependent on the number of fibers stimulated and the frequency of the stimulation. When a muscle fiber is stimulated through a single contraction-relaxation cycle, it is called a twitch. The duration of a twitch is dependent upon the fiber producing the action. Fibers are generally defined as one of two types, fast twitch or slow switch. Fast twitch fibers obviously twitch quickly (10 milliseconds), whereas slow twitch fibers take more time to complete the contraction-relaxation cycle (100 milliseconds) (5). Twitches in a skeletal muscle do not accomplish anything useful. It takes sustained muscle contractions to perform normal movements. Sustained muscle contractions occur when the rate of stimulation is increased to the point that there is no longer a relaxation phase. This is called **complete tetanus,** and is necessary for muscle contractions to produce force. Normal muscle contractions occur due to complete tetanus.

To produce significant tension to accomplish movement, motor units are stimulated within the desired muscle. The greater the number of motor units stimulated, the more fibers are recruited and

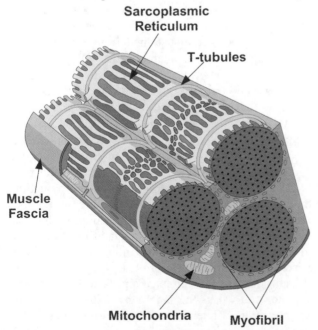

~Quick Insight~

Muscle tone occurs because some of the motor units are always active even when the muscle is not contracted. The motor unit activation does not produce enough tension to cause movement but provides tone or firmness to the tissue. The degree of tone is dependent upon the tension created and number of motor units firing to stabilize the position of the bones and joints. The motor units are stimulated in varying patterns to prevent fatigue. When external forces act on the body, the tension in the tissue provides data to the nervous system via proprioceptors, which better enables the skeletal muscle and tendons to function in response to a sudden change in tension or body position (16). Specialized intrafusal fibers called **muscle spindles** aid in this response by helping the tissue manage forces (13).

Muscle spindles are clusters of specialized muscle tissue (intrafusal fibers) that lie parallel to the normal muscle fibers (extrafusal fibers) (15). The intrafusal fibers relay information to sensory neurons regarding changes in the tissue length and tension. When stretched, these tissues respond using reflex action, called the stretch reflex, to initiate a stronger contraction to reduce the imposed stretch in a shock absorbing fashion. The excitatory impulses activate agonist muscles to contract and antagonist muscles to relax in a process of rapid self-regulation. Recalling from Chapter 1, agonist/antagonist muscles are those that cause opposite movement trajectories across a joint, exemplified by the bicep and tricep muscles at the elbow joint. As the bicep muscle contracts, the triceps muscle must relax and vice versa. The reflex action aids in automatic tone adjustment which supports control of body position and posture. Because it is a reflex, the process does not require input from the brain, but rather, occurs at the level of the spinal cord, allowing for immediate compensatory adjustments during activities requiring balance and coordination. The constant supply of information from the muscle spindles through the stretch reflex is fundamental to mechanisms for neuromuscular regulation (3).

Golgi tendon organs complement muscle spindles in regulating the muscle and connective tissue tension (8). The Golgi tendons are tiny sensory receptors which exist inside the muscle tendons. They rapidly communicate information to the motor neurons in the muscles they serve to prevent excessive tension that could be potentially dangerous to the tissues' integrity. If tension becomes too great, the Golgi tendon organs send inhibitory signals to reduce motor neuron activity and thereby reduce the force of muscular contraction. By inhibiting tension in the muscle the Golgi tendons serve to prevent tissue injury that would likely occur from the excessive tension. An example of this process occurs in the masseter muscle. Contraction of the masseter muscle causes closure of the jaw bone when one chews. The masseter muscle is capable of producing enough force in the jaw to cause fracturing of the teeth. However, the golgi tendon organs in the masseter musculotendon sense the amount of tension in the muscle and prevent the muscle from attaining this level of force, preventing damage to the teeth.

subsequently, the more tension that is produced. The total force exerted by a skeletal muscle is a factor of how many muscle fibers are recruited for the contraction. Peak tension occurs when all the motor units in the muscle are contracting in complete tetanus.

Motor units generally work in a tag team fashion because most work is not performed under peak tension. When maximal outputs are required, all the motor units are recruited at a high rate to produce tension. This level of tension can only occur for a short period of time. The muscle starts to fatigue and peak tension is reduced. When activities require force for prolonged periods, the motor units take turns firing, so some fibers recover while others work. This phenomenon suggests that firing patterns are specific to the demand of the activity (6). High output demands use synchronized firing of fast twitch fibers and high number recruitment patterns, whereas endurance activity uses asynchronous firing patterns of slow twitch fibers which are fatigue resistant to conserve motor unit potential, thereby allowing for longer periods of sustained work.

Muscle force potential as it relates to the motor unit is analogous to a crew team rowing a boat. We have identified that a muscle's peak tension requires sustained tetanus, or the sustained firing of all muscle fibers recruited. This is analogous to everyone on a crew team rowing at a nonstop rate. The more teammates who contribute and the faster they row, the more force they will produce to move the boat across the water. The same idea applies to force production in muscle tissue. The more muscle tissue recruited, the more force potential of the contraction. Similarly, if one can get the rowers to row faster (increased firing rate) the boat will accelerate due to greater force production. If the firing rate in the motor neurons increases so does the resultant force of the muscle contraction. If all of the rowers are recruited to put forth an effort (increased recruitment) and they are coordinated to row at precisely the same time (improved synchronicity) you will attain the best performance and fastest boat speed. The motor unit works the same way. With training, the fibers are more efficiently recruited, firing rates of the motor units are enhanced, and the firing rates occur in unison, creating synchronized tension and greater force outputs. It is an important concept to understand that all of these actions are functions of the nervous system, which becomes more efficient with training experience. The ability to increase force production within a muscle through training is dependent on adaptations that occur to both the muscle fibers and the nervous system together (1).

The example of the crew team rowing a boat explains improvements in maximal tension development. But what if the rowers want to travel long distances rather than moving at an extremely fast rate? In this case, it would make more sense for the rowers to use an alternating rowing pattern and slower stroke. If two rowers perform a synchronized stroke and then recover while two other rowers perform their stroke in an alternating fashion, the boat's momentum will be maintained without any particular rower becoming overly fatigued. This illustrates the motor unit pattern for endurance activities described above. The more synchronized the stroke patterns and rest to work activity ratio, the more efficiently the action will be performed.

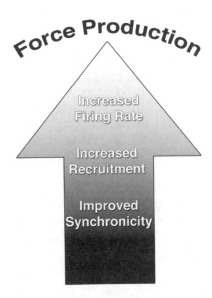

An interesting fact related to the neural influence on force production is that improvements in the development of force can occur even if no new muscle is added. The efficiency changes related to motor unit recruitment make this possible. As the body experiences situations which require force to be produced, it learns the most efficient methods to meet the new demands. This adaptation is often referred to as motor learning. Essentially, the body learns how to maximize the use of the tissue it already has via improved regulation by the nervous system (12). These facts will be explored in more detail later in the text.

Fatigue

The ability to maintain muscle tension is dependent upon several factors, with the most notable being the intensity of the exercise (9). The more force needed, the faster the rate of fatigue. Muscle fatigue results from disruption somewhere along the chain of events in the production of force. Fatigue is defined by an inability to contract despite continued neural stimulation. The cause of fatigue can occur in the central nervous system, peripheral nervous system, at the neuromuscular junction, or in the muscle fiber itself (14). Since the fatigue is intensity-specific, the particular cause will be reflective of the activity. Short-term, high force activities cause neuromuscular fatigue due to several possible mechanisms listed below. During prolonged activities with less force output, the cause of fatigue is most often attributed to the energy supply. Muscle fatigue is cumulative, so as fibers fatigue, they disrupt the motor unit's ability to produce the force necessary to continue the activity at the current rate. As the rate of motor unit fatigue increases, the effect becomes more pronounced, causing performance to decline proportionate to the level of fatigue (4).

Periods of recovery enable a working tissue to avoid fatigue for longer periods of time. This is evidenced by the alternating recruitment patterns used during prolonged activities. In short burst activity, the muscles perform at peak or near peak levels, which leads to rapid fatigue.

~Key Terms~

Skeletal muscle- A type of striated muscle, attached to the skeleton used to facilitate movement, by applying force to bones and joints via contractions.

Cardiac muscle- A type of involuntary mononucleated, or uninucleated, striated muscle found exclusively within the heart.

Smooth muscle- A type of non-striated muscle, found within the "walls" of hollow organs such as the bladder, the uterus, and the gastrointestinal tract. It also lines the lumen of the body, such as in blood vessels. Smooth muscle is fundamentally different from skeletal muscle and cardiac muscle in terms of structure and function.

Capillaries- Tiny blood vessels throughout the body that connect arteries and veins. Capillaries form an intricate network around body tissues in order to distribute oxygen and nutrients to the cells and to remove waste substances.

Sarcoplasmic reticulum- A tubular network that surrounds each individual myofibril and acts as a storage site for calcium within the skeletal muscle.

When the action is temporarily discontinued, the muscle fiber attempts to return to pre-exertion levels. The period of time between repeated actions, such as a sprint or squat performance, is called the rest period or rest interval. During this period of time, the muscle cell's recovery is dependent upon the return of intracellular energy supply, circulatory based cellular by-product removal, and the delivery of oxygen. When the exercise bout is completely discontinued, the cell has a much longer period of time to manage the disruption caused by the activity. This is referred to as the recovery period. During the recovery period, the muscle fibers can rebuild their energy reserves, fix any damage resulting from the production of force, and fully return to normal pre-exertion levels. The duration of the recovery period required to return the cell back to normal depends upon the degree that the muscle fiber was used (7). In cases of sustained high-level output, full recovery may take as long as one week (2). Recovery between exercise bouts is an important consideration in the exercise prescription.

CAUSES OF SHORT-TERM FATIGUE	CAUSES OF LONG-TERM FATIGUE
Exhaustion of ATP/CP reserves	Depleted glycogen and blood glucose levels
Decreased muscle pH	Damage to the sarcoplasmic reticulum
Insufficient oxygen	Depletion of electrolyte ions
Reduced enzyme activity	
Tubular system disturbance	

Types of Muscle Contractions

The muscle contractions produced by the stimulation of motor units contribute to different internal forces within the body. These contractions are categorized by the actions they produce. A tonic action, during which a lengthening or shortening occurs within the muscle, is called an isotonic contraction. The term isotonic is derived from the greek *isotonos* (*iso,* meaning equal, and *tonos,* meaning tension). This term is generally used inexactly when describing dynamic muscle actions because the muscle's effective force production across the joint changes through the movement and is not uniform. These types of contractions are visible in all movements. The shortening phase, called the concentric phase of the contraction, occurs when muscle tension force exceeds the resistance force applied to it, so positive work is attained.

This can be demonstrated with a bicep curl. As the bicep muscle contracts concentrically, the elbow flexes. When the arm returns to the start position of the curl movement, the bicep lengthens as a result of the muscle producing less tension than is necessary to accelerate the resistance in the direction of the force. When the muscle lengthens under tension, it produces an **eccentric contraction** to perform negative work. **Concentric contractions** accelerate joint movements, while eccentric contractions decelerate movements.

If the tension created to accelerate force is equal to the resistance force no movement will occur. Although the motor units fire, the tension in the muscle is insufficient to accelerate the object in the direction of the force. This type of contraction is called an **isometric contraction**. The joint angle does not change even though the attached musculature exerts force. Isometric contractions are not commonly employed in training programs to strengthen prime movers. However, any time the body performs a movement, isometric contractions are necessary. Isometric contractions are used by stabilizing muscles to control movements and prevent undesirable actions of the body. When the body is in a stationary position, for example, the muscles acting on the skeleton must contract isometrically to prevent it from collapsing under the pull of gravity. The same types of contractions maintain posture and joint position during dynamic activities, such as the isometric contractions of the abdominals during the performance of a push-up. In effect, we use and train with isometric contractions all of the time, as they contribute to stability.

~Key Terms~

T-tubules- The tubule that passes in a transverse manner from the sarcolemma across a myofibril of striated muscle, allowing depolarization of the membrane to quickly penetrate to the interior of the cell.

Sarcolemma- A thin polarized membrane enclosing a striated muscle fiber.

Endomysium- The fine connective tissue sheath surrounding a muscle fiber.

Action potential- The wave-like change in the electrical properties of a cell membrane, resulting from the difference in electrical charge between the inside and outside of the membrane, causing the muscle cell to contract.

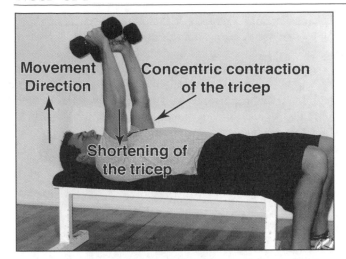

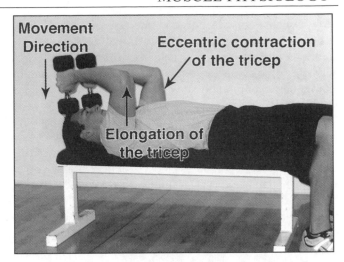

Muscle Fiber Types

The type of muscle fiber recruited to produce a contraction depends upon the amount of force needed for the desired action. Muscle fibers and their respective motor units are classified by their physiologic and mechanical properties. These properties include the fiber contractile speed or twitch characteristics, force output or tension generating capacity, and ability to resist fatigue. The particular characteristics gear the motor units for either power or endurance. Motor units are either classified as fast-twitch fast-fatigue, fast-twitch fatigue-resistant, or slow-twitch- fatigue-resistant. Consistent with the motor unit classification categories there are three skeletal muscle fiber types. The fiber type classifications are sometimes expressed using type distinction abbreviations or labeled according to the energy system they prefer to utilize. The high force producing fibers are called **Type IIb fibers** or fast glycolytic fibers (FG). The intermediate force producing fibers are called **Type IIa fibers** or fast oxidative/glycolytic fibers (FOG). The low power output fibers are called **Type I** or slow oxidative fibers (SO).   The glycolytic or oxidative annotation refers to the type of energy source utilized to generate ATP by the muscle fiber and is described in detail in Chapter 5.

Fast twitch fibers are recognized by their characteristically large diameter size, densely packed myofibrils and large glycogen (consolidated sugar molecules for energy) reserves. They are preferentially recruited for activities requiring high power outputs and are subject to dramatic improvements in size and strength when trained under conditions of short duration and high intensity. They preferentially function using **anaerobic** metabolic systems. On the other end of the spectrum, the slow twitch muscle fibers are 50% smaller than their fast twitch counterparts and produce peak force at one third the rate upon stimulation. They primarily use **aerobic** metabolic systems and are far

better suited for endurance, containing an extensive capillary network and high mitochondrial density. They also have the addition of a notably higher amount of myoglobin, which increases oxygen reserves in the cell. These characteristics make it ideal for activities of prolonged duration.

When an activity requires the combination of elevated force and prolonged duration, the intermediate fibers, Type IIA, become favored. Due to the fact that these fibers maintain properties of both fast and slow fibers, they are well suited to support both anaerobic and aerobic activities. Intermediate fibers are classified as fast twitch fibers because they contain small quantities of **myoglobin**. But, like the slow-twitch fibers, they have an extensive blood supply and are more resistant to fatigue.

In the previous section, we identified that the motor recruitment patterns were based on the tension demands of the muscle. This identifies the fact that the fiber types selected for activation depend upon the speed and magnitude of the tension required for the activity.

~Key Terms~

Neuromuscular junction- The site at which nerve impulses are transmitted to muscles.

Sarcomere- smallest functional unit of a muscle fiber, composed of contractile myofilaments.

Troponin- a protein complex found in both skeletal muscle and cardiac muscle that relays calcium sensitivity to muscle cells.

Tropomyosin- a group of muscle proteins that bind to molecules of actin and troponin to regulate the interaction of actin and myosin.

Motor unit- A motor neuron and all of the corresponding muscle fibers it innervates.

Slow-twitch fibers do not generate tension quickly, so they cannot meet the demand of high power output activities and are therefore selected to serve low level activities of varying force requirements. Activities such as jogging, cycling, and slow speed, light weight lifting involve selective recruitment of the slow-twitch fibers. When the activities are fast and powerful, the selective recruitment adds fast-twitch fibers for a greater magnitude of force production. During activities of varying intensity, such as those found with soccer, basketball, and interval training, slow twitch fibers serve the lower force outputs aerobically, while fast-twitch fibers dominate the high intensity anaerobic segments of the activity. The recruitment patterns match the fiber characteristics.

Fiber Type Distribution

Fiber type distribution is genetically predetermined, so no method exists to manipulate how the fibers are proportionately concentrated in the body. The distribution of fiber types within a particular skeletal muscle can be quite variable. Although certain muscles, such as those used primarily for posture, maintain higher concentrations of slow-twitch fibers. These muscles, including the soleus, deep muscles of the back, and the rectus abdominis must contract continuously to maintain upright posture. They are not designed for rapid, high force output, and therefore experience limited improvements in activities aimed at power or **hypertrophy**.

It has been said, "you don't pick your sport, your sport picks you" suggesting that certain people are designed to succeed in a particular sport, whereas others are not. Fiber type distribution plays a role in this determination. As would be expected, muscle biopsies demonstrate that individuals who perform well in sprint or burst power activities have higher concentrations of fast-twitch fibers in the respective prime mover muscles necessary for their activity. Endurance athletes show higher concentrations of slow-twitch fibers in these same muscle groups. If a highly trained sprinter and marathoner switched roles for a day, neither would be very successful in the other's event. Although training in a particular event will certainly cause anyone to improve in the activity, practice alone is not enough for a person to reach an elite status. Genetic predisposition is a powerful factor. Ultimately, the percentage of any particular fiber type within a muscle is based on the role of the tissue in movement and the genetically determined distribution pattern assigned to the muscle. Among individuals in similar sports, distinctions in performance advantage by muscle fiber type distribution seem to be specific to the most elite athletes. However, fiber distribution patterns determine only a component of performance capacity. Although they do provide an advantage in activities that match the fiber-specific characteristics, they do not define performance outcomes because measurable performance is based on the blend of many physiological systems.

~Key Terms~

Adenosine Triphosphate (ATP)- Serves as the major energy source within a cell to drive a number of biological processes such as muscle contractions and the synthesis of proteins.

Cross bridge- A myosin head that projects from the surface of the thick filament that binds to the surface of a thin filament (actin) in the presence of calcium ions.

Complete tetanus- Sustained skeletal muscle contraction due to repeated stimulation at a frequency which prevents relaxation.

Muscle tone- Unconscious nerve impulses that maintain the muscles in a partially contracted state.

Muscle spindles- A specialized muscle structure innervated by both sensory and motor neuron axons, functioning to send proprioceptive information about the muscle to the central nervous system in response to muscle stretching.

Golgi tendon organs- Kinesthetic receptors situated near the junction of muscle fibers and tendons which act as muscle-tension regulators.

Concentric contraction- A type of muscle contraction in which the muscles apply enough force to overcome the resistive force so that it shortens as it contracts.

Muscle Fiber Diameter

 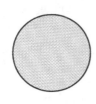 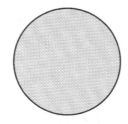

Type I   Type IIa   Type IIb

Training for an activity will cause improvements in many of the physiological systems that affect the performance outcome. In response to the training stress, several components of the motor unit adapt to become better suited to the conditions. The motor units begin to more closely reflect the desired skeletal tissue type through modifications in properties and characteristics. The actual fiber type, however, does not change. In humans a slow-twitch fiber has not been shown to convert to a fast-twitch fiber and vice versa. Changes in patterns of neural stimulation, capillary and mitochondrial density, and enzyme concentration cause the muscle fiber to become better suited to the training stimulus (11). This fact is exemplified by the changes in performance with training.

Although a person may not be born with a muscle fiber type distribution that is best suited for a given activity, through specific training, they can cause changes in the recruitment pattern and muscle fibers that allow them to improve their performance despite their genetic predisposition (10).

All of the information regarding recruitment and fiber characteristics is relevant when creating the exercise prescription. Matching the stimulus to the desired adaptation response is pivotal to successful exercise programming. For instance, increasing strength and muscular size is dependent upon the magnitude and rate of the stimulus. Without employing appropriate methods to maximize these factors, the end adaptation response will be compromised to the degree that the exercise prescription is in error. This is true of any program that does not properly consider the energy system, recruitment patterns, and characteristics of the muscle involved.

~Key Terms~

Eccentric contraction- A type of muscle contraction in which the resistive force is greater than the force applied by the muscle so that the muscle lengthens as it contracts.

Isometric contraction- A contraction in which muscle tension is increased, but the joint angle is not changed because the resistance cannot be overcome. Also known as static contraction.

Type IIb fibers- Largest diameter muscle fiber, characterized by anaerobic metabolism and the greatest maximum tension.

Type IIa fibers- Large diameter muscle fiber, characterized by aerobic and anaerobic metabolism. High maximum tension.

Type I fibers- Smaller diameter muscle fiber characterized by aerobic metabolism and lower maximum tension.

Myoglobin- The oxygen-transporting protein of muscle, resembling blood hemoglobin in function.

FIBER TYPE	FATIGUE POWER/NERVE CHARACTERISTICS	METABOLIC CHARACTERISTICS
TYPE I	Fatigue Resistant/Slow Twitch Low Power Output Small Fiber Diameter	High Oxidative Capacity Low Glycolytic Capacity High Mitochondrial Density
TYPE IIA	Fatigue Resistant/Fast Twitch Intermediate Power Output Intermediate Fiber Diameter	Medium/High Oxidative Capacity High Glycolytic Capacity Moderate Mitochondrial Density
TYPE IIB	Fast Fatigue/Fast Twitch High Power Output Large Fiber Diameter	High Glycolytic Capacity Low Oxidative Capacity Low Mitochondrial Density

Chapter Three References

1. **Akataki K, Mita K and Watakabe M**. Electromyographic and mechanomyographic estimation of motor unit activation strategy in voluntary force production. *Electromyogr Clin Neurophysiol* 44: 489-496, 2004.

2. **Angeli A, Minetto M, Dovio A and Paccotti P**. The overtraining syndrome in athletes: a stress-related disorder. *J Endocrinol Invest* 27: 603-612, 2004.

3. **BERNIER JJ, PAUPE J and DALLOZ JC**. [ILLUSTRATED PHYSIOPATHOLOGY. MEDULLARY REFLEXES AND MUSCLE TONUS. 3. CENTRAL CONTROL OF THE MYOSTATIC REFLEX. 2) REGULATION AT THE UPPER LEVEL.]. *Concours Med* 86: 3075-3076, 1964.

4. **Calder KM, Stashuk DW and McLean L**. Physiological characteristics of motor units in the brachioradialis muscle across fatiguing low-level isometric contractions. *J Electromyogr Kinesiol* 2006.

5. **Dahmane R, Djordjevic S, Simunic B and Valencic V**. Spatial fiber type distribution in normal human muscle Histochemical and tensiomyographical evaluation. *J Biomech* 38: 2451-2459, 2005.

6. **Dahmane R, Djordjevic S and Smerdu V**. Adaptive potential of human biceps femoris muscle demonstrated by histochemical, immunohistochemical and mechanomyographical methods. *Med Biol Eng Comput* 44: 999-1006, 2006.

7. **Hug F, Grelot L, Le Fur Y, Cozzone PJ and Bendahan D**. Recovery kinetics throughout successive bouts of various exercises in elite cyclists. *Med Sci Sports Exerc* 38: 2151-2158, 2006.

8. **Hwang IS and Cho CY**. Muscle control associated with isometric contraction in different joint positions. *Electromyogr Clin Neurophysiol* 44: 463-471, 2004.

9. **Kayser B**. Exercise starts and ends in the brain. *Eur J Appl Physiol* 90: 411-419, 2003.

10. **Kuipers H, Janssen GM, Bosman F, Frederik PM and Geurten P**. Structural and ultrastructural changes in skeletal muscle associated with long-distance training and running. *Int J Sports Med* 10 Suppl 3: S156-S159, 1989.

11. **Kuipers H, Janssen GM, Bosman F, Frederik PM and Geurten P**. Structural and ultrastructural changes in skeletal muscle associated with long-distance training and running. *Int J Sports Med* 10 Suppl 3: S156-S159, 1989.

12. **Park JH and Stelmach GE**. Effect of combined variation of force amplitude and rate of force development on the modulation characteristics of muscle activation during rapid isometric aiming force production. *Exp Brain Res* 168: 337-347, 2006.

13. **Perrin P, Perrin C, Boura M, Uffholtz H and Conraux C**. [Static and dynamic posturography. Application to a population of young athletes]. *Ann Otolaryngol Chir Cervicofac* 106: 463-471, 1989.

14. **Schillings ML, Hoefsloot W, Stegeman DF and Zwarts MJ**. Relative contributions of central and peripheral factors to fatigue during a maximal sustained effort. *Eur J Appl Physiol* 90: 562-568, 2003.

15. **Wicke W, Wasicky R, Brugger PC, Kaminski S and Lukas JR**. Histochemical and immunohistochemical study on muscle fibers in human extraocular muscle spindles. *Exp Eye Res* 2007.

16. **Zhang LQ, Huang H, Sliwa JA and Rymer WZ**. System identification of tendon reflex dynamics. *IEEE Trans Rehabil Eng* 7: 193-203, 1999.

Chapter 4

Endocrine System

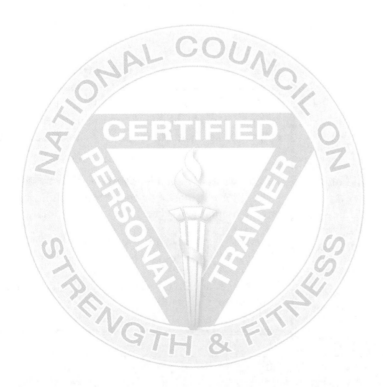

The Endocrine System

The endocrine system is a complex network of integrated organs that communicates and helps regulate all other bodily systems to manage the internal activities and maintain **homeostasis**. Within the body, fine balances exist, with seemingly unlimited cause and effect patterns which occur in response to internal and external variations of environment. Although the systems of the body are often viewed independently, they are actually intimately integrated and cannot function autonomously. The relationship between the muscular system and the nervous system would seem to be a logical example of the interaction of networked systems because, in essence, nerves are the brains behind the machine. A muscle cannot function without neural communication. Additionally, for the musculoskeletal system to function, the gastrointestinal system must supply it with nutrients for energy and building blocks, and the pulmonary system must work cooperatively with the cardiovascular system to deliver nutrients and oxygen, while simultaneously eliminating waste products of cellular metabolism, including CO_2. A not so obvious relationship also exists between the muscular and **endocrine systems**. Most fitness professionals maintain a very limited knowledge of this relationship beyond that it actually exists. Due to the fact that adaptations to exercise depend upon this relationship, trainers must understand how to manipulate the systems to optimize health improvements and maximize performance.

The endocrine system's role is to assist in integrating and controlling bodily functions. It serves to provide internal balance within almost all aspects of human function. A group of small endocrine glands are responsible for the maintenance of homeostasis in every situation the body endures. This function includes reproduction, growth, tissue maintenance and repair, as well as augmenting the physiological actions to manage the application of **eustress** and **distress**. The main endocrine workforce is comprised of the pituitary, thyroid, adrenal, pineal, and thymus glands. Some hormonal providers have other functions in addition to their endocrine role, such as the hypothalamus, pancreas, and gonads (testicles and ovaries). They produce endocrine hormones, in addition to the other jobs they perform.

Hormones

A gland is an organ that produces a secretion for use elsewhere in the body or in a body cavity. When endocrine glands produce and release hormones, they do so for communication purposes. Hormones essentially direct actions of other tissues via chemical messaging. During and following physical activity, these endocrine glands must regulate electrolyte activity, acid/base balance, and manage energy for biological work and recovery. They do so by producing hormones, which enter circulation and are picked up by the appropriate receptor on target cells.

Cellular receptors are small proteins on the outside of cells that bind to hormones and transmit the information into those cells to regulate the cells' behaviors. These receptors are generally specific to a single hormone and not all cell types have every type of receptor. The concentration and location of **hormone receptors** depend upon the specific responsibility of the hormone. Thus only the tissue that is supposed to receive the information gets the information, alleviating confusion within the body. This internal policy of communication is called **target cell specificity**. An easy analogy to make is when you send e-mail. Think of yourself as a gland and the e-mail as the hormone. When you send that e-mail, it travels across the internet which is accessed by millions of people; however, the information on that e-mail is only received by the one or more persons you designate as recipients.

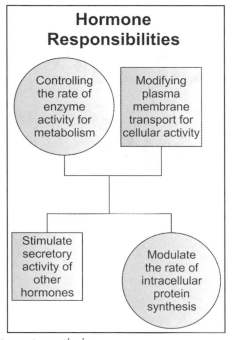

Hormone Responsibilities

- Controlling the rate of enzyme activity for metabolism
- Modifying plasma membrane transport for cellular activity
- Stimulate secretory activity of other hormones
- Modulate the rate of intracellular protein synthesis

~Key Terms~

Endocrine system- Body control system composed of a group of glands that maintain a stable internal environment by producing chemical regulatory substances called hormones.

Homeostasis- The tendency of the body to seek and maintain a condition of balance or equilibrium within its internal environment, even when faced with external changes.

Eustress- A positive, desirable form of stress that influences physical or physiological health.

Distress- A negative form of stress that influences physical or physiological health.

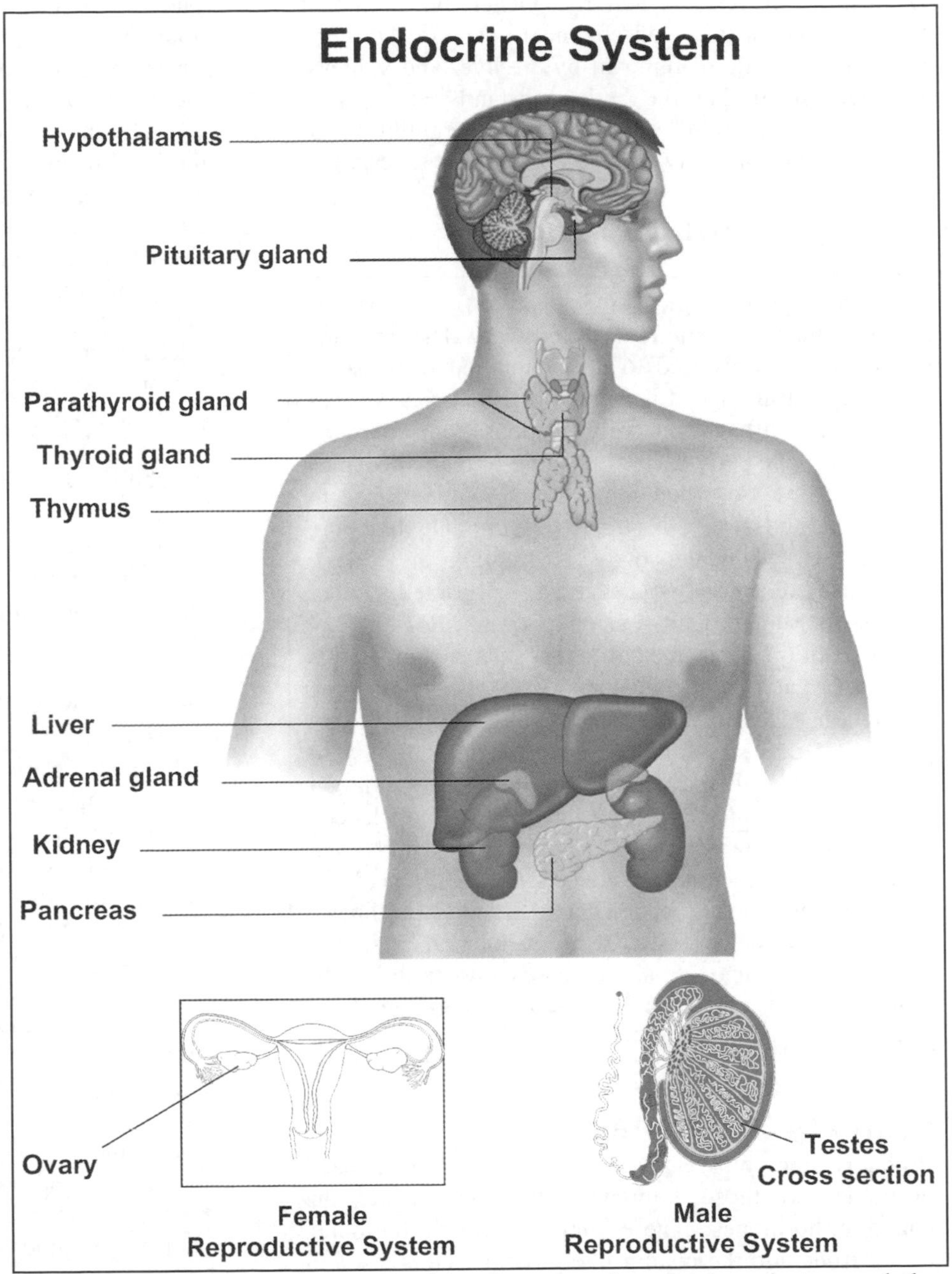

Hormones are categorized into two classes: **steroids** (lipid based) and **polypeptides** (protein based). The type and structural foundation of the hormone is most often related to its message and the tissue that is supposed to receive it.

The intricacy of the specific activity each hormone regulates is often rather sophisticated. The information that a hormone relays to a target tissue depends on the type of tissue it binds to, what other hormones are binding to that tissue at that time, and the cellular environment of the tissue. The endocrine system is further complicated by the fact that certain organs that are not endocrine glands can release hormones. In addition to the hormones of the endocrine glands, at least eight other hormones come from alternate sources, including the stomach, duodenum, kidneys, heart, and plasma membranes of different bodily cells. However, for the purposes of this text, the focus will be specific to hormones and tissues most relevant to physical activity and the consequential adaptations that come from participation in varying types of exercise.

Due to the fact that hormones are not produced at a constant rate, but rather act in a more surge-like manner (in response to variations in physiological and psychological demand), exercise and related stress have a notable effect on hormone activity (9; 28; 45). Most of the endocrine glands do not store a large reserve of hormone, and the amount of hormones synthesized by the respective gland tends to equal the hormone release. Therefore, rapid adjustments in production and excretion must be made to regulate the body's internal conditions when the environment

Endocrine System

- Hypothalamus
- Pituitary gland
- Parathyroid gland
- Thyroid gland
- Thymus
- Liver
- Adrenal gland
- Kidney
- Pancreas
- Ovary
- Testes Cross section

Female Reproductive System

Male Reproductive System

~Key Terms~

Hormone receptors- A receptor protein on the surface of a cell or in its interior that binds to a specific hormone.

Target cell specificity- Hormones circulate to all tissues but influence only certain cells due to the presence of receptors on or in the cells.

Steroid- Any of a group of organic compounds belonging to the general class of biochemicals called lipids, which are easily soluble in organic solvents and slightly soluble in water.

Polypeptides- A small protein typically between 10 and 100 amino acids in length.

changes from rest to activity. Generally, hormonal balance is consistent with chemical uptake of hormone receptors and rate of removal by the liver and kidneys. It would seem that the body constantly attempts to control concentration levels to maintain equilibrium so that hormones are only available to target tissues when needed.

~Quick Insight~

Exercise, psychological stress, physiological stress, and immune function all intertwine. The immune system is closely tied to the adaptation response to physical training. Likewise, psychological stress negatively affects recovery response and immune function. The body can only handle so many demands at one time, so when it is laboring in response to exercise and stress, it suppresses immune function. Likewise, when the body is fighting an illness, exercise response is negatively impacted. Other stressors, such as lack of sleep, poor nutrition, alcohol consumption, and mental stress can magnify this impact. Each factor independently affects immune function and status; therefore a long- term exposure to compound stressors can increase susceptibility to illness and disease. One of the more common illnesses contracted during periods of imbalanced stress and recovery is an upper respiratory tract infection. Often times, exercisers question whether it is detrimental to exercise when affected by an illness. Since exercise suppresses immune function, and post-exercise immune status increases susceptibility to microbe invaders, it would be prudent not to exercise when fighting an illness.

Pituitary Hormones

Probably the most notable and easily recognized hormones to those familiar with exercise are the anabolic hormones. These include growth hormone, testosterone and the insulin-like growth factors, as well as insulin and thyroid hormones. Each plays a role in muscle remodeling and the adaptation effects produced from exercise (14; 35; 65). Growth hormone (GH), also called somatotropin, is excreted by the anterior pituitary gland and is one of the most relevant hormones in the body, as it has extensive responsibilities related to physiological activity (4; 65). It promotes cell division and proliferation throughout the body by facilitating protein synthesis (3). It does this by increasing amino acid (the building blocks of proteins) transport through plasma membranes, stimulating RNA formation, and activating cellular **ribosomes** (2). GH also protects glycogen reserves and carbohydrate breakdown by encouraging the mobilization and utilization of **lipids** for fuel during exercise.

The secretion of GH is regulated by the hypothalamus in the brain. The hypothalamus, which measures bodily stress, sends GH releasing-factor (GH-RF) hormones to the pituitary, which stimulates pituitary secretion of GH. During physical activity, GH is released based on the level of intensity. The more intense the exercise or demand, the greater the secretion and subsequent blood concentration level of GH. The hypothalamus releases GH-RF in response to low blood glucose, increased levels of certain amino acids, and stress, all of which occur during intense exercise. The hypothalamus also releases somatostatin, which inhibits GH secretion in response to high blood glucose common during inactivity. The elevation in GH during acute exercise benefits the active tissue and positively mediates energy metabolism (30). This action allows for prolonged work as the body relies on lipids for fuel, while sparing carbohydrates (29). The quantity of GH released seems to be dependent upon the relative intensity (39). When untrained and trained individuals exercise to exhaustion, similar levels of GH are released. However, untrained individuals show greater concentrations post exercise (50). Likewise, during acute submaximal bouts, untrained individuals, when compared to conditioned individuals, show higher levels of GH (49). These findings suggest that the perceived demand on the body determines the quantity of the GH production in response to exercise intensity (39). The presumed mechanism for increases in GH production and secretion is through stimulation of the hypothalamus, originating from the active tissues. In a practical sense, notable improvements in strength, power, and muscle size require higher intensity training (17). This may sound obvious, but the mechanism is still somewhat unclear to researchers.

The anabolic effect GH has on muscle mass, cartilage formation, and bone through the augmentation of protein synthesis often occurs in conjunction with another hormone, insulin-like growth factor (IGF) (34). The interaction of IGF polypeptides and GH seems to be the main reason muscle fibers adapt, by increasing the magnitude of their protein structures (20). The liver is the organ responsible for IGF secretion, as dictated by the GH stimulation of liver cell DNA (34). The IGF binds to proteins, which transport and supervise the physiological mechanisms of the hormones (19).

Testosterone has often been implicated as the premier anabolic hormone (probably due to the notable effect of steroids), but it seems that the direct effect testosterone has on fiber **hypertrophy** is not as significant as that of IGF (37). IGF directly increases protein synthesis activity. Testosterone's main contribution to muscle hypertrophy is more likely from the effect it has on increasing the quantity of GH released from the pituitary gland and the synergistic augmentation of GH response on target tissues, rather than through its direct effect on muscle cell DNA activity (37).

Gonadal Hormones - Testosterone

Testosterone is produced in the gonadal glands of men and women. It is the primary **androgenic hormone** (dihydrotestosterone) for secondary male characteristics. It is also the primary hormone responsible for muscle tissue interaction, which explains the visual and measurable differences between men and women. Testosterone, though, is not a male or female hormone, as it exists in both men and women alike. There are, though, distinct differences in the concentration of the hormone within the respective genders, as males demonstrate much higher levels of circulating testosterone than women.

Testosterone's contribution to anabolic activity helps characterize the differences in lean mass and strength found between men and women (56). Although the concentration of testosterone in women is ten times less than that in men, concentrations will increase in response to exercise in both genders (40). Similar to testosterone, estrogen is not a gender-specific hormone. Testosterone is converted into estrogen (estradiol) in men and aids in the maintenance of bone throughout a male's lifespan. Estrogen is a key hormone in bone maintenance in both men and women. When men inject testosterone or take testosterone precursors such as **Dehydroepiandrosterone (DHEA), Androstenediol,** or **Androstenedione**, the body perceives excessively high concentrations and thus attempts to re-establish hormonal balance by converting the excess testosterone to estradiol (6; 7). This explains why male steroid users may develop breast tissue called **gynecomastia**.

When testosterone interacts with muscle tissue, it does so through direct and indirect mechanisms. As previously mentioned, testosterone increases pituitary activity, causing the release of GH, which in this case, would be an indirect influence on protein synthesis in the tissue (38). Testosterone does have direct communication with DNA. This relationship identifies the direct path testosterone takes to encourage increased

~Key Terms~

Lipids- A group of organic molecules that includes fats, oils, and waxes:, lipids store energy and form parts of cell structures, such as cell membranes.

Ribosomes- Small particles, present in large numbers in every living cell, whose function is to convert stored genetic information into protein molecules.

protein synthesis. Testosterone also interacts with the nervous system to enhance strength and size via direct influence on neurons and structural protein changes. Increases in testosterone concentrations are attributed to high intensity exercise.

Pancreatic Hormones

The pancreas has two main functions. The first is the production of digestive enzymes that are released into the small intestines to break down fat, carbohydrates, and protein so that they can be absorbed into the blood stream. The second function, which is more important to this discussion, is the regulation of blood sugar levels by the release of two endocrine hormones known as **insulin** and **glucagon**.

When you eat a meal, carbohydrates are broken down primarily into simple sugars so that they can be absorbed by the blood stream. The most common sugar they are broken down to is glucose. When glucose is absorbed into the blood stream, the concentration level is measured by pancreatic receptors as the blood flows through the pancreatic tissue. The total quantity of the glucose is referred to as the glycemic load. This causes insulin to be released into the blood stream from the beta cells in the islet of Langerhans, located in the pancreas. The pancreas attempts to maintain a steady-state level of blood glucose. After a meal, when the blood sugar rises, this release of insulin drives glucose into the muscle and liver cells to be stored as glycogen (8). Insulin also pushes some of the excess sugar into the fat cells where the imported glucose is converted into triglycerides to reduce the blood glucose to normal steady-state levels. When insulin is appropriately regulated, carbohydrate levels in the blood do not surpass the apparent glucose concentration threshold, thereby reducing the propensity of insulin to facilitate fat cell uptake of sugar (8). In the absence of insulin, fat cells mobilize fatty acids to fuel energy demands. This identifies the relevance of lower glycemic loads upon the metabolic system to control insulin release. For optimal fat utilization and a reduced risk of fat storage caused by high blood glucose concentrations, dietary intake of excess calories, simple sugars, and processed carbohydrates should be controlled.

If the body experiences low blood glucose levels, a condition known as hypoglycemia, the alpha cells in the pancreas are stimulated to release glucagon. Glucagon quickly travels to the liver to stimulate the release of stored glucose in the form of glycogen into circulation to raise and stabilize blood glucose levels back to a steady-state level. Blood insulin and blood glucose will decrease as a function of prolonged exercise duration (23). The presence of **catecholamines** cause an

Blood Sugar Regulation

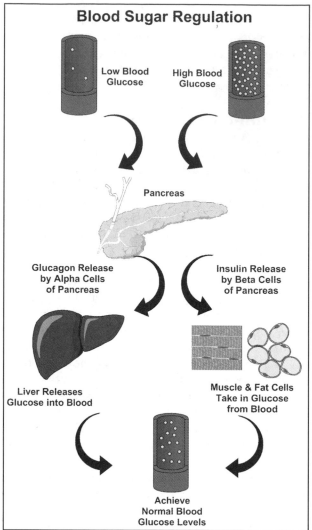

inhibitory effect on beta cells in the pancreas, leading to a reduction in circulating insulin levels (24). This drop in insulin levels is matched by an enhancement of muscle cellular permeability to energy substrates such as glucose and fats. Concurrently, liver cells become more sensitive to glucagon and epinephrine to raise and sustain glucose levels during exercise (41). As the exercise duration increases, so too does the contribution of fatty acids due to a reduced insulin secretion and the progressive decrease in glycogen reserves.

It is important to understand that insulin is anabolic in nature. It is true that the major function of insulin is to regulate glucose metabolism in the tissues through facilitated diffusion, but insulin is more anabolically dynamic than many people realize (5). Glucose carriers located in the cell membrane transport glucose into the cell in the presence of insulin. Without insulin, only trace quantities of glucose enter the cell, explaining why diabetics must inject insulin for proper cellular function. Additionally, the presence of insulin in the muscle cells increases enzyme activity, thereby facilitating heightened protein synthesis. Therefore, insulin is

anabolic both in its effect on the uptake of glucose in lipid and muscle cells, as well as through the promotion of protein synthesis (58).

Thyroid Hormones

The thyroid gland secretes two similar thyroid hormones, thyroxine (T4) and tri-iodothyroxine (T3). T3 is the active form of thyroid hormone (formed from T4) and acts to increase the metabolic rate of all cells (1). High level thyroid activity increases body temperature. T3 serves a permissive role, aiding in the development of lean mass. It does so by facilitating the actions of anabolic hormones and stimulating an increased secretion of GH in the pituitary gland and IGF-1 by the liver. During heavy exercise, thyroxine increases by about 35% (10). This elevation possibly contributes to immediate short-term excess post-exercise oxygen consumption through an increase in the resting metabolic rate of cells, thereby possibly adding to the effect exercise has on weight loss through heightened metabolic activity and increased use of fatty acids for fuel (31; 46; 47).

The Thyroid Gland

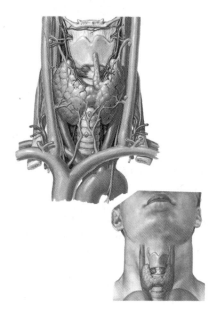

Adrenal Hormones

The adrenal glands produce two categories of hormones, neural and steroidal. Neural and steroidal hormones are made in different parts of the adrenal gland. Steroidal hormones are secreted from the adrenal cortex, and the neural catecholamines are produced in the adrenal medulla. The pituitary gland excretes adrenocorticotropin (ACTH) which stimulates the adrenal cortex to secrete **adrenocortical hormones**. These hormones serve functions such as the regulation of electrolytes and the production of cortisol and androgens. The adrenal medulla is stimulated through neural pathways originating in the brain, which provide a more rapid response, producing the catecholamines epinephrine and norepinephrine. As part of the sympathetic nervous system, the adrenal medulla is responsible for augmenting neural effects.

The adrenal hormones are very important to exercise as they are specifically designed to manage stress (44). Aldosterone plays a key role in regulating ion activity and water balance by reabsorbing or excreting sodium. Aldosterone also contributes to the maintenance of proper mineral balance, which is important for nerve transmission and subsequent motor function. Cortisol is another adrenocortical hormone that contributes to physical activity by way of glucose metabolism and the preservation of storage reserve (43). Cortisol is viewed as a catabolic hormone due to the fact that its presence results in the breakdown of muscle tissue. It does so by increasing proteolytic enzymes, converting amino acids to glucose, and inhibiting protein synthesis in a process to spare glucose in the body. Cortisol inhibits carbohydrate uptake and oxidation in the body by acting as an insulin antagonist (22). In cases of high psychological stress, cortisol is continually produced, leading to significant protein breakdown, thereby causing muscle wasting and a negative **nitrogen balance**. Additionally, sustained high levels of cortisol can suppress the immune function, making one more susceptible to infection (21). This explains how psychological stress inhibits the immune function (42).

The body has a natural defense against the catabolic effects of cortisol. Testosterone can block the genetic element in DNA from cortisol, or insulin can bind in greater numbers to receptors, trumping cortisol's effects on the protein (13; 62). The hormones that dominate the anabolic/catabolic balance determine which gets to apply its will upon the tissue (25; 27).

The hormones of the adrenal medulla are non-steroidal and work rapidly, through neural expression, on force outputs. Epinephrine and norepinephrine serve numerous functions, but in the muscle, they generally serve four categorical functions:

1) Neural, through central motor stimulation
2) Muscular, through enhancement to the enzyme systems of the tissue
3) Vascular, through vasodilation
4) Hormonal, through the augmentation of anabolic hormones

~Key Terms~

Hypertrophy- The increase in the size of an organ due to an increase in cell size. It is most commonly seen in muscle that has been actively stimulated, the most well-known method being exercise.

Androgenic Hormone- A steroid hormone, such as testosterone or androsterone, that controls the development and maintenance of masculine characteristics.

DHEA- Dehydroepiandrosterone, is a natural steroid hormone produced from cholesterol by the adrenal glands.

Androstenediol- An unsaturated steroidal derivative of androstene.

Androstenedione- An unsaturated androgenic steroid that has a weaker biological potency than testosterone.

Gynecomastia- Overdevelopment of the mammary glands in males; male breast development.

Insulin- A natural hormone made by the pancreas that helps control the level of glucose in the blood.

Glucagon- A hormone produced by the pancreas that stimulates an increase in blood sugar levels, opposing the action of insulin.

Catecholamines- Any naturally occurring amine, functioning as a neurotransmitter or hormone, including dopamine, norepinephrine, and epinephrine.

Adrenocortical hormones- Any of the various hormones secreted by the adrenal cortex, especially cortisol, aldosterone, and corticosterone.

Nitrogen Balance- The difference between the amount of nitrogen taken into the body and the amount excreted.

Endocrine Gland	Hormone	Action
Anterior Pituitary	Growth Hormone	Stimulates IGF, protein synthesis, growth and metabolism
Thyroid	Thyroxine	Stimulates metabolic rate, regulates cell growth and activity
Adrenal Cortex	Cortisol Aldosterone	Promotes use of fatty acids and protein catabolism; conserves sugar; maintains blood glucose level Promotes sodium, potassium metabolism and water retention
Adrenal Medulla	Epinephrine Norepinephrine	Increases cardiac output; increases glycogen catabolism and fatty acid release Has properties of epinephrine and constricts blood vessels
Pancreas	Insulin Glucagon	Promotes glucose uptake by the cell, stores glycogen; aids in protein synthesis Releases sugar from the liver into circulation
Liver	Insulin-like Growth Factors	Increase protein synthesis
Ovaries	Estrogen	Stimulates bone remodeling activity; female sex hormone
Testes	Testosterone	Stimulates growth; increases protein anabolism; reduces body fat; male sex hormone

The release of catecholamines is based on the acute stress experienced by the body. As with the other adrenal hormones, prolonged stress leads to reduced return or detrimental outcomes (16). The adrenal gland is tied very tightly to all components of training and recovery, including immuno-related activity (15; 64). This suggests that training needs to be dose-appropriate and balanced with other perceived stresses in the body to insure positive adaptive outcomes.

Hormone Considerations for Training

As the intensity of the training regimen increases, the changes in both the muscular system and endocrine system become more apparent (26; 59). Although a great deal of attention is paid to the cellular activities in the target tissue, it is important to note that the hormones that most often dictate these adaptations also experience improvement in their function in response to the training. The adaptive process within the tissue and glands is a positive feedback loop. The tissues become more efficient as disruptive environments force them to improve in efficiency; consequently changes in the tissue in response to the stress augment the hormonal effect and the glands that secrete them.

Endocrine adaptations are simply improvements in the actions they already perform. For instance, the glands increase the amount of hormones they produce and store. Obviously a greater concentration and secretion of hormones would suggest increased activity in the tissues they act upon. The hormones themselves do not change, but their concentration and effectiveness does. This occurs because more hormones can be transported; larger quantities are sustained in the system for longer periods of time; receptors increase in numbers and sensitivity, causing the magnitude of the signal to be enhanced; and finally, the tissue interactions increase for a more dynamic adaptation response.

The type of training one engages in, and the intensity at which it is performed, dictates the specific response by both the working tissue and the endocrine glands that mediate their actions (36). This is not only true between aerobic and anaerobic training, but also between training techniques within a particular category of training. Simply stated, the type of training one performs dictates the type and level of the hormonal response. For instance, resistance training can be performed for increased force and power output with very little change to the size of the muscle (36). This is due to the fact that tissue adaptations are most influenced by the circulating hormonal levels. As a personal trainer, it is important to understand that exercise prescriptions should be aimed at stimulating specific hormone activity related to the desired adaptation effect.

Identifying what each hormone does and what causes the respective gland or tissue to release it is integral in prescribing exercise designed to harness the desired outcome of the hormone. Due to the fact that muscle tissue is most responsible for physical action, it is noteworthy to analyze its relationship with hormones and the respective training responses. Muscle adaptations are generally viewed as metabolic changes or anatomical changes. The latter suggests that the tissue actually changes in structure. The positive adaptation process that occurs in muscle protein is called muscle remodeling. When the tissue experiences significant physiological stress the consequent disruption and damage to the muscle cell stimulates an inflammatory response (48). The specific method by which the physiological disruption occurs determines the extent of remodeling from neural, hormonal, and immune system influence (53). The hormonal

interaction of GH, testosterone, IGF, T3, and insulin cause the cell to synthesize new protein structures along the sarcomere (51). Starting at the genetic level, cellular stimulation by hormone interactions initiates the action by which the muscle cells lay down new proteins (36). The contractile proteins, actin and myosin and the structural non-contractile proteins all experience protein enhancements, leading to greater size and strength of the tissue. Type II fibers experience a far more dramatic effect in protein synthesis than Type I fibers, which is why they are most often associated with muscle hypertrophy. But the abundance of Type I fibers distributed throughout the muscular system still plays a key role in muscle mass augmentation. Although limited protein synthesis occurs, Type I fibers experience a reduced degradation effect from hormone mediation. This combination of protein synthesis and reduced protein metabolism leads to noticeable gains in muscle tissue over time.

Hormonal Interaction and Exercise

When the motor neurons are activated, the stimuli to the brain cause a reactive communication to the endocrine system to secrete the appropriate hormones to manage the situation. As previously mentioned, the acute hormonal, neural, and immune messengers stimulated from physiological stress and consequent cellular disruption direct hormonal activity specific to the type of stress experienced (48). Therefore, the type of response one experiences from muscular endurance training is different from the response elicited by muscular power training, which is, in turn different then that from aerobic training. Each type of stress and the way the stress is applied has specific communications to how the body should manage the internal environment during and after an exercise session. The neural patterns activate hormonal patterns which shape the adaptive response to the training. Because the physiological environments are consistent in response to the stress of a particular nature, outcomes are very predictive based upon the exercise engaged in, and the intensity, rest interval, and duration employed.

Strength training utilizes heavy resistance loading and near maximal recovery periods (2-5 minutes) between sets with repetition ranges often less than eight. This formula makes the hormone activity very predictive. The training causes an increase in the anabolic hormones, but because the rest periods allow for so much recovery in the tissue and the stimulus is applied for only a short period of time, far less hypertrophic effects are noticed (36). This is explained by acute increases in testosterone without the more notable increases in GH. Recall that IGF, produced by GH influences, is the key protein synthesizer (52).

Therefore, activities that do not encourage the full hormone matrix responsible for muscle remodeling will not significantly increase muscle mass. The testosterone and neural factors contribute to increased force output with less protein synthesis due to a lower concentration of GH (36). It should be noted that heavy cross-joint lifts including squats and deadlifts have the most dramatic effect on circulating testosterone levels in heavy strength training programs.

Resistance Training & Hormone Response

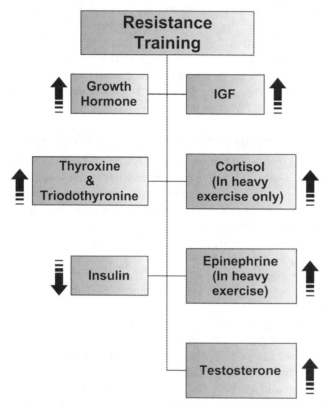

Effects on Hypertrophy

When the training stress is modified so that the volume is high (3-4 sets), the resistance is moderately heavy (70-85% of 1RM), and performed for longer durations (8-12 repetitions) with short, one-minute rest periods, the serum concentrations of GH increase dramatically (36). Classically considered bodybuilding, the collective activity utilizes all the reactive stimuli for muscle growth. Conversely, lower repetition schemes (<8 repetitions) with heavy weight do not stimulate the body in the same manner, so less hypertrophy is experienced. Two notable factors to consider with hypertrophy training are blood lactate and cortisol levels (55). Although both products are considered detrimental to muscle protein in their respective activity, there is a definite link between the stress that causes their presence and the response of the pituitary gland. It is

suggested that the body manages cortisol activity differently in high-demand-resistance-stress environments compared to other stress stimuli by blunting its negative effects (63). High productions of lactic acid with concurrent cortisol released by the adrenal glands in response to high intensity, extended-time-under-tension exercise stimulate greater GH release (36). The higher concentrations of GH released in response to the training stimulates IGF-1 release from the liver adding to the anabolic effects (36). Since high-volume, short-rest periods stimulate both cortisol release and higher concentrations of lactic acid in the blood, but heavy resistance training with low repetition schemes and long rest periods does not, it explains why the heavy strength training causes far less effect on GH and hypertrophy compared to the bodybuilding approach. The most common errors in bodybuilding or activities aimed at hypertrophy are lifting too light, not properly applying high volume isolative overload, and taking too long a rest period between sets and exercises, all of which consequently reduce the magnitude of the hormonal response.

Effects on Aerobic Fitness

Endurance training has a different hormone product response than that experienced during resistance training (60). This is, in part, due to the common employment of steady-state, continuously-applied activities that utilize the repeated action of certain muscle groups. Hormone activity seems to be sensitive to variations of intensity, so when the intensity is sustained, a lower hormone response is observed (60; 61). As would be expected from the previous reading, GH released in response to the endurance activities depends upon intensity (57). High intensity training, particularly that done above lactate threshold, shows the greater increase in GH compared to lower intensity markers (18). Testosterone seems to be suppressed during high intensity aerobic activities, but plasma levels will increase during moderate levels of endurance training (12). Testosterone production during aerobic activities is less when compared to anaerobic exercise at similar intensities. Insulin sensitivity is heightened and glucagon levels will increase slightly as exercise becomes more prolonged (11; 54). Catecholamines seem to remain relatively stabilized, but cortisol will slightly increase. In long endurance bouts, such as running a marathon, cortisol production will increase, as will the release of protein from muscle to promote carbohydrate sparing and help maintain energy stores (32). Due to the limited anabolic hormone activity, endurance training has minimal effect on muscle mass gain and actually will decrease lean mass in high volume programs due to catabolic effects (33).

Chapter Four References

1. **Acheson K, Jequier E, Burger A and Danforth E Jr.** Thyroid hormones and thermogenesis: the metabolic cost of food and exercise. *Metabolism* 33: 262-265, 1984.

2. **Borer KT**. Neurohumoral mediation of exercise-induced growth. *Med Sci Sports Exerc* 26: 741-754, 1994.

3. **Borer KT**. The effects of exercise on growth. *Sports Med* 20: 375-397, 1995.

4. **Borer KT**. The effects of exercise on growth. *Sports Med* 20: 375-397, 1995.

5. **Bracy DP, Zinker BA, Jacobs JC, Lacy DB and Wasserman DH**. Carbohydrate metabolism during exercise: influence of circulating fat availability. *J Appl Physiol* 79: 506-513, 1995.

6. **Broeder CE, Quindry J, Brittingham K, Panton L, Thomson J, Appakondu S, Breuel K, Byrd R, Douglas J, Earnest C, Mitchell C, Olson M, Roy T and Yarlagadda C**. The Andro Project: physiological and hormonal influences of androstenedione supplementation in men 35 to 65 years old participating in a high-intensity resistance training program. *Arch Intern Med* 160: 3093-3104, 2000.

7. **Brown GA, Vukovich MD, Reifenrath TA, Uhl NL, Parsons KA, Sharp RL and King DS**. Effects of anabolic precursors on serum testosterone concentrations and adaptations to resistance training in young men. *Int J Sport Nutr Exerc Metab* 10: 340-359, 2000.

8. **Buczkowska EO and Jarosz-Chobot P**. [Insulin effect on metabolism in skeletal muscles and the role of muscles in regulation of glucose homeostasis]. *Przegl Lek* 58: 782-787, 2001.

9. **Charkoudian N and Joyner MJ**. Physiologic considerations for exercise performance in women. *Clin Chest Med* 25: 247-255, 2004.

10. **Ciloglu F, Peker I, Pehlivan A, Karacabey K, Ilhan N, Saygin O and Ozmerdivenli R**. Exercise intensity and its effects on thyroid hormones. *Neuro Endocrinol Lett* 26: 830-834, 2005.

11. **Coggan AR**. Plasma glucose metabolism during exercise: effect of endurance training in humans. *Med Sci Sports Exerc* 29: 620-627, 1997.

12. **Consitt LA, Copeland JL and Tremblay MS**. Endogenous anabolic hormone responses to endurance us resistance exercise and training in women. *Sports Med* 32: 1-22, 2002.

13. **Daly W, Seegers CA, Rubin DA, Dobridge JD and Hackney AC**. Relationship between stress hormones and testosterone with prolonged endurance exercise. *Eur J Appl Physiol* 93: 375-380, 2005.

14. **Frost RA and Lang CH**. Regulation of insulin-like growth factor-I in skeletal muscle and muscle cells. *Minerva Endocrinol* 28: 53-73, 2003.

15. **Fry AC and Kraemer WJ**. Resistance exercise overtraining and overreaching. Neuroendocrine responses. *Sports Med* 23: 106-129, 1997.

16. **Fry AC and Kraemer WJ**. Resistance exercise overtraining and overreaching. Neuroendocrine responses. *Sports Med* 23: 106-129, 1997.

17. **Godfrey RJ, Madgwick Z and Whyte GP**. The exercise-induced growth hormone response in athletes. *Sports Med* 33: 599-613, 2003.

18. **Godfrey RJ, Madgwick Z and Whyte GP**. The exercise-induced growth hormone response in athletes. *Sports Med* 33: 599-613, 2003.

19. **Goldspink G and Yang SY**. Effects of activity on growth factor expression. *Int J Sport Nutr Exerc Metab* 11 Suppl: S21-S27, 2001.

20. **Goldspink G and Yang SY**. Effects of activity on growth factor expression. *Int J Sport Nutr Exerc Metab* 11 Suppl: S21-S27, 2001.

21. **Gomez-Merino D, Chennaoui M, Burnat P, Drogou C and Guezennec CY**. Immune and hormonal changes following intense military training. *Mil Med* 168: 1034-1038, 2003.

22. **Holm G, Bjorntorp P and Jagenburg R**. Carbohydrate, lipid and amino acid metabolism following physical exercise in man. *J Appl Physiol* 45: 128-131, 1978.

23. **Horton TJ, Grunwald GK, Lavely J and Donahoo WT**. Glucose kinetics differ between women and men, during and after exercise. *J Appl Physiol* 100: 1883-1894, 2006.

24. **Howlett KF, Watt MJ, Hargreaves M and Febbraio MA**. Regulation of glucose kinetics during intense exercise

in humans: effects of alpha- and beta-adrenergic blockade. *Metabolism* 52: 1615-1620, 2003.

25. **Hug M, Mullis PE, Vogt M, Ventura N and Hoppeler H**. Training modalities: over-reaching and over-training in athletes, including a study of the role of hormones. *Best Pract Res Clin Endocrinol Metab* 17: 191-209, 2003.

26. **Izquierdo M, Ibanez J, Hakkinen K, Kraemer WJ, Ruesta M and Gorostiaga EM**. Maximal strength and power, muscle mass, endurance and serum hormones in weightlifters and road cyclists. *J Sports Sci* 22: 465-478, 2004.

27. **Izquierdo M, Ibanez J, Hakkinen K, Kraemer WJ, Ruesta M and Gorostiaga EM**. Maximal strength and power, muscle mass, endurance and serum hormones in weightlifters and road cyclists. *J Sports Sci* 22: 465-478, 2004.

28. **Jorgensen JO, Krag M, Kanaley J, Moller J, Hansen TK, Moller N, Christiansen JS and Orskov H**. Exercise, hormones, and body temperature. regulation and action of GH during exercise. *J Endocrinol Invest* 26: 838-842, 2003.

29. **Jorgensen JO, Krag M, Kanaley J, Moller J, Hansen TK, Moller N, Christiansen JS and Orskov H**. Exercise, hormones, and body temperature. regulation and action of GH during exercise. *J Endocrinol Invest* 26: 838-842, 2003.

30. **Kanaley JA, Dall R, Moller N, Nielsen SC, Christiansen JS, Jensen MD and Jorgensen JO**. Acute exposure to GH during exercise stimulates the turnover of free fatty acids in GH-deficient men. *J Appl Physiol* 96: 747-753, 2004.

31. **Kirkeby K, Sromme SB, Bjerkedal I, Hertzenberg L and Refsum HE**. Effects of prolonged, strenuous exercise on lipids and thyroxine in serum. *Acta Med Scand* 202: 463-467, 1977.

32. **Kraemer WJ, Fleck SJ, Callister R, Shealy M, Dudley GA, Maresh CM, Marchitelli L, Cruthirds C, Murray T and Falkel JE**. Training responses of plasma beta-endorphin, adrenocorticotropin, and cortisol. *Med Sci Sports Exerc* 21: 146-153, 1989.

33. **Kraemer WJ, Patton JF, Gordon SE, Harman EA, Deschenes MR, Reynolds K, Newton RU, Triplett NT and Dziados JE**. Compatibility of high-intensity strength and endurance training on hormonal and skeletal muscle adaptations. *J Appl Physiol* 78: 976-989, 1995.

34. **Kraemer WJ and Ratamess NA**. Hormonal responses and adaptations to resistance exercise and training. *Sports Med* 35: 339-361, 2005.

35. **Kraemer WJ and Ratamess NA**. Hormonal responses and adaptations to resistance exercise and training. *Sports Med* 35: 339-361, 2005.

36. **Kraemer WJ and Ratamess NA**. Hormonal responses and adaptations to resistance exercise and training. *Sports Med* 35: 339-361, 2005.

37. **Kraemer WJ and Ratamess NA**. Hormonal responses and adaptations to resistance exercise and training. *Sports Med* 35: 339-361, 2005.

38. **Kraemer WJ and Ratamess NA**. Hormonal responses and adaptations to resistance exercise and training. *Sports Med* 35: 339-361, 2005.

39. **Kraemer WJ and Ratamess NA**. Hormonal responses and adaptations to resistance exercise and training. *Sports Med* 35: 339-361, 2005.

40. **Kraemer WJ, Staron RS, Hagerman FC, Hikida RS, Fry AC, Gordon SE, Nindl BC, Gothshalk LA, Volek JS, Marx JO, Newton RU and Hakkinen K**. The effects of short-term resistance training on endocrine function in men and women. *Eur J Appl Physiol Occup Physiol* 78: 69-76, 1998.

41. **Lavoie JM**. The contribution of afferent signals from the liver to metabolic regulation during exercise. *Can J Physiol Pharmacol* 80: 1035-1044, 2002.

42. **Mastorakos G, Pavlatou M, Diamanti-Kandarakis E and Chrousos GP**. Exercise and the stress system. *Hormones (Athens)* 4: 73-89, 2005.

43. **Mastorakos G, Pavlatou M, Diamanti-Kandarakis E and Chrousos GP**. Exercise and the stress system. *Hormones (Athens)* 4: 73-89, 2005.

44. **Mastorakos G, Pavlatou M, Diamanti-Kandarakis E and Chrousos GP**. Exercise and the stress system. *Hormones (Athens)* 4: 73-89, 2005.

45. **McMurray RG and Hackney AC**. Interactions of metabolic hormones, adipose tissue and exercise. *Sports Med* 35: 393-412, 2005.

46. **O'Connell M, Robbins DC, Horton ES, Sims EA and Danforth E Jr**. Changes in serum concentrations of 3,3',5'-triiodothyronine and 3,5,3'-triiodothyronine during prolonged moderate exercise. *J Clin Endocrinol Metab* 49: 242-246, 1979.

47. **Refsum HE and Stromme SB**. Serum thyroxine, triiodothyronine and thyroid stimulating hormone after

prolonged heavy exercise. *Scand J Clin Lab Invest* 39: 455-459, 1979.

48. **Rooyackers OE and Nair KS**. Hormonal regulation of human muscle protein metabolism. *Annu Rev Nutr* 17: 457-485, 1997.

49. **Rubin MR, Kraemer WJ, Maresh CM, Volek JS, Ratamess NA, Vanheest JL, Silvestre R, French DN, Sharman MJ, Judelson DA, Gomez AL, Vescovi JD and Hymer WC**. High-affinity growth hormone binding protein and acute heavy resistance exercise. *Med Sci Sports Exerc* 37: 395-403, 2005.

50. **Rubin MR, Kraemer WJ, Maresh CM, Volek JS, Ratamess NA, Vanheest JL, Silvestre R, French DN, Sharman MJ, Judelson DA, Gomez AL, Vescovi JD and Hymer WC**. High-affinity growth hormone binding protein and acute heavy resistance exercise. *Med Sci Sports Exerc* 37: 395-403, 2005.

51. **Sheffield-Moore M and Urban RJ**. An overview of the endocrinology of skeletal muscle. *Trends Endocrinol Metab* 15: 110-115, 2004.

52. **Sheffield-Moore M and Urban RJ**. An overview of the endocrinology of skeletal muscle. *Trends Endocrinol Metab* 15: 110-115, 2004.

53. **Sheffield-Moore M and Urban RJ**. An overview of the endocrinology of skeletal muscle. *Trends Endocrinol Metab* 15: 110-115, 2004.

54. **Silverman HG and Mazzeo RS**. Hormonal responses to maximal and submaximal exercise in trained and untrained men of various ages. *J Gerontol A Biol Sci Med Sci* 51: B30-B37, 1996.

55. **Smilios I, Pilianidis T, Karamouzis M, Parlavantzas A and Tokmakidis SP**. Hormonal Responses after a Strength Endurance Resistance Exercise Protocol in Young and Elderly Males. *Int J Sports Med* 2006.

56. **Staron RS, Karapondo DL, Kraemer WJ, Fry AC, Gordon SE, Falkel JE, Hagerman FC and Hikida RS**. Skeletal muscle adaptations during early phase of heavy-resistance training in men and women. *J Appl Physiol* 76: 1247-1255, 1994.

57. **Stokes KA, Nevill ME, Cherry PW, Lakomy HK and Hall GM**. Effect of 6 weeks of sprint training on growth hormone responses to sprinting. *Eur J Appl Physiol* 92: 26-32, 2004.

58. **Tipton KD and Wolfe RR**. Exercise, protein metabolism, and muscle growth. *Int J Sport Nutr Exerc Metab* 11: 109-132, 2001.

59. **Tremblay MS, Copeland JL and Van Helder W**. Effect of training status and exercise mode on endogenous steroid hormones in men. *J Appl Physiol* 96: 531-539, 2004.

60. **Tremblay MS, Copeland JL and Van Helder W**. Effect of training status and exercise mode on endogenous steroid hormones in men. *J Appl Physiol* 96: 531-539, 2004.

61. **Tremblay MS, Copeland JL and Van Helder W**. Influence of exercise duration on post-exercise steroid hormone responses in trained males. *Eur J Appl Physiol* 94: 505-513, 2005.

62. **Tremblay MS, Copeland JL and Van Helder W**. Influence of exercise duration on post-exercise steroid hormone responses in trained males. *Eur J Appl Physiol* 94: 505-513, 2005.

63. **Urhausen A, Gabriel H and Kindermann W**. Blood hormones as markers of training stress and overtraining. *Sports Med* 20: 251-276, 1995.

64. **Uusitalo AL, Huttunen P, Hanin Y, Uusitalo AJ and Rusko HK**. Hormonal responses to endurance training and overtraining in female athletes. *Clin J Sport Med* 8: 178-186, 1998.

65. **Weber MM**. Effects of growth hormone on skeletal muscle. *Horm Res* 58 Suppl 3: 43-48, 2002.

Chapter 5

Bioenergetics

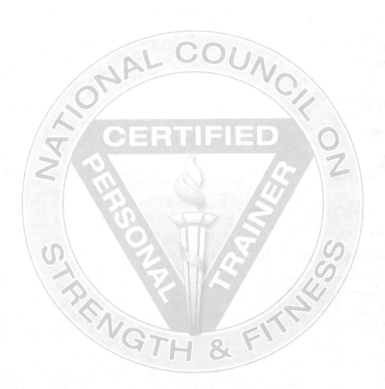

Energy

The first scientific **law of thermodynamics** states that energy cannot be created nor destroyed. Instead, it is transferred from one form to another. All biological functions require energy, and therefore, living matter requires energy to sustain life. For instance, plants use energy from sunlight, water, and CO_2 to form carbohydrates, proteins, and fats using **chlorophyll** in the process of photosynthesis. The energy is stored in the bonds that connect the molecules. Carbohydrates can be manipulated to form proteins and fatty structures in plants and animals. When humans eat plants and animal products, the energy is transferred from one organism to another. The energy transferred in food is called a **calorie**. The calorie represents the quantity of heat necessary to raise the temperature of 1 g of water 1° Celsius. The calorie represents an extremely small measure of energy. If it were used as the unit for food energy on nutritional labels, the energy value per gram of a nutrient would be expressed in the thousands. For this reason the United States uses the **kilocalorie**. The kilocalorie (kcal) represents 1000 calories, or the measurement of heat required to raise 1 kg (1L) of water 1° Celsius. To avoid consumer confusion, the labels use the word calorie, but the value actually reflects kilocalorie units. The international unit of energy is the kilojoule, which is equal to 4.2 kilocalories.

Energy Value of Food

The energy value of food is determined by the respective heat of combustion yielded when it is burned. There are slight variations in the heat created between foods composed of similar energy substrates. For practical purposes, a food's energy value is rounded to a whole number. For instance, fat values vary between animal lipids (mean = 9.5 kcal) and plant lipids (mean = 9.3 kcal). Food labels list fat as containing 9 kcal per gram. Likewise, the arrangement of atoms in carbohydrates determines the net value of the food. Glucose has a very simple molecular structure and therefore is valued at 3.74 kcal per gram, whereas complex carbohydrates such as glycogen and starch are valued at 4.2 kcal per gram. Protein variations in energy value are based on the type and nitrogen content of the particular protein. On average, protein yields 5.65 kcal of energy when burned.

The net energy yielded when foods are consumed by the body sometimes differs from the value identified through **direct calorimetry** (12). This is particularly true for foods containing nitrogen. Nitrogen yields energy when burned, but in the body, it is combined with hydrogen to form urea, which is excreted through urine. For this reason, proteins, which contain nitrogen, actually reflect a value of 4.6 kcal of body energy. Due to the fact that carbohydrates and fats do not contain nitrogen, their respective energy value is consistent between direct calorimetry and the consumed value. The net energy of food is also affected by the digestive and absorption process, referred to as the **coefficient of digestibility**. The coefficient of digestibility reflects the total energy the body has available from the food it consumes. Certain components of food are indigestible and pass through the body as excrement. Fibrous food reduces digestibility by as much as 5-10% in some foods (5). The fiber cannot be broken down and speeds transportation through the intestines, thereby reducing absorption time (37). Plant proteins seem to yield the lowest coefficient of digestibility, whereas animal products seem to yield the highest measured levels (13; 28). In general, 97% of carbohydrate, 95% of lipid and 92% of protein energy is absorbed by the body for fuel.

Atwater general factors represent the value food is assigned for nutritional purposes. The average net value for protein and carbohydrate is set at 4 kcal per gram and dietary fats are valued at 9 kcal per gram. Alcohol also contributes to energy intake when consumed. Pure alcohol is valued at 7 kcal per gram (ml). When the weight of each energy nutrient is

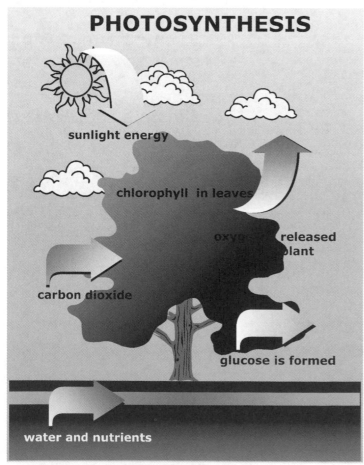

PHOTOSYNTHESIS

sunlight energy

chlorophyll in leaves

oxygen released plant

carbon dioxide

glucose is formed

water and nutrients

known, the calories can be determined for a select food or meal. Food labels attempt to clearly identify the energy value in foods and are expressed in both weight (g) and energy (kcal).

When food is consumed, the body breaks it down through the process of digestion. It then absorbs the energy substrates and either stores the energy in a state of potentiality (potential energy) or uses it to fuel biological activity (kinetic energy). The specific use of the energy is identified when changes in energy demands occur. Biological activity changes the form of energy based on its particular need. For instance, stored energy is released for mechanical work, while some is spared as chemical energy or released as heat energy. Recall, the first Law of Thermodynamics suggests the energy is not lost, it is just transferred as one reaction releases heat and energy (exothermic reaction) and another absorbs heat and energy (endothermic reaction).

ATP

The only form of energy that can be directly used for muscular contractions is Adenosine Triphosphate (ATP). The fuel for mechanical, chemical, and transport work all relies on the energy released from the high energy phosphate bonds within the ATP molecule. When the bonds are broken, energy is released into the system and cultivated for a particular action. ATP can be thought of as being "spring-loaded" with energy that can be released upon enzymatic hydrolysis of the bonds that connect the phosphate molecules. **Enzymes** serve

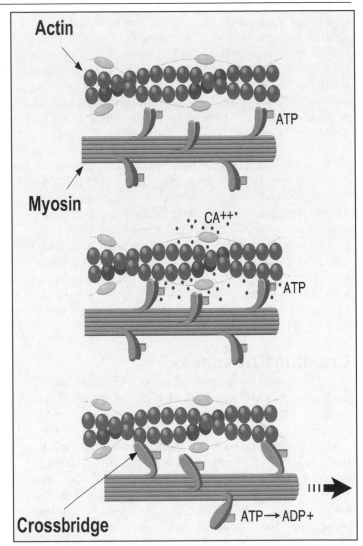

~Key Terms~

Law of Thermodynamics- Describes the specifics for the transport of heat and work in thermodynamic processes.

Chlorophyll- Green pigment that gives most plants their color and enables them to carry on the process of photosynthesis.

Calorie- A unit measuring the energy value of foods, calibrated by the quantity of heat required to raise the temperature of 1 gram of water by one degree Celsius.

Kilocalorie- A unit of energy equal to the amount of heat required to raise the temperature of one kilogram of water by one degree Celsius.

Direct Calorimetry- Is the measurement of heat generated as a result of metabolism.

Coefficient of Digestibility- Represents the actual energy that the body will yield from the foods it consumes; based on how the human body actually digests the food.

Atwater General Factors- Identifies the caloric value for fats, proteins, and carbohydrates.

as biological catalysts and are usually named for the functions they perform. ATPase is the enzyme responsible for the breakdown of the ATP molecule inside the cell. The suffix (–ase) identifies the substance as an enzyme.

When ATP is split for mechanical work, the action takes place deep within the muscle fiber at the level of the myofilaments. Myosin, the thick myofilament, holds the ATPase enzyme. In the presence of calcium, myosin binds with actin, forming crossbridges. When the crossbridges are formed, the catalyst reaction of the enzyme essentially cleaves off the end phosphate ion from the ATP molecule, leaving a by-product of ADP and an inorganic phosphate. The energy released causes the myosin to detach from the actin filament. This permits the movement of the myosin head, so it can expel the energy by-products and reattach to actin further along the filament. This process allows myofilaments within the sarcomeres of muscle fibers to lengthen and shorten to produce force. Thousands of muscle fibers contract within a whole muscle, causing joint action in response to the energy released from the phosphate bonds of ATP. Therefore, calories expended during exercise can serve as an indirect measurement of ATP molecules being split during muscular work and other metabolic processes.

ATP is derived from the metabolism of carbohydrate, fat, and protein fuel substrates. However, ATP for immediate work is stored in small quantities in the cell. This ATP is readily usable and therefore, is the primary source of energy for fast rate, powerful work. The energy potency of the molecule allows for high speed reactions. Maximal muscular work, lasting 1-3 seconds, will exploit stored ATP for energy. Examples of activities relying on stored ATP include a maximal vertical jump, pitching a fast ball, or swinging a driver on the golf course.

Creatine Phosphate

Due to the rapid depletion of stored ATP, the muscle maintains an additional pool of high energy phosphate storage in the form of intracellular creatine. Creatine is phosphorylated with an inorganic phosphate ion to form a high energy bond molecule called **creatine phosphate** (CP). When ATP becomes depleted, the first reaction to replenish the energy needed for continued muscular work is the splitting of CP by the enzyme **creatine kinase (CK).** CK breaks the high-energy creatine phosphate bond, which releases energy to **re-phosphorylate** intracellular ADP molecules. During the re-phosphorylation process, ADP binds with an inorganic phosphate molecule to resynthesize ATP for energy. After this occurs the newly formed ATP molecule is split, and energy to drive the cell continues. Creatine phosphate concentrations in the cell are 4-6x that of ATP, allowing for approximately 10-15 seconds of available high-power energy to drive burst activities, such as 3 maximal repetitions in weight lifting, a 40 yard dash, or a 100 meter sprint.

CP Energy Sequence

1) Creatine Phosphate is split by Creatine Kinase.

2) The liberated phosphate uses the released energy to bind ADP and P.

3) The new ATP molecule is split into ADP and P, and energy is released.

Phosphates are connected with very high energy bonds, and when they are connected in the form of ATP or CP, they are heavy molecules. This explains why the body

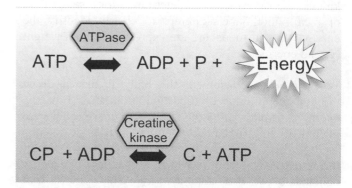

does not maintain high levels of storage. Excessive storage would weigh down the body tissue. Instead, the body resynthesizes ATP after the bonds have been separated by ATPase. Thus, perpetual energy can be formed from lighter molecules rather than storing the weighty ATP in the cell. When exercise discontinues after a single maximal effort, it takes the body at least 90 seconds to fully refuel (64). It does so by rephosphorylating the ADP with the liberated phosphagen ions. When CP is required to fuel the mechanical work being performed, it too is depleted, and consequently, the high-power energy source runs out. CP replenishment can take between 2-5 minutes (63; 66). The phosphorylation periods required to re-establish ATP and CP stores in the muscle ultimately determine rest periods between heavy resistance training and sprinting activities. At maximal lifted loads or running speeds, the period of time between sets equals the time it takes to replenish the energy. Power exercises such as Olympic lifts and plyometrics, as well as heavy strength training, utilize low repetition numbers and longer rest periods to maximize the performance in the phosphagen energy system (65).

Glycolysis

ATP cannot be supplied through blood or other tissues, relying on other energy substrates to form its usable biological structure. It is easy to phosphorylate ATP from CP because the phosphagen is simply being mobilized from one molecule to another. But when phosphagen energy runs out and the body continues to demand ATP for work, the energy has to come from another source. Carbohydrates are the next fuel the body uses to create ATP. However, this energy must be derived from glucose, a 6-carbon sugar molecule, and this process takes several steps and numerous catalysts to accomplish. In fact, the energy derived from sugar requires 10 enzymatic reactions, whereas CP and ATP only use one enzyme. In the **anaerobic** process known as **glycolysis** (sugar-splitting), these ten controlled chemical reactions are required so that ATP can be synthesized and energy metabolites can be made available for ongoing work. Recall, CP can rapidly donate a phosphate to ADP to form ATP; however due to the three step process a level of power drop off occurs. Thus, it makes sense that the ten-step process causes an even greater decline in maximal power output, and that the energy released from ATP produced from glycolytic means is less than the energy provided by immediate sources. This explains why a person is able to lift more weight for five repetitions than he or she can for ten repetitions. The energy system employed determines the maximal force output.

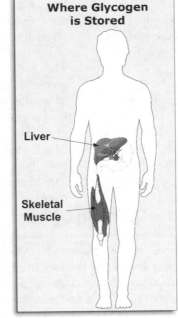

Where Glycogen is Stored

Liver

Skeletal Muscle

The breakdown of carbohydrates, like most reactions, uses water as an assistive catalyst with enzymes to fracture glucose into its respective parts outside of the **mitochondria**. Anaerobic glycolysis is unique in that glucose is the only carbon-fuel nutrient that can be used to yield energy without the use of oxygen. Fats and proteins cannot be used anaerobically. However, fat, protein, and glucose can all be used to produce energy via aerobic metabolism inside the mitochondria. Here, the hydrogen ions are essentially pulled off of the different carbon fuels and transferred to molecular oxygen to make water (H_2O). Since the anaerobic breakdown of glucose through glycolysis occurs without oxygen, water is not made and the liberated hydrogen ions remain free in solution, increasing the acidity of the surrounding environment.

Most of the energy generated through this **exergonic reaction** is not sufficient to form high-bond ATP and is lost to the body as heat. The products of glycolysis include two (2) molecules of ATP and two energy

substrates, **lactic acid** or **pyruvate**. Although the efficiency of the process is only about 33%, significant energy can be derived from anaerobic glycolysis due to the high concentrations of glycolytic enzymes present in the muscle tissue and the speed of the associated reactions (11; 30). The ATP derived from this system is the major contributor to activities of maximal effort lasting up to 90 seconds (11; 16). Therefore, anaerobic glycosis is the primary energy system to fuel the average weight lifting set.

When exercisers experience the onset of a burning sensation in active tissue, it is due to insufficient oxygen, not acid pain. Lactic acid is essentially the buffer for the hydrogen by-product of muscle that has become ischemic, receiving insufficient oxygen supply compared to the oxygen demand (48). Muscle ischemia causes pain, similar to the pain experienced if you placed a rubber band on the end of your finger to occlude blood flow. During moderate levels of activity, where the rate of energy utilization is matched by energy re-synthesis, the cellular pH stays in balance. However, during intense work, ischemia occurs, and the excess hydrogen builds up (59). This leads to a drop in pH which may inhibit enzymatic reactions, alter calcium handling, and lead to intrinsic muscular **fatigue** (60). The lactic acid that is produced can be transferred to a neighboring cell that is not ischemic and can be oxidized to yield additional energy (44). Lactic acid can also be transported in the blood to other skeletal muscles, the liver, or to the heart, where it can be metabolized (47). Although this can occur during exercise, lactic acid utilization is a marked component of the recovery phase.

It would seem that lactic acid is a consequentially detrimental byproduct of glycolysis, but this view would be short-sighted (7). Ongoing exercise requires large amounts of ATP from metabolic sources to sustain the work production. The body has contingency plans for all the substrate byproducts from metabolism. In this way, the body has potential energy stores ready to be converted to kinetic energy as dictated by exercise duration and intensity. Due to the fact that very little ATP is produced from glycolysis and that the

~Key Terms~

Enzymes- A protein that catalyzes a biochemical reaction or change.

Creatine phosphate- An organic compound found in muscle tissue and capable of storing and providing energy for muscular contraction.

Creatine kinase- An enzyme present in muscle and other tissues that catalyzes the reversible conversion of ADP and phosphocreatine into ATP and creatine.

Re-phosphorylate- The process of adding an inorganic phosphate back to a molecule such as ADP.

Anaerobic - The process of energy production in the body in the absence of freely availible oxygen.

Glycolysis- A metabolic process that breaks down carbohydrates and sugars, through a series of reactions to either pyruvic acid or lactic acid, releasing energy for the body in the form of ATP.

carbohydrate substrates pyruvate and lactate are left over from the glycolytic process, the body can utilize the potential chemical energy by converting the carbon skeletons back to glucose in the liver (4). **Lactate** and pyruvate enter a biochemical process of **gluconeogenesis** called the **Cori cycle**. In this process the body can utilize the lactic acid from high-intensity activities to help preserve blood glucose levels which are crucial to physiological function, particularly in the brain, which, despite making up approximately 2% of the body's mass, represents 50% of blood glucose utilization (3). The remanufactured glucose from exercise byproducts can also be used to replenish liver and muscle glycogen stores (51).

To improve exercise performance at high intensities and to reduce the reliance on the lactic acid system, exercisers should specifically train in the glycolytic pathways by recruiting larger and faster motor units. These motor units require near maximal efforts to be recruited and primarily use anaerobic glycolysis to produce ATP to fuel them. With more frequent

recruitment, such as with interval training or more intense resistance training, these muscle fibers will have a greater tolerance to fatigue. This is often referred to as "lactic acid tolerance," which seems somewhat paradoxical since the adaptation results in less lactic acid production at absolute exercise intensities. Analysis of training adaptations of glycolytic (anaerobic) muscle fibers reveals that recruitment of these fibers actually leads to improved aerobic adaptations, including oxygen delivery and utilization (27). Other adaptations include increased oxidation of lactic acid and more efficient lactate removal.

The body maintains ATP levels through metabolic processes that take place either in the cytosol of the cell or in the mitochondria. Anaerobic processes occur in the cytosol and use fuel from phosphocreatine, glucose, glycogen, glycerol (e.g. from triglyceride), and deaminated amino acids. The anaerobic processes can contribute to maximal biological work lasting approximately 3 minutes. For activities lasting beyond 3 minutes, ATP re-synthesis is achieved primarily by

~Quick Insight~

Lactic acid has been blamed for delayed onset muscle soreness (DOMS), cramping, and as an inhibitor to recovery from exercise. It is often considered to be a negative waste product from high intensity work. The reality is that none of these statements is true. Lactic acid is produced when glucose is metabolized. The breakdown leaves lactate and hydrogen ions as by-products. The hydrogen ions may build up under conditions of rapid metabolism and increase the acidity of the environment which may interfere with the electrical signals from motor neurons, slow enzymatic reactions, and impair muscle contractility. To the contrary, the lactate is a treasured fuel (7). It is rapidly produced and easily used by tissue. The heart, slow twitch muscle fibers, and postural muscles thrive on lactate because it is easily shuttled into the cell without insulin (40). Lactate rapidly moves across the cell membrane through a process called facilitated transport, enabling the body to use the lactate without the detrimental effects of insulin in the blood (46).

Lactate is produced in greater quantities when exercise intensity exceeds 50% of VO_2max. The production is linear with the rise in intensity as fast twitch fibers preferentially rely on carbohydrates as the fuel. As the lactate is produced, it is used by the muscle or transported to other tissues via general circulation. The increased blood flow with exercise effectively mobilizes the lactate for use by different tissues. Liver glycogen storage is maintained in part by the gluconeogenic activity to create glycogen for lactate. Equally important, lactate in the blood maintains available energy for working tissues (53). Unlike the liver, muscle tissue cannot free up glycogen stores to aid other working tissues due to a missing enzyme. Lactate can provide the needed assistance via circulatory delivery to muscles that need energy. The transport and use of lactate is often considered the "second wind" because more energy becomes available (49).

If the intensity of exercise becomes too elevated, the hydrogen ions produced inhibit muscle contractions. With quick recovery, the production removal balance is restored and training can continue. Training in the presence of lactic acid improves one's performance through more efficient management of the lactate and removal of the hydrogen (7). Intense resistance conditioning, like plyometrics and sprints, intervals, and hill climbs produce large quantities of lactic acid and stimulate the body to produce enzymes that increase the rate of lactic acid utilization.

Blaming lactic acid for cramps, delayed onset muscle soreness (DOMS), and as an obstacle to recovery is simply ignorant. Cramps are not caused by a sugar metabolite, but more likely, the over-excitation of nerves from fatigue and intra/extracellular electrolyte imbalance. DOMS is an inflammatory response to cellular damage, ischemia, and tonic spasm, not from leftover lactic acid. Likewise, recovery is not inhibited by lactate (9). The body has already used the leftover lactic acid for fuel before the next bout of exercise has even occurred. Lactate is a friend of intensity. If there is a foe, it's the hydrogen ion, and even that has been shown to be important for energy metabolism.

cellular oxidation via the **aerobic system**. This refers to the mitochondrial oxidation of fatty acids (fats), pyruvate from glucose (carbohydrates), and some deaminated amino acids (protein). Cellular oxidation is a process that is the reverse of photosynthesis, where plants take CO_2 and H_2O to produce O_2 and glucose, lipids, and protein.

At the onset of exercise, oxygen consumption undergoes a transitional phase in an attempt to meet the new demand. Physiological actions transpire to equalize the oxygen requirement of the activity and the available oxygen at the cell.

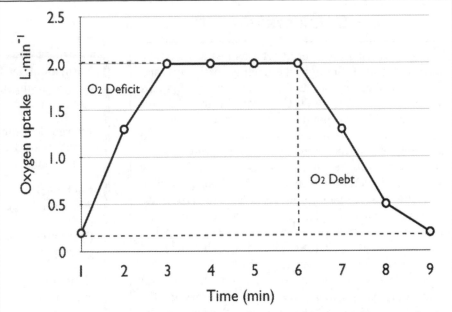

When the utilization of oxygen matches the demand, the body is said to reach metabolic **steady state**. During the transitional process, cells do not have the energy needed from oxygen sources and therefore, must borrow fuel from anaerobic sources in a phase referred to as **oxygen deficit**. This term quantitatively expresses the difference between the total oxygen consumed during an exercise bout and the actual amount of oxygen required. It is important to understand that exercise is not a product of switching on and off different energy systems, but rather a smooth blending and overlap of energy transfer from one pathway to another. With exercise training, the process of energy transfer among pathways becomes smoother, allowing trained individuals to reach steady-state sooner, consequently improving performance.

When exercise stops, the body is in a temporary state of disruption, compared to its normal resting state. **Recovery oxygen consumption** (also referred to as oxygen debt) persists after exercise and represents the excess oxygen consumption needed to recover from the physical activity and return the body to resting homeostasis. For example, after a vigorous set of squats a weight-lifter will be consuming greater levels of oxygen (notice greater ventilation rates following the lift) then those he or she was consuming prior to the set. During short aerobic bouts of exercise at a mild intensity, about 50% of the recovery oxygen will occur within 30 seconds after the exercise is completed. This is termed the "fast component" and is used primarily to re-synthesize high-energy phosphates and replenish oxygen in the body fluids and muscle stores (myoglobin). Intense exercise and exercise of long duration causes an additional, longer lasting phase of excess post-exercise oxygen consumption (EPOC; slow component) which can last up to 24 hours following

exercise (33). It is attributed to: 1) the elevated body temperature persisting post-exercise; 2) ion-leakage across cell membranes, leading to greater reliance on active ionic transport across the membrane to preserve homeostasis; 3) mitochondrial calcium uptake during exercise, reducing aerobic efficiency; 4) increased levels of thermogenic hormones existing post-exercise; 5) the re-synthesis of glycogen in the liver from lactate; and 6) the oxidation of the lactate in the mitochondria. Even transient bouts of high intensity exercise, such as interval training and weight lifting can produce recovery oxygen periods lasting greater than an hour (18).

The work rate, oxygen availability, and enzymatic profile of the muscle cell determines the primary energy system relied on to perform an exercise. Practically, a trainer will be able to observe the effects of work rate (intensity) on energy system demand. If the intensity is too high, aerobic contributions will not be enough to sustain the reaction and the exercise will stop. This explains why heavier resistant loads can only be lifted for a short period of time and for a minimal number of repetitions. If activities are being performed beyond three minutes, the force, expressed as percentage of 1RM, will need to be relatively low. Energy will still be applied anaerobically by glucose, but aerobic activity will be the primary contributor. As the aerobic system contributions increase, the maximal force output will decline. This stems from the inhibitory actions of rising hydrogen ion concentration from the breakdown of glucose, as well as the decline in rapid energy metabolism from the anaerobic system. The number of enzymatic reactions necessary to produce ATP from energy substrates and oxygen slows the speed and degree of force production.

AEROBIC METABOLISM

The previous section identified that the body transitions very smoothly from one energy system to rising contributions from another. With the ongoing performance of activity, the transition from anaerobic metabolism to aerobic metabolism is initiated by the pyruvate left over from glycolysis as it is transferred to the mitochondria in the cell. We know that the mitochondria serve as manufacturing plants, housing enzymes and substrates used to make cellular fuel. When the pyruvate enters the mitochondria, it sparks the reaction called the **Citric Acid Cycle, or Krebs Cycle**. The Krebs cycle refers to the process in which ATP is formed using oxygen and energy substrates or **oxidative phosphorylation**. A simplified way to understand mitochondria would be to view them as blenders. Inside the organelle the body takes glucose, adds in some oxygen, then blends it through 11 reactions and spits out 36 molecules of ATP, water, carbon dioxide, and heat.

The mitochondrial density in the muscle cell directly relates to the amount of energy that can be produced through aerobic means. In aerobic exercise, the three largest determinants of efficiency are 1) the number of mitochondria, 2) the concentration of enzymes inside them, and 3) the amount of oxygen rich blood which can be delivered to the cell. These efficiency factors also represent the adaptations to muscle tissue when aerobic exercise is routinely employed. The metabolic pathway is characterized by the release of hydrogens and carbon dioxide as the carbohydrate and oxygen are transformed through the metabolic process.

The same process can be performed using lipids and proteins. When the body works at lower intensities, lipids are the primary source of energy in aerobic metabolism. For instance, when a person sits on the couch to watch TV or sits at their desk at work on a computer, approximately 70% of the aerobic energy comes from lipid metabolism. One might think this would cause people to lose weight. However, at rest, we burn very few calories per hour, so the contribution is minimal. During exercise, the system works the same way. Low level exercise (40-60% of maximal aerobic output) utilizes fat as the preferred fuel for energy (42). During low to moderate exercise, it takes approximately

10 minutes of continuous movement for lipids to significantly contribute to aerobic energy.

In order for fat to be used as a fuel, it must first be released into its individual parts. **Triglycerides** represent 90% of the fat stored in the body in adipose tissue. **Lipase** is the enzyme which, in the presence of water, splits triglycerides into a glycerol molecule and three **fatty acids** through a process called **lipolysis**. The fatty acids hold the predominance of energy to be used by the muscle cell. These fatty acids bind to plasma **albumin** to form **free fatty acids** (FFA) in the blood stream where they can be transported to working tissue. Lipids can also be delivered by **lipoproteins** and freed to be used as fuel. The more blood flow to the tissue, the greater the propensity for fat to be burned for energy. Individuals who routinely engage in aerobic exercise enhance their ability to use lipids because they have more mitochondria and capillaries. These adaptations improve glucose sparing and increase exercise capacity. Additionally, exercise mediates lipid use through the adrenal hormones epinephrine and contributions from GH and glucagon. In Chapter 4, we learned that hormone augmentation was a factor in training adaptation. This further emphasizes the importance of participating in routine exercise for increased lipid metabolism (41).

When the lipids reach the cell, they have two pathways into oxidative phosphorylation. The glycerol molecule enters the same way glucose does by forming pyruvate. Remember, all these molecules are carbon chains of

~Key Terms~

Citric acid cycle- A series of enzymatic reactions in the mitochondria, involving oxidative metabolism of acetyl compounds, which produce high-energy phosphate compounds (ATP) that are the source of cellular energy.

Oxidative phosphorylation- The formation of ATP from the energy released by the oxidation of various substrates, especially the organic acids involved in the Krebs cycle.

Triglycerides- Consists of a glycerol and three fatty acids bound together in a single large molecule; an important energy source forming much of the fat stored by the body.

hydrogen and oxygen, so they can donate or accept ions to become something else. The triglycerides cannot enter as easily, they have to first enter a process called **beta oxidation** in the mitochondria. Fatty acid molecules must be reduced to smaller components before entering the Krebs cycle as **acetyl CoA**. Beta oxidation continues until the entire fatty acid molecule has been broken down and used. Through the process, a triglyceride molecule can yield 460 ATP, which is 10 times more energy than a glucose molecule can provide. The glycerol contributes to 19 ATP, while the three fatty acids provide 441 ATP. Clearly, lipids are a valuable source of energy for prolonged work.

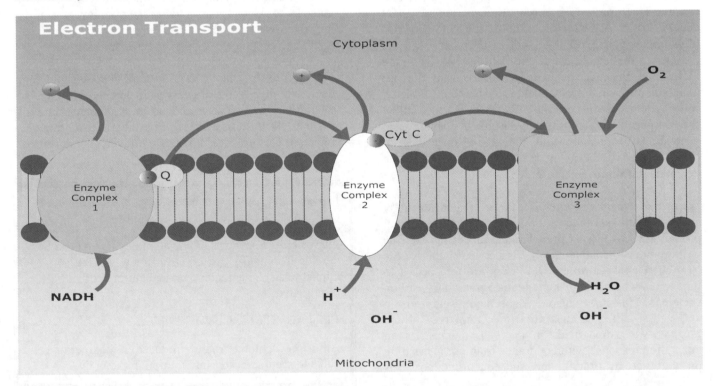

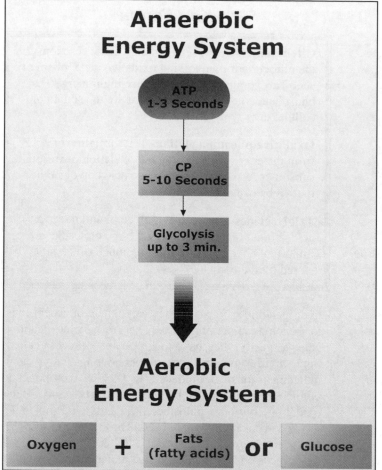

Anaerobic Energy System

ATP
1-3 Seconds

CP
5-10 Seconds

Glycolysis
up to 3 min.

Aerobic Energy System

Oxygen **+** Fats (fatty acids) **or** Glucose

When the work rate increases, the body again shifts to a greater reliance on glucose metabolism through both anaerobic and aerobic pathways, which is faster, and can therefore provide a more efficient and powerful energy source. A person on a Stairmaster who performs high intensity intervals will notice the change as the muscles in the legs begin to burn and fatigue due to the increasing presence of hydrogen ions from glucose metabolism. For improvements in aerobic capacity, carbohydrates are a necessary fuel because they allow for training at higher intensity. Limited physiological adaptations occur at low intensities, and once they do occur, there will be no new improvements unless the demands of exercise increase.

When the demands of exercise are prolonged, the body can also elicit assistance from **amino acids,** freed from protein sources (15). Cortisol released during exercise will remove proteins from tissue, particularly the **branched chain aminos** (61). They are transported to the liver where they are **deaminated** into carbon skeletons. This ability also exists in the muscle itself, in a process called **transamination**. Enzymes, which break down amino acids in the cell, increase as an adaptation response with endurance training. Depending on the type of protein and subsequent amino acids

released, the route to entry into the Krebs cycle can be through several mechanisms (62). Amino acids can be turned into pyruvate, acetyl CoA, or enter through hydrogen ion exchange called **electron transport.** During prolonged exercise, the preferred method is in the form of pyruvate. It should be noted that adequate carbohydrates are needed for protein to positively contribute to carbohydrate reserves. When proteins are deaminated, nitrogen is removed. Therefore, a byproduct of protein metabolism is urea. This increases the fluid intake requirements so urea can be mixed with water and passed from the body as urine.

ENERGY DEPLETION

When exercise intensity is low, it is sustained by lipid metabolism so that glycogen reserves may be spared. When the intensity is elevated to sustained, moderately-high performances or intermittent, high-intensity bouts, glycogen reserves become depleted with increasing exercise duration (16). The particular fiber depletion rate is specific to the intensity of the exercise. Shorter duration bouts, such as one minute sprints or heavy weight training deplete fast-twitch fibers. In contrast, the slow twitch fibers become depleted during continuous bouts of moderately high intensity. As it would be expected, depletion is a factor of recruitment. An interesting fact, related to cellular energy depletion, is that glycogen depletion is more rapid in trained individuals than untrained individuals in short all-out bouts of exercise. This is due to the faster conversion of glucose to lactic acid. Higher lactate levels signify higher power outputs. This emphasizes, again, the relative importance of energy specific training.

Fatigue sets in when the body experiences significant decline in glycogen stores. Even during aerobic exercise where adequate oxygen and fat is available, a lack of sugar in the system will lead to a fatigue condition and impaired performance. It is fairly obvious that during

~Key Terms~

Lipase- An enzyme capable of breaking down a lipid (fat) molecule.

Fatty acids- Form part of a lipid molecule and can be derived from fat by hydrolysis, often with a long aliphatic tail (long chains), either saturated or unsaturated.

Lipolysis- The breakdown of lipids.

Albumin- A blood protein produced in the liver that helps to regulate water distribution in the body.

anaerobic activities, glycogen depletion is related to direct use of the fuel. Since fats and proteins cannot support anaerobic exercise, when the sugars are gone, performance capabilities are lost. But this is also true of submaximal aerobic exercise. Even at levels where oxygen and lipids are adequate to meet the intensity demands of the work, the lack of carbohydrates in the body will cause significant fatigue (14). In endurance sports, this is referred to as hitting the wall. It is likely that the need for glucose to run the nervous system is a key component to the fatigue (19). It is also probable that the slow rate of lipid metabolism and the need for pyruvate to initiate oxidative phosphorylation causes inefficiency in the system (32). Insufficient carbohydrate intake leads to early decline in performance (23).

When inadequate carbohydrate consumption occurs for an extended period of time, the metabolic systems become dysfunctional (17). A lack of carbohydrate means a reduced quantity of pyruvate in the mitochondria (21). The lack of pyruvate means **oxaloacetate** (byproduct of pyruvate metabolism) is not available to bind with acetyl CoA to enter the Krebs cycle. Fatty acid metabolism will only occur when sufficient oxaloacetate is available for acetyl CoA in the process of betaoxidation (20). This presents two problems: 1) lipid metabolism yields only about half the power as that of carbohydrates and 2) when carbohydrates are not available, lipid metabolism is

slowed. With a lack of carbohydrate availability, lipids are predominantly required for ATP formation aerobically. In this environment, central fatigue (neural) occurs, as does peripheral fatigue (muscular) (35). If this is an on-going occurrence due to a low carbohydrate diet or a diet insufficient in calories, it causes a back-up in the system. The delivery of free lipids has nowhere to go, and acetyl CoA does not have a binding partner due to insufficient oxaloacetate to enter the Krebs cycle. This causes the two compounds to build up in the tissue. In response to increasing concentrations, the liver responds by converting these compounds into ketone bodies. These ketones enter circulation and are either excreted in urine or build up and negatively affect the pH levels of body fluid. Extreme cases lead to acidosis.

Acute depletion of anaerobic sources is specific to the intensity and duration of the training as well as pre-exercise storage. Stored ATP and CP depletion is similar in untrained and trained individuals, but as stated earlier, the higher lactate tolerance in trained individuals accounts for the more rapid decline in peripheral glycogen reserves and higher power outputs. In **acute peripheral fatigue**, increased lactic acid formation creates an acidic environment (54). The increasing acidity negatively affects the cellular activity because enzymes function at specific pH levels (55). The low pH inactivates enzymes for energy metabolism and negatively effects contractility, causing the muscles'

~Quick Insight~

The body has natural buffers to counteract the shift in pH which occurs in glycolytic pathways during exercise performance. The declining pH levels adversely affect enzyme activity and likely serve an inhibitory response to contractility. In lower-intensity activities, lactic acid is buffered into its salt lactate and taken to the liver to reformulate glucose. When production of lactic acid is met by equal buffering mechanisms, a fairly static pH equilibrium exists and there are no metabolic consequences. With increasing intensities the tissue produces more lactic acid than can be buffered by normal means. If the body does not compensate, the acid levels in the blood can reach high levels, dropping pH down to 6.8 from its comfortable 7.4. This generally is the point of physical exhaustion. Individuals will suffer nausea, headaches, cramps, and even disorientation (52). At this point, the body shuts down to allow the acid to be buffered in a process to regain homeostasis.

To prevent this from occurring, the body will increase its buffering capabilities through chemical, renal, and ventilatory adjustments. Chemical buffering is enhanced by an increase in bicarbonate formation and phosphate buffers (45; 50). Renal buffering occurs by a shift in the rate of reabsorption of buffering agents with a concurrent increase in the number of hydrogen ions released into urine. Ventilation can also serve to buffer the blood by increasing the rate of carbon dioxide released by the body, consequently reducing carbonic acid concentrations, increasing fluid alkalinity (6; 22).

Some theorize that buffering adaptations may occur in response to near maximal or maximal training efforts lasting 1-2 minutes. This though, has not been clearly established. Additionally, the use of sodium bicarbonate and sodium citrate solutions prior to 1-2 minute all out exercise bouts has been tested in experiments, showing some benefits. More research is needed, but the solutions seem to have a positive effect on hydrogen efflux from the cells. No benefit has been shown in events lasting less than one minute, so it has little implication for traditional strength training.

force output to decline (10). The change in the enzymes' surroundings is not an energy depletion-type of fatigue because a relatively short rest interval will remove the limiting factor. Peripheral fatigue associated with depletion of energy stores occurs relatively quickly during intense exercise because glucose (the primary fuel in intense exercise) is used up fairly rapidly. Performance decline is linear to glycogen decline in the muscle (34). When different muscles are used, as seen in resistance training, the rate of decline is inversely consistent with the amount of tissue used for work. Dispersing the work over many tissue areas avoids rapid depletion in individual muscle groups. Isolated muscle group activity, like repeated sprint training or lower body plyometrics, can only be performed at high intensity for short training bouts due to the localized depletion.

The body attempts to refuel depleted tissues by releasing sugar into the blood from the liver. Muscle stores of glycogen in unused tissues cannot be liberated in the presence of glucagons. Skeletal muscle cells do not contain the enzyme needed for glucose release into the blood (phosphatase), as it is only found in the liver. When excessive sugars are being used, the body will attempt to reserve some glucose for the central nervous system (56). Decline in performance mirrors both glycogen depletion and attempts to reserve glucose by reducing its availability through endocrine mediators and increasing fat substrates as a fuel. When glucose is not available to serve all the actions of exercise, peripheral fatigue will be joined with **central fatigue** (58). The lack of glucose affects the nervous system and communication signals decline in speed and strength (36). Without strong signals from the nervous system, exercise performance notably declines (57). Even though the body can produce glucose through gluconeogenesis in the liver, the by-products of fat metabolism cannot create sugar for the nervous system. Amino acids will support some level of glucose maintenance, but this most often occurs through catabolic means. Once this level has been reached, exercise is futile.

In attempts to maximize exercise performance, the most important component is the fuel available in the body. Although a high carbohydrate low fat meal consumed 3 hours before an event aids in available energy, to promote glycogen storage for subsequent events, it seems it is more important for exercisers to consume adequate energy post-exercise (1; 39). The physiological environment in the tissues causes a notable increase in energy substrate uptake immediately post-exercise. Scientists suggest that cellular permeability and heightened hormone sensitivity allows for increased storage capacity of glucose and protein in the three-hour period post exercise (38). Early literature in this area suggested that high amounts of carbohydrates (up to 500 g) should be consumed in 3-4 post-exercise meals (24; 26; 43). Higher glycemic foods were recommended to allow for glucose availability within the metabolic window following exercise.

The latest findings suggest that post-exercise muscle glycogen storage can be further enhanced with a carbohydrate/protein meal or supplement due to the interaction of the carbohydrate and protein on insulin secretion (2; 29; 70). Studies analyzing carbohydrate-protein recovery mixtures found increases in both carbohydrate and protein uptake occurred above that of the carbohydrate-only solutions (25; 68; 69). Additional research indicates that the rate of recovery is coupled with the rate of muscle glycogen replenishment and suggests that recovery supplements should be consumed to optimize muscle glycogen synthesis as well as fluid replacement post-exercise (31; 67). A key note to post-exercise replenishment is that the quantity of calories should reflect the intensity (8). Low to moderate efforts do not significantly deplete glycogen stores, so increasing post-exercise consumption of calories may not be warranted. In heavy resistance training and endurance bouts, energy and fluid replenishment is very important for subsequent bouts of training.

~Key Terms~

Free fatty acids- When fatty acids are not attached to other molecules, they are known as "free" fatty acids.

Lipoproteins- Compounds of protein that carry fats and fat-like substances, such as cholesterol in the blood.

Beta oxidation- is the process by which fats are broken down in the mitochondria to generate Acetyl-CoA, the entry molecule for the Citric Acid Cycle.

What Happens to Excess Macronutrients

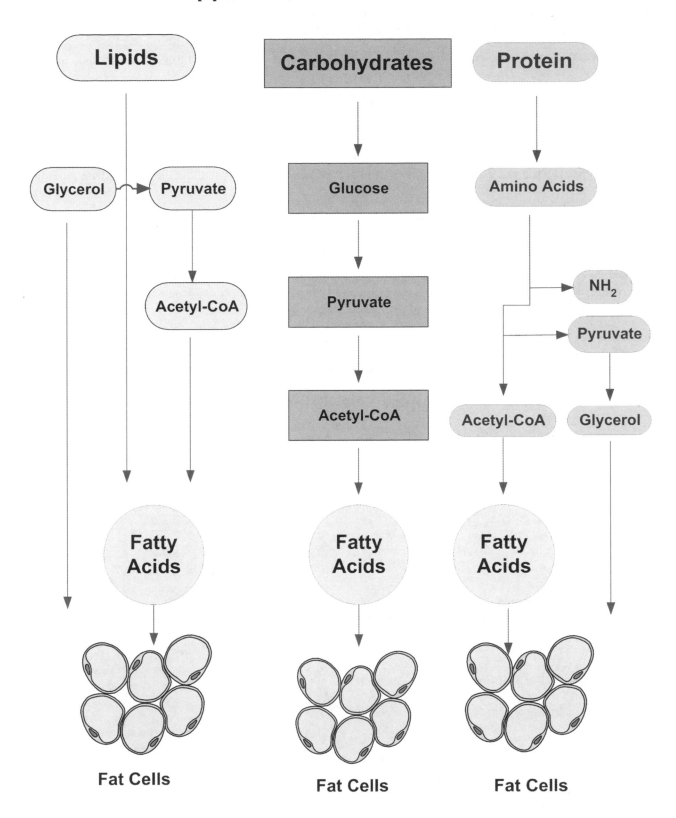

~Key Terms~

Acetyl CoA- A compound that functions as a co-enzyme in many biological acetylation reactions and is formed as an intermediate in the oxidation of carbohydrates, fats, and proteins.

Amino acids- Basic organic molecules consisting of hydrogen, carbon, oxygen, and nitrogen that combine to form proteins.

Branched chain aminos- Including leucine, isoleucine, glutamine, aspartic acid, and valine; used as fuel during long-term exercise bouts.

Deaminate- To breakdown a protein by removing an amino group.

Transamination- The transfer of an amino group from one molecule to another without the intermediate formation of ammonia.

Electron transport- A series of oxidation-reduction reactions during the aerobic production of ATP.

Oxaloacetate- The buffered form of oxaloacetic acid that binds with acetyl-CoA to enter the citric acid cycle.

Acute peripheral fatigue- Fatigue during physical work, caused by an inability of the body to supply sufficient energy to the contracting muscles to meet the increased energy demand. This causes contractile dysfunction that is manifested in the eventual reduction or lack of ability of a single muscle or local group of muscles to do work.

Central fatigue- The central component to fatigue generally described as a reduction in the neural drive or nerve-based motor command to working muscles that results in a decline in the force output.

Chapter Five References

1. **Adamo KB, Tarnopolsky MA and Graham TE**. Dietary carbohydrate and postexercise synthesis of proglycogen and macroglycogen in human skeletal muscle. *Am J Physiol* 275: E229-E234, 1998.

2. **Berardi JM, Price TB, Noreen EE and Lemon PW**. Postexercise muscle glycogen recovery enhanced with a carbohydrate-protein supplement. *Med Sci Sports Exerc* 38: 1106-1113, 2006.

3. **Blomstrand E and Saltin B**. Effect of muscle glycogen on glucose, lactate and amino acid metabolism during exercise and recovery in human subjects. *J Physiol* 514 (Pt 1): 293-302, 1999.

4. **Blomstrand E and Saltin B**. Effect of muscle glycogen on glucose, lactate and amino acid metabolism during exercise and recovery in human subjects. *J Physiol* 514 (Pt 1): 293-302, 1999.

5. **Brighenti F, Casiraghi MC, Ciappellano S, Crovetti R and Testolin G**. Digestibility of carbohydrates from rice-, oat- and wheat-based ready-to-eat breakfast cereals in children. *Eur J Clin Nutr* 48: 617-624, 1994.

6. **Buono MJ and Roby FB**. Acid-base, metabolic, and ventilatory responses to repeated bouts of exercise. *J Appl Physiol* 53: 436-439, 1982.

7. **Cairns SP**. Lactic acid and exercise performance : culprit or friend? *Sports Med* 36: 279-291, 2006.

8. **Costill DL and Hargreaves M**. Carbohydrate nutrition and fatigue. *Sports Med* 13: 86-92, 1992.

9. **Coudreuse JM, Dupont P and Nicol C**. [Delayed post effort muscle soreness]. *Ann Readapt Med Phys* 47: 290-298, 2004.

10. **Davis JA**. Anaerobic threshold: review of the concept and directions for future research. *Med Sci Sports Exerc* 17: 6-21, 1985.

11. **De Feo P, Di Loreto C, Lucidi P, Murdolo G, Parlanti N, De Cicco A, Piccioni F and Santeusanio F**. Metabolic response to exercise. *J Endocrinol Invest* 26: 851-854, 2003.

12. **Emmans GC**. Effective energy: a concept of energy utilization applied across species. *Br J Nutr* 71: 801-821, 1994.

13. **Englyst HN and Cummings JH.** Digestion of polysaccharides of potato in the small intestine of man. *Am J Clin Nutr* 45: 423-431, 1987.

14. **Fitts RH, Booth FW, Winder WW and Holloszy JO.** Skeletal muscle respiratory capacity, endurance, and glycogen utilization. *Am J Physiol* 228: 1029-1033, 1975.

15. **Friedman JE and Lemon PW.** Effect of chronic endurance exercise on retention of dietary protein. *Int J Sports Med* 10: 118-123, 1989.

16. **Gastin PB.** Energy system interaction and relative contribution during maximal exercise. *Sports Med* 31: 725-741, 2001.

17. **Grego F, Vallier JM, Collardeau M, Bermon S, Ferrari P, Candito M, Bayer P, Magnie MN and Brisswalter J.** Effects of long duration exercise on cognitive function, blood glucose, and counterregulatory hormones in male cyclists. *Neurosci Lett* 364: 76-80, 2004.

18. **Haddock BL and Wilkin LD.** Resistance training volume and post exercise energy expenditure. *Int J Sports Med* 27: 143-148, 2006.

19. **Hargreaves M.** Carbohydrates and exercise. *J Sports Sci* 9 Spec No: 17-28, 1991.

20. **Hawley JA.** Symposium: Limits to fat oxidation by skeletal muscle during exercise--introduction. *Med Sci Sports Exerc* 34: 1475-1476, 2002.

21. **Hawley JA.** Symposium: Limits to fat oxidation by skeletal muscle during exercise--introduction. *Med Sci Sports Exerc* 34: 1475-1476, 2002.

22. **Hirakoba K, Maruyama A, Inaki M and Misaka K.** Effect of endurance training on excessive CO_2 expiration due to lactate production in exercise. *Eur J Appl Physiol Occup Physiol* 64: 73-77, 1992.

23. **Holloszy JO and Kohrt WM.** Regulation of carbohydrate and fat metabolism during and after exercise. *Annu Rev Nutr* 16: 121-138, 1996.

24. **Ivy JL.** Glycogen resynthesis after exercise: effect of carbohydrate intake. *Int J Sports Med* 19 Suppl 2: S142-S145, 1998.

25. **Ivy JL.** Dietary strategies to promote glycogen synthesis after exercise. *Can J Appl Physiol* 26 Suppl: S236-S245, 2001.

26. **Ivy JL, Katz AL, Cutler CL, Sherman WM and Coyle EF.** Muscle glycogen synthesis after exercise: effect of time of carbohydrate ingestion. *J Appl Physiol* 64: 1480-1485, 1988.

27. **Jacobs I, Kaiser P and Tesch P.** Muscle strength and fatigue after selective glycogen depletion in human skeletal muscle fibers. *Eur J Appl Physiol Occup Physiol* 46: 47-53, 1981.

28. **Jenkins DJ, Cuff D, Wolever TM, Knowland D, Thompson L, Cohen Z and Prokipchuk E.** Digestibility of carbohydrate foods in an ileostomate: relationship to dietary fiber, in vitro digestibility, and glycemic response. *Am J Gastroenterol* 82: 709-717, 1987.

29. **Jentjens R and Jeukendrup A.** Determinants of post-exercise glycogen synthesis during short-term recovery. *Sports Med* 33: 117-144, 2003.

30. **Jeukendrup AE.** Carbohydrate intake during exercise and performance. *Nutrition* 20: 669-677, 2004.

31. **Khanna GL and Manna I.** Supplementary effect of carbohydrate-electrolyte drink on sports performance, lactate removal & cardiovascular response of athletes. *Indian J Med Res* 121: 665-669, 2005.

32. **Kirwan JP, O'Gorman DJ, Cyr-Campbell D, Campbell WW, Yarasheski KE and Evans WJ.** Effects of a moderate glycemic meal on exercise duration and substrate utilization. *Med Sci Sports Exerc* 33: 1517-1523, 2001.

33. **LaForgia J, Withers RT and Gore CJ.** Effects of exercise intensity and duration on the excess post-exercise oxygen consumption. *J Sports Sci* 24: 1247-1264, 2006.

34. **Layzer RB.** Muscle metabolism during fatigue and work. *Baillieres Clin Endocrinol Metab* 4: 441-459, 1990.

35. **Layzer RB.** Muscle metabolism during fatigue and work. *Baillieres Clin Endocrinol Metab* 4: 441-459, 1990.

36. **Layzer RB.** Muscle metabolism during fatigue and work. *Baillieres Clin Endocrinol Metab* 4: 441-459, 1990.

37. **Leeds AR.** Dietary fibre: mechanisms of action. *Int J Obes* 11 Suppl 1: 3-7, 1987.

38. **Levenhagen DK, Gresham JD, Carlson MG, Maron DJ, Borel MJ and Flakoll PJ.** Postexercise nutrient intake timing in humans is critical to recovery of leg glucose and protein homeostasis. *Am J Physiol Endocrinol Metab* 280: E982-E993, 2001.

39. **Maffucci DM and McMurray RG.** Towards optimizing the timing of the pre-exercise meal. *Int J Sport Nutr Exerc Metab* 10: 103-113, 2000.

40. **Messonnier L, Freund H, Denis C, Feasson L and Lacour JR.** Effects of training on lactate kinetics parameters and their influence on short high-intensity exercise performance. *Int J Sports Med* 27: 60-66, 2006.

41. **Mittendorfer B and Klein S.** Effect of aging on glucose and lipid metabolism during endurance exercise. *Int J Sport Nutr Exerc Metab* 11 Suppl: S86-S91, 2001.

42. **Pagan JD, Geor RJ, Harris PA, Hoekstra K, Gardner S, Hudson C and Prince A.** Effects of fat adaptation on glucose kinetics and substrate oxidation during low-intensity exercise. *Equine Vet J Suppl* 33-38, 2002.

43. **Peters EM.** Nutritional aspects in ultra-endurance exercise. *Curr Opin Clin Nutr Metab Care* 6: 427-434, 2003.

44. **Philp A,** Macdonald AL and Watt PW. Lactate--a signal coordinating cell and systemic function. *J Exp Biol* 208: 4561-4575, 2005.

45. **Philp A, Macdonald AL and Watt PW.** Lactate--a signal coordinating cell and systemic function. *J Exp Biol* 208: 4561-4575, 2005.

46. **Philp A, Macdonald AL and Watt PW.** Lactate--a signal coordinating cell and systemic function. *J Exp Biol* 208: 4561-4575, 2005.

47. **Philp A, Macdonald AL and Watt PW.** Lactate--a signal coordinating cell and systemic function. *J Exp Biol* 208: 4561-4575, 2005.

48. **Philp A, Macdonald AL and Watt PW.** Lactate--a signal coordinating cell and systemic function. *J Exp Biol* 208: 4561-4575, 2005.

49. **Philp A, Macdonald AL and Watt PW.** Lactate--a signal coordinating cell and systemic function. *J Exp Biol* 208: 4561-4575, 2005.

50. **Requena B, Zabala M, Padial P and Feriche B.** Sodium bicarbonate and sodium citrate: ergogenic aids? *J Strength Cond Res* 19: 213-224, 2005.

51. **Robergs RA, Ghiasvand F and Parker D.** Biochemistry of exercise-induced metabolic acidosis. *Am J Physiol Regul Integr Comp Physiol* 287: R502-R516, 2004.

52. **Robergs RA, Ghiasvand F and Parker D.** Biochemistry of exercise-induced metabolic acidosis. *Am J Physiol Regul Integr Comp Physiol* 287: R502-R516, 2004.

53. **Robergs RA, Ghiasvand F and Parker D.** Biochemistry of exercise-induced metabolic acidosis. *Am J Physiol Regul Integr Comp Physiol* 287: R502-R516, 2004.

54. **Robergs RA, Ghiasvand F and Parker D.** Biochemistry of exercise-induced metabolic acidosis. *Am J Physiol Regul Integr Comp Physiol* 287: R502-R516, 2004.

55. **Roecker K, Mayer F, Striegel H and Dickhuth HH.** Increase characteristics of the cumulated excess-CO2 and the lactate concentration during exercise. *Int J Sports Med* 21: 419-423, 2000.

56. **Secher NH, Quistorff B and Dalsgaard MK.** [The muscles work, but the brain gets tired]. *Ugeskr Laeger* 168: 4503-4506, 2006.

57. **Secher NH, Quistorff B and Dalsgaard MK.** [The muscles work, but the brain gets tired]. *Ugeskr Laeger* 168: 4503-4506, 2006.

58. **Secher NH, Quistorff B and Dalsgaard MK.** [The muscles work, but the brain gets tired]. *Ugeskr Laeger* 168: 4503-4506, 2006.

59. **Shulman RG.** Glycogen turnover forms lactate during exercise. *Exerc Sport Sci Rev* 33: 157-162, 2005.

60. **Shulman RG.** Glycogen turnover forms lactate during exercise. *Exerc Sport Sci Rev* 33: 157-162, 2005.

61. **Urhausen A, Gabriel H and Kindermann W.** Blood hormones as markers of training stress and overtraining. *Sports Med* 20: 251-276, 1995.

62. **Wagenmakers AJ.** Muscle amino acid metabolism at rest and during exercise: role in human physiology and metabolism. *Exerc Sport Sci Rev* 26: 287-314, 1998.

63. **Willardson JM.** A brief review: factors affecting the length of the rest interval between resistance exercise sets. *J Strength Cond Res* 20: 978-984, 2006.

64. **Willardson JM.** A brief review: factors affecting the length of the rest interval between resistance exercise sets. *J Strength Cond Res* 20: 978-984, 2006.

65. **Willardson JM.** A brief review: factors affecting the length of the rest interval between resistance exercise sets. *J Strength Cond Res* 20: 978-984, 2006.

66. **Willardson JM and Burkett LN.** The effect of rest interval length on bench press performance with heavy vs. light loads. *J Strength Cond Res* 20: 396-399, 2006.

67. **Williams MB, Raven PB, Fogt DL and Ivy JL.** Effects of recovery beverages on glycogen restoration and endurance exercise performance. *J Strength Cond Res* 17: 12-19, 2003.

68. **Williams MB, Raven PB, Fogt DL and Ivy JL.** Effects of recovery beverages on glycogen restoration and endurance exercise performance. *J Strength Cond Res* 17: 12-19, 2003.

69. **Zawadzki KM, Yaspelkis BB, III and Ivy JL.** Carbohydrate-protein complex increases the rate of muscle glycogen storage after exercise. *J Appl Physiol* 72: 1854-1859, 1992.

70. **Zawadzki KM, Yaspelkis BB, III and Ivy JL.** Carbohydrate-protein complex increases the rate of muscle glycogen storage after exercise. *J Appl Physiol* 72: 1854-1859, 1992.

Chapter 6

Cardiovascular Physiology

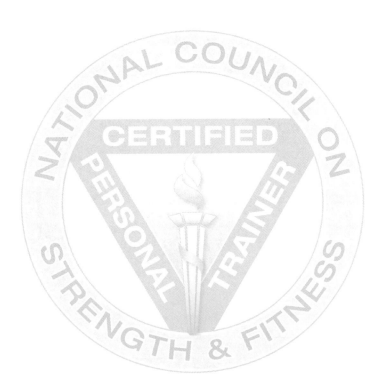

The Heart

The single most important muscle in the body is the heart. By performing continuous synchronized contractions, the heart works as a pump to deliver oxygen-rich blood and nutrients to tissues in the body. The heart is divided into two distinct sides that actually perform different tasks. The right side of the heart pumps deoxygenated blood to the lungs, whereas the left side of the heart sends oxygenated blood to the rest of the body. It accomplishes both responsibilities by functioning with a dual pump action. To manage this, each side of the heart has two distinct chambers, a top chamber called the **atrium** and a bottom chamber called the **ventricle**. The blood flows through the chambers under the force of the contracting tissue.

During cellular respiration, oxygen is used by the cell to perform its normal activities. In the process, oxygen chemically attaches to carbon to form carbon dioxide. The carbon dioxide is shuttled into circulation as **bicarbonate** where it is transported to the heart. It is then pumped to the lungs to be diffused across the alveoli and expired into the air. The deoxygenated blood enters the upper portion of the heart, the right atrium, through a large blood vessel called the **superior vena cava**. Blood fills the right atrium and is prevented from entering the right ventricle by the closed **tricuspid valve**. When the upper portion of the heart contracts both the left and right atria are emptied into their respective ventricles. Upon contraction, the deoxygenated blood is pushed through the tricuspid valve into the right lower chamber, which fills while the ventricle tissue is in a relaxed state. The ventricle relaxation phase is referred to as **diastole**. When the lower portion of the heart contracts it pushes the blood back against the tricuspid valve, forcing it to close. At the same time, the **pulmonary semilunar valve** is pushed open, allowing the blood to pass into the pulmonary artery. The contraction phase of the ventricles is referred to as **systole.** This interaction between the chambers and their corresponding valves is important so that blood flow is maintained in only one direction. The familiar "lub-dub" sound of a heart beating is actually the sound that the valves make when they close. It is

important to understand that while the atria are contracting, the ventricles are relaxed (diastole), allowing them to fill with blood. Conversely, when the ventricles contract (systole), the atrium is relaxed, allowing for them to refill with blood so that the cycle can repeat itself.

The pulmonary trunk transports the blood to the lungs where carbon dioxide is released while freshly inhaled oxygen is picked up. The oxygen diffuses through the lungs' alveoli and attaches to hemoglobin located in the red blood cells. The blood turns red with oxygenation and is transferred back to the heart via the **pulmonary vein**. It re-enters the heart through the left atrium. In the same manner it was pumped out to the lungs, the now oxygen-rich blood is pushed through the **bicuspid valve** (mitral valve)**,** which separates the left atrium from the left ventricle. Contraction of the left ventricle pushes the blood back against the bicuspid valve, closing it, while at the same time forcing the volume of blood through the **aortic valve** to the **aorta**. The aorta then distributes the blood to the rest of the body.

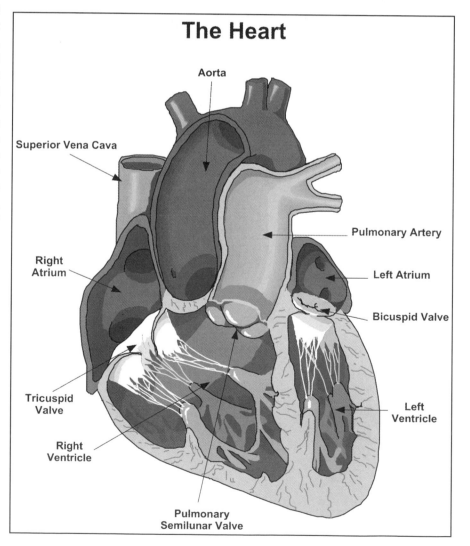

The Heart

Aorta

Superior Vena Cava

Pulmonary Artery

Right Atrium

Left Atrium

Bicuspid Valve

Tricuspid Valve

Left Ventricle

Right Ventricle

Pulmonary Semilunar Valve

Blood Flow Through the Heart

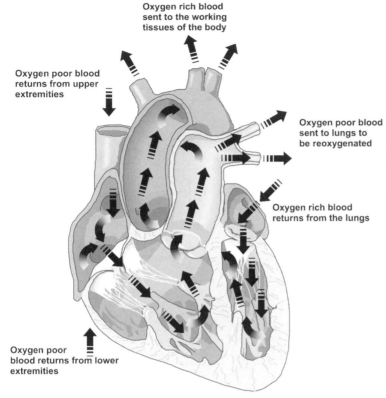

Oxygen rich blood sent to the working tissues of the body

Oxygen poor blood returns from upper extremities

Oxygen poor blood sent to lungs to be reoxygenated

Oxygen rich blood returns from the lungs

Oxygen poor blood returns from lower extremities

~Quick Insight~

Oxygen depleted blood returning from the body enters the right atrium, which fills and contracts. This mobilizes the blood into the right ventricle. The right ventricle then contracts, pushing the blood into the pulmonary artery, which delivers it to the lungs where carbon dioxide is exchanged for oxygen. The oxygen diffuses into the blood across the lungs' **alveoli** and binds to **hemoglobin,** a component of red blood cells that serves as oxygen's transporter throughout circulation. Once oxygenated, the blood returns to the left side of the heart through the pulmonary vein and enters the left atrium, which contracts, pushing the blood into the left ventricle. Completing the heart flow cycle, the left ventricle contracts, driving the blood through the **aorta** out to the rest of the body where oxygen and nutrients are exchanged for carbon dioxide and metabolic waste. All of which is returned back to the right side of the heart, re-initiating this continuous ongoing loop. The left ventricle has to deliver blood to the entire body, so it is not surprising that it is the largest of all the chambers. Furthermore, the wave of depolarization smoothly moves blood through the respective chambers through simultaneous and synchronized contractions. The SA Node dictates pace to the right and left atrium, which contract, pushing the blood into the ventricles, which, in turn, are then stimulated to contract in a likewise synchronized fashion to effectively push blood out from the heart.

~Key Terms~

Atria- The two upper chambers in the heart, which receive blood from the veins and push it into the ventricles.

Ventricle- The two lower chambers of the heart, which receive blood from the atria and pump it into the arteries.

Hemoglobin- A protein in red blood cells that transports oxygen to tissues.

Bicarbonate- A salt of carbonic acid in which one hydrogen atom has been replaced.

Alveoli- A tiny, thin-walled, capillary-rich sac in the lungs where the exchange of oxygen and carbon dioxide takes place.

Superior vena cava- The primary vein collecting blood from the head, chest wall, and upper extremities and draining into the right atrium.

Tricuspid valve- A three-segmented valve of the heart that keeps blood in the right ventricle from flowing back into the right atrium.

Systole- The contraction of the chambers of the heart (especially the ventricles) to drive blood into the aorta and pulmonary artery.

Diastole- The relaxation and dilatation of the heart chambers, especially the ventricles, during which they fill with blood.

Pulmonary semilunar valve- A semilunar valve between the right ventricle and the pulmonary artery which prevents blood from flowing from the artery back into the heart.

Pulmonary vein- A vein that carries oxygenated blood from the lungs to the left atrium of the heart.

Bicuspid valve- A valve of the heart, composed of two triangular flaps, that is located between the left atrium and left ventricle and regulates blood flow between these chambers.

Aortic valve- A heart valve comprising three flaps, which guards the passage from the left ventricle to the aorta and prevents the backward flow of blood.

Aorta- The major artery that carries oxygenated blood from the heart to be delivered by arteries throughout the body.

Cardiac Muscle Tissue

The heart muscle, also called the **myocardium**, is somewhat similar to skeletal muscle but is more specialized for its purpose of repeated, measured contractions. Cardiac muscle tissue, like skeletal muscle tissue, has a sarcoplasmic reticulum for calcium storage and T-tubules to manage action potentials. It also has organized sarcomeres, which contain actin and myosin contractile proteins. However, there are distinct differences between cardiac and skeletal muscle. These differences allow the heart to function in a constant non-stop manner, rather than serving the intermittent, voluntary actions common of skeletal muscle.

Cardiac tissue, like all tissue, relies on ATP for fuel. The heart needs a constant supply of energy and oxygen so it will not fatigue. If the heart were to fatigue under conditions of high stress, it could be lethal because oxygen would no longer reach vital organs, including the brain and the heart's contractile tissue. Cardiac tissue relies heavily on ATP produced from lipids. In the last chapter, lipid metabolism was shown to produce large quantities of ATP at lower intensities. This makes it the ideal fuel for the heart, as the cardiac muscle runs almost exclusively using oxidative metabolism to satisfy its energy demands (9).

In an effort to maximize the efficiency of the aerobic system, cardiac muscle is densely packed with mitochondria and contains an extensive network of capillaries (one capillary per muscle fiber). This arrangement provides a constant flow of oxygen-rich blood to the mitochondria for the production of ATP. Consistent with skeletal muscle, cardiac muscle must utilize carbohydrates to fuel the higher force outputs required during heavy exercise (6). But unlike the skeletal muscle, the heart cannot allow hydrogen ions from lactic acid to build up, as they may inhibit enzyme activity and contractility. To ensure this does not occur, myocardial tissues possess greater capacity to utilize oxygen and blood to increase the rate of lactate conversion, effectively preventing fatigue. Cardiac muscle extracts approximately 75% of the available oxygen, whereas skeletal muscle extracts closer to 25% of the oxygen delivered to the tissue.

Another significant difference between cardiac and skeletal muscle is the conduction system used by the heart to manage an efficient pump mechanism. The **sinoatrial (SA) node** and the **atrioventricular (AV) node** are modified cardiac muscle cells that connect to a conducting bundle. The nodes send electrical impulses that run down the connecting bundle, which braches to the chambers of the heart. Respectively, the branches are identified as the left and right **bundle branches**.

Cross Section of Cardiac Muscle Tissue

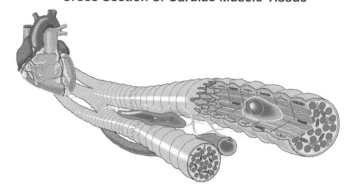

The signals from the nodes dictate the contractile element of the heart. Essentially, the SA and AV nodes communicate to the atria and ventricles when to contract. This eloquent system of conduction allows the atria and ventricles to contract in synchronicity so that the forward flow of blood is maintained.

The initial contractile signal for the heart originates in the SA node. For this reason, the SA node is called the pacemaker, as its chief responsibility is to signal the contractile pace to the atria. It sends a slower signal through the atrial cardiac tissue to stimulate contraction of the right and left atrium and a faster messenger signal to the AV node through preferential pathways to relay the pace to the ventricles (17). The passage of the slower signals across the atrial portion of the heart represents the electrical impulse that drives the atrial contraction. After receiving the signal from the SA node, the AV node transfers these signals to the AV bundle. When the action potential reaches the left and

~Key Terms~

Myocardium- The muscular tissue of the heart.

Sinoatrial (SA) node- A small mass of specialized cardiac muscle fibers that controls the heartbeat.

Atrioventricular (AV) node- A small mass of specialized cardiac muscle fibers between the atria and the ventricles of the heart, which conducts the normal electrical impulse from the atria (SA node) to the ventricles.

Bundle branches- Part of the impulse-conducting network of the heart that rapidly transmit impulses from the atrioventricular node to the ventricles.

Wave of depolarization- Electrical activation of the myocardium. Occurs in the sinoatrial (SA) node; current travels through the tracts of the atria to the atrioventricular (AV) node then through the Bundle of His, which divides into right and left bundle branches.

right bundles, it speeds up to stimulate the contraction of the ventricles. This process of electrical transfer across the heart is called the **wave of depolarization**. The relatively slow transfer time allows the atrium to contract and then relax as the ventricles become stimulated. This conduction system maintains a steady flow of blood through the heart and out to the lungs and circulation.

Conduction System of the Heart

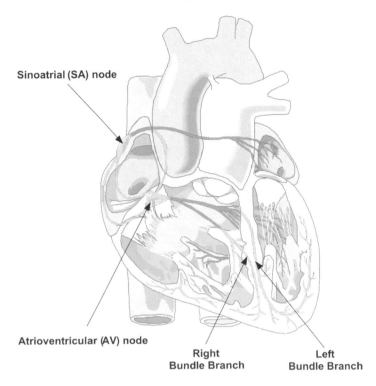

Sinoatrial (SA) node

Atrioventricular (AV) node

Right Bundle Branch

Left Bundle Branch

Cardiac Output

When the heart pumps blood from the left ventricle out to the body's tissues, the volume of blood expelled per contraction is called the **stroke volume (SV)**. The volume expelled depends upon the strength of the cardiac muscular contraction, as well as the volume of the left ventricle. Individuals who engage in endurance training activities increase their capacity to pump blood out to the tissues through adaptations that make the ventricular contraction stronger and the volume of blood expelled out of the aorta larger (18). The rate at which the blood is pumped determines the amount of blood available to the tissue. **Heart rate** describes the number of beats that occur in the heart each minute. When the heart rate is multiplied by the amount of blood expelled per beat (stroke volume), the total volume of blood available per minute can be determined. This value is referred to as the heart's **cardiac output**. Cardiac output is a major determinant of the body's ability to sustain physical activity (12).

CARDIAC OUTPUT = HR X SV

Blood Pressure

Blood leaving the heart enters into peripheral circulation via the left ventricle. Blood from the right ventricle flows to the lungs to be re-oxygenated, while the blood from the left ventricle flows through the systemic vessels and is transported to the body tissues. When the blood reaches the tissue, it deposits oxygen and nutrients and removes the cellular waste. To ensure that the flow of blood to the tissues is maintained at appropriate levels, the circulatory system has regulatory mechanisms that control the pressure exerted on the blood. **Blood pressure** is managed by **baroreceptors** located in the aorta and the carotid arteries. When the body needs oxygen for working tissue, the pressure in the blood vessels is adjusted to meet the demand. Areas of the body which require more oxygenated blood experience expansion in the diameter of their respective vessels called **vasodilation**, while the areas requiring less oxygenated blood experience a narrowing of the vessels referred to as **vasoconstriction**. By changing the diameter of the vessels, blood pressure can be increased or decreased according to relative demands.

Blood pressure is determined by multiplying the cardiac output of the heart and the **peripheral resistance** applied by the vessels. When the body is at rest, the cardiac output is low, so the main determinant of blood pressure is peripheral resistance (20). Peripheral resistance reflects the difficulty with which the blood passes through the vessels. Constricted or compressed

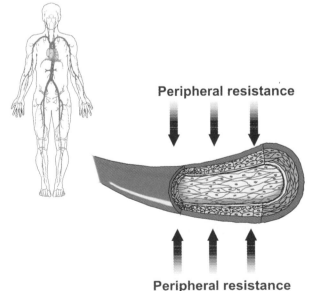

Peripheral resistance

Peripheral resistance

**Blood Pressure =
Cardiac Output x Peripheral Resistance**

vessels or those that have **plaque** built up along the walls make it harder for the blood to pass because the space in the vessel is compromised. When the blood experiences difficulty passing through a vessel, it builds up pressure and becomes turbulent. This is common in individuals who smoke, are obese, or experience a build-up of fat along the vessel wall (16). In small vessels, the stress can lead to artery disease. On the contrary, large vessels and those that provide little resistance pass blood with much less effort and do not cause damaging fluid turbulence.

During exercise or high stress situations, the heart rate is increased, consequently increasing cardiac output. The increase in cardiac output forces blood to flow through the system at a faster rate. The high speed circulation of blood pushes out on the walls of the vessels, increasing the pressure. When this pressure is added to the peripheral resistance of the vessels, it equals the net blood pressure of the body. Due to elevations in heart rate during exercise, blood pressure is always higher than when the body is at rest. At rest, mean arterial pressure (MAP) in the large arteries is about 100 mmHg. During aerobic exercise the MAP will jump to 115-120 mmHg, while during heavy resistance training that number can increase to 200 mmHg (4). When selecting or prescribing exercise modalities for clients, personal trainers should consider blood pressure response, to ensure the exercises reflect the individual's current vascular health. Increasing blood pressure in hypertensive and elderly clients increases risk of vessel wall damage and may exacerbate tissue lesions and arteriosclerosis (2).

Peripheral Circulatory System

To get blood to all the working tissues of the body, an intricate network of vessels of varying sizes is needed. In the same way a tree branches into limbs that further divide into smaller branches, large vessels from the heart branch to smaller vessels that are far reaching throughout the body. Blood leaving the heart enters into large arteries, which branch repeatedly into smaller arteries. The main arteries direct blood to the major sections of the body. Leaving the heart, the ascending aorta branches into the large arteries that deliver blood to the brain, called the carotid arteries, and the brachiocephalic artery, which extends to arteries of the upper extremity, including the brachial artery. The descending aorta travels down the trunk to form the iliac artery, which eventually branches into the femoral arteries. These arteries are responsible for delivering blood to the lower limbs. Along the way, the aorta has branches that extend to the organs and tissues of the trunk.

The large arteries have elastic properties to manage the high pressure in the vessels. They maintain lower amounts of smooth muscle tissue when compared to smaller vessels in part due to their role in delivery and their respective proximity to the heart. Their primary function in the vascular system is to deliver large quantities of blood to the main body segments, which is why they are referred to as **conducting arteries**. Large arteries give way to medium size arteries, which turn

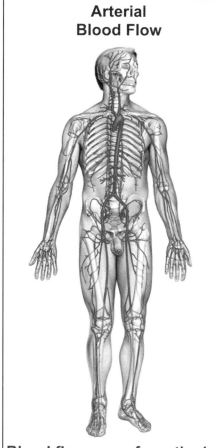

Arterial Blood Flow

Blood flow away from the heart (Generally Oxygen Rich)

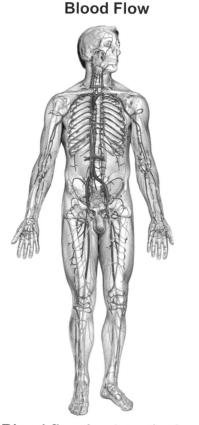

Venous Blood Flow

Blood flow back to the heart (Generally Oxygen Poor)

into smaller branch arteries. As the artery diameter becomes narrower, the amount of elastic tissue is reduced and is replaced by larger amounts of smooth muscle. Medium size arteries are called distributors because they have a regulatory control over what area of the tissue gets the most blood flow through vasodilation and vasoconstrictive controls. During exercise, the medium arteries that supply blood to the gastrointestinal organs, such as the stomach and bowel vasoconstrict, decreasing the blood flow to these areas. Conversely, the medium arteries that distribute blood to muscles vasodilate, effectively shunting a larger amount of blood to the muscles, where more oxygen is required due to increased activity levels. The small arteries further control the flow of blood through a similar process.

Capillaries are the smallest blood vessels and supply the cells with oxygen and nutrients. Because these vessels do not have a muscle layer, the nutrients diffuse across the capillary walls into the interstitial spaces for cellular use. They connect to the arterial system via **arterioles**. The smallest of the arteries, arterioles have only a couple of layers of smooth muscle surrounding the **endothelium**, and they do not have an elastic layer like their larger counterparts. Like the other vessels

How Oxygen is Transported

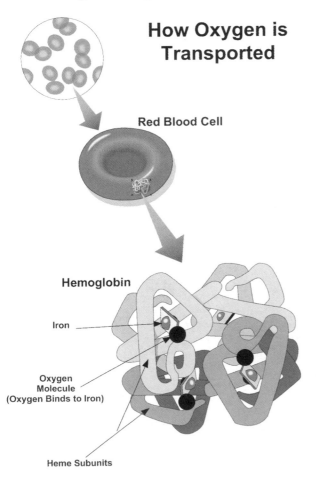

Red Blood Cell

Hemoglobin

Iron

Oxygen Molecule (Oxygen Binds to Iron)

Heme Subunits

surrounded by smooth muscle, arterioles can constrict or dilate dependent upon need to assist in blood flow management.

After the oxygen diffuses into the cells and carbon dioxide is absorbed, the blood travels from the capillaries to **venules** which turn into small **veins**. Venules enable a level of nutrient transport across their walls, but as those walls thicken with smooth muscle cells, (as they turn into small veins) the exchange is

~Key Terms~

Stroke volume- The volume of blood pumped out of the left ventricle of the heart in a single beat.

Heart rate- The number of heart beats per unit of time, usually expressed as beats per minute.

Cardiac output- The volume of blood being pumped by the heart; it is equal to the heart rate multiplied by the stroke volume.

Blood pressure- The pressure exerted by the blood against the walls of the blood vessels, especially the arteries.

Baroreceptors- Detect the pressure of blood, and can send messages to the central nervous system to increase or decrease total peripheral resistance and cardiac output.

Vasodilation- Dilation or expansion in flow width of a blood vessel.

Vasoconstriction- Constriction or reduction in flow width of a blood vessel.

Peripheral resistance- Resistance of the blood vessels in the body.

Plaque- A fat deposit on the inside wall of a blood vessel.

Conducting arteries- Deliver large quantities of blood to different regions of the body.

Capillaries- Tiny blood vessels throughout the body that connect arteries and veins.

Arterioles- One of the small, thin-walled arteries that end in capillaries.

Endothelium- A thin layer of flat epithelial cells that lines blood vessels.

Venules- Small veins that join capillaries to larger veins.

How Oxygen Exchanges with Muscle Tissue

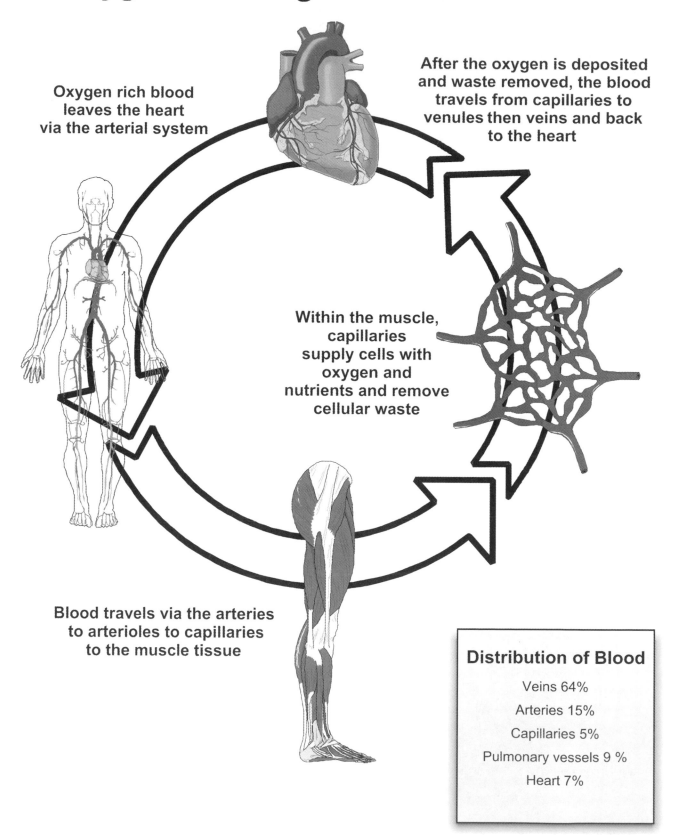

Oxygen rich blood leaves the heart via the arterial system

After the oxygen is deposited and waste removed, the blood travels from capillaries to venules then veins and back to the heart

Within the muscle, capillaries supply cells with oxygen and nutrients and remove cellular waste

Blood travels via the arteries to arterioles to capillaries to the muscle tissue

Distribution of Blood

Veins 64%

Arteries 15%

Capillaries 5%

Pulmonary vessels 9 %

Heart 7%

essentially blocked. The deoxygenated blood travels from small veins to medium-sized veins, like tributaries flowing into a river. The venous system is similar to the arterial system of vessels in size and distribution, but holds significantly more blood. The two circulatory passages run basically parallel to each other throughout the body, which is clearly illustrated by red and blue color distinction. The major difference between veins and arteries is the amount of oxygen in the blood contained within the respective vessels and the way the fluid is moved through circulation.

Arteries have a pulse because the blood that flows through them is pushed by the rhythmic contractions of the heart. The venous return does not have the pressure from cardiac output to drive the fluid back to the heart, and therefore, must use smooth muscle contractions and a system of one-way valves to prevent any back flow as the blood is mobilized to the right atrium and eventually to the lungs to be re-oxygenated. Veins that are larger

~Quick Insight~

When muscle tissue is engaged in hard work, the body floods the area with blood to satisfy the oxygen demands of the activity. The delivery continues until the activity stops. When exercisers engorge the large muscles of the lower body with blood and then do not follow with a cool down of lighter rhythmic activities, the blood remains in the tissue (1). When this occurs, blood can build up around the valves, a condition called blood pooling. The fluid is deoxygenated and high in bicarbonate and other byproducts of exercise metabolism. Due to the fact that approximately 64% of all circulatory blood is located in the systemic veins, transitioning the body from heavy work to rest may impede upon blood flow back to the heart (3). Blood pooling shunts the needed blood away from the heart, which can cause acute ischemia in the tissue and a reduced cardiac output. Blood pooling is often identified by leg heaviness and discomfort, which often makes sleeping difficult.

Blood pooling can be avoided if exercisers routinely engage in cool-down activities following training. Light aerobic exercise increases the flow of blood back to the heart due to the venous mobilization caused by rhythmic muscular contractions. This begins to restore the body to pre-exercise condition. The activity increases by-product removal and conversion, including lactic acid, and sets up the tissue for more successful recovery. Elderly individuals or those with peripheral vascular problems should use longer warm-ups and cool downs to better regulate blood flow, as older or damaged veins have a reduced capacity to return blood to the heart on their own, and an immediate cessation of activity can have negative effects on the vascular system (14).

than 2 mm contain valves that occlude the vessel when the blood attempts to reverse direction. The smooth muscle is stimulated to contract by nervous signals from the autonomic nervous system.

Assessing Pulse

Palpating the area where large arteries are close to the skin, one will feel a rhythmical pulse, caused by the pressure exerted on the arteries when the heart contracts. There are a number of locations at the arms, legs, head and neck at which one can identify the heart's pace. In the head and neck, the superficial temporal artery, facial artery, and common carotid artery can be palpated. The carotid arteries are often easily identified by a strong pulse as they ascend from the aorta. They can be palpated on either side of the larynx just below the jaw. In the arms, the radial pulse is probably the most recognized and is often palpated for exercise pulse rate. In the upper arm, both the axillary artery and brachial artery can be felt with moderately light finger pressure. Although not commonly used for pulse assessment, the leg's femoral artery, popliteal artery, and dorsalis pedis all have a measurable pulse rate.

The tendency of the blood vessel to match pressure with volume is called **compliance**. The more the vessel will stretch when pressure increases, the better its compliance. As pressures increase against the endothelium, elastic vessels expand in compliance to accommodate an increase in blood flow, thereby reducing the pressure. Even small increases in pressure translate into large volume shifts by compliant tissues. The veins have significantly more compliance to variations in blood pressure than arteries. In fact, veins are almost 25 times more compliant than arteries, one of the primary reasons veins have a greater contribution to blood storage. Veins retain almost two-thirds of the blood supply at any given time. The ability of the venous system to hold blood is sometimes detrimental, as blood can build up in the tissues, referred to as **blood pooling**. Elevated levels of blood pooling result in reduced blood flow to the heart, lowering cardiac output.

Aging & Vessel Health

The aging effect plays a role in vessel decline. The elastic properties of the arteries suffer degenerative changes, causing them to lose pliability and compliance and begin to harden. Veins also experience decline in function through a reduced compliance to changes in blood pressure. This process is called hardening of the arteries or **arteriosclerosis**. Layers of the vessel thicken and experience chemical changes in elastic properties. Between the elastic and collagenous fibers, fat deposits

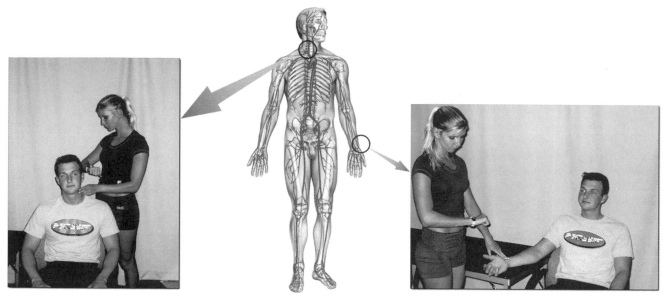

Carotid Pulse

Pulse Locations

Radial Pulse

build up, which begin to impede blood flow. The cholesterol-based materials, eventually add calcium deposits and fibrous material further occluding the flow of blood. This process is called **atherosclerosis**. These mechanisms of vessel dysfunction can dramatically reduce and even stop the flow of blood to tissues, leading to cellular death. Obesity, smoking, high cholesterol, physical inactivity, and hypertension are all related to increased risk for arteriosclerosis.

Degenerative function of the vascular tissues reduces the capacity for the circulatory system to manage exercise. Personal trainers should be cautious when working with hypertensive clients and elderly

populations due to their vascular systems' reduced efficiency at regulating pressures. Rapid changes in body position, particularly from a supine to upright posture can cause **orthostatic hypotension** (19). Caution should also be applied when these exercisers perform activities with intense loads. Individuals with hypertension or reduced vascular compliance should not engage in heavy resistance training.

Varicose Vein

Plaque Formation in Vessels

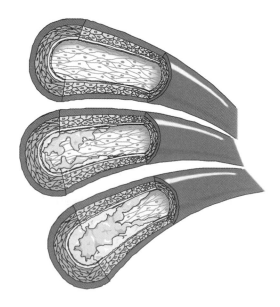

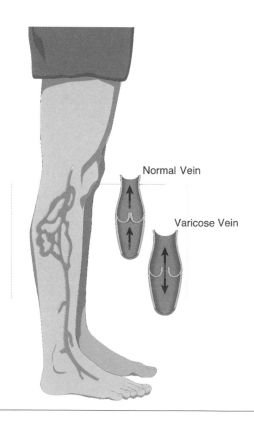

~Quick Insight~

If the veins get stretched, the integrity of the valve system may be compromised. When this occurs, the valves become progressively less capable of preventing backflow. Compromised valves cause the vein to become abnormally dilated in response to the back flow pressure, which causes them to swell. The outcome is a vascular bulge of the superficial vessels, most often observed in the legs. Hyperdilated superficial veins are known as varicose veins.

Most varicose veins do not present a serious medical problem but can sometimes lead to complications. When the flow of blood in the vessel becomes stagnant, clots can form. Unlike blood clots in deep veins, clots in superficial veins rarely travel to the heart or lungs, where they could cause serious blockages. Phlebitis or inflammation of the vein is more of a threat because it may lead to cellular ischemia and gangrenous tissue (13). Surgery may be needed to remove damaged vessels.

Exercisers with varicose veins should avoid heavy resistance training (11). Excessive pressure can increase back flow force, exacerbating the condition and causing pain. Aerobic or rhythmic physical activity is recommended because dynamic muscle contractions increase the propensity for blood to flow back to the heart.

The Role of Blood

During both rest and exercise, the dynamics of the circulatory system depend upon the physics of blood flow and the tissue anatomy of the vessels. Because they must satisfy the blood flow demands of all the tissues in the body, it makes sense that approximately 84% of the blood circulates systemically in the arteries and veins. The other 16% is in the process of oxygenation in the pulmonary vessels or in the heart itself. Blood flows quickly through large arteries and slowly through capillaries because pressure declines as the flow moves from large to small vessels. The pressure in the capillaries averages about 20 mmHg compared to the average aortic pressure of 100 mmHg. This lower pressure in the capillaries results in slower blood velocity, allowing the cellular nutrients and waste products to be exchanged between the arterial entrance and the venous exit.

Capillaries allow fluids containing oxygen and nutrients to diffuse across the vessel's wall. This is possible because capillaries have less smooth muscle compared to veins and arteries. It is the combination of interstitial pressure and blood pressure that drives the exchange. The blood pressure pushes nutrients into surrounding tissues, while the interstitial pressure of the tissues drives metabolic waste from the tissue into the blood. Blood pressure at the beginning, or the arterial side, of the capillary is higher than the pressure at the venous side, which lends itself to the regulatory mechanisms of exchange. Essentially, cellular nutrients leave the vessel at the beginning of the capillary, and waste enters the vessel at the end. Because exercise increases the cellular demand for oxygen and nutrients, as well as the removal of metabolic waste, the body will add capillaries as an adaptive response. Increasing the number of capillaries or capillary density within muscle tissue, occurs mainly in response to repetitive endurance activities. This allows for increased oxygen and nutrient delivery to the muscle cells during exercise, consequently improving performance outcomes.

Function of Blood

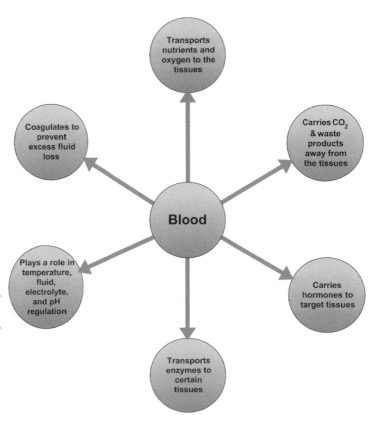

~Quick Insight~

Hemoglobin is a molecule made of proteins that require iron to carry oxygen in the body. Approximately 66% of the four grams of iron contained in humans is found attached to hemoglobin. Females lose iron through menstruation, requiring an increased ingestion of dietary iron above the requirements of males. Research indicates that iron absorption triples in the presence of ascorbic acid (Vitamin C). If iron availability is insufficient, blood hemoglobin levels decrease, leading to a condition known as iron-deficiency anemia. Consequently, the body experiences a reduced availability of oxygen in the blood. Additionally, cigarette smoking affects oxygen transport with hemoglobin. Cigarette smoke produces carbon monoxide, which bonds to hemoglobin, inhibiting the ability of oxygen to be transported in the blood. In its transport form with hemoglobin, carbon monoxide may represent 5-15% of blood and impede on physical capacity during work due to decreased oxygen delivery to working tissue (7).

The blood's ability to deliver nutrients and remove waste is a factor of its transport mechanisms and constitution. Blood is the connecting factor between tissues.

The human body generally maintains 4 to 5 liters of blood in total circulation. Some of the blood is comprised of cells and cell fragments called the **formed element** of blood. The rest is made up of a liquid **plasma** called the fluid matrix. Approximately 95% of the formed element is comprised of **red blood cells.** The remaining 5% is made up of the **white blood cells** and **platelets**. Males have nearly 14% more formed element than females, which makes up approximately 44-54% of the total blood volume in the body. The formed element of blood is referred to as **hematocrit**. The remaining plasma makes up the other 46-56%. Plasma is comprised of mostly water, interspersed with some dissolved or suspended molecules. Due to its high water volume, plasma is often extracted from the blood during periods of dehydration. This is one mechanism by which dehydration causes body dysfunction. During dehydration, the plasma volume, and thus blood volume, decreases. The heart then has to pump harder to maintain blood pressure so that oxygen delivery to tissue is maintained.

At any given time, numerous compounds are contained within the constituents of the blood. Each compound has a specific function and; the measured concentration of each depends upon the internal and external environment the body is exposed to. During exercise, concentrations of dissolved components such as ions, enzymes, hormones, nutrients, and exercise by-products, increase in response to work demands. In addition to the changes in plasma concentrations, erythrocytes (red blood cells) increase in oxygen and carbon dioxide transport during physical activity. Oxygen bonds to hemoglobin contained within the **erythrocytes**. The erythrocytes also contain an enzyme that catalyzes the reaction between carbon dioxide and water to form carbonic acid, which ionizes to form hydrogen and bicarbonate ions. Bicarbonate ions diffuse into the blood plasma, which represents the primary method of carbon dioxide transport to the lungs. Recalling the buffering effect from sugar metabolism, bicarbonate is an important component to the maintenance of blood pH as well.

~Key Terms~

Compliance- A measure of the ease with which a structure may be deformed or distended.

Blood pooling- An accumulation of blood in the venous system that can reduce blood return to the heart.

Arteriosclerosis- A chronic condition, characterized by thickening and hardening of the arteries and the build-up of plaque on the arterial walls.

Atherosclerosis- A stage of arteriosclerosis in which the arteries become clogged by the build-up of fatty substances, which eventually reduces the flow of blood to the tissues.

Orthostatic hypotension- A form of low blood pressure, precipitated by moving from a lying or sitting position to standing up straight.

Plasma- The clear, fluid portion of blood in which cells are suspended.

Red blood cells- Cells in the blood that transport oxygen and carbon dioxide to and from the tissues.

White blood cells- A group of several cell types that occur in the bloodstream and are essential for a properly functioning immune system.

Platelets- A type of blood cell responsible for blood coagulation and for the repair of damaged blood vessels.

Hematocrit- The proportion, by volume, of the blood that consists of red blood cells.

Erythrocytes- Red blood cells.

Circulation During Activity

When the body engages in activities with increasing intensity, the circulatory system increases its capacity to deliver blood to the working tissue. At rest, only 20%-25% of the capillaries in skeletal muscle are open, and the rate of the heart is at its lowest working level. When the body is about to engage in activity, the circulatory system receives signals from the brain preparing it to manage oxygen demands. Heart rate increases before a person even picks up a weight or turns on the treadmill in anticipation of the activity. Concurrently, capillary beds open up to provide oxygen to the tissues they feed. During exercise, 100% of the capillaries in active skeletal muscle are open.

Three mechanisms regulate blood flow to the tissues:

1) Individual tissues can control flow based on metabolic need.

2) The nervous system manipulates blood flow by adjusting the mean blood pressure and shunting the blood from one area of the body to another.

3) Hormonal communications influence the mean blood pressure and the chemical release by tissues that affect blood flow characteristics.

Blood flow is generally proportionate to the metabolic needs of the tissue. Therefore, organs that are not needed during exercise, such as those of the digestive tract, have their blood redirected to active skeletal muscle tissue or metabolic organs. Blood flow to skeletal muscles increases by 15-20 fold. To accommodate the increase in blood needed by the cell, the blood vessels react to vasodilators released into circulation in response to exercise. Lactic acid, carbon dioxide, and potassium ions are key dilators, as their presence signals to the body that there is increased metabolic turnover and greater demand for oxygen in the active tissues. The nervous system interprets the metabolic messages and signals the less metabolically active tissues to vasoconstrict, resulting in shunting and redirection of blood flow. Initially, blood flow to the skin is reduced, but as the body heats up, nervous signals redirect blood flow back to the skin to release the heat created from metabolic activities.

The heart must work harder to accommodate the demand of blood by the tissues. Sympathetic nervous system stimulation of the heart increases the heart rate and stroke volume resulting in greater cardiac output and increased blood pressure by approximately 20-60 mmHg. At the same time,

~Quick Insight~

A natural tendency when lifting or exerting high force is to hold your breath. This action, referred to as the valsalva maneuver increases intra-abdominal pressure, allowing the diaphragm to forcefully contract against the viscera to support the spine. The process of holding your breath during resistance training dramatically increases blood pressure. Exercisers should be conscious to exhale during concentric contractions and inhale during eccentric contractions to reduce the blood pressure response during exercise.

veins constrict to increase the flow of blood back to the heart for gaseous turnover in the lungs. Recall that the pressure response in the vessels is a factor of cardiac output and peripheral resistance; thus the harder the body works, the more the pressure in the vessels will increase. During activities of a rhythmic nature, such as running, swimming, or biking, the blood flow back to the heart is constant and consistent. Venous return is efficiently managed by vasoconstriction through coordinated smooth muscle action. Because the forces being produced are relatively low, and breathing rates are consistent with heart rate, diastolic pressure remains low. Mean systolic blood pressure, like ventilation rates, increases linearly with oxygen consumption due to increases in cardiac output. When assessing exercise blood pressure during aerobic steady-state work, personal trainers should expect to see a rise in systolic

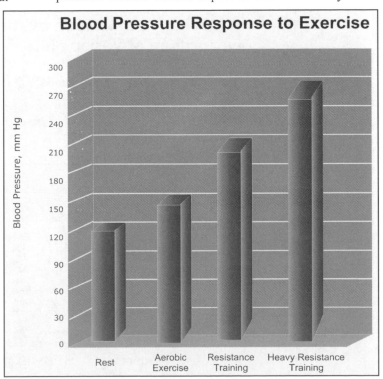

Blood Pressure Response to Exercise

blood pressure consistent with the work rate, but only a slight change in diastolic blood pressure compared to rest.

When activities require greater intra-abdominal pressure for spinal stability and the contracting muscles mechanically compress arteries, peripheral resistance increases. Both diastolic and systolic blood pressure will increase linearly with the intensity of the effort. The magnitude of the response is specific to the amount of muscle tissue employed and the resistive load. Blood pressure is further increased when internal compressive forces are joined by external compressive forces. Exercises such as the back squat and leg press have significant compressing forces from the external load, causing blood pressure to increase dramatically. For this reason, hypertensive clients should avoid heavy lifting exercises, particularly those which apply compression upon the body. Although factors that affect increased exercise blood pressure can work independently, they usually work together to cause an additive effect. Blood pressure factors in resistance training exercises include the **valsalva maneuver**, intra-abdominal pressure, compressive forces from muscle contractions, elevated cardiac output, and external compressive forces.

Exercise is very important for the circulatory system. Regular exercise improves blood pressure response at rest, both immediately post-exercise and as a chronic adaptation to routine aerobic training. It is presumed that alterations in the sympathetic nervous system reduce peripheral resistance, and increase renal secretion of sodium, accounting for the normal 8-11 mmHg decrease following aerobic endurance training (10). The chronic effects of resistance training do not yield the same results, but may provide slight improvement in resting measures. Measured resistance training blood pressure response has shown to decrease with regular participation.

The heightened action of the heart during physical activity, like any other muscle, increases its oxygen demand. However, the heart cannot pull oxygen from the blood in its atria or ventricles, as there are no circulatory channels from inside the chambers. The coronary blood supply leaves the aorta through the main coronary arteries and enters an extensive network of myocardial blood vessels called the **coronary circulation**. The myocardium is densely packed with capillaries and mitochondria, allowing for efficient extraction and utilization of oxygen. At rest, between 70-80% of oxygen is extracted from the 200-250 ml of coronary blood flow every minute. During activity, that value can jump 5-6 times if the activity is performed at a vigorous level (15). The demand of work must be met by proportionate increases in coronary blood flow to maintain cardiac output. As the myocardial tissue increases in metabolic function, the subsequent by-products produced stimulate vasodilation, consequently increasing the flow of blood to the tissue. To estimate the oxygen demand of the heart, systolic blood pressure is multiplied by the heart rate. The product, or myocardial oxygen demand, is called the **rate pressure product**.

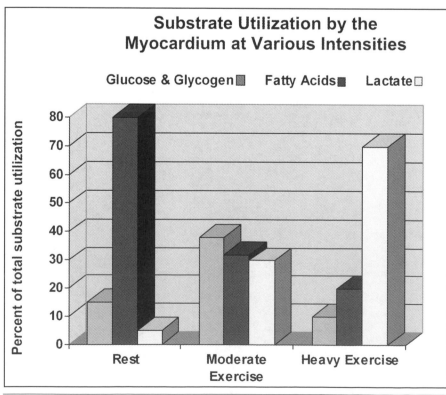

The high demand for oxygen in the heart occurs because the tissue is not efficient at using anaerobic pathways. As previously stated, cardiac muscle tissue is mitochondria dense, deriving its energy almost exclusively from aerobic metabolism. Consequently, cardiac muscle is highly adapted for ATP production using lipid metabolism. The largest majority of the ATP used in the heart during rest, like skeletal tissue, comes from lipid metabolism. During exercise of increasing intensity, energy metabolism comes from glucose, fatty acids, and lactic acid freed from skeletal muscle metabolism. Heavy exercise is mainly fueled by aerobic metabolism of lactic acid due to the heightened availability and increased power response from carbohydrate breakdown when compared to fats. When the exercise is performed using a prolonged steady-state pace, the heart tissue increases lipid metabolism to spare carbohydrates. Trained and untrained individuals are comparable in myocardial metabolic pathways when the work is hard and carbohydrates are used as fuel. When the work is moderate, trained individuals show a greater reliance on myocardial lipid metabolism when compared to their untrained counterparts. Again, the differences reflect carbohydrate sparing in trained individuals.

Ventilation

The increased myocardial vigor is met by increased ventilation rates needed to meet the oxygen demand during exercise. Heart rate alone does not regulate the ventilation response. If it did, breathing rates would noticeably increase when psychological nervousness was experienced or stimulants were present in the body. Physiological control of respiration is multifaceted, based upon chemical and neural mediation. At rest, pulmonary ventilation is largely controlled by factors that affect the chemical state of the blood, including temperature, arterial gas concentrations, and pH. During the onset of exercise or work, body movement stimulates the medulla of the brain through neurogenic means to rapidly increase respiration rates. This abrupt increase is then leveled and begins to more closely reflect the intensity of the exercise. Neurons in the brain and peripheral chemoreceptors in the vessels dictate ventilation rates to ensure adequate oxygen is available in the blood.

During exercise, ongoing ventilation will be controlled by chemoreceptor modulation based on concentrations of blood metabolites, temperature of the blood, and variations in gas exchange and pH. When the exercise is continuous and steady-state, the ventilation is linear to oxygen uptake. When the exercise is intense, the minute ventilation increases disproportionately to the oxygen uptake (5). A dramatic upswing in the rate of breathing corresponds with heightened lactate accumulation in the blood. When lactate threshold is exceeded, ventilation rates increase in an attempt to make more oxygen available to the tissue and to buffer the lactic acid produced by the muscle. Heavy resistance performed in short bouts causes dramatic increases in both heart and ventilation rates due to significant increases in blood lactate (8). This explains rapid post-lift respiration rates in exercises like the squat and deadlift.

Breathing adaptations do occur with training. In maximal measures, the ventilation rates correspond to increases in oxygen consumption, which makes sense due to the increase in oxygen required to meet the tissue demand. The increased turnover of oxygen to carbon dioxide triggers increased ventilation rate to remove the

CO_2 and infuse O_2 back into the blood. During submaximal work, ventilation rates reduce at the same relative intensity in trained individuals compared to the untrained. This is due to a reduced demand on ventilatory musculature and the oxygen not used because of an improved efficiency of exercise breathing that can be used by other tissues.

Trained individuals expire about 3% less oxygen compared to untrained individuals at the same relative intensity. Therefore more oxygen is being used and less respiration is required in trained exercisers compared to the untrained. An improved rate of oxygen extraction from the blood by working tissues occurs in response to endurance adaptations, accounting for the differences between trained and untrained individuals.

~Key Terms~

Valsalva maneuver- A strain against a closed airway combined with muscle tightening, such as when a person holds his or her breath and tries to move a heavy object.

Coronary circulation- Consists of the blood vessels that supply blood to, and remove blood from, the heart muscle itself.

Rate pressure product- The measure of myocardial oxygen consumption.

Chapter Six References

1. **Arbeille PP, Besnard SS, Kerbeci PP and Mohty DM.** Portal vein cross-sectional area and flow and orthostatic tolerance: a 90-day bed rest study. *J Appl Physiol* 99: 1853-1857, 2005.

2. **Bakke EF, Hisdal J, Kroese AJ, Jorgensen JJ and Stranden E.** Blood pressure response to isometric exercise in patients with peripheral atherosclerotic disease. *Clin Physiol Funct Imaging* 27: 109-115, 2007.

3. **Belin dC, Pascaud L, Custaud MA, Capri A, Louisy F, Ferretti G, Gharib C and Arbeille P.** Calf venous volume during stand-test after a 90-day bed-rest study with or without exercise countermeasure. *J Physiol* 561: 611-622, 2004.

4. **Fagard RH and Cornelissen VA.** Effect of exercise on blood pressure control in hypertensive patients. *Eur J Cardiovasc Prev Rehabil* 14: 12-17, 2007.

5. **Haouzi P, Chenuel B and Chalon B.** Control of breathing and muscle perfusion in humans. *Exp Physiol* 86: 759-768, 2001.

6. **Hartil K and Charron MJ.** Genetic modification of the heart: transgenic modification of cardiac lipid and carbohydrate utilization. *J Mol Cell Cardiol* 39: 581-593, 2005.

7. **Huang YC, O'brien SR, Vredenburgh J, Folz RJ and Macintyre NR.** Intrabreath analysis of carbon monoxide uptake during exercise in patients at risk for lung injury. *Respir Med* 100: 1226-1233, 2006.

8. **Kato T, Tsukanaka A, Harada T, Kosaka M and Matsui N.** Effect of hypercapnia on changes in blood pH, plasma lactate and ammonia due to exercise. *Eur J Appl Physiol* 95: 400-408, 2005.

9. **Lopaschuk GD.** Targets for modulation of fatty acid oxidation in the heart. *Curr Opin Investig Drugs* 5: 290-294, 2004.

10. **McDonald AM, Liao YL, Trevisan M, Dyer A, Gosch FC, Stamler R and Stamler J.** Sodium-lithium countertransport and systolic blood pressure response to exercise. *J Hypertens* 8: 129-137, 1990.

11. **Mozes VG.** [Therapeutic exercise in a complex of conservative therapy of the small pelvis varicosity in women of the reproductive age]. *Vopr Kurortol Fizioter Lech Fiz Kult* 24, 2005.

12. **Nagashima J, Musha H, Takada H and Murayama M.** Left ventricular chamber size predicts the race time of Japanese participants in a 100 km ultramarathon. *Br J Sports Med* 40: 331-333, 2006.

13. **Pascarella L and Schmid Schonbein GW.** Causes of telengiectasias, reticular veins, and varicose veins. *Semin Vasc Surg* 18: 2-4, 2005.

14. **Raj SR.** The Postural Tachycardia Syndrome (POTS): Pathophysiology, Diagnosis & Management. *Indian Pacing Electrophysiol J* 6: 84-99, 2006.

15. **Rigo F, Gherardi S, Galderisi M and Cortigiani L.** Coronary flow reserve evaluation in stress-echocardiography laboratory. *J Cardiovasc Med (Hagerstown)* 7: 472-479, 2006.

16. **Shibao C, Gamboa A, Diedrich A, Ertl AC, Chen KY, Byrne DW, Farley G, Paranjape SY, Davis SN and Biaggioni I.** Autonomic contribution to blood pressure and metabolism in obesity. *Hypertension* 49: 27-33, 2007.

17. **Silverman ME, Grove D and Upshaw CB, Jr.** Why does the heart beat? The discovery of the electrical system of the heart. *Circulation* 113: 2775-2781, 2006.

18. **Spirito P, Pelliccia A, Proschan MA, Granata M, Spataro A, Bellone P, Caselli G, Biffi A, Vecchio C and Maron BJ.** Morphology of the "athlete's heart" assessed by echocardiography in 947 elite athletes representing 27 sports. *Am J Cardiol* 74: 802-806, 1994.

19. **Winker R, Barth A, Bidmon D, Ponocny I, Weber M, Mayr O, Robertson D, Diedrich A, Maier R, Pilger A, Haber P and Rudiger HW.** Endurance exercise training in orthostatic intolerance: a randomized, controlled trial. *Hypertension* 45: 391-398, 2005.

20. **Wray DW, Donato AJ, Nishiyama SK and Richardson RS.** Acute sympathetic vasoconstriction at rest and during dynamic exercise in cyclists and sedentary humans. *J Appl Physiol* 102: 704-712, 2007.

Chapter 7

Nutrition: Energy Yielding Nutrients

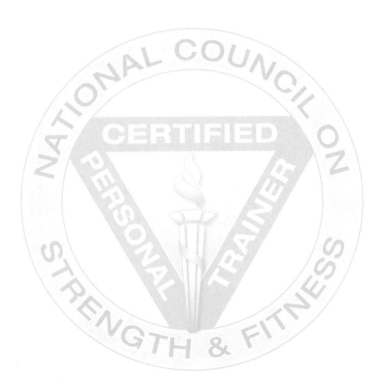

Introduction

An optimal diet is one that supplies the necessary nutrients in adequate amounts to maintain, repair, and grow tissue without providing excess energy that the body stores in the form of adipose tissue. Human nutritional needs are relative to individual genetic predisposition; affected by normal variations in nutrient digestion, absorption, and assimilation; needed to meet specific requirements for energy expenditure of physical activity; and influenced by individual dietary practices and preferences.

These four factors indicate that there is no single, universal diet for optimal nutrition (26; 36; 50; 51). However, careful evaluation of food consumption, coupled with food intake planning in accordance with sound nutritional guidelines, will result in general and specific improvements in overall health, fitness, and performance.

Nutrients are divided into six classes and two subcategories. Carbohydrates (CHO), proteins, and lipids are individually classed and categorized as energy-yielding nutrients. The non-energy-yielding category includes the other three classes of nutrients: vitamins, minerals, and water. Each plays a vital role in the proper function of the human body in response to varying physiological conditions. This chapter will review the energy yielding nutrients.

Energy Yielding Nutrients

Energy yielding nutrients are those nutrients that provide the body tissues with usable energy to form ATP. All of the energy-yielding nutrients contain the chemical element carbon. The carbon atoms are bound together into varying carbon chain skeletons. Carbon chains become linked with atoms of other elements to form lipids, carbohydrates, and proteins. When consumed, the process of digestion breaks food down to its most basic energy form. In the small intestine, the nutrients are absorbed into the blood and transported to tissues to perform their respective jobs throughout the body.

Once the energy is in the blood stream, chemoreceptors identify the nutrients and determine a specific course of action for the energy. The body has the ability to manipulate the energy to meet any particular demand or to store the energy for later use. The metabolic organs determine the outcome of the energy consumed in the diet via hormonal regulation. The liver is the primary metabolic organ that can manipulate the energy form based on the acute internal needs of the body. If needed, the liver can convert proteins

into carbohydrates, or proteins and carbohydrates into fat by arranging the carbon chains and elements to reflect the desired energy substrate. The rearrangement of carbons by the body is an important function, as it supports the ability of the body to reformulate nutrients that are needed but may not be present in necessary quantities. This process allows for energy needs to be met during work and energy to be stored when not currently needed by the body.

Carbohydrates

Although all nutrients are necessary for the body to function properly, carbohydrates are the most important nutrient related to physical activity. They represent the primary fuel source for intense work and are necessary for the formation of ATP used by the central nervous system, making the nutrient an indispensable part of a healthy diet. Carbohydrates fall into three general categories: **monosaccharides, disaccharides,** and **polysaccharides**. Monosaccharides are the most basic form of carbohydrate. They represent a single sugar moiety. Different monosaccharides vary from each other based on their carbon-to-hydrogen-to-oxygen linkage sequences.

These differences in sequence determine a carbohydrate's biochemical characteristics. For example, glucose and galactose are monosaccharides with the same number of carbon, hydrogen, and oxygen atoms, but they are arranged differently, thus making them behave and taste slightly different from each other. Disaccharides, as their name implies, are formed by the joining of two separate sugar molecules (monsaccharides). Lactose is a disaccharide formed by the combination of a glucose molecule with galactose. Both mono- and disaccharides are referred to as simple sugars because they require little manipulation by the cell for use as energy   Finally, polysaccharides are chains of monosaccharides linked together in sequences from as few as three sugars, to as many as several thousand. As the chains of monosaccharides sugars increase in length and diversity, the complexity of the nutrient increases. Polysaccharides are more commonly referred to as **complex carbohydrates** and have chain linkages of tens to thousands of monosaccharide

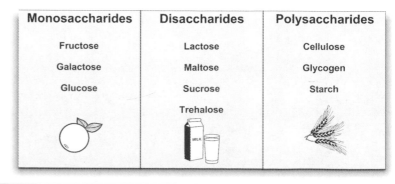

Monosaccharides	Disaccharides	Polysaccharides
Fructose	Lactose	Cellulose
Galactose	Maltose	Glycogen
Glucose	Sucrose	Starch
	Trehalose	

~Key Terms~

Monosaccharides- The simplest form of carbohydrates, comprised of one saccharide molecule.

Disaccharides- A simple form of carbohydrate, comprised of two monosaccharides.

Polysaccharides- A form of carbohydrate, consisting of a number of monosaccharides.

Complex Carbohydrates- Sugar molecules that are strung together in long, complex chains.

Glycogen- The main storage carbohydrate found primarily in the liver and muscles.

residues. These complex chains are classified as either plant or animal polysaccharides depending on their dietary source.

Glycogen and starch are two common forms of polysaccharides in our diets. **Glycogen** is the storage form of carbohydrates in animal tissue, while **starch** is the term used for the storage form of carbohydrates in plants. Starch is the larger component in seeds, corn, potatoes, beans and the various grains that make up common foods like spaghetti, bread, and cereals. Plant starch remains the most important source of carbohydrates for most Americans, accounting for more than 50% of the total carbohydrates consumed. This number has decreased by 30% since the turn of the century, when starches comprised about 80% of carbohydrate sources. This significant decline has been met by an equally significant increase in simple sugar consumption.

Fiber

Fiber is a non-starch polysaccharide, and in the form of cellulose, is the most abundant organic molecule found on earth. It is a tough material that resists enzymatic breakdown, making it indigestible by humans, except for a small portion that is fermented by intestinal bacteria. Fiber is commonly categorized as either **soluble** or **insoluble**. The bacterial breakdown of fiber generally contributes less than 2 kcal per gram, making it an excellent addition to calorie-controlled diets. Its consumption is linked with lower occurrences of several "Western" diseases including obesity, diabetes, hypertension, intestinal disorders, some cancers, and heart disease (1; 19; 55; 61). Due to the fact that most Americans consume far less (12-15g) than the recommended 20-35 grams, the Western diet predisposes consumers to an elevated disease risk (65).

In less industrialized nations, the fiber content of the average diet is between 40-100g per day (17). Not surprisingly, the rate of related diseases is dramatically lower in those countries than in America. Fiber enhances gastrointestinal function and reduces irritation to the intestine wall, mobilizes harmful chemicals and compounds inhibiting their activity, shortens the time for intestinal transport to excretion, decreases the length of time carcinogenic materials stay in the intestines, and slows down the absorption rate of carbohydrates, acting positively on blood glucose dynamics. Additionally, the foods associated with a high fiber diet often support health by being lower in calories and more nutrient-rich (6; 7). For this reason, fiber should be consumed through food sources rather than as a supplement (66). Sample foods high in fiber are whole grain products, fruits, and leafy green vegetables.

Due to the fact that carbohydrates serve as the primary fuel source for physical activity, it makes sense that they represent the largest portion of energy from the diet. The recommended dietary intake for carbohydrates is 55%-60% of the total diet, with the majority being derived from polysaccharide (complex) sources. However, the average American consumes only about 40-50% of their total diet from carbohydrate sources with 50% of those calories being derived from mono- and disaccharides (simple sugars). It has been

Foods High in Fiber

Oat Bran
Whole Wheat Flour
Wheat Germ
Rice Bran
Oatmeal
Almonds
Pumpkin Seeds
Peanuts
Pinto Beans
Lima Beans
Avocado
Pear
Figs
Strawberries
Corn on the Cob
Bran Muffin
Spaghetti, Whole Wheat
Grapefruit
Apple
Chestnuts
Broccoli, Raw
Green Beans
All Bran Cereal

Hidden Calories

One 12 oz. can of soda per day

39 grams of sugar per can x 365 days in a year = 14,235 grams of sugar

14,235 grams sugar = 32 lbs of sugar

estimated that at least 25% of the American diet is simple sugar, a trend that significantly contributes to the increased risk for obesity, diabetes, and heart disease. Most people consume more than 100 lbs. of sugar annually, mainly in the form of sucrose and high fructose corn syrup (23).

Sugars

Sugars fall into the categories of monosaccharides and disaccharides. **Glucose, fructose** and **galactose** are all monosaccharides. They are similar in chemical formula but differ by specific carbon, hydrogen, and oxygen linkage. Glucose is the main monosaccharide used by the body. It can be split for ATP, stored for later use as glycogen, or converted into lipid form following its absorption into the cells. Fructose is nature's fruit sugar. It is the sweetest of the sugars per gram. When ingested, it is converted into glucose by the liver. Galactose is an animal monosaccharide found in dairy products.

The disaccharides include **lactose, maltose, sucrose,** and **trehalose**. Sucrose is the most commonly consumed sugar form, representing up to 25% of some American diets (24). It is commonly consumed in baked products or in the form of table sugar. Lactose is formed from glucose and galactose. It is often referred to as dairy sugar. Many people around the world are lactose intolerant, lacking sufficient enzymes to break the disaccharide down in the body. When two glucose molecules are combined, they form maltose, which is present in cereals, germinating seeds, and beer.

Glycemic Response

When sugars enter the blood, they raise the blood glucose levels. The specific response is based on the amount and type of sugar consumed. The elevation in blood glucose concentrations is quantified using a measurement system called **glycemic indexing**. The glycemic index describes the effect carbohydrate sources have on circulating blood glucose levels by rate and concentration. The rate at which the food increases blood glucose is called the **glycemic response**. The amount of glucose in the blood is referred to as the **glycemic load**.

In low fiber diets, manufacturer processed starches and simple sugars are digested quickly and enter the blood stream at a rapid rate. This causes the release and often over-release of insulin, which heightens hyperinsulinemia (a state of high insulin release by the pancreas) (4; 9; 12; 18). Consistently eating high glycemic foods may lead to reduced insulin sensitivity (3; 6; 7; 9). This reduced insulin sensitivity causes the pancreas to release higher amounts of insulin in response to the blood sugar; this response in

conjunction with obesity is linked to the development of Type II diabetes.

As mentioned earlier, a concern with high amounts of insulin is that abnormally high levels facilitate the conversion of sugar into triglycerides in the liver, which are then stored as fat in adipose tissue. Diets high in sugar are directly linked to an increased risk for obesity. Contrary to this, foods high in dietary fiber and protein slow the absorption rate of the sugars and minimize surges of blood glucose. A reduction in blood sugar causes a decrease in the concentration of insulin secreted into the blood. Additionally, when fat is combined with simple carbohydrates, the glycemic effect is reduced, compared to the effects of the independent sugar source (29; 59). Regular exercise also exerts a notable positive influence on the body's sensitivity to insulin making regular physical activity a key component in the prevention and management of diabetes.

The following glycemic index table identifies foods according to their specific insulin responses. The glycemic value in the table is determined after ingesting 50 grams of a carbohydrate source and comparing the resultant blood sugar levels over a two-hour period to a standard for carbohydrates, usually white bread or glucose, which has an assigned value of 100. The corresponding value expresses the relationship or percentage of total area under the curve set by the reference standard. If white bread represents 100% of the curve, then a food encompassing 45% of the total area would be assigned a glycemic index value of 45. International values for glycemic index do exist, but slight discrepancies arise when comparing specific trials due to variations in the foods used.

~Quick Insight~

Monosaccharides can be broken down to form derivatives which can be used by the body. Sugar acids, sugar alcohols, and amino sugars are formed when monosaccharides are metabolized. Amino sugars and sugar acids are present in connective tissue and assist in supporting the tissue's metabolic needs. Sugar alcohols have become a popular additive to supplements and foods to provide flavor with a decreased energy value. Glycerol and sorbitol, among others, are used in energy bars and foods that attempt to provide reduced sugar content and glycemic effect in the diet (2). They are often not counted under the total carbohydrates measured on the labels of food or they are advertised on the label as "non-impact carbs" for carbohydrate-conscious consumers. They generally provide 1-3 calories and have much less of an effect on blood glucose dynamics (52).

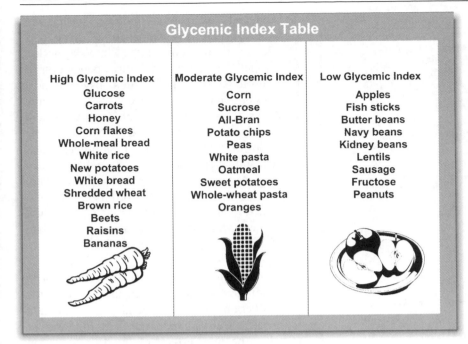

Glycemic Index Table

High Glycemic Index	Moderate Glycemic Index	Low Glycemic Index
Glucose	Corn	Apples
Carrots	Sucrose	Fish sticks
Honey	All-Bran	Butter beans
Corn flakes	Potato chips	Navy beans
Whole-meal bread	Peas	Kidney beans
White rice	White pasta	Lentils
New potatoes	Oatmeal	Sausage
White bread	Sweet potatoes	Fructose
Shredded wheat	Whole-wheat pasta	Peanuts
Brown rice	Oranges	
Beets		
Raisins		
Bananas		

Processed Carbohydrates

The manufacturing process manipulates the biological integrity of some foods and consequently will often affect the glycemic response. For instance, whole grains are processed to create a more desirable consistency, as seen with white flour. The reduction in biochemical complexity increases the glycemic index of the food from its original form. Essentially, the complex chains are broken down to reflect a more simplified food source. The end product from grain processing produces a carbohydrate that is more rapidly digestible and

absorbed into the blood at a faster rate, which can quickly elevate blood glucose levels. This may be good for post-exercise consumption, but for the average, inactive person, this translates to excessive circulating blood sugars, leading to increased fat storage.

Ideally, the body attempts to keep blood sugar concentrations at a constant level throughout the day without dipping too low, which can cause fatigue, or going too high, such as with hyperglycemia. However, most Americans have large fluctuations in their blood glucose levels within a 24-hour period. When plotted on a line graph it looks somewhat erratic, with many peaks and valleys. After meals, especially those high in simple sugars, a quick rise in blood glucose concentration occurs, which is often referred to as "spiking." These large fluctuations occur because most Americans consume the majority of their calories in two to four sittings. The body's blood glucose response from three or four large meals exceeds the stable regulatory functions because the glycemic load is so high. As mentioned earlier, the pancreas releases insulin during periods of high blood sugar to increase glucose uptake by cells. Glucagon is released during low levels of blood sugar, causing the liver to release glucose into the blood stream so that it is constantly available to cells that do not store glycogen,

~Quick Insight~

Certain sugars, such as sucrose and high fructose corn syrup, can wreak havoc on blood glucose stability. These saccharides are collectively identified as dietary troublemakers. Naturally occurring fructose is touted as dietetic, or a more desirable sugar, because of its sweetness and reduced glycemic index (see below), particularly when consumed from non-juiced, whole fruit sources. But unlike naturally occurring fructose, the commercially formulated high-fructose corn syrup is quickly absorbed and causes a rapid rise in the body's blood glucose concentration. Research trials identified increased serum cholesterol and low-density lipoprotein (LDL) concentrations in the blood when 20% of the dietary calories came from this monosaccharide.

It is estimated that the largest part of the American population routinely exceeds 20% of total dietary calories from sucrose and high fructose corn syrup. The high consumption of sugars disrupts normal metabolic pathways due to the response of insulin in attempts to prevent hyperglycemia. The hormones that control the level of circulating blood sugar are regulated by beta- and alpha-cells in the pancreas. Elevated blood glucose causes the pancreas to release insulin in proportion to the rate and quantity of sugar absorption. Insulin facilitates an uptake of the circulating blood sugar into skeletal muscle and the liver, where it is stored as glycogen.

When high amounts of simple sugars are consumed on a regular basis, the body works hard to remove the glucose from the blood. Once glycogen stores are filled, the body may metabolize the sugar as fuel or convert it in the liver into triglycerides. Triglycerides are then stored as fat in adipose cells. Insulin is lipogenic, meaning it increases fat storage. Consistently elevating blood glucose and the consequent release of insulin causes an increased susceptibility to fat gain. This phenomenon is considered a major contributor to weight gain in America.

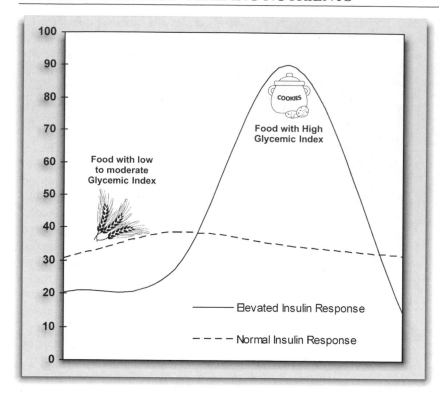

relieved and blood glucose levels are appropriately re-established. If hunger is deferred, it soon turns into **appetite**. Appetite is the psychological perception of caloric need. The brain's psychological discernment of need exceeds the physiological requirements for food and predisposes an individual to over consume calories. Anyone who has ordered and consumed appetizers before the main course at a restaurant probably realized they were not as hungry as they originally thought when the main dish arrived. Avoiding appetite-related eating patterns is important for preventing overeating habits (8).

When carbohydrate selections are made intelligently, they can effectively aid in the reduction of body weight and improve health. Carbohydrates account for most of the **thermic effect of food**, which can represent up to 10% of daily caloric expenditure. As previously stated, complex carbohydrates are nutrient dense and provide dietary fiber, which reduces the risk of digestive disorders, and can be low in calories when

such as the brain. Eating patterns that cause the body to work in constantly fluctuating blood glucose level conditions cause higher concentration release of pancreatic hormones. These conditions manifest themselves in poor utilization of energy nutrients and cause changes in the cellular use of glucose. For the ideal blood glucose situation to occur, we need to take in smaller quantities of food at roughly 90-120 minute intervals, reflecting a grazing style of eating. This suggests the average meal size should be lower in calories to maintain optimal blood glucose levels (20; 62; 67). Grazing animals such as deer follow this eating pattern and maintain low levels of body fat and do not develop type II diabetes, in part because their foods are high in fiber and low in calories, but it is also because regular intake normalizes blood glucose (30). Although 7-9 meals may be unrealistic, many nutritionists recommend eating small meals more frequently throughout the day to mirror the grazing pattern of eating to avoid large spikes in blood glucose levels.

A second benefit to increasing the consumption frequency of carbohydrates and consuming calories in smaller portions is to thwart hunger. When chemical receptors in the tissues identify reduced levels of blood glucose, the hypothalamus stimulates the physiologically controlled **hunger mechanism** to communicate the need for food. When this occurs, the required calorie intake to meet the current need is often low, equal to maybe a couple hundred calories. If food is consumed at this time, the hunger mechanism is

~Key Terms~

Starch- A complex carbohydrate found in seeds, fruits, and stems of plants and more notably, in corn, rice, potatoes, and wheat.

Fiber- Indigestible plant matter, consisting primarily of polysaccharides that when consumed increase water absorption and intestinal peristalsis.

Soluble Fiber Sources- Oats/oat bran, dried beans, nuts, barley, and vegetables such as carrots.

Insoluble Fiber Sources- Dark green/leafy vegetables, fruit skins, corn bran, and seeds.

Glucose- A simple sugar (monosaccharide) used as the primary fuel source by most cells in the body to generate energy.

Fructose- A sweet sugar (monosaccharide) found primarily in fruits.

Galactose- A simple sugar (monosaccharide) found in dairy products.

Lactose-A disaccharide in dairy products that hydrolyzes to yield glucose and galactose.

Maltose- A white sugar formed during the digestion of starch.

consumed from appropriate sources. Likewise, phytochemicals and other compounds found in whole grains can reduce the risk of certain diseases, such as cancer and cardiovascular disease (31; 48). Compliance with the suggested guidelines for carbohydrate consumption seems to be one of the problems with the American diet. Due to the fact that the majority of calories in the average diet come from processed carbohydrates and sugars, the added health benefits from the foods are minimal, and the thermic effect of most diets is low. Authors of diet books have recognized this pattern and recommend reducing carbohydrates to decrease the effects of sugar and processed carbohydrates for weight control. Carbohydrate selection can play a major role in weight management and disease risk when intelligently applied.

The current trend toward cutting carbohydrates should refer to reducing simple sugar and processed carbohydrate consumption, not cutting complex carbohydrates from the diet. The problem lies in the dissemination of information to the general public. In many cases, the popularized low-carbohydrate diets cause weight loss for all the wrong reasons. Cutting carbohydrates reduces the stored glycogen in the body and is often not appropriately replaced. Due to the fact that glucose bonds with water molecules when forming glycogen in the cell, reducing glycogen stores within the body also reduces the body's water content. The body will significantly diminish its carbohydrate stores in about 96 hours under an extended fast, which can account for significant metabolic water loss (21; 54). This mechanism accounts for most of the initial weight loss in low carbohydrate diets. Whereas calorie control and exercise have been touted as the only way to effectively lose weight and keep it off, most low carbohydrate dieters gain the weight back soon after finishing the diet. In fact, attempting to lose weight by diet alone usually is only successful for approximately 2-5% of the population (13; 33). Most dieters gain the weight back within 6-9 months. Additionally, low carbohydrate diets are contrary to the metabolic functions of the body for activity. When glycogen stores are low, so is work capacity. In general, low carbohydrate diets should not be recommended for physically active people. It should be noted that controlling sugar and processed carbohydrates is not the same as a low carbohydrate diet.

~Key Terms~

> **Sucrose**- A disaccharide found in many plants and used as a sweetener, which is more commonly known as table sugar.
>
> **Trehalose**- A sweet tasting disaccharide.
>
> **Glycemic Indexing**- A rating system for evaluating how different foods affect blood sugar levels.
>
> **Glycemic Response**- A measure of the increase of blood sugar after food consumption.
>
> **Glycemic Load**- A ranking system for carbohydrate content in food portions based on their glycemic index and portion size.
>
> **Hunger Mechanism**- A physiological response to hunger controlled by chemical receptors being stimulated by the hypothalamus in response to reducing levels of blood glucose.
>
> **Appetite**- An instinctive physical desire or caloric need.
>
> **Thermic Effect of Food**- The increment in energy expenditure above resting metabolic rate due to the cost of processing food for storage and use.
>
> **Protein-Sparing Mechanism**- The body's preferential utilization of fats and carbohydrates instead of protein for energy.

Carbohydrate Depletion

Carbohydrate availability affects more than energy output alone; it also affects metabolic biochemistry. When carbohydrate consumption is reduced by poor eating habits, high protein diets, reduced energy intake, starvation, or fasting, the body reacts to compensate for the deficit. Reduced glycogen reserves and low plasma glucose concentration trigger glucose synthesis through a process called gluconeogenesis in the liver and, to a lesser extent, in the kidneys. Amino acids and triglyceride molecules are rearranged to form sugar to fuel the body's need. The gluconeogenic conversion breaks down both lean mass and fat mass to augment carbohydrate availability. Normally the body has a natural **protein-sparing mechanism,** maintained by an adequate consumption of carbohydrates and fat. Preferably, the body does not want to use protein for fuel. Even if adequate protein is consumed to meet functional requirements, protein-sparing may not occur because it is regulated by neural and hormonal assessment of carbohydrate stability. Without protein-sparing, amino acids are liberated from lean mass, primarily skeletal muscle, and reformulated into carbohydrates in the liver for energy. Prolonged effects of lean mass catabolism can lower the body's total metabolic rate. This problem is exacerbated by the fact that the body relies on carbohydrates as the primer for fat metabolism. As mentioned earlier, with the by-products of carbohydrate breakdown being reduced,

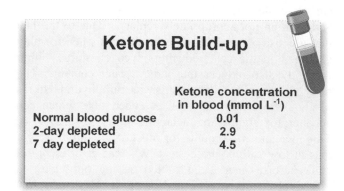

Ketone Build-up

	Ketone concentration in blood (mmol L^{-1})
Normal blood glucose	0.01
2-day depleted	2.9
7 day depleted	4.5

there is an increased fat mobilization and decreased capacity for fat oxidation. Under this state of insufficient carbohydrate metabolism, more fat is mobilized than can be oxidized. This produces an incomplete breakdown of the fat and the build up of acetone byproducts referred to earlier as ketone bodies. For this reason, low carbohydrate diets are also referred to as ketogenic diets. Only consumption of adequate amounts of carbohydrates will prevent this phenomenon from occurring.

Carbohydrate consumption proves to be of further significance due to the fact that the brain and central nervous system require carbohydrates for proper function. Under normal conditions, the brain uses blood glucose almost exclusively for fuel. When the body is deprived of carbohydrates, gluconeogenesis is used to maintain blood glucose concentrations for nerve tissue metabolism and as a fuel for red blood cells. In a low carbohydrate environment, blood glucose can drop to hypoglycemic levels. In extreme situations, this condition can lead to central fatigue and may trigger unconsciousness, and even irreversible brain damage.

Carbohydrate Need
Earlier text indicated that carbohydrates are stored in the liver and muscle tissue in the form of glycogen. When consuming a normal diet, the storage capacity for glycogen is between approximately 300 to 400 grams or 1200-1600 kcal of energy, of which about 80% is stored in the skeletal muscles. When exercise is performed, carbohydrates serve to fuel both high- and moderate-intensity exercise anaerobically, and contribute to a substantial amount

of energy in higher-intensity aerobic training. Energy derived from the breakdown of absorbed glucose, and glycogen stored in the muscles and liver, powers the protein contractile elements during muscle contractions and additionally required biological work. When exercise is intense or prolonged, glycogen stores are rapidly depleted. For physically active people, carbohydrate intake should mirror the training volume on a daily or weekly basis. Low carbohydrate consumption can lead to premature depletion of glycogen, causing the storage volume to become too low to support activity. The following graph illustrates the varying fuel source contribution to glycogen storage and its role in prolonging steady-state exercise.

After analyzing the relationship between energy metabolism and available carbohydrates, it should be obvious that the consumption of carbohydrates is relative to specific need but has a definite lower limit. The exact quantity consumed depends on the amount and type of physical activity an individual engages in on a regular basis. If a person is sedentary, carbohydrate consumption may be as low as 45% of the total diet because the level of activity they routinely engage in is equally low. For individuals who exercise regularly, carbohydrates should comprise roughly 55-60% of the total diet (27; 38; 43). It is recommended that the majority of carbohydrates come from complex sources

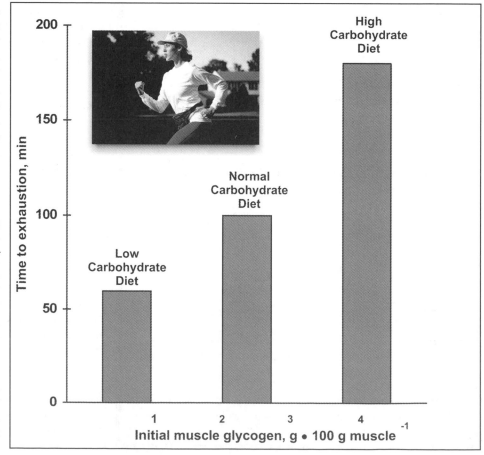

Method One

The following example demonstrates the amount of carbohydrates needed for a 35 year old 5' 5" male, weighing 75 kg, who participates in regular, moderate exercise most days of the week.

Daily Caloric Intake Requirement   2744 kcal

Recommended CHO Intake   60%

Step 1   2744 x 60% = 1646 kcal CHO

Step 2   1646 kcal CHO ÷ 4 kcal/g = 412 g

Step 3   412 g ÷ 75 kg body weight = 5.5 g   CHO per kg of body weight

Method Two

The following example demonstrates the amount of carbohydrates needed for a 35 year old 5' 5" male, weighing 75 kg, who participates in regular, moderate exercise most days of the week.

Daily Caloric Intake Requirement: 2744 kcal

Recommended CHO Intake: 60%

Population	Carbohydrate Requirements
Sedentary Individual	3-4 g/kg of body weight (BW)
Physically Active	4-5 g/kg of BW
Moderate Exercise	5-6 g/kg of BW
Vigorous Exercise	6-8 g/kg of BW

Body weight in kilograms x selected activity status

Step 1   75 kg x 5.5 g = 412 g

Step 2   412 g x 4 kcal = 1648 kcal CHO

Two ways exist to estimate the grams of carbohydrates necessary for daily intake needs. One method is to calculate the value using a predicted daily need and subjective percentage rate. The other method is to use recommended grams per kilogram of body weight, based on estimations of activity status. Based on the prediction outcomes, the two are similar in predictability when calculated correctly.

This number will vary as relative carbohydrate needs change based on current activity status. If training volume and intensity are increased or decreased, the CHO intake should reflect the shifts in training.

Fats

Fats, also known as dietary lipids, are the other primary source of energy the body uses to fuel biological work. Lipid molecules have the same structural elements as carbohydrate molecules (carbon, oxygen and hydrogen), but differ in the way the atoms are linked. This marked difference determines the way lipids are metabolized and stored in the body. Like carbohydrates, lipids differ in chain length and molecular complexity, which places them in three distinct categories: **simple lipids**, **compound lipids**, and **derived lipids**. The following table identifies the specific characteristics related to each category.

Lipids are necessary for normal function of the body. Most people view fat as a negative constituent of the diet because of the perceived link to obesity. But this is unwarranted, as fat actually serves many important functions in the body.

The aforementioned roles that fat plays in the body identify the importance of adequate consumption in the diet. Problems with fat in the diet occur when more fat

with no more than 10% derived from simple sugar. Total carbohydrate intake recommendation jumps to 70% for individuals who engage in regular intense training (3; 56). The idea behind "carb-loading," which is the intake of high amounts of carbohydrates prior to a race, is to optimize glycogen reserves, much like topping off the fuel tank of a car before a trip (22; 34; 57). Frequently, however, athletes overeat the amount of carbohydrates required, with the excess amount being stored as fat (58). Additionally, diets that over emphasize protein often fail to meet the carbohydrate needs of most physically active individuals.

Lipid Function

- Providing energy to the body
- Transporting molecules in the blood
- Storing nutrients, including vitamins
- Serving as conduction canals in the nervous system
- Forming hormones
- Protecting organs
- Serving in temperature regulation
- Communicating energy needs
- Forming cell membranes

is consumed than is required. Fat is high in calories and therefore, accounts for a good part of the over consumption predicament experienced by many Americans. At 9 kcal per gram, the energy in fat is more than twice that of carbohydrates and protein, a characteristic that can contribute significantly to a positive caloric balance. Additional problems occur because fats are more easily stored as adipose tissue throughout the body than their carbohydrate and protein counterparts. Unlike carbohydrates, where stores are limited and oxidation occurs rapidly, fat storage goes relatively unregulated because the human body has an almost unlimited ability to store lipids. Additionally, biological mechanisms promote fat storage in situations where high amounts of calories are consumed.

In the average American diet, lipids represent approximately 35% of total caloric intake (64). About 34% of the dietary fats consumed come from non-animal sources while the majority, 66%, comes from animal sources. Dietary fat is classified as either unsaturated or saturated fatty acids. **Monounsaturated** and **polyunsaturated fatty acids** are commonly found in plant sources of fat. Animal sources of fat often contain higher amounts of **saturated fats**. It is generally recommended that 30% of a individual's diet be derived from fat sources, with less than 7-10% from saturated fat (40). On average, approximately 15% of total calories are consumed as saturated fatty acids by Americans everyday (39). This is very relevant, as a relationship exists between fat intake, specifically saturated fat, and coronary heart disease (16). Diets high in saturated fats lead to a pronounced change in the blood lipid profile, particularly in **LDL cholesterol**, whereas a diet higher in **monounsaturated fats** has been linked with lower coronary heart disease risk (37; 63).

Unsaturated and saturated fats differ by the structural bonds and respective carbon element make-up. Saturated fatty acids do not have double bonds between the carbons, which maximizes the hydrogen attachment sites (making them saturated with hydrogen). Monounsaturated fatty acids have a single double bond within the carbon chain, and polyunsaturated fatty acids have multiple double bonds, thereby reducing the number of hydrogen attachments. Additionally, the location of the double bond plays a role in the dynamics of the fatty acid. For instance, when the first double bond is next to the sixth carbon, the fatty acid is an omega-6, and when the first double bond is next to the third carbon it is referred to as an omega-3 fatty acid. The amount of hydrogen and double bond number and site all play a role in how the fatty acid reacts in the body. The following illustration demonstrates the chemical differences between saturated and unsaturated fats. Notice the differences in the bonds and hydrogen concentration.

When fatty acids are consumed in the diet, they enter in varying proportion based on the type and quantity of foods consumed. Fatty acids enter circulation through the intestine and are picked up by lipoproteins called **chylomicrons**. The lipids are transported to the liver where they are metabolized, attached to **very low density lipoproteins (VLDL)**, and delivered to fat

~Key Terms~

Simple Lipids- Oils or fats containing one or two different types of compounds.

Compound Lipids- Phospholipids and glycol-lipids, which frequently contain three or more chemical identities.

Derived Lipids- Includes sterols and fatty acids.

Monounsaturated Fatty Acids- Any of a large group of monobasic acids found in animal and vegetable fats and oils.

Polyunsaturated Fatty Acids- An unsaturated fatty acid with a carbon chain containing more than one double or triple valence bond per molecule.

Saturated Fats- A fat, most often of animal origin, that is solid at room temperature, which contains chains of saturated fatty acids.

LDL Cholesterol- A complex of lipids and proteins that functions as a transporter of cholesterol in blood, which, at high levels, is associated with an increased risk of atherosclerosis and coronary heart disease (CHD).

Monounsaturated Fats- Fatty acids with one double bonded carbon in the molecule.

cells to be stored or utilized as fuel in the form of triglycerides. The VLDL gives up the transported lipids and is turned into a **low density lipoprotein (LDL)**. The density of the lipoprotein refers to the protein to fat ratio. VLDLs are 95% fat. LDL cholesterol circulates in the blood en route back to the liver where it can form bile. LDL is considered to be hazardous cholesterol because it is so small it can collect on the lining of damaged arteries. This affinity for the cells of the arterial wall increases risk of oxidation and the proliferation of smooth muscle cells, thereby adding to plaque in the artery, known as atherosclerosis (see Chapter 12). **High density lipoprotein (HDL)** has a protective role, inhibiting arterial plaque formation, making HDL the more desirable cholesterol in circulation.

Cholesterol is produced in the body, but it is also found in food products. The body produces about 70% of its approximately 1000 mg need per day. The remaining 300 mg comes from dietary sources (35; 71). Cholesterol is needed to perform complex bodily functions, including the formation of plasma membranes and hormones. It also works in digestive functions, forming bile and serves as a precursor for vitamin D. Although an important lipid in the body, it can also be problematic if consumed in abundance in the diet. For this reason the American Heart Association recommends consuming no more than 300 mg per day (35). For individuals at higher risk for heart disease, that recommendation drops to between 150 and 200 mg. Dietary cholesterol is common in animal products that contain higher amounts of fat. One egg yolk, for instance, contains the full daily amount of cholesterol. Likewise, red meat, shell fish, and dietary liver are also high in cholesterol.

Trans Fatty Acids

Identifying which fats to consume has become increasingly difficult due to the manipulation of fats in processed food. Saturated fats are solid at room temperature, whereas unsaturated fats are liquid. Scientists working on ways to improve upon the dynamics of fatty acids when manufacturing food products created a specialized fat that takes advantage of the desirable chemical components of both saturated and unsaturated fats. **Trans fatty acids** have become an ever-present component in many manufactured food

Monounsaturated	Polyunsaturated	Saturated
Avocados Canola oil Olive oil Peanut oil and other nuts	Safflower oil Sunflower oil Corn oil Cottonseed oil Soybeans Fish	Whole milk Cream Ice cream Cheeses Butter Lard Palm oil Palm kernel Coconut oil Cocoa butter Red meats

compounds. The molecular manipulation, called **hydrogenation**, occurs when one hydrogen atom of the cis-monounsaturated fatty acid is moved from its naturally occurring position to the opposite side of the double bond that separates two carbon atoms. In doing so, food manufacturers create more desirable texture consistencies for foods like margarine, cookies, and ice cream. Consequently, this change in the molecular structure changes the way the lipids act in the body. Trans fatty acids have a profound effect on serum lipoproteins and can have possible adverse health affects by increasing LDL cholesterol and triglycerides, while at the same time reducing HDL cholesterol (45-47). Trans fatty acids do not occur in nature, and their intake may have other unknown detrimental effects. The CDC estimates that trans fatty acids account for at least 30,000 deaths annually from heart disease. In 2006, the American Heart Association recommended that 0% of the diet come from trans fat sources (68).

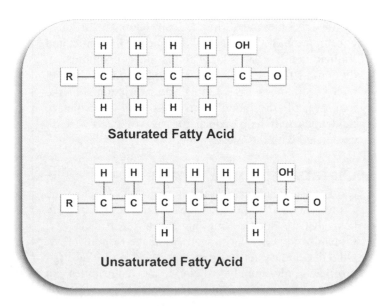

Saturated Fatty Acid

Unsaturated Fatty Acid

Not all lipids have detrimental effects for coronary artery disease. Studies performed on Eskimos have shown a low incidence of coronary heart disease associated with the omega-3 fatty acids found in the high quantities of fish they consume. Polyunsaturated fatty acids may benefit the blood lipid profile by reducing triglycerides and reducing risk for heart disease (15; 25; 69; 70). Theoretically, the cold water fish oils reduce the formation of clots on the arterial wall in conjunction with decreasing plasma triglycerides levels. Monounsaturated fats have also been implicated as a healthier fat choice. Mediterranean diets are often high in monounsaturated fat, such as found in olive oil, representing sometimes more than 50% of the dietary fat consumed. Even though the average person in Greece consumes at least 40% of their diet from fat, they experience a much lower incidence of heart disease (14; 42). It is important to note that the Mediterranean diet is low in animal products and high in vegetables, fruits, olives, and legumes. Scientists are not clear whether the Mediterranean diet itself is the cause or if the elevated amounts of monounsaturated fat is an independent variable. Most conclude it is the totality of the dietary consumption which is important.

Even with the beneficial effects some fats have on reducing coronary risk factors, these fats still need to be consumed in moderation. Dietary fats can be converted to adipose tissue very efficiently when the diet is too rich in lipid consumption (5; 49). Fat intakes that exceed 30% of the total diet increase the risk for developing many diseases, even if the diet is within recommended caloric intake for the individual. To the contrary, cutting fats out of the diet is not a prudent decision either. Diets that drop dietary fat below 20% of the recommended intake can cause insufficient consumption of the **essential** fatty acids, **linolenic,** and **linoleic acids** (28; 41). This is not uncommon in dieting, as most people prefer to reduce fat in the diet over practicing a balanced calorie restriction. For the majority of the population, following the dietary guidelines will help reduce the risk of heart disease associated with the Western diet.

Dietary Fat and Disease

Cardiovascular disease is the number one killer in the United States. Although other factors contribute to heart disease, such as smoking and physical inactivity, fat tends to claim a large segment of the responsibility. Directly, dietary fat has a strong effect on blood lipid profiles. Additionally, dietary fat contributes to increases in fat mass and risk for obesity, which is

---

Determining Fat Intake

Daily caloric need x recommended percentage of fat in the diet = Calories of fat in diet

Calories of fat in diet ÷ 9 cal per gram = Grams of fat in the diet

Grams of fat in the diet ÷ Kilograms of body weight = Grams of fat per kg of bodyweight

Example
220 lb   Male
2744   Calorie per day diet
30%   Recommended calories from fat

2744 cal x 30% = 823 calories of fat in diet

823 ÷ 9 cal per gram = 91 Grams of fat in the diet

91 ÷ 100 Kilogram of body weight = .91 Grams of fat per kg bodyweight

---

linked to both heart and metabolic diseases. A high amount of saturated fat in the diet increases blood cholesterol dramatically, which can lead to coronary artery disease. This is further compounded by an excessive consumption of dietary fat, trans fatty acids, and cholesterol. When high amounts of fat are consumed on a regular basis, body fat is often increased, and the risk for disease is further elevated. For this reason, the recommendation is to consume less than 30% of total calories from fat. Categorizing the fat intake is a useful step that can further serve dietary improvement.

The American Heart Association suggests a ratio of fatty acids of 10:10:10. A healthier split of 30% dietary fat intake may be 15% monounsaturated, 10% polyunsaturated, and 5% or less from saturated sources (11; 53). This recommendation alone would drastically reduce the risk of coronary artery disease in many people.

~Quick Insight~

When excess fat accumulates in the body, the risk for cardiovascular disease dramatically increases. For this reason, manufacturers produce fat-replacers, which serve as tasty substitutes for the higher calorie lipids. These replacers have actually caused more problems in the American diet than they have solved. People seem to confuse fat-free foods with calorie-free foods and consume larger volumes of the food product than they would if real fat was an ingredient. This leads to excessive caloric intake and a positive caloric balance. Although the percentage of fat in the diet has declined from just over 40% in the early eighties to approximately 36% today, the total amount of fat has increased because many diets are higher in calories. Additionally, higher sugar intake is common because sugar is used to improve the taste lost from the removal of the fat, further contributing to the problem. In most cases, moderation of fat and non-fat products will help reduce the chances of over eating calories.

Lipid Characteristics & Examples

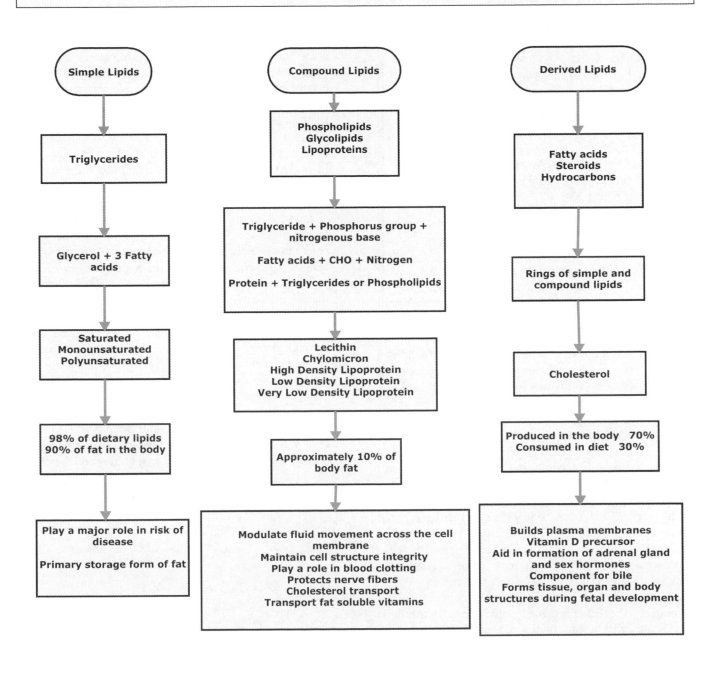

Simple Lipids	Compound Lipids	Derived Lipids
Triglycerides	Phospholipids Glycolipids Lipoproteins	Fatty acids Steroids Hydrocarbons
Glycerol + 3 Fatty acids	Triglyceride + Phosphorus group + nitrogenous base Fatty acids + CHO + Nitrogen Protein + Triglycerides or Phospholipids	Rings of simple and compound lipids
Saturated Monounsaturated Polyunsaturated	Lecithin Chylomicron High Density Lipoprotein Low Density Lipoprotein Very Low Density Lipoprotein	Cholesterol
98% of dietary lipids 90% of fat in the body	Approximately 10% of body fat	Produced in the body 70% Consumed in diet 30%
Play a major role in risk of disease Primary storage form of fat	Modulate fluid movement across the cell membrane Maintain cell structure integrity Play a role in blood clotting Protects nerve fibers Cholesterol transport Transport fat soluble vitamins	Builds plasma membranes Vitamin D precursor Aid in formation of adrenal gland and sex hormones Component for bile Forms tissue, organ and body structures during fetal development

~Key Terms~

Chylomicrons- One of the microscopic particles of fat occurring in chyle and in the blood, especially after a meal high in fat.

Very Low Density Lipoproteins (VLDL)- A lipoprotein containing a very large portion of lipids which carry most of the cholesterol from the liver to the tissues.

Trans Fatty Acids- An unsaturated fatty acid produced by the partial hydrogenation of vegetables oils.

Hydrogenation- The act of combining with hydrogen

Essential Fatty Acids- Any of the polyunsaturated fatty acids which are required in the diet of mammals.

Linolenic Acids- An Omega-3 unsaturated fatty acid considered essential to the human diet.

Linoleic Acid- An Omega-6 unsaturated fatty acid, considered essential to the human diet.

Protein

Proteins serve thousands of functions within the human body, representing the primary structural components of non-bone tissues. Proteins are made up of building blocks called **amino acids**. In the same way many monosaccharides are chained together to form a complex carbohydrate, multiple amino acids are also linked together in a chain to form a protein. Amino acids are substances composed of carbon, hydrogen, and oxygen, much like the other two energy nutrients, but amino acids also have nitrogen added to form an amine group (NH_2) and side chains which give each amino acid a unique identity. Proteins are comprised of different amino acid sequences, making up approximately 50,000 different protein-containing compounds in the body. The order and number of the amino acids in a protein give the protein its unique properties. There are not many physiological reactions that occur within the body that do not require the presence of a protein at some point during the process.

As mentioned above, biochemical function and the properties of each protein differ by how the amino acids are structurally arranged. Twenty (20) different amino acids are currently recognized, each differing from the side chains that attach to the amine group and associated carbon skeleton. The side chains dictate the

particular characteristics of the molecule and the role they will serve in the body. The body can combine elements to create amino acids and combine the amino acids to form an almost infinite number of proteins. As is clear from the following picture, amino acids are carbon chains with different linkage options, which ultimately determine the type of amino acid and their specific characteristics.

The body can synthesize almost all of the 20 different amino acids from other amino acids. However, there are eight amino acids that the body cannot synthesize. These are labeled **essential amino acids** and must be consumed through the diet. They are isoleucine, leucine, lysine, methionine, phenylalanine, threonine, tryptophan, and valine. Infants and children have additional essential amino acid needs because infants cannot synthesize histidine, and children have been identified to have a reduced capacity to form arginine, lysine, histidine and cysteine (32). The source of the amino acid does not matter, so the proteins can be consumed as animal or plant foods. A protein termed **complete** is considered to be higher quality because it contains all eight essential amino acids in appropriate quantity and correct ratio to maintain nitrogen balance, whereas an **incomplete protein** lacks one or more of the essential amino acids.

Animal sources generally receive the highest rating among dietary proteins. For the average American, animal proteins account for up to 70% of the total dietary protein consumed (60). This is an increase of 20% from the early 1900's. One problem associated with the increased intake of animal proteins is that they are often accompanied by higher amounts of saturated fats and cholesterol. Plant proteins, although often incomplete, can supply all the essential proteins when

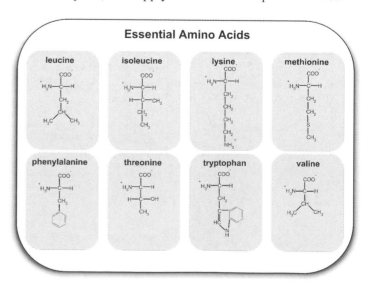

Essential Amino Acids

leucine   isoleucine   lysine   methionine

phenylalanine   threonine   tryptophan   valine

consumed through a variety of sources and often contain fiber and other beneficial nutrients. This suggests that vegetarians can get adequate protein from the foods they consume, as long as their diets maintain a variety of plant food sources that together provide the eight essential amino acids. Dietary recommendations established by the Food and Nutrition Board of the National Research Council and National Academy of Science reflect the nutritional needs of the total population, not an individual's specific requirements. The recommendation of 0.8-0.9 grams per kilogram of bodyweight meets the protein requirements for most individuals. Those who are physically active may require increased intake. For most active people, the increased need for protein is already met by the higher caloric intakes associated with extra calories consumed to meet the heightened energy needs. Individuals who engage in high volume resistance programs or participate in endurance training programs often need more protein to meet the tissue re-synthesis requirements associated with recurring microtrauma, or in the case of the endurance athlete, protein lost to energy metabolism.

Protein Intake Guidelines

Population	Protein Intake
Sedentary Individual	0.8 g-0.9g/kg of body weight (BW)
Physically Active	1.0 - 1.2 g/kg of BW
Endurance Athlete	1.3 - 1.5 g/kg of BW
Bodybuilding & Strength Training	1.6 - 2.0 g/kg of BW
Children	up to 2 g/kg of BW
Pregnant Female	Add 20g to total daily requirements Add 10g if nursing

The chart above identifies recommended intake options for different activities and physiological demands.

It should be noted that protein consumption beyond 1.6 grams per kilogram of body weight has been associated with increased risk of elevated saturated fat in the diet due to higher amounts of animal foods consumed and renal and liver distress due to excessive nitrogen in certain individuals.

Individual requirements are based on the frequency, duration, and intensity of exercise. High intensity endurance and resistance training activities increase protein requirements significantly, compared to sedentary and low level physical activity participation. To calculate the estimated protein requirements of an individual use the formula on the next page and the previous protein intake chart.

Protein intakes above 2.0 g/kg of bodyweight often cause increased renal stress due to the high quantities of nitrogen (10; 44). Protein consumption that exceeds requirements for anabolic processes can force the body into additional work to deal with the overflow. Protein is degradated into amino acids during digestion. Deamination occurs in the liver where the amino acid loses its nitrogen group to form urea. When protein is needed in the body, the deaminated amino acids formulate into new amino acids. Excessive protein intakes can cause the deaminated amino acid to formulate carbohydrates or fat, depending on the physiological environment. When protein is over-consumed, the kidneys and liver must process the excess, and therefore, become stressed from additional biochemical reactions. Furthermore, the kidneys require more water to create urine when the solute concentration of urea is high. This can lead to increased fluid loss and dehydration. Excessive protein consumed over an extended period of time can be detrimental to the body.

~Quick Insight~

Most people consume two times the protein they need for the day. If Americans complied with the recommended 10-15% of total calories coming from protein they would likely find their nutritional needs would be met. The American diet relies heavily on protein as a staple to most meals, making the diet rich in nitrogen. For most exercisers, additional protein is not warranted based on their current consumption level and relative intensity of the activities they regularly complete. Many new exercisers want to buy protein supplements to encourage muscle gain. Increasing protein alone will add no new benefits and is likely to contribute to weight gain from a positive caloric balance. Likewise, increasing protein intake requires an equal increase in water consumption to manage excess nitrogen. If protein supplements are deemed necessary to meet training demands, many experts recommend whey protein as a first choice.

A 175 lb. male with 15% body fat, training four days a week and using moderate resistance training would have a recommended protein intake of approximately 110 grams and a total calorie requirement of 2912 kcal per day. His protein needs can easily be met by consuming 15% of his calories from protein.

3000 calorie diet x 10-15% = 300-450 kcal or 75-113 grams

Determining Protein Needs

Body weight in lbs ÷ 2.2 lbs per kg = Kilograms of body weight

Kilograms of body weight x desired grams of protein per kilogram = Daily protein requirement in grams

Daily protein requirement in grams x 4 kcals per gram = Total protein calorie requirement

Example

220 lb Male
Population: Physically Active

220 lbs ÷ 2.2 lbs per kg = 100 kg

100 kg x 1.1 grams per kg = 110 grams of protein

110 grams of protein x 4 kcal per gram = 440 kcals of protein

Recommended DRI

10% - 15% Protein
≤ 30% Fat
55% - 60 % Carbohydrates

When manipulating protein intake for weight gain or weight loss some key recommendations should be followed. As described earlier, a high protein diet does not increase rate of weight loss, compared to balanced diets of similar calorie content. Most early weight loss is due to dehydration from the loss of water. Protein diets do offer some fat loss, but again, the weight reduction is due to calorie control, not the specific energy involved. To ensure adequate protein is consumed during dietary restriction, protein should be consumed at approximately 15% of the total calories.

If weight gain is intended, the additional calories can come from protein sources. In general, adding 30-50 grams (120-200 kcal) of protein is recommended as long as the total amount reflects a value less than 2.0 grams per kilogram of body weight. Additional calories beyond a positive caloric balance of 200 kcal per day may lead to fat gain in many individuals by the conversion of excess proteins into carbohydrates and fat. If protein supplements are consumed, the appropriate time is post-exercise. Cellular use of protein is heightened as is cellular uptake of carbohydrates in the presence of insulin.

~Key Terms~

Essential Amino Acids- Eight of the 20 amino acids that the body cannot synthesize that must be consumed in a diet.

Complete Protein- A food source that contains adequate amounts of the essential amino acids.

Incomplete Proteins- A food source that does not contain adequate amounts of the essential amino acids.

~Quick Insight~

Nitrogen balance occurs when the amount of nitrogen in the protein consumed equals the nitrogen excreted by the body. When nitrogen balance is positive, the amount of nitrogen intake exceeds the amount of nitrogen excreted. Positive nitrogen balance occurs when the tissues utilize the largest amount of protein for anabolic processes, such as growth, maintenance and repair. This is commonly seen during the stages of developmental growth, pregnancy, illness and with resistance-trained individuals through protein synthesis. When the nitrogen balance becomes negative, the output of nitrogen exceeds the intake, and protein is utilized as an energy source. Inadequate consumption of carbohydrates and fats can lead to negative nitrogen balance, even in the presence of adequate protein intake. Low carbohydrate diets, inadequate nutrition, or excessive exercise have all been implicated in negative nitrogen balance and consequential loss of lean mass proteins.

CHAPTER SEVEN REFERENCES

1. High fiber intake may reduce progression of coronary artery disease. *Mayo Clin Womens Healthsource* 10: 3, 2006.

2. **Aaltonen AS, Suhonen JT, Tenovuo J and Inkila-Saari I.** Efficacy of a slow-release device containing fluoride, xylitol and sorbitol in preventing infant caries. *Acta Odontol Scand* 58: 285-292, 2000.

3. **Applegate EA.** Nutritional considerations for ultraendurance performance. *Int J Sport Nutr* 1: 118-126, 1991.

4. **Aston LM.** Glycaemic index and metabolic disease risk. *Proc Nutr Soc* 65: 125-134, 2006.

5. **Barnea M, Shamay A,** Stark AH and Madar Z. A high-fat diet has a tissue-specific effect on adiponectin and related enzyme expression. *Obesity (Silver Spring)* 14: 2145-2153, 2006.

6. **Bazzano LA, Serdula MK and Liu S.** Dietary intake of fruits and vegetables and risk of cardiovascular disease. *Curr Atheroscler Rep* 5: 492-499, 2003.

7. **Bazzano LA, Song Y, Bubes V, Good CK, Manson JE and Liu S.** Dietary intake of whole and refined grain breakfast cereals and weight gain in men. *Obes Res* 13: 1952-1960, 2005.

8. **Berthoud HR.** Homeostatic and non-homeostatic pathways involved in the control of food intake and energy balance. *Obesity (Silver Spring)* 14 Suppl 5: 197S-200S, 2006.

9. **Black RN, Spence M, McMahon RO, Cuskelly GJ, Ennis CN, McCance DR, Young IS, Bell PM and Hunter SJ.** Effect of eucaloric high- and low-sucrose diets with identical macronutrient profile on insulin resistance and vascular risk: a randomized controlled trial. *Diabetes* 55: 3566-3572, 2006.

10. **Brouhard BH.** The role of dietary protein in progressive renal disease. *Am J Dis Child* 140: 630-637, 1986.

11. **Buse JB, Ginsberg HN, Bakris GL, Clark NG, Costa F, Eckel R, Fonseca V, Gerstein HC, Grundy S, Nesto RW, Pignone MP, Plutzky J, Porte D, Redberg R, Stitzel KF and Stone NJ.** Primary prevention of cardiovascular diseases in people with diabetes mellitus: a scientific statement from the American Heart Association and the American Diabetes Association. *Circulation* 115: 114-126, 2007.

12. **Buyken AE and Liese AD.** Dietary glycemic index, glycemic load, fiber, simple sugars, and insulin resistance: the Inter99 Study: response to Lau et al. *Diabetes Care* 28: 2986-2987, 2005.

13. **Christiansen T, Bruun JM, Madsen EL and Richelsen B.** Weight loss maintenance in severely obese adults after an intensive lifestyle intervention: 2- to 4-year follow-up. *Obesity (Silver Spring)* 15: 413-420, 2007.

14. **de Lorgeril M and Salen P.** The Mediterranean diet in secondary prevention of coronary heart disease. *Clin Invest Med* 29: 154-158, 2006.

15. **DeFilippis AP and Sperling LS.** Understanding omega-3's. *Am Heart J* 151: 564-570, 2006.

16. **Denke MA.** Dietary fats, fatty acids, and their effects on lipoproteins. *Curr Atheroscler Rep* 8: 466-471, 2006.

17. **Eaton SB.** The ancestral human diet: what was it and should it be a paradigm for contemporary nutrition? *Proc Nutr Soc* 65: 1-6, 2006.

18. **Elliott SS, Keim NL, Stern JS, Teff K and Havel PJ.** Fructose, weight gain, and the insulin resistance syndrome. *Am J Clin Nutr* 76: 911-922, 2002.

19. **Erkkila AT and Lichtenstein AH.** Fiber and cardiovascular disease risk: how strong is the evidence? *J Cardiovasc Nurs* 21: 3-8, 2006.

20. **Farshchi HR, Taylor MA and Macdonald IA.** Regular meal frequency creates more appropriate insulin sensitivity and lipid profiles compared with irregular meal frequency in healthy lean women. *Eur J Clin Nutr* 58: 1071-1077, 2004.

21. **Fery F, Plat L and Balasse EO.** Mechanisms of whole-body glycogen deposition after oral glucose in normal subjects. Influence of the nutritional status. *J Clin Endocrinol Metab* 83: 2810-2816, 1998.

22. **Forgac MT.** Carbohydrate loading--a review. *J Am Diet Assoc* 75: 42-45, 1979.

23. **Gaby AR.** Adverse effects of dietary fructose. *Altern Med Rev* 10: 294-306, 2005.

24. **Gaby AR.** Adverse effects of dietary fructose. *Altern Med Rev* 10: 294-306, 2005.

25. **Galli C and Marangoni F.** N-3 fatty acids in the Mediterranean diet. *Prostaglandins Leukot Essent Fatty Acids* 75: 129-133, 2006.

26. **Gibney MJ.** Optimal macronutrient balance. *Proc Nutr Soc* 58: 421-425, 1999.

27. **Gonzalez-Gross M, Gutierrez A, Mesa JL, Ruiz-Ruiz J and Castillo MJ.** [Nutrition in the sport practice: adaptation of the food guide pyramid to the characteristics of athletes diet]. *Arch Latinoam Nutr* 51: 321-331, 2001.

28. **Hamilton C, Austin T and Seidner DL.** Essential fatty acid deficiency in human adults during parenteral nutrition. *Nutr Clin Pract* 21: 387-394, 2006.

29. **Hare-Bruun H, Flint A and Heitmann BL.** Glycemic index and glycemic load in relation to changes in body weight, body fat distribution, and body composition in adult Danes. *Am J Clin Nutr* 84: 871-879, 2006.

30. **Hoffman RM, Kronfeld DS, Cooper WL and Harris PA.** Glucose clearance in grazing mares is affected by diet, pregnancy, and lactation. *J Anim Sci* 81: 1764-1771, 2003.

31. **Hu FB.** Plant-based foods and prevention of cardiovascular disease: an overview. *Am J Clin Nutr* 78: 544S-551S, 2003.

32. **Imura K and Okada A.** Amino acid metabolism in pediatric patients. *Nutrition* 14: 143-148, 1998.

33. **Jehn ML, Patt MR, Appel LJ and Miller ER, III.** One year follow-up of overweight and obese hypertensive adults following intensive lifestyle therapy. *J Hum Nutr Diet* 19: 349-354, 2006.

34. **Juhn MS.** Ergogenic aids in aerobic activity. *Curr Sports Med Rep* 1: 233-238, 2002.

35. **Katsilambros N, Liatis S and Makrilakis K.** Critical review of the international guidelines: what is agreed upon--what is not? *Nestle Nutr Workshop Ser Clin Perform Programme* 11: 207-218, 2006.

36. **Knowler WC.** Optimal diet for glycemia and lipids. *Nestle Nutr Workshop Ser Clin Perform Programme* 11: 97-102, 2006.

37. **Kratz M.** Dietary cholesterol, atherosclerosis and coronary heart disease. *Handb Exp Pharmacol* 195-213, 2005.

38. **Lambert CP, Frank LL and Evans WJ.** Macronutrient considerations for the sport of bodybuilding. *Sports Med* 34: 317-327, 2004.

39. **Lichtenstein AH, Appel LJ, Brands M, Carnethon M, Daniels S, Franch HA, Franklin B, Kris-Etherton P, Harris WS, Howard B, Karanja N, Lefevre M, Rudel L, Sacks F, Van Horn L, Winston M and Wylie-Rosett J.** Diet and lifestyle recommendations revision 2006: a scientific statement from the American Heart Association Nutrition Committee. *Circulation* 114: 82-96, 2006.

40. **Lichtenstein AH, Appel LJ, Brands M, Carnethon M, Daniels S, Franch HA, Franklin B, Kris-Etherton P, Harris WS, Howard B, Karanja N, Lefevre M, Rudel L, Sacks F, Van Horn L, Winston M and Wylie-Rosett J.** Diet and lifestyle recommendations revision 2006: a scientific statement from the American Heart Association Nutrition Committee. *Circulation* 114: 82-96, 2006.

41. **Ling PR, Ollero M, Khaodhiar L, McCowen K, Keane-Ellison M, Thibault A, Tawa N and Bistrian BR.** Disturbances in essential fatty acid metabolism in patients receiving long-term home parenteral nutrition. *Dig Dis Sci* 47: 1679-1685, 2002.

42. **Mackenbach JP.** The Mediterranean diet story illustrates that "why" questions are as important as "how" questions in disease explanation. *J Clin Epidemiol* 60: 105-109, 2007.

43. **Manore MM.** Exercise and the Institute of Medicine recommendations for nutrition. *Curr Sports Med Rep* 4: 193-198, 2005.

44. **Martin WF, Armstrong LE and Rodriguez NR.** Dietary protein intake and renal function. *Nutr Metab (Lond)* 2: 25, 2005.

45. **Matthan NR, Welty FK, Barrett PH, Harausz C, Dolnikowski GG, Parks JS, Eckel RH, Schaefer EJ and Lichtenstein AH.** Dietary hydrogenated fat increases high-density lipoprotein apoA-I catabolism and decreases low-density lipoprotein apoB-100

catabolism in hypercholesterolemic women. *Arterioscler Thromb Vasc Biol* 24: 1092-1097, 2004.

46. **Matthan NR, Welty FK, Barrett PH, Harausz C, Dolnikowski GG, Parks JS, Eckel RH, Schaefer EJ and Lichtenstein AH.** Dietary hydrogenated fat increases high-density lipoprotein apoA-I catabolism and decreases low-density lipoprotein apoB-100 catabolism in hypercholesterolemic women. *Arterioscler Thromb Vasc Biol* 24: 1092-1097, 2004.

47. **Mauger JF, Lichtenstein AH, Ausman LM, Jalbert SM, Jauhiainen M, Ehnholm C and Lamarche B.** Effect of different forms of dietary hydrogenated fats on LDL particle size. *Am J Clin Nutr* 78: 370-375, 2003.

48. **McCullough ML and Giovannucci EL.** Diet and cancer prevention. *Oncogene* 23: 6349-6364, 2004.

49. **Milagro FI, Campion J and Martinez JA.** Weight gain induced by high-fat feeding involves increased liver oxidative stress. *Obesity (Silver Spring)* 14: 1118-1123, 2006.

50. **Millward DJ.** Optimal intakes of protein in the human diet. *Proc Nutr Soc* 58: 403-413, 1999.

51. **Prentice A, Schoenmakers I, Ann LM, de Bono S, Ginty F and Goldberg GR.** Nutrition and bone growth and development. *Proc Nutr Soc* 65: 348-360, 2006.

52. **Robertson MD, Bickerton AS, Dennis AL, Vidal H and Frayn KN.** Insulin-sensitizing effects of dietary resistant starch and effects on skeletal muscle and adipose tissue metabolism. *Am J Clin Nutr* 82: 559-567, 2005.

53. **Rosamond W, Flegal K, Friday G, Furie K, Go A, Greenlund K, Haase N, Ho M, Howard V, Kissela B, Kittner S, Lloyd-Jones D, McDermott M, Meigs J, Moy C, Nichol G, O'Donnell CJ, Roger V, Rumsfeld J, Sorlie P, Steinberger J, Thom T, Wasserthiel-Smoller S and Hong Y.** Heart disease and stroke statistics--2007 update: a report from the American Heart Association Statistics Committee and Stroke Statistics Subcommittee. *Circulation* 115: e69-171, 2007.

54. **Ryan T, Coughlan G, McGing P and Phelan D.** Ketosis, a complication of theophylline toxicity. *J Intern Med* 226: 277-278, 1989.

55. **Saito YA, Locke GR, III, Weaver AL, Zinsmeister AR and Talley NJ.** Diet and functional gastrointestinal disorders: a population-based case-control study. *Am J Gastroenterol* 100: 2743-2748, 2005.

56. **Serfass RC.** Nutrition for the athlete. *N Y State J Med* 78: 1824-1825, 1978.

57. **Sharman IM.** Glycogen loading: advantages but possible disadvantages. *Br J Sports Med* 15: 64-67, 1981.

58. **Sharman IM.** Glycogen loading: advantages but possible disadvantages. *Br J Sports Med* 15: 64-67, 1981.

59. **Shikany JM, Thomas SE, Henson CS, Redden DT and Heimburger DC.** Glycemic index and glycemic load of popular weight-loss diets. *MedGenMed* 8: 22, 2006.

60. **St Jeor ST, Howard BV, Prewitt TE, Bovee V, Bazzarre T and Eckel RH.** Dietary protein and weight reduction: a statement for healthcare professionals from the Nutrition Committee of the Council on Nutrition, Physical Activity, and Metabolism of the American Heart Association. *Circulation* 104: 1869-1874, 2001.

61. **Suter PM.** Carbohydrates and dietary fiber. *Handb Exp Pharmacol* 231-261, 2005.

62. **Terpstra J, Hessel LW, Seepers J and van Gent CM.** The influence of meal frequency on diurnal lipid, glucose and cortisol levels in normal subjects. *Eur J Clin Invest* 8: 61-66, 1978.

63. **Thijssen MA and Mensink RP.** Fatty acids and atherosclerotic risk. *Handb Exp Pharmacol* 165-194, 2005.

64. **Thompson FE, Midthune D, Subar AF, McNeel T, Berrigan D and Kipnis V.** Dietary intake estimates in the National Health Interview Survey, 2000: methodology, results, and interpretation. *J Am Diet Assoc* 105: 352-363, 2005.

65. **Thompson FE, Midthune D, Subar AF, McNeel T, Berrigan D and Kipnis V.** Dietary intake estimates in the National Health Interview Survey, 2000: methodology, results, and interpretation. *J Am Diet Assoc* 105: 352-363, 2005.

66. **Trepel F.** [Dietary fibre: more than a matter of dietetics. I. Compounds, properties, physiological effects]. *Wien Klin Wochenschr* 116: 465-476, 2004.

67. **Westerterp-Plantenga MS, Kovacs EM and Melanson KJ.** Habitual meal frequency and energy intake regulation in partially temporally isolated men. *Int J Obes Relat Metab Disord* 26: 102-110, 2002.

68. **Woodside JV and Kromhout D.** Fatty acids and CHD. *Proc Nutr Soc* 64: 554-564, 2005.

69. **Zadak Z, Hyspler R, Ticha A, Solichova D, Blaha V and Melichar B.** Polyunsaturated fatty acids, phytosterols and cholesterol metabolism in the Mediterranean diet. *Acta Medica (Hradec Kralove)* 49: 23-26, 2006.

70. **Zarraga IG and Schwarz ER.** Impact of dietary patterns and interventions on cardiovascular health. *Circulation* 114: 961-973, 2006.

71. **Zello GA.** Dietary Reference Intakes for the macronutrients and energy: considerations for physical activity. *Appl Physiol Nutr Metab* 31: 74-79, 2006.

Chapter 8

Nutrition: Non-Energy Yielding Nutrients

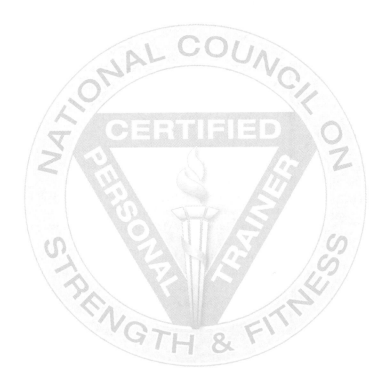

In This Chapter

Vitamins

Dietary Reference
Intakes

Minerals

Electrolytes

Water

Exercise and Fluid Loss

Acclimation

Food Guide Pyramid

Food Labels

Food Descriptors

Vitamins

Unlike carbohydrates, fats, and proteins, vitamins do not provide energy to the body. They function primarily as metabolic catalysts that release energy from food consumed and help maintain homeostasis within the body. There are currently thirteen different vitamins classified as either water-soluble or fat-soluble. **Water-soluble vitamins** regulate metabolic reactions, control the process of tissue synthesis, aid in the protection of the cell's plasma membrane and facilitate proper tissue function. **Fat-soluble vitamins** function to enhance tissue formation and integrity, prevent cell damage, and serve as constituents of certain compounds.

Vitamin requirements are generally met by the consumption of a well balanced diet. Unlike carbohydrates and protein structures, the body cannot reassemble vitamins from other chemical compounds, with the exception of vitamin D, and therefore must be consumed in the diet. Some vitamins, such as A, D, niacin, and folic acid require activation from an inactive precursor known as a pro-vitamin. A common example of a pro-vitamin is beta-carotene, the precursor for vitamin A.

Water-Soluble

Water-soluble vitamins largely act as **coenzymes**, which participate directly in chemical reactions. Because they are water-soluble, these vitamins disperse in the body's fluid without being stored in any appreciable quantity. They generally exist in the body at usable potency between 8 to 14 hours, which suggests that they should be consumed periodically throughout the day (13; 35; 88). Excess consumption is usually excreted in the urine but toxicity is possible in rare situations. When daily consumption of water-soluble vitamins falls to approximately 50% of the recommended value, deficiencies can develop in as little as four weeks time (12; 100).

Fat-Soluble

Fat-soluble vitamins are dissolved and stored in the liver and adipose tissue. Metabolic demands cause the vitamins to mobilize in lipids, allowing them to be transported to the body's tissues from the liver. Without the lipids, the vitamins do not have a transport mechanism. Excess consumption of fat-soluble vitamins can cause toxicity, particularly with vitamins A and D (63; 99). Diets that are very low in fat can accelerate deficiencies but are relatively uncommon. Although fat-soluble vitamins do not need to be consumed everyday, regular intake is useful in maintaining homeostasis.

Fat Soluble Vitamins	Water Soluble Vitamins
A K E D	C B Complex

A well-balanced diet will usually meet most individuals' requirements, regardless of age and physical activity level. For those who are highly active, a multi-vitamin may be warranted to provide any additional nutrient needs from vitamins (14; 89). This may be particularly important for individuals who do not consume enough vitamin C and folic acid. Additionally, folic acid and B_6 may provide added protection against heart disease (7; 20). They reduce high blood **homocysteine** levels that have been linked to coronary heart disease (18; 30). Other beneficial actions of certain vitamins include their role as **antioxidants**. During both aerobic and anaerobic metabolism, **free radical** formation can occur, caused by electron leakage along the electron transport chain. Under normal metabolic conditions, as much as 2-5% of oxygen used by the body forms oxygen-containing free radicals (28; 42; 79). These highly chemically reactive molecules increase the potential for cellular damage and can increase the oxidation of LDL cholesterol, accelerating the process of atherosclerosis (25; 69; 81). Free radical production is associated with cigarette smoke inhalation, environmental pollutants, and even exercise. They have been linked with oxidative stress leading to advanced aging, cancer, diabetes, heart disease and a decline in the immune system. Vitamins A, C, E, and the vitamin precursor beta-carotene can serve protective function against free radical activity, notably lowering risks of cancer and heart disease (24; 68; 80).

~Key Terms~

Water-soluble Vitamins- Consist of the B-vitamins and vitamin C and are stored in the body for a brief period of time before being excreted.

Fat-soluble Vitamins- Consist of the vitamins A, D, E and K. These vitamins are stored in fat cells.

Coenzymes- A non-protein, organic substance that usually contains a vitamin or mineral and combines with a specific protein, the apoenzyme, to form an active enzyme system.

Homocysteine- An amino acid normally used by the body in cellular metabolism and in the manufacturing of proteins. Elevated concentrations in the blood are thought to increase the risks for heart disease.

Vitamin	Adult RDA[a]		Functions	Sources	UL[o]
	Men	Women			
Thiamin(B1)	1.2 mg	1.1 mg	Part of a coenzyme used in energy metabolism, supports normal appetite and nervous system functions	Occurs in all nutritious foods in moderate amounts; pork, bacon, ham, whole grains, nuts, legumes	ND
Riboflavin(B2)	1.7 mg	1.3 mg	Part of a coenzyme used in energy metabolism, supports normal vision and skin health	Milk, yogurt, cottage cheese, meat, green leafy vegetables, and whole grains	ND
Niacin	16 mg	14 mg	Part of a coenzyme used in energy metabolism, supports health of skin, nervous system, and digestive system	Milk, eggs, meat, poultry, fish, whole-grain and enriched breads & cereals, nuts	35 mg
B6	2.0 mg	1.6 mg	Part of a coenzyme used in amino acid and fatty acid metabolism, helps convert tryptophan to niacin, helps make red blood cells	Green and leafy vegetables, meats, fish, poultry, shellfish, legumes, fruits, whole grains	100 mg
Pantothenic acid	5 mg*	5 mg*	Part of a coenzyme used in energy metabolism	Whole-grain cereals, bread, dark green vegetables	ND
Folic Acid	400 µg	400 µg	Functions as coenzyme in synthesis of nucleic acids and protein	Green vegetables, beans, whole-wheat products	1000 µg
B12	2.4 µg	2.4 µg	Part of a coenzyme used in new cell synthesis, red blood cell formation, helps maintain nerve cells	Animal products such as meat, fish, poultry, milk, cheese, eggs	ND
Biotin	30 µg	30 µg	Part of a coenzyme used in the synthesis of fatty acids and glycogen	Egg yolk, dark green vegetables	ND
C	90 mg	75 mg	Intracellular maintenance of bone, capillaries, and teeth	Citrus fruits, green peppers, tomatoes	2000 mg
A	900 µg	700 µg	Vision, skin health, bone and tooth growth, reproduction, hormone synthesis and regulation, immunity	Retinol: Fortified milk, cheese, carrots, butter, fortified margarine, eggs, liver	3000 µg
D	5 µg*	5 µg*	Mineralization of bones, calcium absorption	Fortified milk, margarine, butter, cereals, eggs	50 µg
E	15 mg	15 mg	Antioxidant, stabilization of cell membranes, regulation of oxidation reactions	Polyunsaturated plant oils, green and leafy vegetables, wheat germ, whole grain products, nuts, seeds	1000 mg
K	120 µg*	90 µg*	Synthesis in blood clotting proteins and a protein that binds calcium in the bones	Bacterial synthesis in the digestive tract, green leafy vegetables, cabbage-type vegetables, potatoes	ND

[a]Values are Recommended Daily Allowance (RDA) for adults 19 to 50 years of age, unless marked with an asterisk. The requirements may vary for children, older adults, and pregnant or lactating women. *Values are Adequate Intakes (AI), indicating that sufficient data to set the RDA are unavailable.

[o]Tolerable Upper Intake Levels (UL) for adults 19 to 50 years of age. Intakes above the UL may lead to negative health consequences. ND = not yet determined.

Adapted from Franks and Howley, 1989, and Institute of Medicine

To ensure adequate consumption of the micronutrients, the American government funds an expert committee of the Food and Nutrition Board of the National Academy of Sciences' Institute of Medicine to establish recommendations and guidelines for nutrient intake. In 1995, a Standing Committee on the Scientific Evaluation of Dietary Reference Intakes was established to review scientific research on nutrients and recommend levels that would prevent deficiency and chronic diseases, as well as estimate intake levels that may be hazardous to health. Collectively the values are called the **Dietary Reference Intakes (DRI)**.

Vitamin Overdose Effects	
Vitamin C	Increases serum uric acid and may cause gout and kidney stones
Vitamin B6	May cause liver and nerve damage
Riboflavin (B2)	May impair vision
Niacin	May cause flushing of the skin, headache, fatigue, nausea, and possible liver dysfunction
Pyridoxine	May cause skin lesions and nerve damage
Vitamin E	May cause headache, fatigue, blurred vision, gastrointestinal disorders, muscular weakness, and low blood sugar
Vitamin A	May cause hair loss, dry skin, headache, bone and muscle pain, liver damage, bone abnormalities, nervous system toxicity, and possible death
Vitamin D	May cause nausea, elevated blood pressure, kidney damage, and failure

Dietary Reference Intakes (DRI)

The DRI's encompass four categorical sets of reference values including the **Estimated Average Requirements (EAR), Recommended Daily Allowance (RDA), Adequate Intakes (AI), and the Tolerable Upper Intake Level (UL)**. Although not enough research exists to cover every nutrient in each category, significant information exists to provide values for the large majority of nutrients. The DRI's are based on the bioavailability of the nutrient, which takes into account the actual quantity absorbed by the intestines, not just the amount ingested. Essentially, the nutrient recommendations establish a range that consumers can follow to meet their individual nutritional needs. Individuals who exercise or are ill often have additional nutrient requirements above the needs of the sedentary population. Therefore, nutritional experts may assign a consumption value near the tolerable upper intake level of particular nutrients for these individuals. On the contrary, individuals who do not engage in physical activity may only need to consume the nutrient quantities reflected by the RDA. The RDAs are evidence-based estimates of what intakes are necessary to support good health and lower risk for disease.

Estimated Average Requirements (EAR) – The amount of each nutrient that meets the requirements of half of healthy people in a particular life-stage and gender group.

Recommended Daily Allowance (RDA) – The amount of each nutrient that meets the needs of 97% of healthy people in a particular life-stage and gender group. The RDAs are determined using the EARs. Therefore, if an estimated average has not been determined for a nutrient, it will not be assigned a value in the RDAs.

Adequate Intakes (AI) – The average intake of each nutrient needed to sustain health, based on studies of people in a particular life-stage and gender group. AI's are used when an RDA does not exist.

Tolerable Upper Intake Level (UL) – The upper limit of safe, daily intake for a nutrient. Exceeding the UL may lead to adverse health effects.

The concept of "more is better" often does not apply in nutrition. Due to the fact that physiological homeostasis depends upon biochemical reactions, adding more of a particular element or compound will not necessarily increase the level of the reaction. High intakes of vitamins cause increased chemical concentrations once the enzyme systems are saturated. The additional circulating compounds impact system function. In fact, adding excessive amounts of most nutrients causes adverse effects. Megadosing vitamins can cause irreversible damage even if the vitamin is water soluble (63; 101).

~Quick Insight~

Food manufacturers are conscious of the nutrients in the foods they sell. When nutrients are lost during the manufacturing process, a practice of replacing the lost nutrients to improve the food's nutritional quality called "enrichment" is utilized. In some cases, the manufacturer will add nutrients that exist in small quantities or are not present in the food at all. Fortified foods have nutrients added into the product to improve the overall nutritional value. Common examples are Vitamin D fortified milk or orange juice fortified with calcium.

~Key Terms~

Free Radicals- An unstable molecule that causes oxidative damage by stealing electrons from surrounding molecules, thereby disrupting activity in the body's cells.

Dietary Reference Intakes (DRI) - A comprehensive set of nutrient reference values for healthy populations that can be used for assessing and planning diets.

Although a daily vitamin is often recommended to ensure adequate nutritional status, when combined with other supplements and normal dietary consumption, the intake values may rise above the upper limit for safe consumption.

Minerals

Roughly 4% of total body mass is composed of minerals. These inorganic compounds are mainly metallic elements that serve as constituents of enzymes, hormones, and vitamins. **Minerals** are often incorporated into structures and chemicals in the body. Their functions include:

1. Providing components for bone and teeth.

2. Regulation of cellular metabolism, actions of the heart, muscle, and nervous system.

3. The maintenance of acid base balance.

4. Regulation of cellular fluid balance.

Minerals play an extensive role in the catabolic and anabolic processes of the cell, activating the numerous reactions necessary to release energy from the breakdown of energy-yielding nutrients. Minerals also help assist with the synthesis of the metabolic compounds, which enables the biological nutrient formation of glycogen, triglycerides, and protein from glucose, fatty acids, and amino acids. Minerals are fundamental in most activities of the body, and although they are consumed in small amounts, play a significant role in physiological homeostasis.

Calcium

The average American diet usually meets the nutritional requirements for every mineral except iron and calcium (48; 62). **Calcium** is the most abundant mineral in the body, carrying out numerous roles to support normal biological processes. It is involved in muscle contractions, the transmission of nerve impulses, serves as an activator for several enzymes, and helps transport fluids across cell membranes. Calcium combines with phosphorus in the body to form bone and teeth, which represents about 75% of the total mineral content found in humans. Due to its role in bone formation, calcium deficiencies significantly impact bone health.

A common misconception is that bones are static, when in fact they are actually very dynamic, going through constant changes. Earlier, we learned bones are continuously being broken down and rebuilt in a process known as bone remodeling. Bone remodeling is controlled by two types of bone cells, **osteoclasts** and **osteoblasts**. This catabolic/anabolic relationship allows the bone to remain healthy and facilitates repair of damage. When the main construction material, calcium, is unavailable, the process of remodeling becomes impaired. Bones represent the largest storage pool of calcium in the body. When inadequate amounts of calcium are taken in through the diet, the body pulls calcium from the bone and transfers it to the blood stream in order to maintain other biological processes. When calcium is used for other purposes, the restorative balance becomes disproportionate, leading to osteopenia and eventually, osteoporosis. The average adult female consumes approximately half of the recommended 1000-1500 mg per day (86; 90), which supports the trend of osteoporosis reaching near-epidemic numbers.

Recommended Calcium Intakes by Age & Gender

Life Stage	Age	Males(mg/day)	Females(mg/day)
Infants	0-6 months	210	210
Infants	7-12 months	270	270
Children	1-3 years	500	500
Children	4-8 years	800	800
Children	9-13 years	1,300	1,300
Adolescents	14-18 years	1,300	1,300
Adults	19-50 years	1,000	1,000
Adults	51 years and older	1,200	1,200
Pregnancy	18 years and younger		1,300
Pregnancy	19 years and older		1,000
Breastfeeding	18 years and younger		1,300
Breastfeeding	19 years and older		1,000

Mineral	Adult RDA[a] Men	Women	Functions	Sources	UL[c]
Calcium	1000 mg*	1000 mg*	The principal mineral of bones and teeth. Normal muscle contraction and relaxation, nerve function, blood clotting, blood pressure, immune defenses	Milk and milk products, oysters, sardines, tofu (bean curd), greens, legumes	2500 mg
Chloride	750 mg	750 mg	Nerve and muscle function water balance(with sodium)	Table salt	ND
Magnesium	420 mg	320 mg	Bone mineralization, building of protein, enzyme action, normal muscular contraction, transmission of nerve impulses, and maintenance of teeth	Nuts, legumes, whole grains, dark green vegetables, seafood, chocolate, cocoa	350 mg^
Phosphorus	700 mg	700 mg	Important in cells' genetic material, in cell membranes as phospholipids, bones and teeth	All animal tissues	4000 mg
Potassium	2000 mg	2000 mg	Nerve and muscle function	All whole foods: meats, milk, fruits, vegetables, grains, legumes.	ND
Sodium	500 mg*	500 mg*	Maintains cells' normal fluid balance and acid-base balance in the body; nerve impulse transmission	Salt, soy sauce, processed foods	ND
Chromium	35 µg*	25 µg*	Associated with insulin and required for the release of energy from glucose	Meat, unrefined foods, fats, vegetable oils	ND
Copper	900 µg	900 µg	Necessary for the absorption and use of iron in the formation of hemoglobin; part of several enzymes	Meat, nuts, seafood	10,000 µg
Fluoride	4 mg	3 mg	An element involved in the formation of bones and teeth; helps to make the teeth resistant to decay	Drinking water, tea, seafood	10 mg
Iodine	150 µg	150 µg	Thyroid hormone function	Iodized salt, seafood	1100 µg
Iron	8 mg	18 mg	Part of the proteins hemoglobin and myoglobin, necessary for the utilization of energy	Red meats, fish, poultry, shellfish, eggs, legumes, dried fruits	45 mg
Manganese	2.3 mg*	1.8 mg*	Enzyme function	Whole grains, nuts, fruits, vegetables	11 mg
Molybdenum	45 µg	45 µg	Energy metabolism in cells	Whole grains, organ meats, peas, beans	2000 µg
Selenium	55 µg	55 µg	Works with vitamin E	Meat, fish, whole grains, eggs	400 µg
Zinc	11 mg	8 mg	Part of the hormone insulin and many enzymes; involved in making genetic materials and proteins, immune reactions	Meats, fish, shellfish, poultry, grains, vegetables	40 mg

[a]Values are Recommended Daily Allowance (RDA) for adults 19 to 50 years of age, unless marked with an asterisk. The requirements may vary for children, older adults, and pregnant or lactating women.
*Minimum estimated daily intake requirement
[c]Tolerable Upper Intake Levels (UL) for adults 19 to 50 years of age. Intakes above the UL may lead to negative health consequences.
^This refers to pharmacological agents only, and not amounts contained in food and water. No evidence of ill effects from ingestion of naturally occurring amounts in food and water.
ND= not yet determined
Adapted from Franks and Howley, 1989, and Institute of Medicine

~Quick Insight~

Osteopenia is characterized by a reduction in bone mineral density. The disorder affects almost 40% of adult women over the age of fifty (105). Osteopenia is the precursor for the disease osteoporosis. Characterized by significant bone loss, the diagnostic criteria for osteoporosis is a loss of bone equivalent to 2.5 standard deviations below the average measured bone mineral density for a given age range. Caucasian and Asian women present the highest incident of osteoporosis. Osteoporosis increases risk of bone fracture and commonly afflicts the bones of the hip, vertebral column, and wrist. Adequate nutrition and resistance training using weight-bearing exercise can significantly reduce the risk for developing the disease.

It is estimated that more than 50% of all women eventually develop the disease (43).

Studies have shown that bone mass decreases through the third decade of life without proper nutrition and exercise (39; 84), but this action can be significantly reduced with adequate consumption of calcium and load-bearing exercise, such as resistance training. Females may lose as much as 1% of bone mineral density a year after the age of 35 (38; 85). This loss is aggravated by menopause, a time during which estrogen production is dramatically reduced, and calcium absorption is decreased, thereby causing as much as a 3-6% loss of bone mass annually for the five years following menopause (41). Estrogen is a vital hormone in calcium regulation. It facilitates intestinal absorption of calcium, reduces calcium excretion, and enhances calcium retention by the bone in both men and women. Adequate calcium, vitamin D, and exercise can reverse the developmental process of osteoporosis (29).

Iron

Iron deficiency is the most common nutrient deficiency in the world (52). **Iron** serves as the key mineral in the formation of oxygen carrying materials, including hemoglobin and myoglobin. In these molecules, iron is responsible for the binding of oxygen. It is also an important component of many enzyme systems and physiological processes. The intestinal absorption of iron is consistent with the type of iron source consumed.

Approximately 2-10% of the iron from plant-based foods (non-heme iron) is absorbed, compared to the 10-30% of the heme-iron found in animal products (34; 53). In fact, non-heme iron absorption increases when consumed with heme forms. Likewise, heme iron sources are absorbed at significantly higher rates than supplemental iron.

Inadequate iron consumption is another problem for female population groups. Iron loss during menstrual cycles can be as high as 45 mg (5-45 mg) (37). This loss is compounded by the fact that heme iron consumption is often lower in females than in male populations. This problem leads to insufficient iron levels in approximately 30-50% of the adult female population (55). Due to the role iron plays in the formation of hemoglobin, insufficient consumption reduces hemoglobin in the blood, consequently affecting oxygen transport. Iron-deficiency anemia occurs when iron levels drop too low. Common signs and symptoms of iron-deficiency anemia include fatigue, loss of appetite, and reduced capacity to perform activity. Individuals with iron-deficiency anemia will find a noticeable decline in performance associated with a reduced capacity to transfer oxygen. To avoid iron-deficiency anemia, those at the greatest risk should consume more

Recommended Dietary Allowances For Iron

Population	Age, years	Iron, mg
Children	1-3	7
	4-8	10
Males	9-13	8
	14-18	11
	19-30	8
	31-50	8
	50-70	8
	>70	8
Females	9-13	8
	14-18	15
	19-30	18
	31-50	18
	50-70	8
	>70	8
Pregnancy	≥ 16	27
Lactation	≤ 18	10
	> 18	9

Dietary Reference Intakes for Iron 2001, National Academy of Sciences, Institute of Medicine. Food and Nutrition Board.

~Key Terms~

Minerals- Any of a group of inorganic elements that are essential to humans and animals for normal body function.

Calcium- A mineral essential in building and maintaining bone, blood clotting, and muscle contractions.

Osteoclasts- A type of bone cell that removes bone tissue by removing the bone's mineralized matrix.

Osteoblasts- A cell from which bone develops.

Iron- A key mineral in the formation of oxygen binding material, including hemoglobin and myoglobin.

Electrolytes- Salts and minerals that produce electrically charged particles (ions) in body fluids and are an important component in maintaining proper hydration status.

iron-rich foods, particularly animal source iron, to enhance absorption capabilities. As mentioned earlier, eating meat increases iron status more effectively than iron supplements, even when consumed with vitamin C (triples iron absorption rate) (87). Exercise can also augment iron absorption when supported by proper nutrition (54; 77; 94).

Electrolytes

Some additional minerals are of particular interest for the fitness professional due to their role in fluid balance. **Electrolytes** are electrically charged ions that come from the minerals sodium, potassium, and chlorine. Sodium and chlorine represent the main minerals contained in blood plasma and extracellular fluid, while potassium regulates actions from inside the cell. The electrolytes play a very important role by modulating fluid exchange between the cell and the extracellular environment. The balance is maintained by a well-regulated electrical gradient that enables all the cellular

activities required for biological homeostasis to occur. Nervous transmissions, muscle contractions, glandular function, and the regulation of pH balance all depend on the electrical balance control of the electrolytes. Imbalances associated with poor intake of electrolytes in the diet can lead to serious physiological problems. Of major concern is the thermoregulatory system, which depends upon the regulation of water balance to function properly. When the system becomes impaired, heat illness can result, and the possibility of death becomes a relevant issue. Excessive fluid loss from exercise will contain electrolytes. Proper diet and water consumption should be maintained to ensure adequate intake of electrolytes and proper hydration. Beverages containing electrolytes can be a viable re-hydration option.

Electrolytes

Sodium	Na$^+$
Potassium	K$^+$
Chloride	Cl$^-$

Water

Water constitutes nearly 75% of muscle weight and approximately 50% of fat weight (70). It is the most abundant and important nutrient in the body. Without any water, life can only be sustained for three to five days. It plays a role in almost all the functions of the body as a constituent of compounds, transporter, reactant, and as a principal of gaseous diffusion. As a functional component, water lubricates joints, protects moving organs, provides body volume and form, thermoregulates, and is used in chemical balance and as an ingredient in cellular metabolism. It serves more roles than any other single nutrient in the body. If water consumption does not meet requirements and dehydration occurs, the body fails to function properly.

An important relationship exists between water and minerals within the body, which makes their daily consumption vital for health. Minerals need water to form electrolytes in the body. In turn, water needs minerals to maintain fluid balance inside and outside of the cell membrane. Body water is generally categorized into two compartments: intracellular and extracellular fluids. Most water is found inside of the cells as intracellular fluid, while approximately one-third of body water exists outside of the cell as extracellular fluid. Extracellular fluid includes blood plasma, the water found between the cells (interstitial fluid), lymph, saliva, fluid secreted by glands and organs, as well as the fluids that hydrate the spinal cord. Cells of the body are permeable, so

Heme Iron Sources	Non-heme Iron Sources
Tuna	Oatmeal
Chicken	Spinach
Clams	Soy Protein
Beef	Dried Figs
Oysters	Beans
Liver	Raisin
	Lima Beans
	Prune Juice

~Quick Insight~

The **Female Triad** is a combination of disordered eating, amenorrhea, and osteoporosis. It is estimated that 25% or more of female athletes are at risk of suffering the consequences of estrogen imbalance due to insufficient caloric intake and excessive exercise stress. Body fat levels below essential requirements disrupt menstrual activity, causing a reduction in circulating estrogen concentrations (31). The reduced level of estrogen causes calcium regulation to become dysfunctional. When combined with restricted diets that are low in calcium, the risk for osteoporosis is dramatically elevated (64). Common characteristics, signs, and symptoms of the female triad include (11):

- Young adult females
- Lean or low body mass
- Recurrent stress fractures
- Exercise fanatic
- Low self-esteem
- Self critical
- Hard-driving personality
- Highly competitive
- Signs of depression
- Emotional highs and lows

water moves relatively easily through the cellular membrane as needed by the current physiological environment. This mobility allows the body to maintain a system that prevents cells from losing too much fluid or becoming over saturated. Minerals play an important role in facilitating this regulatory mechanism.

When minerals dissolve in water, they become ions or electrolytes. As stated earlier, the term electrolyte is given to these ions because they have an electrical charge and conduct electricity. When these electrical conductors are maintained in correct concentration within the cell and outside of the cell, water balance is maintained. The electrolyte responsible for maintenance of intracellular fluid volume is potassium, while extracellular fluid is regulated by sodium and chlorine. Magnesium also contributes to the action both inside and outside of the cell but is rarely identified with the other electrolytes (104).

When the cellular environment is disturbed through excess fluid loss, fluid and electrolyte imbalances occur. Individuals experiencing excessive fluid loss through exercise, heat, vomiting, or diarrhea can reach a hazardous state of dehydration (22; 103). When

extracellular fluid is lost due to any of these physiological agitators, the reduction of extracellular fluid draws intracellular fluid from the cell in an attempt to restore balance. Exacerbating the problem, electrolytes are also lost during this process. This creates a hazardous situation because the fluid regulatory mechanism is compromised, which in extreme cases, increases potential risk for kidney and heart failure (10; 97; 102). Immediate fluid replenishment is imperative to restore fluid balance once it is lost. In severe cases of dehydration, intravenous therapy is used to increase fluid volumes. In less severe cases, water and electrolyte solutions should be consumed orally. The following charts illustrate normal fluid intake and fluid output pathways.

Water Input

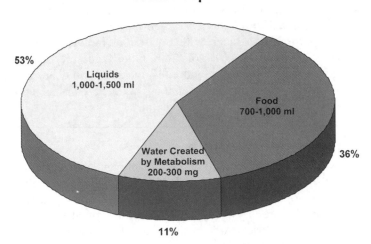

Water Output

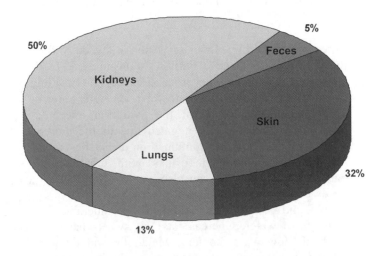

~Quick Insight~

The **sodium-potassium relationship** is very important in the maintenance of homeostasis (59). Together, the electrolyte ions regulate the fluid balance in tissues by establishing the proper electrical gradient across cell membranes. When excess salt is consumed in the diet, it increases the excretory function of the kidneys by decreasing aldosterone, the hormone that increases sodium re-absorption. In some cases the excess sodium cannot be adequately regulated, causing too much sodium to remain in the body. The excess sodium pulls water into the blood, causing the blood to become hyperhydrated, thereby increasing the blood pressure. Sodium-induced hypertension occurs in approximately 33% of the individuals who are diagnosed with hypertension (26; 106).

The average American consumes twice the recommended intake of salt in the diet. The high intake is not often met by appropriate balance with potassium. Individuals who have an elevated risk for high blood pressure should reduce salt in their diet and consume adequate quantities of potassium. Tomatoes, potatoes, oranges, bananas, and meat are good sources of potassium.

Daily Fluid Intake

Daily fluid intake is important to prevent dehydration and heat illness. Most people do not consume enough water to meet their daily requirements, particularly when they are physically active. Fluid is gained and lost through a variety of mechanisms. For the average, sedentary person living in normal environmental conditions, 2.5 L of water should be adequate daily consumption (96). When the environment becomes heated and activity is increased in duration and intensity, the physiological demand for water increases dramatically. Fluid intake volumes may increase to 5 L or as much as 10 L under more extreme physiological stress (49; 95).

Three primary sources can serve to satisfy daily fluid intake requirements: liquids consumed, foods consumed, and metabolic processes (see graph). Fluid consumption should attempt to focus on pure water or electrolyte drinks. Some of the hydration effects of soda, coffee, and tea are negated due to the diuretic effects of the caffeine contained in these beverages. Additionally, supplement drinks with creatine, mahuang, or ephedrine can also negatively affect water balance. Healthy food sources, particularly fruits and vegetables, contain considerable amounts of water, whereas fats and sweets have relatively low water content. Metabolic water is created when food molecules are catabolized for energy-forming carbon dioxide and water. This metabolic water provides about 25% of daily water requirements for a sedentary person. During physical activity, carbohydrate breakdown supplies additional water when glycogen liberates the water that bonds with glucose. Each gram of glycogen contains 2.7 grams of water, accounting for more than 1,000 grams of water maintained inside the body when glycogen stores are at full capacity.

Fluid Loss

Water output from the body is a relatively efficient process. The four primary mechanisms for fluid loss include urine, water loss through the skin, water loss as water vapor during respiration, and water lost in feces. Fluid loss through urine is determined by the re-absorption rate of the kidneys, as well as the amount of solute that passes through the kidneys each day. The average re-absorption rate of water is about 99%, leaving roughly 1000-1500 ml of fluid to be excreted as urine each day (9; 32; 78). This fluid loss is increased when protein is used as energy, which accelerates the dehydration rate of the body. The excretory function of removing fecal matter also requires water. To ensure the matter moves easily through the large intestine, water constitutes approximately 70% of the total volume of human excrement (100-200 ml of water). This becomes increasingly relevant when an individual suffers from diarrhea, which can cause a fluid loss between 1500-5000 ml (19).

Water lost from the skin and through respiration accounts for the rest of the fluid lost each day. Water vapor leaves the body with each breath, and accounts for about 250-300 ml of water lost each day through normal respiration. When under the stress of exercise, fluid loss increases due to increased ventilatory requirements and can equal approximately 2 to 5 ml per minute of vigorous exercise, depending on the environment (33; 98). Interestingly, this rate is highest in colder climates and higher altitudes because the body must release water to moisten inspired air to help it move through the pulmonary airways (6; 27; 57).

The skin also experiences increased fluid loss during exercise. Under normal conditions, the skin will lose about 350 ml of fluid per day to "insensible perspiration." This perspiration occurs as water seeps from deeper tissues out to the skin. Water can also be

Metabolic Water Produced From Energy Substrate Breakdown

Energy Nutrient (100g)	Metabolic Water (grams)
Carbohydrates	55 g
Protein	100 g
Fats	107 g

excreted from sweat glands that lie beneath the skin's surface. Generally, the body will lose between 500-750 ml of water to normal daily sweating. Sweating serves as a refrigeration mechanism to help cool the body. As the body produces sweat, it is evaporated from the skin, causing a cooling effect. This is the body's best defense against overheating. A heat acclimated body can produce as much as 12 L of sweat in one day at a rate of 1 L per hour during prolonged intense exercise (67).

In addition to the aforementioned conditions and physiological functions of the body, fluid output can be affected by several other factors as well. High protein intake, low-calorie diets, pregnancy and lactation, high sodium consumption, higher fiber diets, and the consumption of moderates, such as alcohol and caffeine all increase the need for additional water intake (21; 93). Each particular factor requires a specific amount of water to compensate for the added fluid lost through one of the four fluid loss mechanisms. Determining how much additional water is necessary requires understanding what facilitated the loss in the first place. Examining each mechanism and its relative mean fluid-loss value will help to determine how much more water must be ingested in order to meet daily need.

Exercise and Fluid Loss

Exercise exacerbates the effects of water loss mechanisms due to cardiovascular adjustments and evaporation. The dissipation of metabolically-generated heat can cause excessive sweating, which may lead to an accompanying reduction of plasma volume, which, in turn, causes fluid shifts out of the intercellular and interstitial compartments. When the environmental climate includes high heat and humidity, the cardiovascular system is taxed by the physiological demands of heat dissipation. During these conditions, the blood must transfer metabolic heat to the periphery for cooling. This requirement reduces the amount of available blood for the delivery of oxygen and is one reason why relative intensity is affected by heated conditions. In addition, exercising in the heat lowers absolute VO_2 because the reduced amount of available blood directly lowers stroke volume. The heart rate increases in an attempt to compensate for the decrease in stroke volume and thereby, produces higher heart rates at all submaximal exercise levels. At maximal aerobic capacity, the heart rate cannot make up for the reduced stroke volume and VO_2max is reduced.

During exercise, the body experiences rapid internal temperature changes. Heat generated by the active muscles will lead to an elevated core temperature. A modest rise in core temperature creates the optimal thermal environment for physiologic and metabolic function. Although this response is normal, the thermodynamics of the body still requires a well-regulated heat dissipation response. The hypothalamus in the brain contains the central coordinating center for the regulation of temperature within the body. It is responsible for the thermoregulatory adjustments made in response to deviations in temperature. Heat regulating mechanisms become activated by signals from thermal receptors in the skin and by the temperature of blood, both of which directly stimulate the thermoregulatory center. In response to this information, the body mobilizes fluid for a cooling effect. Evaporation provides the major physiological defense against overheating during rest and activity. When environmental heat and internal heat activated by physical activity are experienced simultaneously, the response is handled primarily by increased perspiration. This results in a decrease of body fluid and leads to rapid dehydration.

Dehydration

The primary controller of hydration status is thirst. Unfortunately, the threshold for the initiation of thirst occurs at a point where a person may already be mildly dehydrated (8; 66; 83). For most people, basing water consumption on thirst will likely lead to inadequate water consumption. This is a particular concern for the elderly as the thirst mechanism becomes impaired due to attenuation of central volume receptors (65; 82). **Dehydration** occurs at a loss of 1.0% or greater of body weight due to fluid loss and occurs when fluid output is greater than fluid intake. As indicated earlier, water is lost from multiple body functions, and all metabolic activity requires water in some capacity. On average, we replace all of the water in our bodies about once every 10-12 days. Athletes in heavy training generally replace all of their water about once every six days. Whenever fluid dynamics become output dominated, body functions become impaired ($\geq$2% loss of body weight) (46). Moderate exercise can cause a fluid loss of 0.5 to 1.5 L $\bullet$ hour^{-1}. This number significantly increases up to 3 L $\bullet$ hr^{-1} when conditions become more strenuous, either through increased physical exertion or environmental factors (16; 73; 76). Fluid loss can reach life-threatening levels in a very short period of time, and accumulative fluid loss can be just as dangerous. Consistently losing water over an extended period of time without adequate replenishment can cause a normal bout of exercise to become a significant hazard due to poor hydration status.

The risk of heat related illness, such as a stroke, is greatly increased when the body is dehydrated. This same problem occurs with prolonged exercise.

~Quick Insight~

To be well hydrated, the average sedentary adult male should consume at least 2.5-3.0 liters of fluid per day, while the average sedentary adult female should consume at least 2.2-2.6 liters of fluid per day (45). The fluid should be in the form of non-caffeinated, non-alcoholic beverages, soups, and foods. Water in its pure form is the most readily used by the body. Drinking tea, coffee, and other soft drinks can over-stimulate the central nervous system, and at the same time, increase risk of dehydration due to the strong diuretic action of caffeine on the kidneys, which causes increased urine production. Persons who regularly drink coffee or sodas without additional adequate water intake can in fact cause mild dehydration without participating in any physical activity whatsoever.

Chronic dehydration has been linked to the development of numerous major health problems. It is generally thought that the prevalence of kidney stones increases in populations with low urinary volume. Decreased fluid intake leads to low urine volume and increased concentrations of all stone-forming salts. Recommendations for individuals at risk for urinary stone formation, as well as patients with stones, include the consumption of at least 250 ml of fluid with each meal, between meals, before bedtime, and when they wake up in the morning (44). This pattern ensures that fluid intake is spread throughout the day and that the urine doesn't become concentrated. These measures decrease the chance for kidney stone development.

Low fluid consumption may increase the incidence of certain cancers. There seems to be a link between patients with urinary tract cancer (bladder, kidney, prostate, and testicle) and low fluid consumption (2; 5). No association with specific fluid volumes has been found, but one study found women who drank more than five glasses of water per day had a 45% decreased risk of colon cancer compared with those who drank two or fewer glasses. Among the men, there was a 32% decrease in risk with increased water consumption (1; 4). This finding is probably due to the fact that fecal mobility is increased with proper fluid intake. It is thought that higher fecal mobility reduces the duration of time carcinogenic toxins sit in the large intestine.

Water also plays a primary role in fat metabolism. One of the many functions of the liver is to mobilize stored fat for energy utilization. Water is a key ingredient in this metabolic process. In times of water shortage, the kidneys cannot perform to the levels required for waste removal. This results in the liver being called upon to aid the kidneys in their efforts, resulting in less efficient metabolism. Additionally, water serves to further aid in reducing dietary caloric content. As opposed to juices and sodas, water is calorie-free. People who consume regular amounts of water experience feelings of satiety (fullness) by maintaining a higher gastric volume. With more contents in the stomach, there is a tendency to eat less. Adequate water intake can take the edge off hunger, reducing the caloric peaks and valleys that many people experience when eating large meals.

Hypovolemia and sweat gland fatigue can occur once hydration status reaches a fluid loss greater than 5% of body mass(61). Since most of the fluid lost from sweat is supplied by blood plasma, cardiovascular function is impaired due to a reduced availability of oxygen and a lower cardiac output. This reduction in cardiac output can cause kidney dysfunction, heart dysfunction and possibly death from stroke. Additionally, the reduced blood plasma volume further compromises the body's thermoregulatory capacity(61) These thermoregulatory and physiologic functions experience decreased efficiency with almost any level of dehydration. The fact that dehydration can occur when swimming, exercising in colder environments, and in higher altitudes is often overlooked (36; 60). Diuretic use also contributes to dehydration status by decreasing the amount of water recycled by the kidneys and thus, increasing urine output. The fluid excreted through urine from diuretic consumption also comes from blood plasma. As mentioned earlier, individuals who consistently consume soda, coffee, or other diuretic-containing beverages instead of water may be impairing their hydration status. The same is true for alcohol consumption.

Maintaining Proper Hydration

Fluid replacement is the key to maintaining healthy body dynamics. When proper hydration combines with adequate acclimation to the training and environment, the synergistic effect greatly reduces the risk for dehydration and heat related illnesses.

Acclimation

For individuals with proper acclimation to training stress and environment, plasma volumes are higher; there is an earlier onset of sweating; the body experiences greater sweat distribution; there is an increased release of antidiuretic hormone (ADH) and **aldosterone** to conserve electrolytes and increase

Early Signs of Dehydration

Fatigue
Headache
Heat Intolerance
Dry Mouth or Cough
Flushed Skin
Appetite Loss
Sensation of Being Light-Headed
Dark Urine with Strong Odor

recycling of water in the kidneys; and there is improved cutaneous blood flow. The effects of acclimation must be complemented with regularly scheduled fluid consumption throughout the day and during activity. Ingesting fluids during exercise increases blood flow to the skin, causing a more effective cooling process. Strictly following an adequate water replacement schedule prevents dehydration and its consequences, particularly hyperthermia. Fitness professionals must remain diligent about keeping scheduled fluid intakes throughout their client's training regimens. Most exercisers and athletes under consume their recommended fluid intake when left to monitor their own intake (23). A fully hydrated individual will experience improvements in performance compared to their efforts during a state of compromised hydration status.

Pre-Exercise Hydration

Pre-exercise hydration can help provide added protection against heat stress due to delayed dehydration and a decrease in core temperature changes (72; 75). This consumption can start 24 hours before the exercise bout or competition and should continue up to 20 minutes before the training begins. Pre-exercise fluid consumption should be approximately 400-600 ml of water, which serves to increase stomach volume and optimizes gastric emptying (51; 61; 71; 74). This pre-exercise hydration can be very important for endurance

Fluid Loss	Recommended Fluid Intake	Rate of Consumption
1000 ml per hour	250 ml	Every 15 min
>1000 ml per hour	250 ml	Every 10 min

activities and training in hot climates where it is difficult to balance intake with output.

Hydration During & Post-Exercise

To maintain proper hydration, fluid should be consumed throughout the exercise regimen. Fitness professionals can ensure that hydration status is optimized by tracking urine composition and bodyweight changes. In a well hydrated individual, urine should typically be produced in large volumes, have a limited odor, and exhibit a light coloration. Urine that is dark and gives off noticeable odor suggests the body is dehydrated. Likewise, changes in pre- and post-exercise bodyweight indicate fluid lost during the training bout. Charting training weight differences enables the fitness professional to gauge the normal fluid loss for each client. This provides clear data for fluid replacement quantities. On average, one pound of weight loss equates to 450 ml (15 oz) of water loss.

Time intervals for replenishment are also important factors in maintaining proper hydration status. For fluid loss of 1000 ml per hour, 250 ml of water should be consumed every 15 minutes (50; 61). For fluid loss in excess of 1000 ml per hour the same quantity should be consumed every 10 minutes (67). Identifying the actual amount of fluid lost is the first step to adequately replacing the lost contents.

Rehydration fluid intake does not have to be limited to water. Palatable carbohydrate-electrolyte solutions (4-8% CHO solution) can serve to facilitate more complete hydration than plain water alone (17; 91). This facilitated hydration can be used both during and following exercise and competition. Beverages containing 20-60 mmol/L have shown to increase recovery hydration and electrolyte balance post-exercise (40; 92). Additionally, small amounts of potassium 2-5 mmol/L may enhance the retention of water in intracellular space and may diminish any extra potassium loss from sodium retention by the kidneys (67).

Immediately post-exercise, pure water is quickly absorbed and dilutes the plasma sodium concentration to the point that it decreases plasma **osmolarity**. This, in turn, increases urine production and inhibits the sodium-dependent stimulation process that initiates the thirst mechanism in the brain. When the fluids have the correct concentration of sodium, plasma sodium concentrations remain elevated, which sustains the thirst sensation, promotes the retention of ingested fluid, and speeds up plasma volume restoration during rehydration (3; 47; 56). Carbohydrate-electrolyte drinks contribute to the ideal solution for activity and recovery hydration. The glucose solutions stimulate both sodium and water absorption in the intestines. Carbohydrate-electrolyte drinks have proven to be effective in aiding fluid replenishment (15; 58). However, when carbohydrate concentrations are too high, gastric emptying and the rate of intestinal fluid absorption is negatively effected. The total gastric volume plays an important role in the rate of gastric emptying. Higher gastric volumes increase the rate of gastric emptying. Due to the fact that many people experience discomfort when exercising with greater gastric volumes, the carbohydrate concentration is very important if a sports drink is used for hydration.

Sport drinks are intended for individuals who exercise at levels that compromise water balance. Many individuals do not reach the exercise intensities or durations that warrant carbohydrate-electrolyte solutions. The glucose solutions do contain calories in the form of sugar. Over-consuming replenishment drinks can contribute to a positive caloric balance. Water alone does not have any calories and, for low to moderate exercise is probably adequate for the majority of participants.

Selecting Dietary Sources

Knowing what to eat and how much of any given nutrient to consume on a daily basis confuses many people. Trends toward increased rates of obesity and related disease in America warrant the serious concerns held by health organizations. Despite constant advancements in knowledge and medicine, a steady decline in the overall health of the nation continues;

~Key Terms~

Sodium-Potassium Relationship- The establishment of a proper electrical gradient across cell membranes which helps to regulate fluid balance in the tissues thus maintaining homeostasis.

Chronic Dehydration- A condition in which the body is in constant deprivation of fluids necessary for the maintenance of homeostasis and can result in debilitating conditions such as gastritis, heartburn, arthritis, kidney stones, and accelerated aging.

Dehydration- Excessive loss of water from the body or from an organ or a body part.

Hypovolemia- A decrease in the volume of blood plasma.

Aldosterone- A steroid hormone secreted by the adrenal cortex that regulates the salt and water balance in the body.

Osmolarity- The osmotic concentration of a solution, expressed as osmoles of solute per liter of solution.

evidenced by the increased rate of obesity and related disease. The problems seem to come from a combination of sources, which include:

1. Sound nutritional practices are not reaching the general public in a way that is effective in reducing the rate of weight gain. Many people do not know what nutrients are in what foods, even with clear labels to help them understand food products.

2. Americans are impacted by time and pressure demands, citing them as excuses for poor nutritional choices.

3. The amount of physical activity engaged in does not match the energy being consumed.

4. Manufacturers have developed numerous pitfalls and obstacles to sound nutrition practices by promoting and endorsing quick-fix solutions and by taking advantage of a natural tendency for convenience.

5. The media presents incomplete or incorrect information and no regulatory body sanctions what is being communicated to consumers through print or digital sources.

The government does provide outlets for quality information, but in many cases, it is still very confusing for consumers to use appropriately. The USDA developed the food guide pyramid as an easy tool to provide Americans with a practical approach to good nutrition. The food guide pyramid provides simple guidelines as to where nutrient sources should be derived, as well as the recommended servings from each category. If followed correctly, the pyramid will meet the nutritional needs of approximately 90% of the population.

Food Guide Pyramid

The **food guide pyramid** should be an easy answer for many of the dietary questions that face Americans. However, it has come under harsh criticism for its effectiveness and practicality, particularly for individuals engaging in weight loss programs. The reasons that some estimates for obesity in the U.S. have broached the 35% mark are a lack of physical activity and the failure of most individuals to eat well-rounded, calorie-controlled diets as suggested by the food guide pyramid. Due to the fact that many Americans maintain low activity levels, consume a diet relatively high in fat and sugar, and commonly ingest more calories then they expend, it is obvious the food guide

Activity
Activity is represented by the steps and the person climbing them, as a reminder of the importance of daily physical activity

Gradual Improvement
Gradual improvement is encouraged. It suggests that individuals can benefit from taking small steps to improve their diet and lifestyle each day.

Personalization
Personalization is shown by the person on the steps.

Variety
Variety is symbolized by the six bands representing the five food groups of the pyramid and oils. This illustrates that foods from all groups are needed each day for good health.

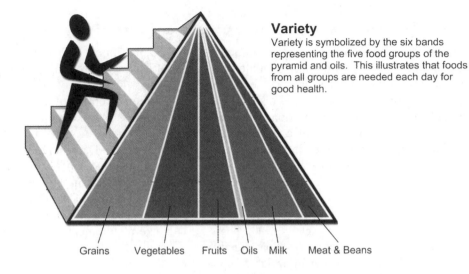

Grains   Vegetables   Fruits   Oils   Milk   Meat & Beans

Proportionality
Proportionality is shown by the different widths of the food group bands. The widths suggest how much food a person should choose from each group. The widths are just a general guide, not exact proportions.

Moderation
Moderation is represented by the narrowing of each food group from bottom to top. The wider base stands for foods with little or no solid fats or added sugar. These should be selected more often. The narrower top area stands for foods containing more added sugar and solid fats. The more active you are, the more of these foods can fit into your diet.

---

system is not, by itself, adequate to manage America's nutritional needs. If individual diets consisted of mainly fruits, vegetables, lean meats, and whole grains in the appropriate serving sizes, as defined by the pyramid, obesity would not be such a pressing health issue in the United States.

A drawback to the pyramid system of eating is that most people do not differentiate between smart food choices and poor food selections from each section of the pyramid. For instance, choosing processed carbohydrate sources over whole grain products is very common because few people recognize the difference. Additionally, for many people there is a tendency to select foods that are higher in calories from each group due to taste.

Attempting to follow the food guide pyramid is also challenging because of the time and convenience factor. The reason for this phenomenon is three-fold: 1) it is difficult to monitor food when eating out, 2) convenience foods selected by many people are often high in fat and sugar, and 3) very few people recognize correct serving sizes. Quite often foods at restaurants are served in portions 2 to 4 times that of the

recommended amount. In addition, the serving sizes defined by the USDA are much smaller than what is normally consumed in the average household. So, even though someone may believe they are following the pyramid, they are actually over-consuming foods from every category, except the fruit and vegetable groups.

Food Labels
Learning how to read a food label and developing an understanding of serving size portions is the first step to being able to effectively use the pyramid. Actually presenting clients with appropriate serving sizes and portion examples can help them realize dietary intake quantities that fulfill their relative need. The chart describes what a typical serving size should look like from each category.

When foods are purchased in a prepared form rather than individually measurable, reading the labels on the container provides insight into the contents, nutrients, and caloric breakdown of the product; however, knowing the information in a single serving is only useful if the number of servings can be determined from the portion consumed. Individuals often inappropriately

Grain Products Group	Vegetable Group	Fruit Group	Dairy Group	Meat and Bean Group	Fats, Oils, Sweets
1 slice bread 1/2 cup pasta 1/2 cup cereal	½ cup chopped vegetables 1 cup leafy vegetables	1 medium apple ¾ cup fruit juice 1 med. orange	8 oz milk 1 oz cheese ½ cup yogurt	3 oz meat 1 egg ½ cup nuts ½ cup beans	Use sparingly <10% sugar <10% sat.fat

apply the single serving content information to the total amount eaten, even though the portion may be multiple servings. Part of this problem lies in the serving containers used for eating. Plates, bowls, and dishes are often large enough to hold numerous portions. It is a natural tendency to cover a plate or fill a bowl with food. People wind up consuming the entire quantity of food served even if their caloric requirements would be met by a smaller portion.

The food label provides specific information required by the Nutrition Education Labeling Act of 1990. The ingredients are required to be on the label for packaged foods and are listed in descending order by weight. The **Nutritional Facts Panel** is also required. It identifies the number of servings per container and reflects the amount of food by weight or volume that constitutes a single serving. The serving size is the portion that contains the nutrient amounts listed on the label. The following nutrient information is required of each label:

The nutritional label attempts to provide additional clarity by expressing the portion list through Daily Values. The **Daily Values** are represented by the nutritional content of one serving by weight as it applies to both a 2000 kcal and 2500 kcal diet. Although it is unlikely that a person will consume exactly 2000 calories, the Daily Values provide some insight to the nutritional value of the food in the diet. Additionally, the total energy in the diet is listed next to each nutrient by percentages of the Daily Value. This is used to assist consumers in meeting their energy and nutritional intake requirements by the recommended percentage in the diet.

Sample Food Label

Nutrition Facts
Serving Size 1 cup
Servings Per Container 4

Amount Per Serving	
Calories 230	Calories from Fat 90

	% Daily Value*
Total Fat 10g	15%
Saturated Fat 5g	22.5%
Cholesterol 24mg	8%
Sodium 730mg	36.5%
Total Carbohydrates 26g	9%
Dietary Fiber 1g	5%
Sugars 9g	
Protein 9g	

Vitamin A 5%	Vitamin C 0%
Calcium 25%	Iron 6%

Percent Values are based on a 2,000 calorie diet. Your Daily values may be higher or lower depending on your calorie needs:

		Calories	2,000
Total fat	Less than		65g
Sat fat	Less than		20g
Cholesterol	Less than		300mg
Sodium	Less than		2,400mg
Total Carbohydrates			300g
Fiber			25g

Calories per gram:
Fat 9   Carbohydrate 4   Protein 4

Nutritional Facts Panel

Serving Size
Servings Per Container
Total Calories
Calories from Fat
Total Fat
Saturated Fat
Cholesterol
Sodium
Total Carbohydrates
Sugar
Fiber
Protein
Vitamin A
Vitamin C
Calcium
Iron

Percentage of calories from carbohydrates, fats, and proteins seem like a reasonable way to track energy nutrients, but the actual implementation methodology required to correctly track energy intake this way is very difficult. Essentially, a person would have to know their total caloric intake, the specific number of calories from each energy source, and know how to convert the energy value into a percentage. Obviously exact serving sizes and knowledge of every food consumed would be required for true accuracy. This is not a reasonable method for tracking dietary intake because it is much too difficult to employ, requires specific competencies in math conversions, and would require knowledge of all food contents ingested. Below is the conversion method used to convert energy nutrient weight into the percentage of dietary calories.

Converting Grams to Percentages

125 grams of fat consumed through a 2700 kcal diet.

125 ~~gram~~ x 9 kcal ~~gram~~ = 1125 kcal from fat

1125 kcal from fat ÷ 2700 kcal diet = 41% fat

Food description terminology can also become confusing. For most consumers looking to avoid adding extra pounds, boxes labeled light, low-fat, non-fat, and reduced-calorie all look very appealing, but very few people recognize what the terms actually mean.

Nutrient content descriptors are used to market foods based on improved consumer health awareness. The FDA and Food Safety and Inspection Service of the USDA regulate the specific descriptive information found on food labels. The following terms are commonly found on many food product labels.

Consumers can rely on the descriptors because they are properly regulated, but some confusion still exists as to when they are appropriate. For instance, a jelly bean package advertises itself as fat-free, but the food is basically pure sugar. True, the product does not contain fat, but jelly beans never have contained fat, so labeling the package fat-free is obviously done to confuse consumers into thinking it is a healthier food. Personal trainers need to educate their clients to appropriate food selection and make them aware of how to use the food labels and recognize the meaning of the labeling descriptors.

~Key Terms~

Food Guide Pyramid- A diagram used in nutrition education which shows the suggested quantity of food from each food group that an individual should consume each day.

Nutritional Facts Panel- A label on consumer products that identifies servings per container, amount of food by weight or volume that constitutes a single serving, and relevant nutritional information.

Daily Values- Indicates the amount of a nutrient that is provided by a single serving of a food item.

Food Description- Terminology in describing food as light, low-fat, non-fat, and reduced calorie.

Nutrient Content- Descriptions used to market foods based on improved consumer standards.

Food Descriptors

Free - often associated with fat-free or sugar-free, means the product contains no amount of, or only trivial quantities of, the referred components. Less than 0.5 g per serving or less than 5 kcal per serving.

Low - can be used if the foods can be consumed regularly without causing excessive intakes of its referred components.

Low-Calorie - less than 40 kcal per serving.

Low-Fat - less than 3g per serving.

Low-Cholesterol - less than 20 mg per serving.

Low-sodium - less than 140 mg per serving.

Light - has three possible meanings: 1) 1/3rd fewer calories or half the fat, 2) the sodium content of a low calorie, low fat food has been reduced by 50%, 3) the term describes the color, texture or other property as long as it explains intent e.g. "light brown sugar."

Reduced - the contents contain at least 25% less of the component than the referenced product.

Lean - less than 10g fat, 4.5g or less saturated fat, and less than 95 mg of cholesterol per serving and per 100 g.

Extra Lean - less than 5 g of fat, less than 2 g of saturated fat, less than 95 mg of cholesterol per serving.

Good Source - 10-19% of the Daily Value.

High In - 20% or more of the Daily Value.

Extra - at least 10% more than the Daily Value in the reference food.

Very Low Sodium - 35 mg or less sodium.

Sodium Free - less than 5 mg per serving.

High Fiber - 5g or more per serving.

Chapter Eight References
6.

1. **Altieri A, La Vecchia C and Negri E**. Fluid intake and risk of bladder and other cancers. *Eur J Clin Nutr* 57 Suppl 2: S59-S68, 2003.

2. **Altieri A, La Vecchia C and Negri E**. Fluid intake and risk of bladder and other cancers. *Eur J Clin Nutr* 57 Suppl 2: S59-S68, 2003.

3. **Armstrong LE and Epstein Y**. Fluid-electrolyte balance during labor and exercise: concepts and misconceptions. *Int J Sport Nutr* 9: 1-12, 1999.

4. **Bar DY, Gesundheit B, Urkin J and Kapelushnik J**. Water intake and cancer prevention. *J Clin Oncol* 22: 383-385, 2004.

5. **Bar DY, Gesundheit B, Urkin J and Kapelushnik J**. Water intake and cancer prevention. *J Clin Oncol* 22: 383-385, 2004.

6. **Bartsch P, Swenson ER, Paul A, Julg B and Hohenhaus E**. Hypoxic ventilatory response, ventilation, gas exchange, and fluid balance in acute mountain sickness. *High Alt Med Biol* 3: 361-376, 2002.

7. **Bazzano LA, Reynolds K, Holder KN and He J**. Effect of folic acid supplementation on risk of cardiovascular diseases: a meta-analysis of randomized controlled trials. *JAMA* 296: 2720-2726, 2006.

8. **Blair-West JR, Burns P, Denton DA, Ferraro T, McBurnie MI, Tarjan E and Weisinger RS**. Thirst induced by increasing brain sodium concentration is mediated by brain angiotensin. *Brain Res* 637: 335-338, 1994.

9. **Blanker MH, Bernsen RM, Bosch JL, Thomas S, Groeneveld FP, Prins A and Bohnen AM**. Relation between nocturnal voiding frequency and nocturnal urine

production in older men:a population-based study. *Urology* 60: 612-616, 2002.

10. **Broqvist M, Dahlstrom U, Karlsson E and Larsson J**. Muscle water and electrolytes in severe chronic congestive heart failure before and after treatment with enalapril. *Eur Heart J* 13: 243-250, 1992.

11. **Brunet M**. Female athlete triad. *Clin Sports Med* 24: 623-36, ix, 2005.

12. **Bruno EJ, Jr. and Ziegenfuss TN**. Water-soluble vitamins: research update. *Curr Sports Med Rep* 4: 207-213, 2005.

13. **Bruno EJ, Jr. and Ziegenfuss TN**. Water-soluble vitamins: research update. *Curr Sports Med Rep* 4: 207-213, 2005.

14. **Bruno EJ, Jr. and Ziegenfuss TN**. Water-soluble vitamins: research update. *Curr Sports Med Rep* 4: 207-213, 2005.

15. **Burke LM**. Nutrition for post-exercise recovery. *Aust J Sci Med Sport* 29: 3-10, 1997.

16. **Burke LM**. Nutritional needs for exercise in the heat. *Comp Biochem Physiol A Mol Integr Physiol* 128: 735-748, 2001.

17. **Burke LM**. Nutritional needs for exercise in the heat. *Comp Biochem Physiol A Mol Integr Physiol* 128: 735-748, 2001.

18. **Cesari M, Rossi GP and Pessina AC**. Homocysteine-lowering treatment in coronary heart disease. *Curr Med Chem Cardiovasc Hematol Agents* 3: 289-295, 2005.

19. **Chongbanyatcharoen P**. Acute diarrhea's recommendations on oral rehydration therapy and feeding. *J Med Assoc Thai* 88 Suppl 1: S30-S34, 2005.

20. **Clarke R, Lewington S, Sherliker P and Armitage J**. Effects of B-vitamins on plasma homocysteine concentrations and on risk of cardiovascular disease and dementia. *Curr Opin Clin Nutr Metab Care* 10: 32-39, 2007.

21. **Clarkson PM and Thompson HS**. Drugs and sport. Research findings and limitations. *Sports Med* 24: 366-384, 1997.

22. **Costill DL, Cote R and Fink W**. Muscle water and electrolytes following varied levels of dehydration in man. *J Appl Physiol* 40: 6-11, 1976.

23. **Coyle EF**. Fluid and fuel intake during exercise. *J Sports Sci* 22: 39-55, 2004.

24. **Czernichow S, Blacher J and Hercberg S**. Antioxidant vitamins and blood pressure. *Curr Hypertens Rep* 6: 27-30, 2004.

25. **Czernichow S, Blacher J and Hercberg S**. Antioxidant vitamins and blood pressure. *Curr Hypertens Rep* 6: 27-30, 2004.

26. **Delgado MC**. Potassium in hypertension. *Curr Hypertens Rep* 6: 31-35, 2004.

27. **Evans TM, Rundell KW, Beck KC, Levine AM and Baumann JM**. Airway narrowing measured by spirometry and impulse oscillometry following room temperature and cold temperature exercise. *Chest* 128: 2412-2419, 2005.

28. **Finaud J, Lac G and Filaire E**. Oxidative stress : relationship with exercise and training. *Sports Med* 36: 327-358, 2006.

29. **Francis RM**. Calcium, vitamin D and involutional osteoporosis. *Curr Opin Clin Nutr Metab Care* 9: 13-17, 2006.

30. **Genser D, Prachar H, Hauer R, Halbmayer WM, Mlczoch J and Elmadfa I**. Homocysteine, folate and vitamin b12 in patients with coronary heart disease. *Ann Nutr Metab* 50: 413-419, 2006.

31. **Goodman LR and Warren MP**. The female athlete and menstrual function. *Curr Opin Obstet Gynecol* 17: 466-470, 2005.

32. **Grenon SM, Sheynberg N, Hurwitz S, Xiao G, Ramsdell CD, Ehrman MD, Mai CL, Kristjansson SR, Sundby GH, Cohen RJ and Williams GH**. Renal, endocrine, and cardiovascular responses to bed rest in male subjects on a constant diet. *J Investig Med* 52: 117-128, 2004.

33. **Grucza R, Szczypaczewska M and Kozlowski S**. Thermoregulation in hyperhydrated men during physical exercise. *Eur J Appl Physiol Occup Physiol* 56: 603-607, 1987.

34. **Hallberg L and Hulthen L**. Perspectives on iron absorption. *Blood Cells Mol Dis* 29: 562-573, 2002.

35. **Halsted CH**. Absorption of water-soluble vitamins. *Curr Opin Gastroenterol* 19: 113-117, 2003.

36. **Hamad N and Travis SP**. Weight loss at high altitude: pathophysiology and practical implications. *Eur J Gastroenterol Hepatol* 18: 5-10, 2006.

37. **Harvey LJ, Armah CN, Dainty JR, Foxall RJ, John LD, Langford NJ and Fairweather-Tait SJ**. Impact of menstrual blood loss and diet on iron deficiency among women in the UK. *Br J Nutr* 94: 557-564, 2005.

38. **Hosoi T**. [Calcium requirement for the maintenance of bone mass]. *Clin Calcium* 11: 163-167, 2001.

39. **Hosoi T**. [Calcium requirement for the maintenance of bone mass]. *Clin Calcium* 11: 163-167, 2001.

40. **Jeukendrup AE, Jentjens RL and Moseley L**. Nutritional considerations in triathlon. *Sports Med* 35: 163-181, 2005.

41. **Kamel HK**. Postmenopausal osteoporosis: etiology, current diagnostic strategies, and nonprescription interventions. *J Manag Care Pharm* 12: 4-9, 2006.

42. **Kanter M**. Free radicals, exercise and antioxidant supplementation. *Proc Nutr Soc* 57: 9-13, 1998.

43. **Kennedy E and Meyers L**. Dietary Reference Intakes: development and uses for assessment of micronutrient status of women--a global perspective. *Am J Clin Nutr* 81: 1194S-1197S, 2005.

44. **Kleiner SM**. Water: an essential but overlooked nutrient. *J Am Diet Assoc* 99: 200-206, 1999.

45. **Kleiner SM**. Water: an essential but overlooked nutrient. *J Am Diet Assoc* 99: 200-206, 1999.

46. **Kleiner SM**. Water: an essential but overlooked nutrient. *J Am Diet Assoc* 99: 200-206, 1999.

47. **Kleiner SM**. Water: an essential but overlooked nutrient. *J Am Diet Assoc* 99: 200-206, 1999.

48. **Kontic-Vucinic O, Sulovic N and Radunovic N**. Micronutrients in women's reproductive health: II. Minerals and trace elements. *Int J Fertil Womens Med* 51: 116-124, 2006.

49. **Koulmann N, Banzet S and Bigard AX**. [Physical activity in the heat: physiology of hydration recommendations]. *Med Trop (Mars)* 63: 617-626, 2003.

50. **Latzka WA and Montain SJ**. Water and electrolyte requirements for exercise. *Clin Sports Med* 18: 513-524, 1999.

51. **Latzka WA and Montain SJ**. Water and electrolyte requirements for exercise. *Clin Sports Med* 18: 513-524, 1999.

52. **Lopez MA and Martos FC**. Iron availability: An updated review. *Int J Food Sci Nutr* 55: 597-606, 2004.

53. **Lopez MA and Martos FC**. Iron availability: An updated review. *Int J Food Sci Nutr* 55: 597-606, 2004.

54. **Magnusson B, Hallberg L, Rossander L and Swolin B**. Iron metabolism and "sports anemia". I. A study of several iron parameters in elite runners with differences in iron status. *Acta Med Scand* 216: 149-155, 1984.

55. **Malczewska J, Raczynski G and Stupnicki R**. Iron status in female endurance athletes and in non-athletes. *Int J Sport Nutr Exerc Metab* 10: 260-276, 2000.

56. **Marlin DJ, Scott CM, Mills PC, Louwes H and Vaarten J**. Rehydration following exercise: effects of administration of water versus an isotonic oral rehydration solution (ORS). *Vet J* 156: 41-49, 1998.

57. **Mason NP and Barry PW**. Altitude-related cough. *Pulm Pharmacol Ther* 2006.

58. **Maughan RJ, Owen JH, Shirreffs SM and Leiper JB**. Post-exercise rehydration in man: effects of electrolyte addition to ingested fluids. *Eur J Appl Physiol Occup Physiol* 69: 209-215, 1994.

59. **Morris RC, Jr., Schmidlin O, Frassetto LA and Sebastian A**. Relationship and interaction between sodium and potassium. *J Am Coll Nutr* 25: 262S-270S, 2006.

60. **Murray R**. Fluid needs in hot and cold environments. *Int J Sport Nutr* 5 Suppl: S62-S73, 1995.

61. **Naghii MR**. The significance of water in sport and weight control. *Nutr Health* 14: 127-132, 2000.

62. **Oliveras Lopez MJ, Nieto GP, Agudo AE, Martinez MF, Lopez Garcia de la Serrana and Lopez Martinez MC**. [Nutritional assessment of a university population]. *Nutr Hosp* 21: 179-183, 2006.

63. **Omaye ST**. Safety of megavitamin therapy. *Adv Exp Med Biol* 177: 169-203, 1984.

64. **Papanek PE**. The female athlete triad: an emerging role for physical therapy. *J Orthop Sports Phys Ther* 33: 594-614, 2003.

65. **Phillips PA, Johnston CI and Gray L.** Disturbed fluid and electrolyte homoeostasis following dehydration in elderly people. *Age Ageing* 22: S26-S33, 1993.

66. **Porth CM and Erickson M.** Physiology of thirst and drinking: implication for nursing practice. *Heart Lung* 21: 273-282, 1992.

67. **Rehrer NJ.** Fluid and electrolyte balance in ultra-endurance sport. *Sports Med* 31: 701-715, 2001.

68. **Riccioni G, Bucciarelli T, Mancini B, Di Ilio C, Capra V and D'Orazio N.** The role of the antioxidant vitamin supplementation in the prevention of cardiovascular diseases. *Expert Opin Investig Drugs* 16: 25-32, 2007.

69. **Riccioni G, Bucciarelli T, Mancini B, Di Ilio C, Capra V and D'Orazio N.** The role of the antioxidant vitamin supplementation in the prevention of cardiovascular diseases. *Expert Opin Investig Drugs* 16: 25-32, 2007.

70. **Sarvazyan A, Tatarinov A and Sarvazyan N.** Ultrasonic assessment of tissue hydration status. *Ultrasonics* 43: 661-671, 2005.

71. **Sawka MN and Montain SJ.** Fluid and electrolyte supplementation for exercise heat stress. *Am J Clin Nutr* 72: 564S-572S, 2000.

72. **Sawka MN and Montain SJ.** Fluid and electrolyte supplementation for exercise heat stress. *Am J Clin Nutr* 72: 564S-572S, 2000.

73. **Sawka MN and Montain SJ.** Fluid and electrolyte supplementation for exercise heat stress. *Am J Clin Nutr* 72: 564S-572S, 2000.

74. **Sawka MN, Montain SJ and Latzka WA.** Hydration effects on thermoregulation and performance in the heat. *Comp Biochem Physiol A Mol Integr Physiol* 128: 679-690, 2001.

75. **Sawka MN, Montain SJ and Latzka WA.** Hydration effects on thermoregulation and performance in the heat. *Comp Biochem Physiol A Mol Integr Physiol* 128: 679-690, 2001.

76. **Sawka MN, Montain SJ and Latzka WA.** Hydration effects on thermoregulation and performance in the heat. *Comp Biochem Physiol A Mol Integr Physiol* 128: 679-690, 2001.

77. **Schmid A, Jakob E, Berg A, Russmann T, Konig D, Irmer M and Keul J.** Effect of physical exercise and vitamin C on absorption of ferric sodium citrate. *Med Sci Sports Exerc* 28: 1470-1473, 1996.

78. **Schmidt F, Shin P, Jorgensen TM, Djurhuus JC and Constantinou CE.** Urodynamic patterns of normal male micturition: influence of water consumption on urine production and detrusor function. *J Urol* 168: 1458-1463, 2002.

79. **Schroder H, Navarro E, Tramullas A, Mora J and Galiano D.** Nutrition antioxidant status and oxidative stress in professional basketball players: effects of a three compound antioxidative supplement. *Int J Sports Med* 21: 146-150, 2000.

80. **Schroder S.** [Is the supplementation with antioxidants effective in the treatment of atherosclerosis?]. *Dtsch Med Wochenschr* 129: 321-326, 2004.

81. **Schroder S.** [Is the supplementation with antioxidants effective in the treatment of atherosclerosis?]. *Dtsch Med Wochenschr* 129: 321-326, 2004.

82. **Stachenfeld NS, DiPietro L, Nadel ER and Mack GW.** Mechanism of attenuated thirst in aging: role of central volume receptors. *Am J Physiol* 272: R148-R157, 1997.

83. **Stachenfeld NS, DiPietro L, Nadel ER and Mack GW.** Mechanism of attenuated thirst in aging: role of central volume receptors. *Am J Physiol* 272: R148-R157, 1997.

84. **Sugimoto T.** [Calcium intake and bone mass]. *Clin Calcium* 11: 193-197, 2001.

85. **Sugimoto T.** [Calcium intake and bone mass]. *Clin Calcium* 11: 193-197, 2001.

86. **Sugimoto T.** [Calcium intake and bone mass]. *Clin Calcium* 11: 193-197, 2001.

87. **Teucher B, Olivares M and Cori H.** Enhancers of iron absorption: ascorbic acid and other organic acids. *Int J Vitam Nutr Res* 74: 403-419, 2004.

88. **Thompson J.** Vitamins, minerals and supplements: part two. *Community Pract* 78: 366-368, 2005.

89. **Thompson J.** Vitamins, minerals and supplements: part two. *Community Pract* 78: 366-368, 2005.

90. **Villar J, Abdel-Aleem H, Merialdi M, Mathai M, Ali MM, Zavaleta N, Purwar M, Hofmeyr J, Nguyen TN, Campodonico L, Landoulsi S, Carroli G and Lindheimer M.** World Health Organization randomized trial of calcium supplementation among low calcium intake pregnant women. *Am J Obstet Gynecol* 194: 639-649, 2006.

91. **Von Duvillard SP, Braun WA, Markofski M, Beneke R and Leithauser R**. Fluids and hydration in prolonged endurance performance. *Nutrition* 20: 651-656, 2004.

92. **Von Duvillard SP, Braun WA, Markofski M, Beneke R and Leithauser R**. Fluids and hydration in prolonged endurance performance. *Nutrition* 20: 651-656, 2004.

93. **Warren LK, Lawrence LM, Brewster-Barnes T and Powell DM**. The effect of dietary fibre on hydration status after dehydration with frusemide. *Equine Vet J Suppl* 30: 508-513, 1999.

94. **Weight LM, Byrne MJ and Jacobs P**. Haemolytic effects of exercise. *Clin Sci (Lond)* 81: 147-152, 1991.

95. **Wertli M and Suter PM**. [Water--the forgotten nutrient]. *Schweiz Rundsch Med Prax* 95: 1489-1495, 2006.

96. **Wertli M and Suter PM**. [Water--the forgotten nutrient]. *Schweiz Rundsch Med Prax* 95: 1489-1495, 2006.

97. **Wester PO**. Electrolyte balance in heart failure and the role for magnesium ions. *Am J Cardiol* 70: 44C-49C, 1992.

98. **Westerterp KR, Plasqui G and Goris AH**. Water loss as a function of energy intake, physical activity and season. *Br J Nutr* 93: 199-203, 2005.

99. **Youngkin EQ and Thomas DJ**. Vitamins: common supplements and therapy. *Nurse Pract* 24: 50, 53, 57-50, 53, 60, 1999.

100. **Youngkin EQ and Thomas DJ**. Vitamins: common supplements and therapy. *Nurse Pract* 24: 50, 53, 57-50, 53, 60, 1999.

101. **Youngkin EQ and Thomas DJ**. Vitamins: common supplements and therapy. *Nurse Pract* 24: 50, 53, 57-50, 53, 60, 1999.

102. **Yu-Yahiro JA**. Electrolytes and their relationship to normal and abnormal muscle function. *Orthop Nurs* 13: 38-40, 1994.

103. **Yu-Yahiro JA**. Electrolytes and their relationship to normal and abnormal muscle function. *Orthop Nurs* 13: 38-40, 1994.

104. **Yu-Yahiro JA**. Electrolytes and their relationship to normal and abnormal muscle function. *Orthop Nurs* 13: 38-40, 1994.

105. **Yukawa H and Suzuki T**. [Dietary calcium and women's health]. *Clin Calcium* 11: 157-162, 2001.

106. **Zhou MS, Adam AG, Jaimes EA and Raij L**. In salt-sensitive hypertension, increased superoxide production is linked to functional upregulation of angiotensin II. *Hypertension* 42: 945-951, 2003.

Chapter 9

Nutritional Supplementation

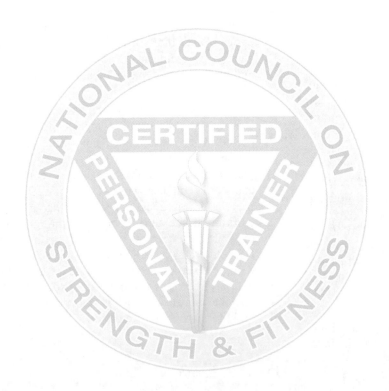

Introduction

The nutritional requirements of every person may differ in some capacity due to the broad number of factors that affect the nutritional needs of an individual. When greater physiological and psychological stress acts upon the body, the need for supportive nutrients increases. The specific type of demand dictates the change in nutritional needs. When the increased stress is from physical activity, the mode, intensity, and duration all become relevant factors in determining the correct nutritional make up of the diet. For instance, heavy resistance training requires different nutritional adjustments than long distance running. The amount of energy used during activity and the physiological recovery and repair mechanisms differentiate the nutrition for optimal performance.

Glycogen Storage

During high-volume, heavy resistance training, glycogen stores in the muscle provides the largest portion of calories for work. For this reason, it is important to maximize glycogen stores before engaging in this type of exercise bout. Cellular glycogen saturation is best initiated immediately following the previous exercise bout. The heightened metabolic environment created from physical exertion causes the depleted cells to more efficiently absorb nutrients. During the three hours immediately post-exercise, cells have an increased permeability to cellular nutrients and an increased sensitivity to anabolic hormones, including insulin (77; 135; 152). Consuming a mixture of protein (6-10 grams) and carbohydrates increases both glycogen saturation and protein synthesis in the muscle tissue under optimal conditions (18; 78).

The quantity of carbohydrates consumed should reflect the caloric expenditure of the previous exercise bout (76). Research suggests that within the first hour following exercise, 1-2 grams of carbohydrate should be consumed for each kilogram of body weight (75; 78). Several studies suggest that during intense training programs, the total replenishment of carbohydrates should reach up to 10 g of carbohydrate per kilogram of body weight and be consumed over the course of several hours following each exercise bout (23; 80). A key factor in glycogen replenishment is the total energy utilized from carbohydrates versus other sources (i.e. fat, protein) during exercise. When glycogen is significantly depleted, it becomes more difficult to fully refuel for the next event.

Immediately following an exercise bout, high glycemic foods (foods with a carbohydrate component that is quickly absorbed into the blood stream) are an ideal choice for carbohydrate replenishment (25). The internal biological environment makes better use of the energy, which quickly enters circulation. Cellular availability of nutrients is very important to the post-exercise metabolic process. This is true for both stop-and-go anaerobic activities typical of resistance training, as well as sustained aerobic exercise events (24; 102; 131). Research trials consistently found that inadequate carbohydrate consumption in the hours following exercise led to reduced performance in subsequent training bouts. Based on these findings, many athletes and high intensity exercisers utilize post-exercise recovery drinks. Carbohydrate-electrolyte solutions can contribute to replenishment, but are often inadequate in calories to fully satisfy the recovery demands. Additional carbohydrate sources should be consumed to reflect adequate caloric intake of the appropriate nutrients.

Recovery beverages or commercially blended meal replacement drinks can be ideal alternatives to regular food due to their easy digestibility and convenience. The actual energy breakdown of the beverages varies by manufacturer and the particular intention of the product. Protein drinks consumed immediately after exercise can contribute to tissue recovery, but are generally too low in carbohydrates to replenish glycogen stores and are excessive for protein synthesis stimulation. Fluid energy mixtures which provide both carbohydrates and protein can be an ideal solution for post-exercise energy consumption when appropriate food sources are not available. Possible benefits include increased digestibility and absorption rates compared to many whole food choices and the convenience of the supplemental energy, providing a practical alternative to the labor and time requirements of meal preparation.

Glycogen storage can also be enhanced by pre-exercise food consumption. Following sleep or any 8-12 hour period when eating does not occur, glycogen stores become reduced. Pre-activity fuel should be mainly in the form of carbohydrates to encourage adequate energy for intense work. Consuming a meal high in protein or fat does not satisfy the energy needs of working tissue during heavy training and slows the digestion process when mixed with carbohydrates. Carbohydrates consumed approximately 3 hours before the exercise bout provide adequate time for digestion and absorption of the nutrients. Adequate fluid should also be consumed during this period to prepare the body for activity participation.

Supplements and Ergogenic Aids

To further enhance physical performance, many exercisers and athletes use supplements in addition to their dietary intake of nutrients. The term **supplement** simply means replacing nutrients that are required for proper nutrition but are not being met through normal dietary intake. When supplements are taken above what is necessary for normal homeostasis with the intention of performance enhancement, they are classified as **ergogenic aids**. Dietary ergogenic aids are supplemental nutrients or compounds that are consumed for the purpose of enhancing a physiological or psychological effect via improvements by one or more functions of the body. The most common dietary supplements are multi-vitamin mineral pills. They represent the largest portion of the dietary supplement industry and are estimated to cover 70-90% of all supplements marketed (3; 91; 136). According to the American Dietetic Association, more than 50% of adults have taken or currently take vitamin pills in addition to their normal dietary intakes. Many exercisers also believe that taking additional vitamins is necessary for improved performance and health (119).

~Key Terms~

Supplement- A substance added to the diet to make up for a deficiency.

Ergogenic Aids- Any external influences which can positively affect physical performance or mental focus.

Goals of Fluid Replacement Drinks

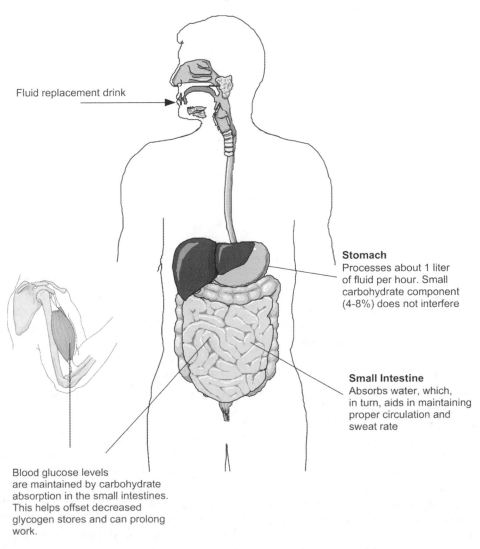

Fluid replacement drink

Stomach
Processes about 1 liter of fluid per hour. Small carbohydrate component (4-8%) does not interfere

Small Intestine
Absorbs water, which, in turn, aids in maintaining proper circulation and sweat rate

Blood glucose levels are maintained by carbohydrate absorption in the small intestines. This helps offset decreased glycogen stores and can prolong work.

Common Sports Drinks

Drink	Carbohydrate Type	Carbohydrate Grams	Calories	Sodium	Potassium
Gatorade	Sucrose, Glucose, & Fructose	14	50	110	30
Powerade	High fructose corn syrup & Glucose Polymers (Maltodextrins)	19	70	55	30
All-Sport	High fructose corn syrup	19	70	55	55
Hydrafuel	Glucose, Glucose polymers, & Fructose	16	66	25	50
1st Ade	High fructose corn syrup, Glucose, Fructose, & Sucrose	16	60	55	25
Coca-Cola	High fructose corn syrup	27	103	69	0
Orange Juice	Sucrose, Fructose, & Glucose	25	104	6	436

For many people, the hardest concept to accept is that "more is not always better." If adequate nutrition is attained in the diet, additional intake of supplements simply adds chemical agents to the body. Over 50 years of research concludes that additional supplementation above adequate nutritional intake values for the individual will not provide exercise performance enhancement. For most people, ingesting additional vitamin and minerals above the recommended dietary upper limit required by the body will simply cause any excess to be excreted in the urine or become processed by the liver and add an increase risk of toxicity poisoning in tissues (2; 4; 74; 157; 165). Will a single multi-vitamin hurt? Certainly not, but caution should be taken when consuming mega-vitamins, particularly when also consuming other supplements (27; 139; 166)

Exercise does increase the nutrient demands of the body, so intense exercisers should be mindful to track their intake of vitamins and minerals, particularly antioxidants (141; 160). Again, the Upper Tolerable Intake Limit should provide the ceiling for prudent ingestion. A variety of food sources, particularly plant-based foods, should be used to meet the majority of vitamin and mineral needs of the body (34; 161).

Vitamins and minerals are not the only supplements used for performance enhancement. Numerous nutrients, compounds, and chemical agents are purported to enhance most performance-related physiological functions. They are generally categorized by the specific "claimed" effect the supplement is supposed to have on the body. The following list includes the most popular categories found in most nutrition stores.

~Quick Insight~

The supplement industry is a "buyer beware" market. The FDA regulates dietary supplements under a different set of regulations than those covering "conventional" foods and drug products (prescription and over-the-counter). Under the Dietary Supplement Health and Education Act of 1994 (DSHEA), the dietary supplement manufacturer is responsible for ensuring that a dietary supplement is safe before it is marketed. The FDA is responsible for taking action against any unsafe dietary supplement product after it reaches the market. Generally, manufacturers do not need to register their products with the FDA or get FDA approval before producing or selling dietary supplements. Manufacturers must make sure that product label information is truthful and not misleading.

The self-regulation of the supplement industry has created an environment where almost anything goes, just as long as the label of the product being sold does not make a medical claim or suggest that the product can cure or prevent a disease. These loose reins on the billion dollar supplement industry have opened the gates to unethical "health hustling." A limited number of supplements reviewed by scientifically sound research trials have shown efficacy in performance enhancement or effective weight loss.

The labels are also of concern when buying supplements. Numerous well-controlled studies have found inconsistencies in the potency and implied or listed concentrations of the active ingredients on supplement labels. Companies manufacturing and selling supplements are not necessarily scrutinized for quality control practices. If supplements are purchased, they should come only from reputable companies.

Beware of advertising and marketing that uses testimonials, "independent research" trials, celebrity endorsements, guarantees of quick results, and "secret" ingredients. Other suspicious marketing buzzwords include "Doctor recommended" or "physician approved," amazing results, pharmaceutical label appearances, or free trial give-away offers. Likewise, when the findings do not match the conventional wisdom of science or governmental recommendations and the research is not published in peer-reviewed journals, this evidence points directly at a questionable approach. Scientifically valid information is extremely welcome and exchanged amongst the top scientists and researchers. This lends itself to question why supplement "research" is often done independently of these prestigious circles if it is actually valid.

Popular Nutrition Store Categories

Muscle Gain

Weight Loss

Anti-aging

Improved Energy/Endurance

Pro Hormones

Sports Performance

Multi-vitamin

Herbs

Hundreds of products fall within these categories. The claims associated with the consumption of the dietary supplements range dramatically. Some products are purported to offer numerous health benefits, while others advertise that consumption will improve a single function of the body. Due to the vastness in product offerings and limited peer-reviewed literature supporting the claims, only the most popular supplements are reviewed below.

Mass and Strength Gains

When the emphasis of the training focuses on muscle hypertrophy, many exercisers and body builders ingest compounds that supposedly aid in the formation of new muscle mass. The most common ergogenic aids include **creatine monohydrate**, supplemental protein, branch chain amino acids, **glutamine**, **nitric oxide**, and **HMB**. The proposed mechanism for improving muscle mass is not the same in each of the dietary supplements. In many cases, individuals ingest several of these supplements to take advantage of a possible synergistic effect.

Creatine

Creatine was first identified by a French scientist in the 1800's. It is a naturally occurring protein that serves as an anaerobic source of immediate energy. The majority (60%) of the creatine in the body is stored in the skeletal muscle as phosphocreatine, with the other 40% found in the free unphosphorylated creatine form.

Creatine is also found in the muscle of animals, so foods such as meat, poultry, and fish provide natural dietary sources. These foods contain approximately 4 to 5 g of creatine per kg of food.

In the human body, the liver, kidneys, and pancreas produce creatine from the non-essential amino acids arginine, glycine, and methionine. The body only synthesizes about 1 to 2 g of creatine a day, which is utilized during physical activity. The molecular structure of creatine makes it heavy; therefore, the body does not maintain large stores, preferring instead to re-phosphorylate the molecule into its active form as dictated by energy demands. Although creatine concentrations are greatest in fast-twitch fibers, slow-twitch fibers more efficiently re-phosphorylate the molecule. No significant differences distinguish the creatine in males and females nor does exercise increase one's storage capacity. Creatine is the primary energy used for immediate high-force output exercise and is also involved in acid buffering, as well as glycolysis regulation.

Creatine monohydrate is the supplement form of creatine formed from sarcosine and cyanamide. Studies have shown that the supplementation of 20-25 g per day for 3-5 days increases intramuscular creatine (10-30%) and phosphocreatine (the phosphorylated active form) stores (10-40%) (14). The magnitude of the concentration enhancements correlate to initial levels of creatine in the body prior to supplementation. The increased concentrations are associated with improved short-term performance of intense exercise and rate of resynthesis back into the active form during rest intervals (13; 97; 123). In addition to improvements in immediate energy availability, creatine also associates with an increase in body mass, which may be due to increases of fat-free mass and/or fluid retention (100). Currently, there are mixed views as to the causes of the mass gains (150). No conclusive evidence suggests that creatine supplementation aids in long-duration activities, such as running (41). It is important to note that scientific investigations have reported equivocal results, with fairly equal numbers of significant and non-significant findings supporting creatine's efficaciousness.

Creatine is usually consumed in cycles of loading and maintenance phases. The loading phase usually requires an individual to consume 20 to 30 g of creatine for 5 to 6 days (132). It appears that an upper limit for total creatine is approximately 160 mmol/kg of dry muscle (4). After a specific amount of creatine storage is attained, the excess is excreted in the urine. The maintenance phase uses a smaller dosage to maintain creatine stores after the loading phase. This

Proposed Mechanism of How Creatine Enhances Performance

1. **Increased intramuscular creatine and phosphocreatine content**

2. **Greater resynthesis of phosphocreatine**

3. **Increased metabolic efficiency**

4. **Enhanced adaptations with training**

phase usually uses consumption rates of 2-5g per day, which reflect two times the turnover rate by the body (133).

Anecdotal reports of side effects associated with creatine supplementation have included abdominal cramping, muscle cramping, stiffness, and strains. These case studies, though, do not represent well-controlled trials, so no causal relationship between creatine supplementation and these side-effects has yet been established. Since activities associated with creatine as the primary fuel are short duration, high intensity, these types of activities alone may result in these types of symptoms. Abdominal cramping or diarrhea may also occur when consuming excessive amounts of creatine, particularly during the loading phases. The current research does not provide evidence of clinically significant side effects (62; 117; 140). Long-term studies may be necessary to determine if excessive amounts of creatine will have adverse effects on the liver, kidneys, or cardiac muscle. Individuals taking creatine should be educated regarding proper dosages. Additionally, caffeine ingestion with creatine has been shown to negate creatine's ergogenic effects.

Protein

Without question, protein is the key component in forming and repairing muscle tissue. Protein plays an integral role in muscle growth and remodeling through protein synthesis. In muscle tissue, amino acids interact with one another to form structural and contractile proteins, aiding in the muscle's production of force. These contractile proteins increase in size and number with appropriate resistance training, therefore causing an increase in the cross sectional area of the muscle, contributing to muscle hypertrophy.

The Recommended Daily Allowance (RDA) for protein and amino acids is 0.9 gram of protein per kilogram of body weight in sedentary populations or 12-15 % of the calories in the total daily diet. The average American diet easily supplies this amount of protein, with most people exceeding their requirements

(151; 169). Depending on the type of activity they engage in, individuals with increased activity levels may have higher requirements for proteins than the RDA recommendation (168). Studies suggest that the highest recommended intake of protein is 2.0 g/kg of body weight (106; 107). This level of protein intake only appears beneficial for competitive power lifters and body builders (101).

The consumption of excessive amounts of protein has not been shown to create additional muscle growth (39). The effect of greater protein synthesis efficiency negates the increased protein recommendations set by other research. Exercise has been shown to increase the efficiency with which the body utilizes protein, making it unnecessary to increase protein consumption above relative need for the maximal protein synthetic response (19; 118; 137). Routine protein consumption above the recommended levels can place added stress on the liver and kidneys, and the excess is either converted and stored as triglycerides and carbohydrates, or excreted in part via urine (114).

Making sure the body has readily available protein is the key to protein synthesis. Without the appropriate amount of available protein, a catabolic environment is created. This is not the optimal situation for gains in muscle size or strength. Protein consumption prior to, and post-exercise, optimizes muscle hypertrophy (17; 36; 159). Consuming protein within three hours post-workout creates the best anabolic environment. The most effective absorption is seen with a protein and carbohydrate mix. This combination likely enhances nutrient uptake via hormonal mechanisms. This mix may be as simple as a glass of milk (87). Post-exercise insulin concentrations stimulated by carbohydrate intake speed the movement of amino acids into muscle cells, thus promoting muscle hypertrophy or muscle repair (167).

No evidence confirms the effectiveness of consuming dietary protein supplements over quality protein sources found in food such as beef, fish, poultry, eggs, and milk. The protein source seems to play a role in its effectiveness. Complete proteins derived from animal sources seem to be more effective than plant sources. Of the supplemental proteins, whey protein has been argued to be a better form than other sources, particularly those derived from plants (33).

Whey Protein

Whey is a high-quality protein with vast nutritional properties that occurs naturally in cow's milk. Whey protein is a complete protein containing all eight essential amino acids. It is extracted and purified in the

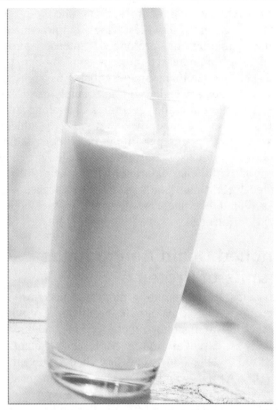

Whey and Casein proteins occur naturally in cow's milk.

cheese making process. Protein synthesis is positively affected by the fast-absorbing whey protein, yielding the greatest benefits (32). Consumption should occur within an hour of an exercise bout due to the rapid absorption and permeability of the cell membrane. Whey also contains glutathione, a powerful antioxidant that boosts immune function. This may provide an additional benefit for strength training athletes, who may compromise their immune systems through intense training (22; 31; 64). Whey protein in its pure form contains very little fat, cholesterol, or lactose (making it an excellent milk substitute for lactose intolerant individuals).

Casein Protein

Casein is also a high quality protein and represents the highest percentage of protein found in milk. Casein has a slower release of amino acids and is not ideal for rapid protein replacement post-exercise. Glutamine, an anti-catabolic amino acid, is found in high concentrations in casein. Due to the body's slow digestion rate of casein, it should be consumed in the evening during rest. Casein does contain a small amount of lactose or milk sugar that could cause a problem for lactose intolerant individuals. The theory that consuming excess protein facilitates greater gains in muscle size is false, as is the theory that body builders require 1 g of protein per pound of body weight to support muscle function during heavy training. Energy intakes are activity and body size specific. In general, activities which employ intense resistance training or prolonged, intense aerobic exercise warrant increased protein consumption (38; 61; 108). Most dietitians suggest that 1.6 grams per kilogram of body weight will adequately meet any protein demand, but higher quantities of protein can be tolerated for competitive strength athletes; approximately 2 grams per kilogram of body weight (60; 109). Individuals who exceed this value are likely consuming additional calories, which may lead to unwanted weight gain and in some cases, cause renal distress due to the increase demand on the kidneys from excess nitrogen.

Branched Chain Amino Acids– Subunits of Proteins

Amino acids are the building blocks of proteins. The body requires approximately 20 amino acids, of which eight (nine in infants and sometimes older adults) are classified as essential amino acids that cannot be synthesized by the body. The branched chain amino acids (BCAA) are essential amino acids that must be consumed in the diet. Valine, isoleucine, and leucine are the BCAAs that account for one third of the protein in muscle tissue. This significant contribution makes them important for muscle remodeling and functioning of the muscle cells.

Long duration endurance activities use protein as a fuel source when glucose is depleted. Branched chain amino acids easily convert to fuel, sparing other amino acids (53; 104). This process decreases the catabolic effect by sparing other proteins (16).

Whey protein contains a high concentration of BCAAs. This group of amino acids also serves as precursors to other muscle building amino acids such as glutamine and **alanine** (70; 103). Glutamine is a non-essential amino acid that aids in the recovery and rebuilding of muscle. Strength training depletes the concentrations of

Branched Chain Amino Acids

Valine	Isoleucine	Leucine
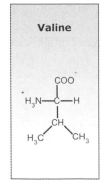	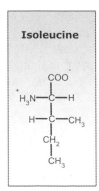	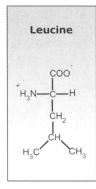

Creatine Monohydrate- A nitrogenous organic acid that is found in the muscle tissue in the form of phosphocreatine and supplies energy for muscle contraction.

HMB- A compound that minimizes the breakdown of protein and damage to muscle cells.

Glutamine- A non-essential amino acid that occurs widely in proteins, blood, and other tissues.

Nitric Oxide- A powerful smooth muscle relaxant involved in oxygen transport to the tissues, the transmission of nerve impulses, and other physiological activities.

Alanine- An amino acid that is a constituent of many proteins.

glutamine and alanine, but due to the fact that these amino acids are non-essential, they are resynthesized within the body from the BCAA.

Additional consumption or supplementation of amino acids over what the body requires does not increase strength or endurance (54). If an activity decreases the concentration of essential amino acids, replenishment is necessary, but excessive amounts do not have an added benefit, other than contributing to a positive caloric balance.

Increased amounts of amino acids in the body can actually cause adverse effects (52). Similar to the discussion regarding minerals, balance is the key to function. Excessive amounts of one type of amino acid can cause biochemical competition for other amino acids. Any imbalance can lead to a deficiency. Digestion of excessive amounts of BCAA may cause gastrointestinal discomfort and/or place added stress on the liver or kidneys (51).

Glutamine

Glutamine is a non-essential, naturally occurring amino acid found within the muscle cell. During prolonged exercise, proteins are used as fuel source for muscle contractions. Amino acids, such as glutamine, are used as precursors for gluconeogenesis in the formation of glycogen. Muscular contractions release glutamine into the blood stream, which is taken to the liver to form glucose for energy during exercise. This process reduces the catabolic effect or protein degradation during exercise recovery (162).

Supplementing glutamine is thought to increase post-exercise glycogen stores and reduce the amount of protein degradation from **glucocorticoids**, positively affecting muscle size (7). Other claims include protein sparing and increased buffering capacity of lactic acid, consequently increasing the time until fatigue. This would allow for a longer and more intense training session and greater gains with decreased recovery times. Furthermore, some evidence exists to support glutamine in the reduction of upper respiratory infections during long duration activities (144).

The premise behind glutamine supplementation is to reduce functional changes in muscle tissue and negative nitrogen metabolism. Increasing glutamine is intended to decrease the use of protein for fuel, decreasing the catabolic effect of muscle wasting (11). Some data on animals shows that glutamine infusion effectively counteracts glucocorticoid-induced muscle atrophy. **Atrophy** attenuation appears related to the maintenance of muscle glutamine levels, which in turn, may limit the glucocorticoid-mediated down regulation of myosin heavy chain synthesis (116; 138). However, studies have not shown that glutamine supplementation has a direct effect on protein sparing and/or decreases in muscle wasting in humans in response to normal exercise. It has shown some promise in excessive stress states, such as burn victims and later stage HIV (AIDS) patients, but not in normally trained individuals consuming adequate nutrients (1; 28). Glutamine supplementation and resistance training during a six

week study showed no difference in strength, torque, or lean body mass compared to a placebo (26; 42).

Although glutamine seems to be ineffective when consumed by healthy individuals that meet their protein requirements, it may have merit when mixed with other amino acids (30). One study examining the use of supplemental protein, a mixture of whey protein and glutamine, showed an increase in muscle strength with consumption (29). When mixed with creatine similar benefits were found (105). This data suggest that a supplement containing key amino acids may contribute positively to an improvement in training efficiency through positive effects on muscle integrity and **hematopoiesis.** The key question is the role glutamine plays, when used within a supplement mixture.

L-arginine

L-arginine (arginine) is a semi-essential or conditional amino acid produced naturally in the body that is purported to have numerous beneficial effects. The normal functions of arginine include aiding in protein synthesis, increasing immune and nervous system function, increasing oxygen delivery to the heart, and regulating growth hormone levels. For athletes and body builders, the claim that arginine plays a role in growth hormone stimulation is of particular interest. Increasing growth hormone levels promotes strength, lean body mass, and the reduction of body fat. Laboratory results do show an increase in growth hormone with very large doses of arginine. However, arginine does not have the same effects when used at the recommended over-the-counter dosages as it does with laboratory dosages that would be clearly unsafe for use by the general population. Therefore, L-arginine remains a non-essential amino acid, falsely promoted as enhancing the secretion of growth hormone, the breakdown of fat, and the development of muscle when dietary intakes are sufficient.

Another claim that is of interest to athletes is that arginine may have a positive impact on protein synthesis when coupled with other amino acids (126). The evidence that arginine supplementation increases strength gains and lean body mass are inconclusive. Abel et al. reported increases in strength gains

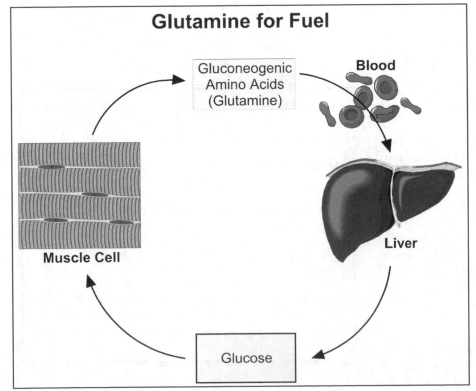

Glutamine for Fuel

Gluconeogenic Amino Acids (Glutamine)

Blood

Liver

Muscle Cell

Glucose

and lean body mass, whereas Marcell et al. stated that arginine did not increase growth hormone levels at rest or with resistance training (6; 112). Supplementation did increase plasma concentrations of glucagon, urea, and somatotrophic hormone with ingestion of 15 g of arginine daily for 14 days prior to a marathon. This study did not show any increase in plasma creatine kinase activity, insulin, ammonia, or respiratory exchange ratio accompanying arginine use (124). Research also has shown that arginine supplementation in some clinical settings involving trauma, such as burn injuries and sepsis, may maintain lean muscle mass and functional capacity (125). However, there is little data to support that arginine has the same effect in healthy individuals. Though arginine is a precursor for nitric oxide and creatine, the effects of supplemental arginine as an ergogenic aid have been inconclusive (5).

As mentioned above, arginine serves as a precursor to the vasodilator, nitric oxide. The function of nitric oxide allows for increased oxygen delivery to the myocardium of the heart. Scientific evidence exists supporting arginine's role in increased myocardial blood flow associated with nitric oxide. Arginine's **vasodilating** and decreased atherosclerotic properties seem to improve the exercise abilities in patients with coronary blood flow issues such as coronary artery disease (9; 113). Ingestion of 6 g of arginine per day for 3 days has been shown to increase exercise tolerance due to increased coronary blood flow in patients with compromised coronary arteries (12). Improved immune function may occur with supplementation in diseased subjects (8; 43). The key is to remember these are patients in a clinical setting with cardiovascular diseases and that similar evidence does not exist connecting these effects with healthy individuals consuming adequate nutrients.

Arginine can be synthesized in sufficient amounts from the average diet. The recommended daily intake of arginine is 3.5 to 5 grams, and the average diet contains approximately 3-6 g of arginine. High amounts of arginine can be found in walnuts, peanuts, and even chocolate. Foods high in protein also contain significant amounts of arginine. There are no significant adverse effects with consumption levels under 25 g per day. Diabetics should not consume high amounts of arginine due to its effect on insulin production.

Nitric Oxide

The vasodilator nitric oxide is synthesized from l-arginine in almost all cells in the body. Nitric oxide is a strong vasodilator and has been shown to assist in the

metabolic regulation of glucose, fatty acids, and amino acids. Nitric oxide signals smooth muscle to relax, causing the arteries to dilate, thereby increasing blood flow. Nitric oxide is the most potent muscle relaxant in the body. It is released from the endothelium or the inner lining of the blood vessels, increasing blood flow capabilities. The endothelium increases the release of vasodilating substances, such as nitric oxide with aerobic training to accommodate increased blood flow and oxygen delivery to muscle (59).

Training improves the tissues' ability to secrete nitric oxide (58; 93; 143). This training adaptation has also been shown to occur in cardiac patients who experience increases in nitric oxide release with aerobic training participation (57; 94; 142). In fact, cardiac medications dependent upon nitrate, such as nitroglycerin, work on the principle of blood vessel dilation. In the case of nitroglycerin, dilation is aimed specifically at the coronary artery to increase blood flow to the myocardial tissue.

Fitness enthusiasts are now using supplemental nitric oxide to increase blood flow during exercise. The premise is to provide greater availability of oxygen and nutrients during the exercise bout as well as to enhance recovery immediately following exercise. Individuals who take nitric oxide experience an enhanced "pump" during exercise due to an increased blood flow to active tissues. However, there is currently no conclusive evidence that nitric oxide increases performance in normal exercise bouts or augments post-exercise

~Key Terms~

Glucocorticoids- A group of anti-inflammatory steroid-like compounds, such as hydrocortisone, that are produced by the adrenal cortex.

Atrophy- A wasting away or decrease in the size of an organ or tissue of the body.

Hematopoiesis- The formation of blood or blood cells in the living body.

L-arginine- An amino acid obtained from the hydrolysis or digestion of protein.

Vasodilator- Something such as a nerve or drug that causes the blood vessels in the body to become wider following the relaxation of the smooth muscle in the vessel wall.

recovery. Physicians warn that experimenting with high levels of nitric oxide as a supplement may be hazardous due to the numerous other roles that this substance plays in the body.

Beta-hydroxy Beta-Methylbutyrate (HMB)

Beta-hydroxy beta-methylbutyrate (HMB) is a bioactive metabolite of the amino acid leucine. HMB is thought to be anti-catabolic, decreasing the breakdown of protein resulting from intense exercise (54; 54; 146; 149). The body naturally produces small amounts of HMB depending on diet. The normal bodily synthesis is between 0.3-1.0 g daily. The recommended daily dosage for the supplement is 3 g/day taken in doses of 1 g, three times a day.

Research concerning the benefits of HMB is inconclusive (54; 148; 149). A literature review of the ergogenic effects of HMB showed minimal or no gains with supplementation (122; 128). One study suggests that **delayed onset muscle soreness** (DOMS) is reduced after 14 days of consecutive HMB supplementation in untrained exercisers (158). Whereas another contradicts these findings (127). It has been suggested that creatine and HMB can increase lean body mass and strength and that the effects are additive (83; 84). Although not definitive, these results suggest that creatine and HMB act by different mechanisms, which may complement each other. Again, more research is necessary to verify these results.

The research is inconclusive as to any actual decreases in protein breakdown in trained individuals. Limited data has shown a decrease in catabolism in untrained individuals. The fact that untrained individuals experience reduced catabolism with HMB supplementation but trained individuals do not could be due to the fact that trained individuals may already suppress protein breakdown as an adaptation to exercise. In conclusion, there have been a variety of studies that have been inconclusive for change in body composition or strength with HMB supplementation in trained individuals (98; 145; 147). To date, there have been no adverse effects associated with HMB.

Androgenic-Anabolic Steroids

Androgenic-anabolic steroids (AAS) is an official definition for all male sex steroid hormones, their synthetic derivatives, and their active metabolites. Although anabolic steroids are drugs with specific therapeutic purposes, they are more commonly used for non-therapeutic effects in a large number of healthy individuals. Steroids have reached the public spotlight

due to their heavy presence in professional and Olympic sports. Athletes use steroids to enhance performance and increase recovery from high volumes of physical exertion due to training, practice, and competitions. The use of steroids is well documented in body building and power sports, but there has been a significant rise in the use of anabolic steroids by recreational exercisers for the purposes of vanity. Additionally, steroid use in adolescent populations has risen significantly with estimates climbing to nearly 3 million users (47; 55; 81).

The lure of the drug is fairly obvious. Increases in mass, reductions in body fat, and notable increases in strength are all very desirable for athletes, those that are vanity driven, and individuals who experience issues related to insecurity or low self-confidence. Dissatisfaction with the body and low self-esteem associate with the so-called reverse anorexia syndrome that often predisposes some individuals to use steroids. Early research trials suggested that anabolic steroids offered little benefit as an ergogenic aid, likely due to low dose administration. Today, supra-dosage analysis shows conclusive evidence of several-measure efficacy. Scientific literature has documented that short-term administration can increase strength and bodyweight when used in conjunction with resistance training. Strength gains between 5-20% above starting value and lean mass gains of 2-5 kg have been observed. Increases in red blood cell counts and hemoglobin concentrations have been documented with anabolic steroid use. However, no effect on endurance performance has been observed. Although limited research exists, it is quite likely that anabolic steroids will yield improvements in recovery and subsequent performance in response to any event that stresses tissue to the point of micro-trauma. Endurance events, including the Tour de France, have shown that steroids have found their place in all sports, regardless of the related metabolic energy system employed.

The abuse of anabolic steroids is linked with various adverse effects. The degree of the side effects seems to be dose related. High level doses commonly used for body building and athletic enhancement can lead to serious and irreversible organ damage, primarily to the liver and cardiovascular system (163). These adverse effects stem from documented increased rates of hypertension and atherosclerosis, blood clotting dysfunction, **jaundice**, **hepatic neoplasms** and **carcinoma**, tendon damage, as well as psychiatric and behavioral disorders (86; 120). The primary negative effects of short- and long-term anabolic steroid abuse self-reported by males include the occurrence of acne vulgaris, increased body hair, **gynecomastia**, as well as anger and aggressive behavior (130). Women and

Physical Risks of Taking Steroid Hormone Drugs

Mind
Extreme aggression, mood swings, anxiety, dizziness, drowsiness, psychotic depression, suicidal thoughts

Face and Hair
Swollen appearance, greasy skin, severe acne, mouth and tongue soreness, male-pattern hair loss, increased growth of face and body hair

Voice
Irreversible deepening of voice

Chest
In males, breathing difficulty, breast development
In females, breast atrophy

Heart
Heart disease, heart attack, stroke, hypertension, increased LDL, drastic reduction in HDL

Abdominal Organs
Nausea, vomiting, bloody stool, liver tumors, liver damage, kidney stones

Blood
Blood clots, high risk of blood poisoning, risk of contracting blood born pathogens

Reproductive System
In males, shrinkage of testes, prostate enlargement with increased risk of cancer, sexual dysfunction, loss of fertility
In females, loss of menstruation and fertility, permanent enlargement of external genitalia

Muscles, Bones, and Connective Tissue
Increased susceptability to injury, cramps, tremors

young adolescents may additionally experience a masculinization (82). Due to the increased presence of testosterone in the blood, the natural production of testosterone and **gonadotrophins** is switched off. The reduced or halted production of testosterone from gonad glands may persist for months after use of the drug has stopped (153).

As indicated above, deleterious cardiovascular alterations can occur with anabolic steroid use, including elevation of blood pressure, **myocardial hypertrophy**, and depression of serum high-density lipoprotein (HDL) (85). Anabolic steroid induced arterial hypertension can cause increases in left ventricular muscle mass (left ventricular hypertrophy), and other **cardiomyopathies** (48; 92). Additionally, blood clotting and **fibrinolysis** are negatively affected, and several case studies of thrombus formation (blood clots that can cut off the blood supply to downstream organs) exist in young strength athletes using anabolic steroids. Sudden death is also a serious possibility with

steroid abuse (37; 45). Many case reports exist of sudden cardiac events leading to death in seemingly healthy subjects. In fatal and non-fatal myocardial infarctions associated with steroid abuse, coronary arteries demonstrated significant atherosclerotic plaque (40; 44; 46).

Anabolic androgenic steroids are illegal in the United States, and therefore, users must buy them illegally, like any illicit drug. In attempts to get the steroid effect without the risk of a jail sentence, many exercisers have used prohormone supplements. Androstenedione is an anabolic androgenic steroid used to increase blood testosterone levels for the purposes of increasing strength, lean body mass, and sexual performance. Research on androstenedione and its related compounds, including androstenediol, have not shown any evidence that the supplementation of **prohormones** works to increase strength or lean body mass in humans (54; 115). The long-term health effects of prolonged androstenedione supplementation are unknown and prohormones are linked with some of the same negative side effects as steroids. **Dehydroepiandrosterone (DHEA)** has also been used to elevate testosterone levels in attempts to enhance muscle mass and strength. DHEA is a weak androgen purported to provide anti-aging effects, including improved libido, vitality, and immunity levels. Research demonstrates that DHEA supplementation does not increase serum testosterone, nor provide any of the touted effects. In fact, prohormones are often converted to estradiol increasing male estrogen levels (21; 35).

The recent availability of the designer steroid **tetra-hydro-gestrinone** (THG) has brought the issue of performance enhancement to the forefront of the public

~Quick Insight~

Psychological and personality adjustments are well documented with steroid abuse. Anabolic steroids can cause aggression, hostility, and anger as well as depression. Mood disturbances are likely to be dose and drug dependent. Other adverse effects include disturbances within the endocrine and immune systems, liver dysfunction and damage, alterations of the urogenital tract, and the sebaceous system of the skin. It is likely that additional effects occur but are not documented or are underestimated because scientific studies use administrations of relatively low dosages. The mechanism of action is specific to the steroid molecule and its affinity to androgen receptors. Therefore, side effects can differ between compounds.

spotlight. Increased public awareness and questions as to implications in professional sports have caused more rigorous screening and more extensive bans on prohormones and related compounds in sanctioned competition. Supplements and drugs used to modify or replace endogenous endocrine activity are associated with disruption of normal hormone homeostasis, leading to subsequent dangerous adverse effects.

Weight Loss Supplements

Weight loss supplement sales generate well over one billion dollars annually. There are currently more than 50 individual dietary supplements and over 125 commercial formulas sold for weight loss purposes. Weight loss supplements appeal to consumers as a "quick fix" solution without the labors of exercise or dieting. Although very few products show any level of effectiveness, very few people investigate whether evidence based efficacy exists beyond the claims of the manufacturer. Weight loss supplements are of particular popularity due to the social stigma associated with obesity and the difficulties most people experience when attempting to lose weight through diet and exercise. Weight loss supplements are classed by their purported biological mechanism. The five general categories of dietary weight loss supplements contain chemicals or compounds that function in one of the following ways:

- Increase energy expenditure

- Modulate carbohydrate metabolism

- Suppress appetite

- Increase fat oxidation or reduce fat synthesis

- Block dietary fat absorption

Clinical data to support the effectiveness of most weight loss supplements is limited. Chemical agents that affect the sympathetic nervous system seem to be the only type of supplements that have shown any level of effectiveness in research. The two most investigated sympathetic agents are caffeine and ephedra, both commonly consumed in a mixture with other compounds. The sale of ephedra alkaloids was banned by the FDA in 2004 due to reports of negative cardiovascular effects associated with its ingestion. Caffeine is currently a regulated chemical, tested for in many sports.

Caffeine

Caffeine is a naturally occurring substance that is widely consumed in a variety of forms. It is a common

Caffeine Consumption

Over-Consumption Symptoms	Physiological Effects
Sweating	Increased heart rate
Nervousness	Increased blood pressure
Feeling of uneasiness	Vasoconstriction
Anxiety	Increased fatty acids in blood
	Increased production of gastric acid

ingredient found in coffee, tea, soda, chocolate, and nutritional supplements. It produces multiple physiologic effects throughout the body which are likely mediated mainly through action at centrally-located adenosine receptors. Caffeine's stimulant effects are used for both weight loss and performance enhancement.

Caffeine improves concentration, reduces fatigue, and enhances alertness. It has been studied for its potential use as an ergogenic aid. Several studies have demonstrated an improvement in exercise performance in submaximal endurance activities (89; 121; 129). Its potential ergogenic effect in acute, high-intensity

~Key Terms~

Delayed Onset Muscle Soreness (DOMS) - The pain or discomfort often felt 24 to 72 hours after exercising, which subsides generally within 2 to 3 days.

Androgenic Anabolic Steroids (AAS) - A class of natural and synthetic steroid hormones that promote cell growth and division, resulting in growth of several types of tissues, especially muscle and bone.

Jaundice-Yellow discoloration of the whites of eyes, skin, and mucous membranes caused by deposits of bile salts in these tissues, occurring as a symptom of various diseases such as hepatitis, that affect the processing of bile.

Hepatic Neoplasm and Carcinoma- Damage and development or onset of liver cancer.

Gynecomastia- Abnormal enlargement of the male mammary glands.

Gonadotrophin- A hormone that stimulates the growth and activity of the gonads.

Myocardial Hypertrophy- An enlargement of the cardiac muscle.

exercise is less clear. It is relatively safe and has no known negative performance effects, nor does it cause significant dehydration or electrolyte imbalance during exercise. Because of its potential use as an ergogenic aid, its use in sports is regulated by most sanctioning bodies. Pre-competition quantities are regulated in athletes participating in IOC and NCAA sanctioned events (79).

The level of caffeine necessary to produce an ergogenic effect is 250 to 700 mg (88; 154). By comparison, a drip method cup of coffee has between 110 to 150 mg of caffeine. Anything above these levels could lead to disqualification from an NCAA or IOC event. Over-consumption of caffeine may lead to symptoms such as sweating, nervousness, and an overall feeling of uneasiness associated with anxiety. These side affects are due to increases in heart rate, blood pressure, vasoconstriction, increased amounts of fatty acids in the blood, and increased production of gastric acid. Excessive consumption may cause an upset stomach and even vomiting. Additionally, routine caffeine consumption may lead to tolerance or dependence, and abrupt discontinuation produces irritability, mood shifts, headache, drowsiness, or fatigue (155).

Ephedra

Ephedra alkaloids are commonly used for weight loss or enhanced athletic performance. They come from a plant containing sympathomimetic compounds. Ephedra is sold commercially as a **bronchodilator,** but is most commonly used as a weight loss supplement. Ephedra supplementation is usually coupled with caffeine or botanical caffeine from **guarana** and sometimes aspirin (69). The mixture is intended to cause stimulation of the sympathetic nervous system with subsequent vasodilation. Ephedra has been shown to work as an appetite suppressant, likely from the stimulant effects associated with its ingestion. Meta-analysis of research trials which used ephedra containing substances showed a consistent weight loss of 0.9 kg per month compared to placebo. Although its use for weight loss seems to be efficacious, the serious risks associated with its consumption were cited for its ban in 2004.

Data collected from 50 trials of the supplementation of ephedra yielded estimates of 2.2- to 3.6-fold increases in the likelihood of psychiatric, autonomic, or gastrointestinal symptoms, and heart palpitations (90). It is estimated that a consequential response occurs in one in every thousand people that use the supplement (56). Reports of adverse events associated with the use of this non-prescription supplement raised concerns in

the United States regulatory community (15). A review of FDA-collected data of adverse effects from ephedra between 1997 and 1999 identified episodes of hypertension, arrhythmias, myocardial infarction, stroke, and seizures (10). At least ten deaths and thirteen permanent disabilities stemmed from these episodes, and 40% of the incidences occurred at recommended dosages in persons without pre-existing cardiovascular conditions.

Although ephedra sales represented less than 1% of all supplement sales in the U.S. in 2001, 64% of all adverse effects from herbal supplements were linked to its use. Many studies have shown positive effects without harm, but the reported risks are sufficient to shift the risk-benefit ratio against ephedra use (20; 164).

Bitter Orange

Following the ban of ephedra-containing supplements in February 2004, many manufacturers were forced to change the chemical formulas of their weight loss supplements. Most quickly substituted the herb bitter orange (citrus aurantium) for ephedra and marketed the products as "ephedra-free" supplements, suggesting that these supplements promote the same desired effects, including energy enhancement, weight loss, and appetite suppression (134). Citrus aurantium extract contains the botanical adrenergic amines **synephrine** and **octopamine**. Synephrine is structurally similar to epinephrine, and like ephedra, it is a sympathomimetic alkaloid. There is little evidence that products containing bitter orange are an effective aid to weight loss, which may be due to the limited research on the product (67). Some authorities question the likelihood of bitter orange working as an effective weight loss supplement at all because synephrine has **lipolytic effects** in human fat cells only at high doses, and octopamine does not yield lipolytic effects in human **adipocytes** (49; 66).

Like ephedra, bitter orange may also have the potential to cause adverse health effects(96). Due to the fact that synephrine increases blood pressure in humans and has the potential to increase cardiovascular events, the supplement likely comes with the same risks as ephedra (50; 65). The few reports of individuals experiencing an adverse event that they attributed to the supplement came from interviews and most indications suggest that the severity of the event was fairly mild. One research trial indicated that ephedra-free weight-loss supplements have significant cardiovascular stimulant actions, similar to ephedra but concluded that these effects are not likely caused by citrus aurantium alone (134). The conclusion was

Evidence Summary and Clinical Stance for Individual Weight-Loss Supplements

Supplement	Product Quality	Product Safety	Product Efficacy	Clinical Stance
Bitter Orange	Uncertain	Uncertain	Uncertain	Uncertain
Chitosan	Uncertain	Low Risk	None	Discourage
Chromium	Present	Uncertain	Uncertain	Caution and Monitor
Conjugated linoleic acid	Uncertain	Uncertain	Uncertain	Caution and Monitor
Ephedra alkaloid-caffeine combinations	Uncertain	Risk	Present	Discourage
Ginseng	Uncertain	Uncertain	Uncertain	Caution and Monitor
L-carnitine	Present	Present	Uncertain	Caution and Monitor
Pyruvate	Uncertain	Uncertain	Uncertain	Caution and Monitor
St. John's Wort	Uncertain	Uncertain	Uncertain	Caution and Monitor

based on the fact that an eight-fold higher dose of synephrine (Advantra Z) had no effect on blood pressure. The increased risk for cardiovascular incident is likely attributed to the synergistic effects of bitter orange and caffeine along with the other stimulants in the multi-component formulation.

Weight Loss Drugs

The prevalence of obesity in America has caused physicians to turn to pharmacological therapy to manage cases of significant obesity. Weight loss drugs differ from over-the-counter supplements in that they require a doctor's prescription for their use. In most cases, a person must have a BMI above 30, or greater than 27, with the addition of coronary risk factors to qualify for medication. Obesity medications primarily have three goals: weight loss, the maintenance of

weight loss, and reductions in cardiovascular and metabolic disease risk. Drug interventions focus specifically on weight loss, with changes in body fat composition and a reduction of health risks as secondary end-points.

Several drugs and pharmacologic interventions have been used to fight obesity, including thyroid hormone, **amphetamines, phentermine, amfepramone** (diethylpropion), **phenylpropanolamine, mazindol, fenfluramines, sibutramine,** and **orlistat**. The purposed mechanisms for the weight loss agents include decreased appetite, reduced absorption of fat, or increased energy expenditure (111). Most pharmacotherapies have shown to be effective at reducing body weight compared to placebo when used in conjunction with a calorie-controlled diet or lifestyle intervention in short-term trials (99; 111). Only

~Key Terms~

Cardiomyopathies- Diseases or disorders of the heart muscle, especially of unknown cause.

Fibrinolysis- The process where a fibrin clot, the product of coagulation, is broken down.

Prohormones- An intraglandular precursor of a hormone.

Dehydroepiandrosterone (DHEA)- A natural steroid hormone produced from cholesterol by the adrenal glands.

Tetra-hydro-gestrinone- A designer anabolic steroid banned by The Food and Drug Administration.

Caffeine- An alkaloid often found in tea or coffee, and used chiefly as a stimulant.

Bronchodilator- A drug that widens the air passages of the lungs and eases breathing by relaxing bronchial smooth muscle.

Guarana- A natural substance similar to caffeine.

Synephrine- A dietary supplement aimed at encouraging fat loss.

Octopamine- A compound used as an adrenergic drug.

Lipolytic Effects- Breakdown of fats.

Adipocytes- Any of various connective tissue cells found in the adipose tissue, specialized for the storage of fat.

Amphetamines- Any one of a group of drugs that are powerful central nervous system stimulants.

Phentermine- A drug that suppresses the appetite by altering the body's metabolism.

Amfepramone- Comparable to amphetamine with similar effects.

Phenylpropanolamine- An androgenic drug that acts as a vasoconstrictor and is used as a nasal decongestant, a bronchodilator, an appetite suppressant, and mild stimulant.

Mazindol- A drug used to control appetite and decrease weight.

Fenfluramines- A drug that is used in the treatment of obesity.

Sibutramine- A drug that suppresses appetite by inhibiting the reuptake of the neurotransmitters norepinephrine and serotonin.

Orlistat- A drug that prevents the digestion and absorption of dietary fats.

Dopamine- A neurotransmitter formed in the brain by the decarboxylation of dopa, which is essential to the normal functioning of the central nervous system.

Norepinephrine- A substance, both a hormone and neurotransmitter, secreted by the adrenal medulla and the nerve endings of the sympathetic nervous system to cause vasoconstriction and increases in heart rate, blood pressure, and the sugar level of the blood.

Serotonin- An organic compound formed in the tissue, especially the brain, blood serum, and gastric mucous membranes, and active in vasoconstriction, stimulation of the smooth muscles, transmission of impulses between nerve cells, and regulation of cyclic body processes.

sibutramine and orlistat have shown evidence of long-term efficacy with acceptable levels of adverse effects (63). Consequently, these are the only currently approved drugs for the long-term management of obesity in adults.

Sibutramine is sold under the name Meridia. It works as an appetite suppressant by inhibiting the reuptake of **dopamine**, **norepinephrine**, and **serotonin**. In doing so, it enhances satiety and reduces the appetite in users.

Compared to placebo use in clinical trials, sibutramine (10-15 mg daily) users experienced an average weight loss of 4.3 kg after one year (68; 110; 156). Increases in blood pressure and resting heart rates were reported in clinical trials and makers suggest that individuals with risks for cardiovascular complications should not take the drug (156). Other side effects may include headache, insomnia, dry mouth, and constipation.

Orlistat is a fat absorption blocker sold under the

Common Weight-Loss Drugs

Generic Name	Trade name(s)	Action	Possible side effects	Comments
Phentermine	Adipex-P®, Fastin®, Obenix®, Obephen®, Obernine®, Obestin®, Phentamine®, Phentride®, T-Diet®, Zantryl®.	Appetite Suppressant (catecholaminergic)	Nervousness, irritability, insomnia, headache	May increase risk of primary pulmonary hypertension
Diethylproprion hydrochloride	Tenuate®, Tenuate Dospan®.	Appetite Suppressant (catecholaminergic)	Nervousness, irritability, insomnia	Safer than other drugs for people with moderate hypertension
Mazindol	Mazanor®, Sanorex®	Appetite Suppressant (catecholaminergic)	Nervousness, irritability, insomnia, dry mouth, constipation	
Phenylpropanol-amine	Active ingredient in many products, including Acutrim®, and Dexatrim®	Appetite Suppressant (catecholaminergic)	Nervousness, insomnia, headache, dry mouth, dizziness	Should be used cautiously in coronary artery disease and high blood pressure
Fluoxetine	Prozac®	Antidepressant with anorectic effects(serotonergic)	Lack of energy, insomnia, nausea, diarrhea	May adversely react with herbal supplements, such as St. John's Wort and tryptophan
Sibutramine	Meridia®	Appetite Suppressant (catecholaminergic and serotonergic)	Headache, insomnia, dry mouth, constipation, elevated blood pressure	Risk of physical and psychological dependence; blood pressure must be checked regularly
Orlistat	Xenical®	Fat absorption blocker(lipase inhibitor)	Gas, rectal leaking, diarrhea, fecal urgency	Vitamin supplementation recommended to prevent fat-soluble vitamin deficiency

name Xenical. Its weight loss mechanism works by blocking up to 30% of the fat in the diet from entering circulation through the intestines. Meta-analysis showed individuals that consumed Orlistat lost an average of 2.7 kg compared to placebo (71; 110). Other positive outcomes associated with Orlistat treatments include lower systolic blood pressure, decreased waist circumference, and a reduction of LDL cholesterol, fasting serum glucose, and insulin levels (73; 95). Due to its function, Orlistat causes unpleasant gastrointestinal side effects including gas, rectal discharge, fatty bowel movements, and fecal urgency (72; 156). Over-consuming fat when using Orlistat causes diarrhea and rectal leakage, which often teaches users to follow a reduced-fat diet. Additionally, users must consume adequate fat-soluble vitamins because the fat blocking mechanism prevents some absorption of the vitamins A, D, E, and K, which are transported by lipids.

Weight loss drugs are not a desirable choice as the first intervention to losing body fat due to the possible acute side effects and lack of information pertaining to long-term use. For individuals experiencing moderate to severe obesity, the drugs may be effective in the reduction of their body weight, subsequently reducing their risk for disease. The use of weight loss medications should be closely monitored by a physician and should only be used in conjunction with a healthy diet and lifestyle. Due to the risk for injury, personal trainers should be familiar with the side effects of the medications their clients use and closely monitor their exercise participation.

Chapter Nine References

1. New supplement treats AIDS wasting successfully. *AIDS Alert* 14: 41-43, 1999.

2. National Institutes of Health State-of-the-science conference statement: multivitamin/mineral supplements and chronic disease prevention. *Ann Intern Med* 145: 364-371, 2006.

3. National Institutes of Health State-of-the-Science Conference Statement: multivitamin/mineral supplements and chronic disease prevention. *Am J Clin Nutr* 85: 257S-264S, 2007.

4. NIH State-of-the-Science Conference: Multivitamin/Mineral Supplements and Chronic Disease Prevention, May 15-17, 2006, Bethesda, Maryland, USA. *Am J Clin Nutr* 85: 251S-327S, 2007.

5. **Abel T, Knechtle B, Perret C, Eser P, von Arx P and Knecht H**. Influence of chronic supplementation of arginine aspartate in endurance athletes on performance and substrate metabolism - a randomized, double-blind, placebo-controlled study. *Int J Sports Med* 26: 344-349, 2005.

6. **Abel T, Knechtle B, Perret C, Eser P, von Arx P and Knecht H**. Influence of chronic supplementation of arginine aspartate in endurance athletes on performance and substrate metabolism - a randomized, double-blind, placebo-controlled study. *Int J Sports Med* 26: 344-349, 2005.

7. **Antonio J and Street C**. Glutamine: a potentially useful supplement for athletes. *Can J Appl Physiol* 24: 1-14, 1999.

8. **Appleton J**. Arginine: Clinical potential of a semi-essential amino. *Altern Med Rev* 7: 512-522, 2002.

9. **Appleton J**. Arginine: Clinical potential of a semi-essential amino. *Altern Med Rev* 7: 512-522, 2002.

10. **Arditti J, Bourdon JH, Spadari M, de Haro L, Richard N and Valli M**. [Ma Huang, from dietary supplement to abuse]. *Acta Clin Belg Suppl* 34-36, 2002.

11. **Balzola FA and Boggio-Bertinet D**. [The metabolic role of glutamine]. *Minerva Gastroenterol Dietol* 42: 17-26, 1996.

12. **Bednarz B, Wolk R, Chamiec T, Herbaczynska-Cedro K, Winek D and Ceremuzynski L**. Effects of oral L-arginine supplementation on exercise-induced QT dispersion and exercise tolerance in stable angina pectoris. *Int J Cardiol* 75: 205-210, 2000.

13. **Bemben MG, Bemben DA, Loftiss DD and Knehans AW**. Creatine supplementation during resistance training in college football athletes. *Med Sci Sports Exerc* 33: 1667-1673, 2001.

14. **Bemben MG and Lamont HS**. Creatine supplementation and exercise performance: recent findings. *Sports Med* 35: 107-125, 2005.

15. **Bent S, Tiedt TN, Odden MC and Shlipak MG**. The relative safety of ephedra compared with other herbal products. *Ann Intern Med* 138: 468-471, 2003.

16. **Bianchi G, Marzocchi R, Agostini F and Marchesini G**. Update on nutritional supplementation with branched-chain amino acids. *Curr Opin Clin Nutr Metab Care* 8: 83-87, 2005.

17. **Bird SP, Tarpenning KM and Marino FE**. Independent and combined effects of liquid carbohydrate/essential amino acid ingestion on hormonal and muscular adaptations following resistance training in untrained men. *Eur J Appl Physiol* 97: 225-238, 2006.

18. **Bird SP, Tarpenning KM and Marino FE**. Independent and combined effects of liquid carbohydrate/essential amino acid ingestion on hormonal and muscular adaptations following resistance training in untrained men. *Eur J Appl Physiol* 97: 225-238, 2006.

19. **Bolster DR, Pikosky MA, McCarthy LM and Rodriguez NR**. Exercise affects protein utilization in healthy children. *J Nutr* 131: 2659-2663, 2001.

20. **Boozer CN, Daly PA, Homel P, Solomon JL, Blanchard D, Nasser JA, Strauss R and Meredith T**. Herbal ephedra/caffeine for weight loss: a 6-month randomized safety and efficacy trial. *Int J Obes Relat Metab Disord* 26: 593-604, 2002.

21. **Brown GA, Vukovich MD, Sharp RL, Reifenrath TA, Parsons KA and King DS**. Effect of oral DHEA on serum testosterone and adaptations to resistance training in young men. *J Appl Physiol* 87: 2274-2283, 1999.

22. **Burke DG, Chilibeck PD, Davidson KS, Candow DG, Farthing J and Smith-Palmer T**. The effect of whey protein supplementation with and without creatine monohydrate combined with resistance training on lean tissue mass and muscle strength. *Int J Sport Nutr Exerc Metab* 11: 349-364, 2001.

23. **Burke LM**. Nutrition for post-exercise recovery. *Aust J Sci Med Sport* 29: 3-10, 1997.

24. **Burke LM**. Nutrition for post-exercise recovery. *Aust J Sci Med Sport* 29: 3-10, 1997.

25. **Burke LM**. Nutrition for post-exercise recovery. *Aust J Sci Med Sport* 29: 3-10, 1997.

26. **Candow DG, Chilibeck PD, Burke DG, Davison KS and Smith-Palmer T**. Effect of glutamine supplementation combined with resistance training in young adults. *Eur J Appl Physiol* 86: 142-149, 2001.

27. **Castano G, Etchart C and Sookoian S**. Vitamin A toxicity in a physical culturist patient: a case report and review of the literature. *Ann Hepatol* 5: 293-395, 2006.

28. **Clark RH, Feleke G, Din M, Yasmin T, Singh G, Khan FA and Rathmacher JA**. Nutritional treatment for acquired immunodeficiency virus-associated wasting using beta-hydroxy beta-methylbutyrate, glutamine, and arginine: a randomized, double-blind, placebo-controlled study. *JPEN J Parenter Enteral Nutr* 24: 133-139, 2000.

29. **Cribb PJ, Williams AD, Carey MF and Hayes A**. The effect of whey isolate and resistance training on strength, body composition, and plasma glutamine. *Int J Sport Nutr Exerc Metab* 16: 494-509, 2006.

30. **Cribb PJ, Williams AD, Carey MF and Hayes A**. The effect of whey isolate and resistance training on strength, body composition, and plasma glutamine. *Int J Sport Nutr Exerc Metab* 16: 494-509, 2006.

31. **Cribb PJ, Williams AD, Carey MF and Hayes A**. The effect of whey isolate and resistance training on strength, body composition, and plasma glutamine. *Int J Sport Nutr Exerc Metab* 16: 494-509, 2006.

32. **Cribb PJ, Williams AD, Carey MF and Hayes A**. The effect of whey isolate and resistance training on strength, body composition, and plasma glutamine. *Int J Sport Nutr Exerc Metab* 16: 494-509, 2006.

33. **Cribb PJ, Williams AD, Carey MF and Hayes A**. The effect of whey isolate and resistance training on strength, body composition, and plasma glutamine. *Int J Sport Nutr Exerc Metab* 16: 494-509, 2006.

34. **Darmon N, Darmon M, Maillot M and Drewnowski A**. A nutrient density standard for vegetables and fruits: nutrients per calorie and nutrients per unit cost. *J Am Diet Assoc* 105: 1881-1887, 2005.

35. **Dayal M, Sammel MD, Zhao J, Hummel AC, Vandenbourne K and Barnhart KT**. Supplementation with DHEA: effect on muscle size, strength, quality of life, and lipids. *J Womens Health (Larchmt)* 14: 391-400, 2005.

36. **De Palo EF, Gatti R, Cappellin E, Schiraldi C, De Palo CB and Spinella P**. Plasma lactate, GH and GH-binding protein levels in exercise following BCAA supplementation in athletes. *Amino Acids* 20: 1-11, 2001.

37. **Di Paolo M, Agozzino M, Toni C, Luciani AB, Molendini L, Scaglione M, Inzani F, Pasotti M, Buzzi F and Arbustini E**. Sudden anabolic steroid abuse-related death in athletes. *Int J Cardiol* 114: 114-117, 2007.

38. **Dohm GL**. Protein nutrition for the athlete. *Clin Sports Med* 3: 595-604, 1984.

39. **Dohm GL**. Protein nutrition for the athlete. *Clin Sports Med* 3: 595-604, 1984.

40. **Du Toit EF, Rossouw E, Van Rooyen J and Lochner A**. Proposed mechanisms for the anabolic steroid-induced increase in myocardial susceptibility to ischaemia/reperfusion injury. *Cardiovasc J S Afr* 16: 21-28, 2005.

41. **Engelhardt M, Neumann G, Berbalk A and Reuter I**. Creatine supplementation in endurance sports. *Med Sci Sports Exerc* 30: 1123-1129, 1998.

42. **Falk DJ, Heelan KA, Thyfault JP and Koch AJ**. Effects of effervescent creatine, ribose, and glutamine supplementation on muscular strength, muscular endurance, and body composition. *J Strength Cond Res* 17: 810-816, 2003.

43. **Field CJ, Johnson I and Pratt VC**. Glutamine and arginine: immunonutrients for improved health. *Med Sci Sports Exerc* 32: S377-S388, 2000.

44. **Fineschi V, Baroldi G, Monciotti F, Paglicci RL and Turillazzi E**. Anabolic steroid abuse and cardiac sudden death: a pathologic study. *Arch Pathol Lab Med* 125: 253-255, 2001.

45. **Fineschi V, Riezzo I, Centini F, Silingardi E, Licata M, Beduschi G and Karch SB**. Sudden cardiac death during anabolic steroid abuse: morphologic and toxicologic findings in two fatal cases of bodybuilders. *Int J Legal Med* 121: 48-53, 2007.

46. **Fineschi V, Riezzo I, Centini F, Silingardi E, Licata M, Beduschi G and Karch SB**. Sudden cardiac death during anabolic steroid abuse: morphologic and toxicologic findings in two fatal cases of bodybuilders. *Int J Legal Med* 121: 48-53, 2007.

47. **Foley JD and Schydlower M**. Anabolic Steroid and Ergogenic Drug Use by Adolescents. *Adolesc Med* 4: 341-352, 1993.

48. **Fritzsche D, Krakor R, Asmussen G, Widera R, Caffier P, Berkei J and Cesla M**. Anabolic steroids (metenolone) improve muscle performance and hemodynamic characteristics in cardiomyoplasty. *Ann Thorac Surg* 59: 961-969, 1995.

49. **Fugh-Berman A and Myers A**. Citrus aurantium, an ingredient of dietary supplements marketed for weight loss: current status of clinical and basic research. *Exp Biol Med (Maywood)* 229: 698-704, 2004.

50. **Fugh-Berman A and Myers A**. Citrus aurantium, an ingredient of dietary supplements marketed for weight loss: current status of clinical and basic research. *Exp Biol Med (Maywood)* 229: 698-704, 2004.

51. **Garlick PJ, McNurlan MA and Patlak CS**. Adaptation of protein metabolism in relation to limits to high dietary protein intake. *Eur J Clin Nutr* 53 Suppl 1: S34-S43, 1999.

52. **Garlick PJ, McNurlan MA and Patlak CS**. Adaptation of protein metabolism in relation to limits to high dietary protein intake. *Eur J Clin Nutr* 53 Suppl 1: S34-S43, 1999.

53. **Garlick PJ, McNurlan MA and Patlak CS**. Adaptation of protein metabolism in relation to limits to high dietary protein intake. *Eur J Clin Nutr* 53 Suppl 1: S34-S43, 1999.

54. **Gleeson M**. Interrelationship between physical activity and branched-chain amino acids. *J Nutr* 135: 1591S-1595S, 2005.

55. **Gomez JE**. Performance-enhancing substances in adolescent athletes. *Tex Med* 98: 41-46, 2002.

56. **Gordon JS**. Banning ephedra: good call, poor vision. *Altern Ther Health Med* 10: 18-19, 2004.

57. **Graham DA and Rush JW**. Exercise training improves aortic endothelium-dependent vasorelaxation and determinants of nitric oxide bioavailability in spontaneously hypertensive rats. *J Appl Physiol* 96: 2088-2096, 2004.

58. **Graham DA and Rush JW**. Exercise training improves aortic endothelium-dependent vasorelaxation and determinants of nitric oxide bioavailability in spontaneously hypertensive rats. *J Appl Physiol* 96: 2088-2096, 2004.

59. **Graham DA and Rush JW**. Exercise training improves aortic endothelium-dependent vasorelaxation and determinants of nitric oxide bioavailability in spontaneously hypertensive rats. *J Appl Physiol* 96: 2088-2096, 2004.

60. **Grandjean A**. Nutritional requirements to increase lean mass. *Clin Sports Med* 18: 623-632, 1999.

61. **Grandjean A**. Nutritional requirements to increase lean mass. *Clin Sports Med* 18: 623-632, 1999.

62. **Groeneveld GJ, Beijer C, Veldink JH, Kalmijn S, Wokke JH and van den Berg LH**. Few adverse effects of

long-term creatine supplementation in a placebo-controlled trial. *Int J Sports Med* 26: 307-313, 2005.

63. **Gursoy A, Erdogan MF, Cin MO, Cesur M and Baskal N**. Comparison of orlistat and sibutramine in an obesity management program: efficacy, compliance, and weight regain after noncompliance. *Eat Weight Disord* 11: e127-e132, 2006.

64. **Ha E and Zemel MB**. Functional properties of whey, whey components, and essential amino acids: mechanisms underlying health benefits for active people (review). *J Nutr Biochem* 14: 251-258, 2003.

65. **Haaz S, Fontaine KR, Cutter G, Limdi N, Perumean-Chaney S and Allison DB**. Citrus aurantium and synephrine alkaloids in the treatment of overweight and obesity: an update. *Obes Rev* 7: 79-88, 2006.

66. **Haaz S, Fontaine KR, Cutter G, Limdi N, Perumean-Chaney S and Allison DB**. Citrus aurantium and synephrine alkaloids in the treatment of overweight and obesity: an update. *Obes Rev* 7: 79-88, 2006.

67. **Haaz S, Fontaine KR, Cutter G, Limdi N, Perumean-Chaney S and Allison DB**. Citrus aurantium and synephrine alkaloids in the treatment of overweight and obesity: an update. *Obes Rev* 7: 79-88, 2006.

68. **Halford JC**. Clinical pharmacotherapy for obesity: current drugs and those in advanced development. *Curr Drug Targets* 5: 637-646, 2004.

69. **Haller CA, Duan M, Benowitz NL and Jacob P, III**. Concentrations of ephedra alkaloids and caffeine in commercial dietary supplements. *J Anal Toxicol* 28: 145-151, 2004.

70. **Haymond MW and Miles JM**. Branched chain amino acids as a major source of alanine nitrogen in man. *Diabetes* 31: 86-89, 1982.

71. **Henness S and Perry CM**. Orlistat: a review of its use in the management of obesity. *Drugs* 66: 1625-1656, 2006.

72. **Hollander P**. Orlistat in the treatment of obesity. *Prim Care* 30: 427-440, 2003.

73. **Hsieh CJ, Wang PW, Liu RT, Tung SC, Chien WY, Chen JF, Chen CH, Kuo MC and Hu YH**. Orlistat for obesity: benefits beyond weight loss. *Diabetes Res Clin Pract* 67: 78-83, 2005.

74. **Huang HY, Caballero B, Chang S, Alberg AJ, Semba RD, Schneyer C, Wilson RF, Cheng TY, Prokopowicz G, Barnes GJ, Vassy J and Bass EB**. Multivitamin/Mineral supplements and prevention of chronic disease: executive summary. *Am J Clin Nutr* 85: 265S-268S, 2007.

75. **Ivy JL**. Glycogen resynthesis after exercise: effect of carbohydrate intake. *Int J Sports Med* 19 Suppl 2: S142-S145, 1998.

76. **Ivy JL**. Glycogen resynthesis after exercise: effect of carbohydrate intake. *Int J Sports Med* 19 Suppl 2: S142-S145, 1998.

77. **Ivy JL**. Glycogen resynthesis after exercise: effect of carbohydrate intake. *Int J Sports Med* 19 Suppl 2: S142-S145, 1998.

78. **Ivy JL**. Dietary strategies to promote glycogen synthesis after exercise. *Can J Appl Physiol* 26 Suppl: S236-S245, 2001.

79. **Jacobson BH and Kulling FA**. Health and ergogenic effects of caffeine. *Br J Sports Med* 23: 34-40, 1989.

80. **Jeukendrup AE, Jentjens RL and Moseley L**. Nutritional considerations in triathlon. *Sports Med* 35: 163-181, 2005.

81. **Johnson MD**. Anabolic steroid use in adolescent athletes. *Pediatr Clin North Am* 37: 1111-1123, 1990.

82. **Johnson MD**. Anabolic steroid use in adolescent athletes. *Pediatr Clin North Am* 37: 1111-1123, 1990.

83. **Jowko E, Ostaszewski P, Jank M, Sacharuk J, Zieniewicz A, Wilczak J and Nissen S**. Creatine and beta-hydroxy-beta-methylbutyrate (HMB) additively increase lean body mass and muscle strength during a weight-training program. *Nutrition* 17: 558-566, 2001.

84. **Jowko E, Ostaszewski P, Jank M, Sacharuk J, Zieniewicz A, Wilczak J and Nissen S**. Creatine and beta-hydroxy-beta-methylbutyrate (HMB) additively increase lean body mass and muscle strength during a weight-training program. *Nutrition* 17: 558-566, 2001.

85. **Kam PC and Yarrow M**. Anabolic steroid abuse: physiological and anaesthetic considerations. *Anaesthesia* 60: 685-692, 2005.

86. **Kam PC and Yarrow M**. Anabolic steroid abuse: physiological and anaesthetic considerations. *Anaesthesia* 60: 685-692, 2005.

87. **Karp JR, Johnston JD, Tecklenburg S, Mickleborough TD, Fly AD and Stager JM**. Chocolate

milk as a post-exercise recovery aid. *Int J Sport Nutr Exerc Metab* 16: 78-91, 2006.

88. **Keisler BD and Armsey TD**. Caffeine as an ergogenic aid. *Curr Sports Med Rep* 5: 215-219, 2006.

89. **Keisler BD and Armsey TD**. Caffeine as an ergogenic aid. *Curr Sports Med Rep* 5: 215-219, 2006.

90. **Keisler BD and Hosey RG**. Ergogenic aids: an update on ephedra. *Curr Sports Med Rep* 4: 231-235, 2005.

91. **Kelly JP, Kaufman DW, Kelley K, Rosenberg L, Anderson TE and Mitchell AA**. Recent trends in use of herbal and other natural products. *Arch Intern Med* 165: 281-286, 2005.

92. **Kindermann W**. [Cardiovascular side effects of anabolic-androgenic steroids]. *Herz* 31: 566-573, 2006.

93. **Kingwell BA and Jennings GL**. The exercise prescription: focus on vascular mechanisms. *Blood Press Monit* 2: 139-145, 1997.

94. **Kingwell BA and Jennings GL**. The exercise prescription: focus on vascular mechanisms. *Blood Press Monit* 2: 139-145, 1997.

95. **Kiortsis DN, Filippatos TD and Elisaf MS**. The effects of orlistat on metabolic parameters and other cardiovascular risk factors. *Diabetes Metab* 31: 15-22, 2005.

96. **Klontz KC, Timbo BB and Street D**. Consumption of dietary supplements containing Citrus aurantium (bitter orange)--2004 California Behavioral Risk Factor Surveillance Survey (BRFSS). *Ann Pharmacother* 40: 1747-1751, 2006.

97. **Kocak S and Karli U**. Effects of high dose oral creatine supplementation on anaerobic capacity of elite wrestlers. *J Sports Med Phys Fitness* 43: 488-492, 2003.

98. **Kreider RB, Ferreira M, Wilson M and Almada AL**. Effects of calcium beta-hydroxy-beta-methylbutyrate (HMB) supplementation during resistance-training on markers of catabolism, body composition and strength. *Int J Sports Med* 20: 503-509, 1999.

99. **Kushner RF and Manzano H**. Obesity pharmacology: past, present, and future. *Curr Opin Gastroenterol* 18: 213-220, 2002.

100. **Kutz MR and Gunter MJ**. Creatine monohydrate supplementation on body weight and percent body fat. *J Strength Cond Res* 17: 817-821, 2003.

101. **Lambert CP, Frank LL and Evans WJ**. Macronutrient considerations for the sport of bodybuilding. *Sports Med* 34: 317-327, 2004.

102. **Langfort J, Zarzeczny R, Pilis W, Nazar K and Kaciuba-Uscitko H**. The effect of a low-carbohydrate diet on performance, hormonal and metabolic responses to a 30-s bout of supramaximal exercise. *Eur J Appl Physiol Occup Physiol* 76: 128-133, 1997.

103. **Laviano A, Muscaritoli M, Cascino A, Preziosa I, Inui A, Mantovani G and Rossi-Fanelli F**. Branched-chain amino acids: the best compromise to achieve anabolism? *Curr Opin Clin Nutr Metab Care* 8: 408-414, 2005.

104. **Laviano A, Muscaritoli M, Cascino A, Preziosa I, Inui A, Mantovani G and Rossi-Fanelli F**. Branched-chain amino acids: the best compromise to achieve anabolism? *Curr Opin Clin Nutr Metab Care* 8: 408-414, 2005.

105. **Lehmkuhl M, Malone M, Justice B, Trone G, Pistilli E, Vinci D, Haff EE, Kilgore JL and Haff GG**. The effects of 8 weeks of creatine monohydrate and glutamine supplementation on body composition and performance measures. *J Strength Cond Res* 17: 425-438, 2003.

106. **Lemon PW**. Protein and amino acid needs of the strength athlete. *Int J Sport Nutr* 1: 127-145, 1991.

107. **Lemon PW**. Protein and amino acid needs of the strength athlete. *Int J Sport Nutr* 1: 127-145, 1991.

108. **Lemon PW**. Protein and amino acid needs of the strength athlete. *Int J Sport Nutr* 1: 127-145, 1991.

109. **Lemon PW**. Protein and amino acid needs of the strength athlete. *Int J Sport Nutr* 1: 127-145, 1991.

110. **Leung WY, Thomas GN, Chan JC and Tomlinson B**. Weight management and current options in pharmacotherapy: orlistat and sibutramine. *Clin Ther* 25: 58-80, 2003.

111. **Li Z, Maglione M, Tu W, Mojica W, Arterburn D, Shugarman LR, Hilton L, Suttorp M, Solomon V, Shekelle PG and Morton SC**. Meta-analysis: pharmacologic treatment of obesity. *Ann Intern Med* 142: 532-546, 2005.

112. **Marcell TJ, Taaffe DR, Hawkins SA, Tarpenning KM, Pyka G, Kohlmeier L, Wiswell RA and Marcus R**. Oral arginine does not stimulate basal or augment exercise-

induced GH secretion in either young or old adults. *J Gerontol A Biol Sci Med Sci* 54: M395-M399, 1999.

113. **Marcell TJ, Taaffe DR, Hawkins SA, Tarpenning KM, Pyka G, Kohlmeier L, Wiswell RA and Marcus R.** Oral arginine does not stimulate basal or augment exercise-induced GH secretion in either young or old adults. *J Gerontol A Biol Sci Med Sci* 54: M395-M399, 1999.

114. **Martin WF, Armstrong LE and Rodriguez NR.** Dietary protein intake and renal function. *Nutr Metab (Lond)* 2: 25, 2005.

115. **Maughan RJ, King DS and Lea T.** Dietary supplements. *J Sports Sci* 22: 95-113, 2004.

116. **Max SR.** Glucocorticoid-mediated induction of glutamine synthetase in skeletal muscle. *Med Sci Sports Exerc* 22: 325-330, 1990.

117. **Mayhew DL, Mayhew JL and Ware JS.** Effects of long-term creatine supplementation on liver and kidney functions in American college football players. *Int J Sport Nutr Exerc Metab* 12: 453-460, 2002.

118. **Millward DJ.** Protein and amino acid requirements of adults: current controversies. *Can J Appl Physiol* 26 Suppl: S130-S140, 2001.

119. **Morrison LJ, Gizis F and Shorter B.** Prevalent use of dietary supplements among people who exercise at a commercial gym. *Int J Sport Nutr Exerc Metab* 14: 481-492, 2004.

120. **Mottram DR and George AJ.** Anabolic steroids. *Baillieres Best Pract Res Clin Endocrinol Metab* 14: 55-69, 2000.

121. **Nehlig A and Debry G.** Caffeine and sports activity: a review. *Int J Sports Med* 15: 215-223, 1994.

122. **Nissen SL and Sharp RL.** Effect of dietary supplements on lean mass and strength gains with resistance exercise: a meta-analysis. *J Appl Physiol* 94: 651-659, 2003.

123. **Okudan N and Gokbel H.** The effects of creatine supplementation on performance during the repeated bouts of supramaximal exercise. *J Sports Med Phys Fitness* 45: 507-511, 2005.

124. **Paddon-Jones D, Borsheim E and Wolfe RR.** Potential ergogenic effects of arginine and creatine supplementation. *J Nutr* 134: 2888S-2894S, 2004.

125. **Paddon-Jones D, Borsheim E and Wolfe RR.** Potential ergogenic effects of arginine and creatine supplementation. *J Nutr* 134: 2888S-2894S, 2004.

126. **Paddon-Jones D, Borsheim E and Wolfe RR.** Potential ergogenic effects of arginine and creatine supplementation. *J Nutr* 134: 2888S-2894S, 2004.

127. **Paddon-Jones D, Keech A and Jenkins D.** Short-term beta-hydroxy-beta-methylbutyrate supplementation does not reduce symptoms of eccentric muscle damage. *Int J Sport Nutr Exerc Metab* 11: 442-450, 2001.

128. **Palisin T and Stacy JJ.** Beta-hydroxy-beta-Methylbutyrate and its use in athletics. *Curr Sports Med Rep* 4: 220-223, 2005.

129. **Paluska SA.** Caffeine and exercise. *Curr Sports Med Rep* 2: 213-219, 2003.

130. **Parkinson AB and Evans NA.** Anabolic androgenic steroids: a survey of 500 users. *Med Sci Sports Exerc* 38: 644-651, 2006.

131. **Peters EM.** Nutritional aspects in ultra-endurance exercise. *Curr Opin Clin Nutr Metab Care* 6: 427-434, 2003.

132. **Preen D, Dawson B, Goodman C, Beilby J and Ching S.** Creatine supplementation: a comparison of loading and maintenance protocols on creatine uptake by human skeletal muscle. *Int J Sport Nutr Exerc Metab* 13: 97-111, 2003.

133. **Preen D, Dawson B, Goodman C, Beilby J and Ching S.** Creatine supplementation: a comparison of loading and maintenance protocols on creatine uptake by human skeletal muscle. *Int J Sport Nutr Exerc Metab* 13: 97-111, 2003.

134. **Preuss HG, DiFerdinando D, Bagchi M and Bagchi D.** Citrus aurantium as a thermogenic, weight-reduction replacement for ephedra: an overview. *J Med* 33: 247-264, 2002.

135. **Reilly T and Ekblom B.** The use of recovery methods post-exercise. *J Sports Sci* 23: 619-627, 2005.

136. **Rock CL.** Multivitamin-multimineral supplements: who uses them? *Am J Clin Nutr* 85: 277S-279S, 2007.

137. **Rodriguez NR, Vislocky LM and Gaine PC.** Dietary protein, endurance exercise, and human skeletal-muscle protein turnover. *Curr Opin Clin Nutr Metab Care* 10: 40-45, 2007.

138. **Salehian B, Mahabadi V, Bilas J, Taylor WE and Ma K**. The effect of glutamine on prevention of glucocorticoid-induced skeletal muscle atrophy is associated with myostatin suppression. *Metabolism* 55: 1239-1247, 2006.

139. **Schrijver J and van den BH**. [Nutrition and health--vitamins and vitamin supplements]. *Ned Tijdschr Geneeskd* 147: 752-756, 2003.

140. **Schroder H, Terrados N and Tramullas A**. Risk assessment of the potential side effects of long-term creatine supplementation in team sport athletes. *Eur J Nutr* 44: 255-261, 2005.

141. **Sen CK**. Antioxidants in exercise nutrition. *Sports Med* 31: 891-908, 2001.

142. **Shen W, Zhang X, Zhao G, Wolin MS, Sessa W and Hintze TH**. Nitric oxide production and NO synthase gene expression contribute to vascular regulation during exercise. *Med Sci Sports Exerc* 27: 1125-1134, 1995.

143. **Shen W, Zhang X, Zhao G, Wolin MS, Sessa W and Hintze TH**. Nitric oxide production and NO synthase gene expression contribute to vascular regulation during exercise. *Med Sci Sports Exerc* 27: 1125-1134, 1995.

144. **Shephard RJ and Shek PN**. Heavy exercise, nutrition and immune function: is there a connection? *Int J Sports Med* 16: 491-497, 1995.

145. **Slater G, Jenkins D, Logan P, Lee H, Vukovich M, Rathmacher JA and Hahn AG**. Beta-hydroxy-beta-methylbutyrate (HMB) supplementation does not affect changes in strength or body composition during resistance training in trained men. *Int J Sport Nutr Exerc Metab* 11: 384-396, 2001.

146. **Slater G, Jenkins D, Logan P, Lee H, Vukovich M, Rathmacher JA and Hahn AG**. Beta-hydroxy-beta-methylbutyrate (HMB) supplementation does not affect changes in strength or body composition during resistance training in trained men. *Int J Sport Nutr Exerc Metab* 11: 384-396, 2001.

147. **Slater GJ and Jenkins D**. Beta-hydroxy-beta-methylbutyrate (HMB) supplementation and the promotion of muscle growth and strength. *Sports Med* 30: 105-116, 2000.

148. **Slater GJ and Jenkins D**. Beta-hydroxy-beta-methylbutyrate (HMB) supplementation and the promotion of muscle growth and strength. *Sports Med* 30: 105-116, 2000.

149. **Slater GJ and Jenkins D**. Beta-hydroxy-beta-methylbutyrate (HMB) supplementation and the promotion of muscle growth and strength. *Sports Med* 30: 105-116, 2000.

150. **Spriet LL and Gibala MJ**. Nutritional strategies to influence adaptations to training. *J Sports Sci* 22: 127-141, 2004.

151. **St Jeor ST, Howard BV, Prewitt TE, Bovee V, Bazzarre T and Eckel RH**. Dietary protein and weight reduction: a statement for healthcare professionals from the Nutrition Committee of the Council on Nutrition, Physical Activity, and Metabolism of the American Heart Association. *Circulation* 104: 1869-1874, 2001.

152. **Stevenson E, Williams C and Biscoe H**. The metabolic responses to high carbohydrate meals with different glycemic indices consumed during recovery from prolonged strenuous exercise. *Int J Sport Nutr Exerc Metab* 15: 291-307, 2005.

153. **Strauss RH**. Anabolic steroids. *Clin Sports Med* 3: 743-748, 1984.

154. **Tarnopolsky MA**. Caffeine and endurance performance. *Sports Med* 18: 109-125, 1994.

155. **Tarnopolsky MA, Atkinson SA, MacDougall JD, Sale DG and Sutton JR**. Physiological responses to caffeine during endurance running in habitual caffeine users. *Med Sci Sports Exerc* 21: 418-424, 1989.

156. **Thearle M and Aronne LJ**. Obesity and pharmacologic therapy. *Endocrinol Metab Clin North Am* 32: 1005-1024, 2003.

157. **Troppmann L, Gray-Donald K and Johns T**. Supplement use: is there any nutritional benefit? *J Am Diet Assoc* 102: 818-825, 2002.

158. **van Someren KA, Edwards AJ and Howatson G**. Supplementation with beta-hydroxy-beta-methylbutyrate (HMB) and alpha-ketoisocaproic acid (KIC) reduces signs and symptoms of exercise-induced muscle damage in man. *Int J Sport Nutr Exerc Metab* 15: 413-424, 2005.

159. **Volek JS**. Strength nutrition. *Curr Sports Med Rep* 2: 189-193, 2003.

160. **Volpe SL**. Micronutrient requirements for athletes. *Clin Sports Med* 26: 119-130, 2007.

161. **Weisburger JH**. Mechanisms of action of antioxidants as exemplified in vegetables, tomatoes and tea. *Food Chem Toxicol* 37: 943-948, 1999.

162. **Williams BD, Chinkes DL and Wolfe RR**. Alanine and glutamine kinetics at rest and during exercise in humans. *Med Sci Sports Exerc* 30: 1053-1058, 1998.

163. **Windsor RE and Dumitru D**. Anabolic steroid use by athletes. How serious are the health hazards? *Postgrad Med* 84: 37-3, 47, 1988.

164. **Worley C and Lindbloom E**. Ephedra and ephedrine: modest short-term weight loss, at a price. *J Fam Pract* 52: 518-520, 2003.

165. **Yetley EA**. Multivitamin and multimineral dietary supplements: definitions, characterization, bioavailability, and drug interactions. *Am J Clin Nutr* 85: 269S-276S, 2007.

166. **Youngkin EQ and Thomas DJ**. Vitamins: common supplements and therapy. *Nurse Pract* 24: 50, 53, 57-50, 53, 60, 1999.

167. **Zawadzki KM, Yaspelkis BB, III and Ivy JL**. Carbohydrate-protein complex increases the rate of muscle glycogen storage after exercise. *J Appl Physiol* 72: 1854-1859, 1992.

168. **Zello GA**. Dietary Reference Intakes for the macronutrients and energy: considerations for physical activity. *Appl Physiol Nutr Metab* 31: 74-79, 2006.

169. **Zello GA**. Dietary Reference Intakes for the macronutrients and energy: considerations for physical activity. *Appl Physiol Nutr Metab* 31: 74-79, 2006.

Chapter 10

Body Composition

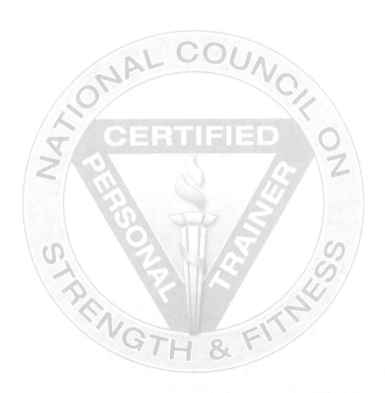

Obesity: A Worldwide Health Issue

Obesity has been labeled a pandemic due to the prevalence of high body fat in the American population and the rising occurrence of weight gain throughout the world (63). According to the World Health Organization, 1 billion people world-wide are overweight and 300 million are clinically classified as obese, using **BMI** criteria (37). The health consequences of maintaining elevated levels of body fat are significant. Obesity is independently classified as a disease, but it is more commonly considered to be a comorbity, meaning it is linked with the development of other diseases. According to the Department of Health and Human Services, the incidence of heart disease including heart attack, congestive heart failure, sudden cardiac death, angina or chest pain, and abnormal heart rhythm increases in persons who are overweight or obese (BMI > 25) (4; 20). For individuals who are obese (BMI > 30) there is a 50% - 100% increased risk of premature death from all causes, compared to individuals with a healthy weight (3; 19; 35). Estimates suggest that 300,000 deaths per year may be attributable to obesity, with the risk of death increasing proportionately with gains in fat mass. Moderate weight gain of even 10-20 lbs. increases the risk of death, particularly among adults aged 30 to 64 years (30).

Body Composition

Body composition is a component of physical fitness and an important part of an individual's overall health profile. It is defined as the ratio of fat mass to fat-free mass, suggesting that the relationship of fat-free mass to fat mass is more relevant than the independent measure of adiposity (the total amount of fat) when expressed in pounds. For instance, a 200 lb. man with 40 lbs. of body fat experiences a higher risk for disease than a man who weighs 220 lbs. and maintains the same quantity (40 lbs.) of fat on his body because the ratio is less.

Body composition is most commonly expressed as the percentage of body weight composed of fat. Using the same example as above, the 200 lb. man has a body fat of 20%, whereas the 220 lb. man has a body fat of 18%. The percentage of fat is categorized

into health risk by gender. The need for body fat differs between men and women, with males requiring less total body fat mass for normal physiological function than females. The reason that females require more fat relates to child birth and the endocrine regulations of their body functions.

Essential Body Fat Levels

Men and women have minimal values of body fat required to facilitate important physiological activities. The lowest level of body fat for proper homeostasis is referred to as essential body fat. Essential levels are necessary for key body functions.

Essential body fat levels for males are between 3% and 5%. When levels drop below these values, increased problems with thermoregulation and metabolic functions occur. Females generally need between 11%-14% body fat to maintain normal menstrual cycles. Endocrine disturbances associated with low female body fat include oligo- and amenorrhea (64). This reduction impairs homogenous estrogen levels and may

Body Fat Facts

High blood pressure is twice as common in adults who are obese than in those who are at a healthy weight.

Obesity is associated with elevated triglycerides (blood fat) and decreased HDL cholesterol ("good cholesterol").

A weight gain of 11 to 18 pounds increases a person's risk of developing type 2 diabetes to twice that of individuals who have not gained weight.

Over 80% of people with diabetes are overweight or obese.

Overweight and obesity are associated with an increased risk for some types of cancer, including endometrial (cancer of the lining of the uterus), colon, gall bladder, prostate, kidney, and postmenopausal breast cancer.

Women gaining more than 20 pounds from age 18 to midlife double their risk of postmenopausal breast cancer, compared to women whose weight remains stable.

Sleep apnea (interrupted breathing while sleeping) is more common in obese persons.

Obesity is associated with a higher prevalence of asthma.

For every 2-pound increase in weight, the risk of developing arthritis increases by 9% to 13%.

Obesity during pregnancy is associated with increased risk of death in both the baby and the mother and increases the risk of maternal high blood pressure by a factor of 10.

In addition to many other complications, women who are obese during pregnancy are more likely to have gestational diabetes and problems with labor and delivery.

Obesity during pregnancy is associated with an increased risk of birth defects, particularly neural tube defects, such spina bifida.

Role of Fat

- **Transports and stores vitamins and lipids**

- **Forms cell membranes**

- **Provides insulation and protection**

- **Aids functions of the nervous system**

- **Assists formation of hormones**

cause increased risk of osteoporosis and other problems. The standards for essential fat are derived from population norms. Some individuals are able to function on low levels of body fat due to genetic differences.

Body Fat Distribution

Body fat and distribution are both gender and genetically dependent. Often referred to as fat depots, significant evidence suggests that fat storage distribution may be a more important determinant than the degree of adiposity for predicting health risks. Where adipose tissue is stored on the body depends on several variables which include genetic predisposition, age, gender, and level of fat (31; 39; 82).

Body Types

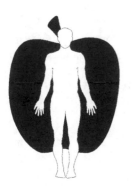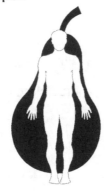

| Android | Gynoid |

Categorically, fat storage is subject to reference by regional distribution or body tissue sectioning. When analyzed using tissue sections, fat storage is viewed by subcutaneous and visceral locations. The storage of fat is most prevalent between the skin and muscle tissue, representing approximately 50-70% of total fat stored on the body. The fat stored in this region is referred to as **subcutaneous fat**. Fat stored below the muscle layer, in and around the organs, is called **visceral fat**. The differences between these storage areas are rather noteworthy. Visceral adipocity is associated with numerous cardiovascular pathologies as well as

metabolic disease (11). Individuals with large stores of visceral fat have an elevated risk for obesity-related health problems. Subcutaneous fat also associates with an elevated risk when the storage is centrally located. Referred to as central adiposity, large fat depots above the waist compound the risks associated with visceral fat storage.

When fat distribution is viewed by region of the body, obesity related to the central storage of fat is referred to as **android obesity** (12; 46). Commonly, android storage is associated with the apple-shape physique. Gynoid storage reflects a greater distribution of fat in the lower region of the body (below the waist) (10). Often viewed as female fat patterning, **gynoid obesity** is synonymous with a pear-shaped body. As stated, the region of the body where the fat is most prevalent relates to the degree of health risk. Upper body fat storage is associated with **hyperinsulinemia**, elevated blood lipids, and hypertension (10; 34; 83). Lower body fat storage is associated with reduced health complications until excessive amounts accumulate in the region. The cellular dynamics are explained by the fat cell characteristics of each respective area.

The Role of Hormones

Several differences exist in the actual fat cells located in the different regions of the body (45; 89). It is likely most differences exist due to the androgenic hormone concentrations in the body. Each area has a hormone sensitivity and acts in response to endocrine mediation. Gynoid fat patterning is enhanced by estrogen in women, whereas testosterone and other androgens affect android storage characteristics in males (6).

~Key Terms~

Body Mass Index (BMI) - A measure which takes into account a person's weight and height to gauge health risk for disease.

Essential Body Fat- Fat required for normal physiological functioning.

Subcutaneous Fat- Fat found just below the skin.

Visceral Fat- Fat stored in and around the organs.

Android Obesity- Male pattern or abdominal fat storage associated with an "apple-shaped" physique (higher risk of heart disease).

Gynoid Obesity- Female pattern or gluteal fat storage associated with a "pear-shaped" physique (lower risk of heart disease).

Cross-Section of the Abdominal Region

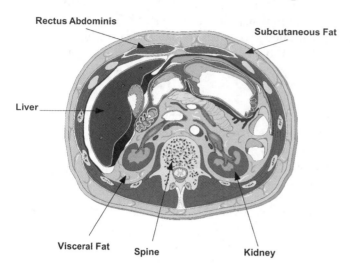

Increased testosterone concentrations during and following puberty are accompanied by increased abdominal fat storage. Likewise, females increase in gynoid body storage with increasing estrogen and progesterone levels following the hormonal shifts related to puberty.

When the regions are compared by lipolytic behavior (fatty acid release), additional differences become evident (8; 74; 77). Males have elevated **beta-adrenergic receptors** in lower body fat cells, which increase the release of free fatty acids from lower body storage in response to catecholamines. Females have higher concentrations of **alpha-adrenergic receptors** in lower body fat stores, which reduce the lipolytic response to catecholamines (1; 13; 81). This suggests that lower body fat stores in females resist freeing fatty acids into circulation for oxidation, making it harder to lose lower body fat in females compared to males (1; 14; 16; 76; 79).

Catecholamine mediated release in upper body fat cells is somewhat comparable between sexes; however, males have a higher free fatty acid release from subcutaneous abdominal fat in response to exercise, although some equivocal data exists (7; 15; 17; 78). Additionally, there are indications that basal fat oxidation, when adjusted for fat free mass, is lower in females as compared to males, partially explaining the higher fat storage in women (18). When compared by internal layer distribution, women commonly show higher levels of subcutaneous fat storage, where males have shown greater susceptibility to visceral fat storage (80). This information suggests that both males and females can change their abdominal storage with appropriate exercise and diet, but females will experience difficulty in reducing gluteofemoral (around

the hips, buttocks and legs) storage due to a natural resistance to fat mobility (9; 38).

Another obstacle to lower body weight loss is that fat patterning in this region tends to be more attributed to hyperplasia of mature adipocytes and therefore, increases in the number of fat cells. Since mature fat cells contain lipids, whereas preadipocytes do not, larger numbers of cells increase one's propensity to store more fat in a particular region. In contrast, abdominal fat deposition increases primarily via hypertrophy of the cell and does not seem to proliferate in response to increased energy balance and fat storage. Therefore, android male-fat patterning is altered more easily with exercise and dietary strategies than gluteofemoral fat stores.

The measures of fat mass, distribution, and risk for disease can be determined using several indirect methods. Since disease risk is the greatest consequence of obesity, identifying total fat mass and regional distribution is important to predict risk and need for intervention. The methods of assessing body fat by mass and distribution range from simple to complex techniques. In some cases, the assessment techniques use anthroprometric measures to provide predictions. Included in this category are height-weight tables and stature-weight indexes.

Height Weight Tables

Height-weight tables (HWT) were originally designed to predict mortality rates associated with a person's size for insurance premiums. If a person was short and heavy their predicted risk was elevated and so were

Muscle Cross-Section

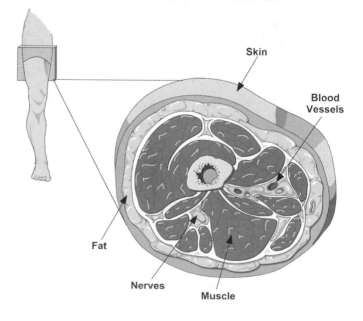

their insurance costs. Data collected in the 1940's and 50's was used to identify the most desirable weight for each height related to the lowest mortality rates. The 1959 tables established weight ranges for different frame sizes to better identify the weight composition with respect to bone thickness. In more recent years, height-weight tables have established a criterion method to determine frame size using elbow breadth. The frame size measures were determined from the first two National Health and Nutrition Examination Studies and tabled by gender for reference. The United States Department of Agriculture also publishes height-weight ranges as part of the Dietary Guidelines for Americans, but the table fails to identify frame size and does not separate gender in the weight ranges.

Height-weight tables have significant deficiencies for health guidance because they incorporate far too many assumptions. Likewise, valuable data that cannot be collected using a scale and a ruler is important to exercise prescription and behavior modification. When using Metropolitan Life height-weight tables, it is important to consider the following:

BMI Formulas

$$BMI = \text{Weight in kilograms} \div \text{Height in meters}^2$$

$$BMI = (\text{Weight in pounds} \div \text{Height in inches}^2) \times 703$$

Height/Weight Tables (HWT) Considerations

- HWT do not identify level of fat content

- Lean mass negatively affects the prediction

- Age variations are not factored into the tables

- The predominant population in the studies used to determine the ranges were middle-aged caucasians

- The tables are based on lowest mortality ,not disease or negative health conditions associated with weight

- The studies only used the weight taken at the time the policy was written and did not measure the weight at any other time before their death. The study would not reflect if the individual died at a much higher weight

- A single weight is not ideal for everyone of the same height

Body Mass Index (BMI)

Another stature weight index that has all but replaced height-weight tables is the Body Mass Index (BMI). BMI is the ratio of body weight to height squared. BMI is more practical because it utilizes anthropometric measures to predict risk for disease and health complications rather than all-cause mortality. Similar limitations to the HWT exist due to the fact that body composition is not assessed. Muscular individuals, for instance, may have lean measures of body fat but may

be considered very high risk due to their height to weight ratio. On the contrary, someone with very little lean mass may present as low risk, when they actually have an unhealthy body composition. Certain height ranges also decrease the accuracy of prediction. Individuals measured at less than five feet in height often have higher BMI scores than their mass represents.

BMI may have some downsides, but it certainly holds some level of merit for health assessment purposes. BMI is more accurate at predicting risk than weight alone and is relatively easy to calculate, even for the nonprofessional (66). Males and females use the same table, so predictive values are somewhat universal, and it takes very little time to calculate and track changes. Ideal values (lowest mortality) for BMI are 22 kg/m^2 for males and 21 kg/m^2 for females (65). Values between 18.5 and 24.5 kg/m^2 are considered to be within the healthy weight range. Once BMI becomes greater than 25 kg/m^2, health risk increases, with values over 27 kg/m^2 reflecting the greatest number of related health complications. A BMI less than 18.5 kg/m^2 is defined as underweight, 25-29.9 kg/m^2 is considered the overweight range, and a measure of 30 kg/m^2 or greater is considered obese. BMI is the reference value used when population segments are defined by percentage of people who are over weight or obese. In the United States, more than one third of the population has a BMI greater or equal to 30 kg/m^2 (72). It is important to understand that BMI predicts risk within a population but may over or underestimate risk for a given individual.

Although stature weight assessments offer a degree of usefulness for predicting risk of disease, circumference measures add value to the prediction by evaluating regional distribution. Abdominal girth and waist-to-hip ratio provide data regarding central adipocity and also contribute to the prediction of body composition. Combining the height-weight data with circumference

Classification of Weight by Body Mass Index (BMI), Waist Circumference, and Associated Disease Risks

Category	BMI (kg/m²)	DISEASE RISK RELATIVE TO NORMAL WEIGHT AND WAIST CIRCUMFERENCE	
		Men<102 cm (40 in.) Women<88 cm (35 in.)	Men >102 cm (40 in.) Women >88cm (35 in.)
Underweight	<18.5	—	—
Normal	18.5-24.9	—	—
Overweight	25.0-29.9	Increased	High
Obese Class I	30.0-34.9	High	Very high
Obese Class II	35.0-39.9	Very high	Very high
Obese Class III	> 40.0	Extremely high	Extremely high

values can better identify risk and demonstrate any predictive weakness with either measure when used independently.

Waist Circumference

Waist circumference has recently gained support for predicting obesity-related risk for disease. The correlation between abdominal adipocity and disease outcomes has made this simple assessment measure quite valuable for identifying need for weight management intervention strategies (71). For certain populations, including Caucasian males, waist circumferences are even more useful when used in conjunction with BMI to predict disease risk (75). Likewise, the measure assists BMI interpretation because large abdominal circumference is not related to muscle mass hypertrophy and therefore, makes a distinction between fat mass and muscle mass (70). Waist circumference is an important reference because it shows behavior-related fat storage. Visceral fat associates with lower levels of physical activity and behavior traits more than genetic predisposition. Waist circumference values above 102 cm (40 inches) for males and 88 cm (34.5 inches) for females are associated with a high risk for cardiovascular and metabolic disease.

Relationship Between Body Mass Index and Percentage Body Fat

Adult Males

Age	Increased Risk (BMI < 18.5)	Healthy (BMI 18.5-24.9)	Increased Risk (BMI 25-29.9)	High Risk (BMI 30+)
20-39	< 7.9%	8-19.9%	20-24.9%	> 25%
40-59	< 10.9%	11-21.9%	22-27.9%	> 28%
60-79	< 12.9%	13-24.9%	25-29.9%	> 30%

Adult Females

Age	Increased Risk (BMI < 18.5)	Healthy (BMI 18.5-24.9)	Increased Risk (BMI 25-29.9)	High Risk (BMI 30+)
20-39	< 20.9%	21-28.9%	29-31.9%	> 32%
40-59	< 22.9%	23-29.9%	30-32.9%	> 33%
60-79	< 23.9%	24-31.9%	32-34.9%	> 35%

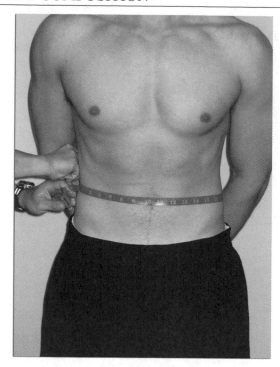

Abdominal circumference measure

Abdominal circumference measures are taken from the side of the body with the subject standing in an upright posture with feet located under the hips. The reference site for abdominal circumference measurement is the horizontal line of the umbilicus (belly button). The assessment should be performed against bare skin with the tape lying taut and parallel to the floor. The tightness of the measure should be enough to prevent folds in the tape but should not cause cutaneous indentations.

Waist-to-Hip Ratio

Waist-to-Hip ratio (WHR) is another circumference measure that predicts risk for negative health consequences. The predictive value of WHR is better than BMI, but may be not as good as waist circumference because additional variables reduce the assessment's ability to identify the level of central adipocity (60). This occurs because the measurement is expressed as a comparison between hip girth and waist girth. If a person maintains high amounts of fat through the hips, the subcutaneous fat mass makes the waist

mass less evident. Since lower body storage is not as detrimental to health as visceral fat storage, the ability of the test to detect changes in visceral fat accumulation is reduced. Similarly, excessive fat in both the stomach and lower body regions may cause reduced identification of visceral fat mass storage (22). Pre-pubescent children cannot be accurately assessed using waist-to-hip ratio due to the fact that hormonally mediated storage has not yet occurred. Additionally, individuals who engage in resistance training may have larger hip measurements due to muscle hypertrophy, which can reduce predictive value.

Waist-to-hip ratio is measured like the abdominal assessment, but unlike the waist circumference measurement, there is no single, universal standard for the measurement sites. The World Health Organization recommends measuring the waist circumference midway between the lower rib margin and the iliac crest of the pelvis. For the hip measurement, they suggest using the widest point over the greater trochanter. The Anthropometric Standardization Reference Manual recommends using the narrowest part of the torso for the waist measurement and the level of the largest part of the buttocks. Since the norms for WHR were formed from the Anthropometric Standardization Reference Manual, it makes logical sense to use their reference sites.

The ratio is calculated by dividing the waist measurement by the hip measurement. The closer the value is to 1.00, the greater indication of central adiposity and greater determination for risk. Although ranges exist which are age and gender specific, values above 0.9 for men and 0.8 for women seem to present the greatest increase in risk for negative health outcomes.

Body Composition Assessment

Assessment of **body composition** provides compartment specific data that categorizes tissue by relative percentage of body weight. This type of measurement identifies the actual fat mass by predicting body density. The advantage of body composition over stature weight and circumference references is that it

Waist-to-Hip Ratio Norms for Men and Women

Risk for Heart Disease	Low		Moderate		High		Very High	
Age (y)	Men	Women	Men	Women	Men	Women	Men	Women
20-29	<0.83	<0.71	0.83-0.88	0.71-0.77	0.89-0.94	0.78-0.82	>0.94	>0.82
30-39	<0.84	<0.72	0.84-0.91	0.72-0.78	0.92-0.96	0.79-0.84	>0.96	>0.84
40-49	<0.88	<0.73	0.88-0.95	0.73-0.79	0.96-1.00	0.80-0.87	>1.00	>0.87
50-59	<0.90	<0.74	0.90-0.96	0.74-0.81	0.97-1.02	0.82-0.88	>1.02	>0.88
60-69	<0.91	<0.76	0.91-0.98	0.76-0.83	0.99-1.03	0.84-0.90	>1.03	>0.90

compartmentalizes lean mass and fat mass. Since lean mass contributes positively to metabolism, it is important to distinguish lean mass from fat mass. Excess fat mass becomes deleterious when stored in abundance. Identifying the actual amount of fat on the body can help to determine health risk and the adjustments necessary to reduce the risk that is associated with excess fat storage.

Body composition assessment also allows personal trainers to track the specific changes in the tissue when weight loss or gain occurs. When combined with circumference values, the predictability of disease risk is dramatically enhanced. Total body fat and regional distribution can be evaluated, and the data can be used to provide direction to the formulation of the exercise prescription and identify any need for dietary changes.

Body composition assessments use different measures to ascertain the body's density. Once body density has been determined, regression equations predict body fat. The tests generally fall into two categories: clinical assessments and field tests. Clinical assessments require precision instruments and controlled clinical settings to measure body density. Common clinical tests include hydrostatic weighing, air displacement plesthsmography, and Dual X-ray absorptiometry. Field tests require less sophisticated equipment and are generally easier to implement. Common field tests include girth measurements, skinfold assessment, bioelectrical impedance, and near-infrared interactance.

Hydrostatic Weighing

Clinical assessments are not commonly used in traditional personal training settings due to the equipment costs, technician expertise required, and labor involved. A brief review of each is warranted because they are often used as the criterion reference value by which standard estimation error is determined for field tests. Both hydrostatic weighing and air displacement plethysmography (ADP) are densitometric methods which estimate body density from the ratio of body mass to body volume. Hydrostatic weighing uses Archimedes principle of buoyancy to calculate density. Fat mass is less dense than water, and therefore it floats. Individuals who maintain more fat mass weigh less underwater. The assessment method has the test subject exhale maximally before being submerged and weighed on an underwater scale. Adjustments for water density are made based on the temperature and residual air in the body. The weight lost under water is proportional to the volume of water displaced by the body volume. Calculations determine body density, which is then converted to body fat percentage using a population-specific conversion formula.

Air Displacement Plethysmography

Air displacement plethysmography (ADP), as the name implies, uses air displacement instead of water to estimate volume. This method requires minimal time, client compliance, and technical skill. The Bod Pod is the most recognized commercial whole body plethysmography chamber. It works via a pressure-volume inverse relationship in accordance with Boyle's law, which is used to calculate total volume displacement. The predictability of body density using the Bod Pod correlates with hydrostatic weighing, but has shown to under-predict percent body fat compared to multi-component methods and Dual X-ray Absorptiometry (24).

~Quick Insight~

Body composition is often viewed as a psychologically uncomfortable assessment. It is very common for a person to be self-conscious of their body when being evaluated by a personal trainer. With roughly 65% of America being overweight, body image becomes a relevant consideration in fitness training and assessment. People are usually not comfortable wearing tight fitness clothes or participating in assessment techniques that require some level of disrobement. Likewise, very few people want someone to grab and acknowledge the amount of fat on their body. This fact becomes even more evident when the amount of fat a person carries is significant.

The assessment a personal trainer uses should reflect the client's size, age, and fitness level and be considerate of the psychological stress the assessment may cause. Using skinfold measurement on an obese client makes very little sense. Skinfold measurement accuracy is inversely proportionate to the person's level of fatness. Obese people cannot be accurately measured using this technique. Likewise, what benefit would exist from using such an invasive measure on people who are likely embarrassed about their weight. If a person is visibly overweight, use circumference measures or consider bioelectrical impedance with correction factors.

In some cases, it does not make sense to measure fat at all. For some people, the stress of the experience is not worth the data. A visibly obese person is obviously overfat and both the trainer and client know this information. Why subject them to an assessment that will tell you that an exercise prescription aimed at safe weight loss is recommended? For overweight people, clothing fit can be the best assessment to identify body fat changes.

Dual X-ray Absorptiometry

Dual X-ray Absorptiometry (DXA) is commonly used in research settings to assess multiple compartments including bone mineral, fat, and lean tissue. The assessment operates on the principle that the attenuation of X-rays with different photon energies is measurable and depends upon tissue characteristics, including thickness, density, and chemical composition. The body tissues weaken the high and low X-ray energies at different magnitudes based on density and chemical composition called attenuation ratios. The attenuation is measured and the tissue composition is identified. Some researchers suggest that DXA is more accurate than hydrostatic weighing and very close to multi-component estimates, making it a popular method for clinical trials (23; 61; 62).

Personal trainers are far more likely to utilize field tests due to their ease of implementation in practical

~Key Terms~

Hyperinsulinemia- A condition in which there are excessive levels of circulating insulin in the blood.

Beta-adrenergic Receptors- Cell receptors, more prevalent in males, which increase the release of free fatty acids from lower body storage in response to catecholamines.

Alpha-adrenergic Receptors- Cell receptors, more prevalent in females' lower body fat stores, which reduce the lipolytic response to catecholamines.

Height Weight Tables (HWT) - An assumptive, guidance table, originally designed to predict mortality rates based upon a person's size.

Waist-to-Hip Ratio (WHR) - A tool that helps determine overall health risks by calculating waist/hip measurements.

Body Composition- Used to describe the percentages of fat, bone, and muscle in human bodies: the relationship of fat mass to fat free mass.

Dual X-ray Absorptiometry (DXA) – A body composition technique in which X-rays are generated at two energies that help estimate three body compartments, consisting of fat mass, lean body mass, and bone mass.

Circumference Measurements- An estimation of body composition employed by measuring select locations to predict body fat.

environments. Field tests vary by assumption and principle, and therefore have specific procedures for employment. The measurement techniques and equipment needs for each method of assessment are subject to the evaluation protocol. The decision to use a particular assessment should be based on the capabilities of the trainer and the population segment being assessed.

Circumference Measurements

Circumference estimation of body composition employs measurements of select locations to predict body fat. The methods are easy to perform and require minimal equipment. The assessment device is often no more than a common linen or plastic measuring tape. Often referred to as "girth measurements" this technique simply requires the **circumference measurement** of specific sites on the body. The measured values are then charted, graphed, or equated based on the particular protocol being used. Depending upon the estimation model, girth measurements can predict body composition and help determine regional fat storage. The estimations are based on the positive linear relationship between the circumference values of particular anatomical areas and the amount of body fat a person carries.

Girth measurements are very practical assessment methods for fitness professionals. When performed correctly with the appropriate prediction equation, circumference estimations of body fat can have a standard error of the estimate (*SEE*) of as little as $\pm$ 2.5%-4% (85; 87). They also provide useful information about fat distribution patterns as well as body fat changes during weight loss. Clients can see and understand the quantifiable differences found between measurements, which often serve as a motivator even when body weight remains unchanged. Additionally, the methods are far more useful for measuring and predicting the body fat of obese individuals, where calipers and other methods have a less accurate predictive value (47; 86). One downside is body fatness in muscular individuals may be over-predicted (67).

Skinfold Measurements

Subcutaneous fat is the lipid mass that lies between the skin and the muscle tissue. Technicians can "pinch" select sites using the thumb and index finger to create a fold of skin and fat with equal parallel sides referred to as a skinfold. Skinfolds at specific locations can be measured and summed to predict body density specific to a particular population (59). There are large inter-individual differences in the patterning of subcutaneous adipose tissue. This is true both within and between genders. Skinfolds can be used because a linear relationship exists among homogeneous groups. This relationship decreases over a wide range, which suggests that the equations used to convert skinfold into a body density must reflect the population being measured (28; 51; 54).

The sum of skinfolds offers a fairly accurate prediction of fat mass when the regression model is appropriate. Regression equations are either quadratic (generalized) or linear (population specific). Jackson and Pollock developed a generalized model which categorizes large segments of gender specific groups varying by age and level of fat mass (53; 57). Age needs to be factored into the equation because variations in storage patterns are seen when comparing the young and the old (5). As a person ages, their storage of subcutaneous fat is replaced by visceral fat storage. Therefore, regression equations applied to older populations should be adjusted to match the population.

Clinical data from criterion measures using hydrostatic weighing suggests that skinfold estimation error is approximately 3.5% (21; 52). Skinfold error is most commonly attributed to testing error by the technician. This may be due to inexperience, variations in tissue consistency, too much fat mass at the site, or incorrect site identification. A trainer should perform numerous individual measurements under supervision of an expert before using skinfold assessment to measure body fat on a client to ensure accuracy.

When deciding on the sites and protocols for skinfold assessment, it is important to realize that accuracy does not necessarily increase with more test sites. Slight error on each measurement of a seven-site assessment may add up to a significant inaccuracy. What may be of more value is how well the assessment identifies and exploits total body storage (36). Using the Jackson-Pollock generalized equation, three site assessment allows for measures at each region of the body (58). This can identify a high storage depot that may be missed when using other skinfold models. A good rule of thumb is that the assessment should at least measure one of the primary storage areas related to gender specific storage. For women, a lower body site should be included in the assessment, while assessment on males should include either the abdominal or subscapular site due to the propensity for regional storage.

Skinfold assessment should be performed on individuals who are not visibly obese. Individuals who maintain excessive fat mass or those who have large fat depots at select sites are difficult to assess. This is particularly true when they are also muscular. In some cases, accurate folds cannot be made due to high levels of fat

mass or the tightness of the skin, making it difficult to create a fold. If the assessment cannot be performed with accuracy, the data is of little use. In this case, an alternate assessment technique should be used (84). Skinfold predictability can be complemented using additional girth measurements (27). For purposes of reliability, the same tester and test should be used during any follow-up evaluations.

There are numerous calipers on the market for skinfold assessment. They range in price from under $20 to over $300. The pressure of the calipers should be calibrated to 10 g/mm^2 (56). The particular brand used is often based on professional preference and budget. It is not recommended to use calipers that require the tester to manually pinch the fold with the instrument due to tension variations which may over or under-compress the fold (55).

~Quick Insight~

Cellulite is not a special fat as many people seem to believe. It is characterized by a dimpled or wrinkled appearance that occurs when the tissue pressure is increased from compression (sitting) or muscle contractions. Cellulite is simply subcutaneous fat that has herniated into the dermal layer of the skin beneath the epidermis (2). Irregularities in the connective tissue border between the dermis and the fat cells resulting from tissue weakness allow the fat mass to migrate through the border into the superficial layer.

Although cellulite is commonly visible on obese individuals, it can also affect the non-obese. It is estimated to affect 80-90% of females (2). The thighs and buttocks of females are of particular susceptibility due to the quantity of fat stored in that region. Since cellulite is based on connective tissue attachment and compressive pressure, the only way to effectively reduce its appearance is to lower total body fat. Many creams and ointments can be purchased to hyperhydrate the area to temporarily mask cellulite, but no over-the-counter or prescription remedies exist to remove it (2).

Skinfold Guidelines

1. Be sure the test subject did not apply skin cream to the sites, or the skin will be come slippery and assessment error may occur.

2. Correctly identify the gender specific sites, and mark the fold location for reliable subsequent measures. Generally, the right side of the body is used for assessment.

3. Using the left hand with a thumb down position, straddle the marked site with the index and thumb and push into the fat mass until the underlying muscle can be felt.

4. Firmly grasp the skinfold and pull away from the muscle. The skinfold should have parallel sides. The pinch width is specific to the amount of fat mass.

5. Holding the calipers in the right hand pull the trigger to open the calipers and place th caliper arms on either side of the fold about ½ an inch below the fingers in the center of the fold. The caliper arms should be held at a level that forms a 90 degree angle perpendicular to the fold.

6. Maintaining the pressure on the fold with the index finger and thumb release the caliper trigger and assess the measurement within 4 seconds. Do not let go of the fold until the reading has been made and the calipers are withdrawn from the fold.

7. Record the value.

8. Measure each site at least twice for accuracy, allowing at least 15 seconds between subsequent measures of the site. If values differ by more than 1-2 mm, reassess a third time. Average the measures.

9. Add the sum of skinfolds and apply the score to the population specific equation, or chart to identify the predicted percentage of body fat.

Site Locations	Fold Orientation	Fold Description
Abdomen	Vertical	Taken 2 cm (approximately 1 in.) to the right of the umbilicus.
Chest (*Males only*)	Diagonal	The site is one half the distance between the anterior axillary line and the nipple.
Thigh	Vertical	On the front of the thigh, midway between the hip (inguinal crease) and the superior aspect of the patella (kneecap).
Triceps	Vertical	Located halfway between the acromion process (shoulder) and the inferior part of the elbow on the rear midline of the upper arm.
Suprailiac	Diagonal	Taken with the natural angle of the iliac crest at the anterior axillary line immediately superior to the iliac crest.
Midaxillary	Vertical	Fold is taken on the midaxillary line at the height of the xiphoid (end of sternum).
Subscapular	Diagonal	Just below the lowest angle of scapula, taken on a 45 degree angle toward the right side.
Medial Calf	Vertical	Seated with the right knee flexed and sole of the foot on the floor. The fold is taken on the medial side of the calf at its greatest circumference.

Skinfold Sites

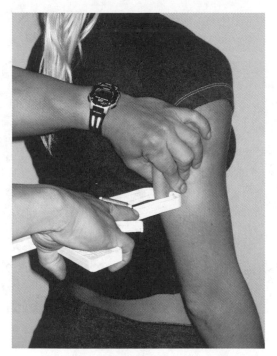

Triceps

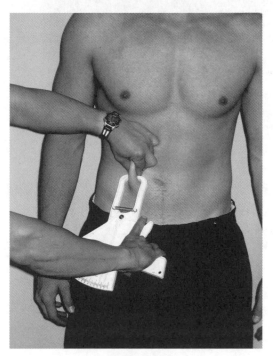

Abdomen

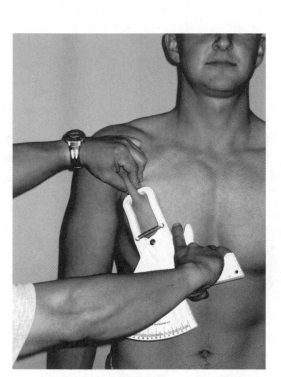

Chest

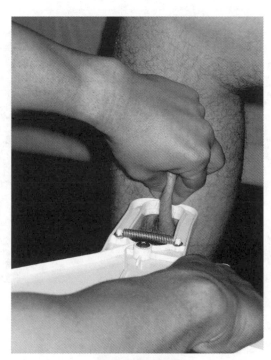

Medial Calf

Skinfold Sites Continued

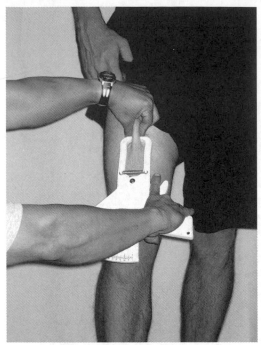

Thigh

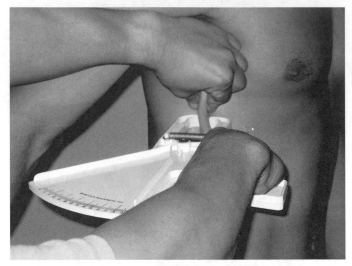

Midaxillary

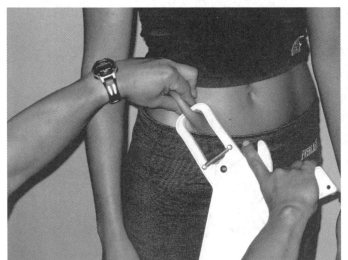

Suprailiac

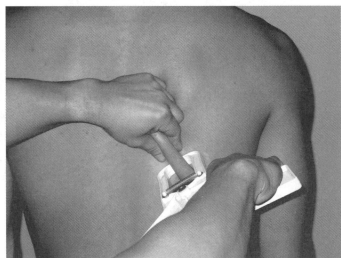

Subscapular

Generalized Body Composition Equations

Males

7-Site Formula (chest, midaxillary, triceps, subscapular, abdomen, suprailiac, thigh)

Body density
$1.11200000 - 0.00043499$ (sum of seven skinfolds) $+ 0.00000055$ (sum of seven skinfolds)$^2 - 0.00028826$ (age)

4-Site Formula (abdomen, suprailiac, tricep, thigh)

Percent body fat
0.29288 (sum of four skinfolds) $- 0.0005$ (sum of four skinfolds)$^2 + 0.15845$ (age) $- 5.76377$

3-Site Formula (chest, abdomen, thigh)

Body density
$1.1093800 - 0.0008267$ (sum of three skinfolds) $+ 0.0000016$ (sum of three skinfolds)$^2 - 0.0002574$ (age)

Body density (chest, triceps, subscapular)

$1.1125025 - 0.0013125$ (sum of three skinfolds) $+ 0.0000055$ (sum of three skinfolds)$^2 - 0.0002440$ (age)

Percentage body fat (abdomen, suprailiac, triceps)

0.39287 (sum of three skinfolds) $- 0.00105$ (sum of three skinfolds)$^2 + 0.15772$ (age) $- 5.18845$

Females

7- Site Formula (chest, midaxillary, triceps, subscapular, abdomen, suprailiac, thigh)

Body density
$1.0970 - 0.00046971$ (sum of seven skinfolds) $+ 0.00000056$ (sum of seven skinfolds)$^2 - 0.00012828$ (age)

4-Site Formula (abdomen, suprailiac, tricep, thigh)

Percent body fat
0.29669 (sum of four skinfolds) $- 0.00043$ (sum of four skinfolds)$^2 + 0.02963$ (age) $- 1.4072$

3- Site Formula (triceps, abdomen, suprailiac)

Percent body fat (triceps, abdomen, suprailiac)
0.41563 (sum of three skinfolds) $- 0.00112$ (sum of three skinfolds)$^2 + 0.03661$ (age) $+ 4.03653$

Body Density
$1.0994921 - 0.0009929$ (sum of three skinfolds) $+ 0.0000023$ (sum of three skinfolds)$^2 + 0.0001392$

Percent Fat in Men and Women

Risk Category	Men (% Body Fat)	Women (% Body Fat)
Essential	3-5	11-14.9
Lean	6-10.9	15-18.9
Fitness	11-15.9	19-22.9
Healthy	16-19.9	23-26.9
Moderate Risk	20-24.9	27-31.9
High Risk	>25	>32

Percent Fat in Children 6-17 Years Old

Risk Category	Boys(% Body Fat)	Girls(% Body Fat)
Very Low	<6	12
Low	7-10	13-15
Optimal Range	11-19	16-25
Moderately High	20-24	26-30
High	25-30	31-35
Very High	>31	>35

Bioelectrical Impedance

Developed in the 1970's, **bioelectrical impedance analysis (BIA)** assesses body fatness based on water conductivity. Due to the fact that fat contains less water than muscle, the speed of conductivity of an electrical impulse provides information on the magnitude of fat in the body. BIA uses a weak 50 kHz electrical current run through the body to identify resistance to the electrical flow referred to as impedance. Numerous instruments, techniques, and population specific equations exist for BIA. Clinical assessments using BIA have been shown to be the most accurate (SEE 4%) (88). The protocol requires the subject to lie in a supine position with electrodes placed on the top of the right hand and foot. Using this technique, outcomes compare favorably to the standard error of estimation for skinfold measurement. Other techniques of BIA have not shown the same level of accuracy, particularly in obese persons (32; 43; 49; 73). Hand-held devices and scales show pronounced differences in accuracy and measurement consistency. Even similar equipment has shown variations among manufacturers (42).

Numerous factors affect the accuracy and precision of BIA (41). Equipment, environmental factors, client factors, and equation appropriateness are all factors influencing error. Because of the variations in equipment prediction, the same measurement instrument should be used each time in order to maximize reliability. Even if the measurement is incorrect when compared to more accurate protocols, it should still reliably show change between pre- and post-tests on the same subject. To maintain reliability and enhance accuracy of the assessment, certain client factors should be considered. Client hydration state needs to be regulated because an increase or decrease in water volume creates variation in the measure. Likewise, the environment needs to be controlled because cold skin temperatures cause underestimation of fat mass. Additionally, the skin thickness at the point of the electrodes influences the assessment. Measurements performed in the original clinical trials are accurate because the electrodes are placed on the back of the hand and top of the foot, where the skin is not conditioned from friction and consequently more permeable to the current. The bottom of the feet and palms of the hands are the most frictionally conditioned parts of the body, and therefore, are not the best sites for electrode placement. Ironically, almost all devices manufactured for BIA use these undesirable locations for electrode placement.

BIA certainly has its share of short comings, but it can be used to track changes effectively outside of clinical environments (40). The assessments are non-threatening and pinpoint accuracy is not completely necessary. When used in conjunction with girth measures, BIA is a viable solution for certain populations. Taking the steps to enhance accuracy is important if the data is to be used effectively. Closely observing the testing protocols and using the correct equation reduces error. Adding client specific data, including age, gender, height, weight, and activity status can also improve accuracy (29). Some devices, including the Omron hand-held BIA analyzer have a computer that adjusts for client specific data.

Testing Guidelines for BIA

1. No eating or drinking within 4 hours of test

2. No exercise or strenuous work within 12 hours of the test.

3. No alcohol consumption for more than 24 hours.

4. Void the bowel and bladder before assessment if possible.

5. Avoid testing during female menstruation.

6. Diuretic medications will invalidate the test.

Near Infrared Light Interactance

Near-infrared (NIR) light interactance was originally used by the USDA to identify food compositions. It has been employed as an easy method to analyze the fat and protein mass of cattle. NIR indirectly measures tissue composition through light absorption and reflection, called optical density (25). Typically performed at the site of the bicep, the NIR emits light into the tissue and measures the amount reflected back. Body fat absorbs the light, while lean mass reflects it. Therefore, the more light emitted back, the leaner the mass. Currently one company, Futrex, makes several commercial instruments with costs in the thousands (69). Claims of accuracy from the manufacturer differ significantly from those found in clinical trials using the NIR device when compared to hydrostatic weighing (44). Standard estimation of error may be as high as 5-8% (26; 33; 48; 68). New equations may improve the prediction accuracy, but more research is needed (50). When the standard estimation of error is added to the cost of the equipment, NIR is not the most practical choice for body composition analysis.

Body Composition Continuum

Body composition values fall along the continuum of health and physical fitness. As a health related component of fitness, various body compositions associate with a range of positive and negative health outcomes. There does appear to be a threshold where, beyond a certain point, the amount of fat mass on the body begins to negatively affect the biological function of other tissues. Although identifying the exact body fat that is ideal for all men and women has been somewhat elusive for researchers, there seems to be a reasonable cut off value for each gender. Values above 20% for men and above 30% for women are more associated with negative health outcomes than values below these body fat percentages (2). This, of course, considers body fat as an independent variable for health risk. When physical activity, diet, and smoking are factored in, the ideal values may fluctuate based on the additional information. A 35 year-old male who smokes and has a body fat of 17% is at much greater risk for disease than a 35 year-old male with 20% body fat who does not smoke. Likewise, a female who has 29% body fat, but routinely eats a healthy diet and performs aerobic exercise most days of the week will likely have a lower risk than a sedentary female with a body fat of 25%. Body fat can be viewed the same way as aerobic fitness, only the relevant numbers are inversed. In aerobic fitness, very low numbers increase risk for disease; with fat the high numbers associate with negative health consequences. Maintaining values that are moderate, in conjunction with appropriate health and fitness behaviors will dramatically reduce risk for possible health problems.

Body fat values can be used for more than predicting health risk. When the values are accurately assessed they can be used in the development and evaluation of the exercise prescription. This is accomplished by converting the weight of fat into caloric value. The Target Body Weight Formula identifies fat weight changes associated with changes in body fat. If the desired body fat is placed in the formula, the end value reflects the new appropriate weight for a client at that particular body fat percentage. This calculation can determine the number of calories that need to be expended and can help clients to realize weight loss goals.

The formula can assist in setting short- and long-term weight loss goals for a client, as well as aid in tracking program effectiveness and identifying errors in balance between diet and energy expenditure. Using the predicted value, correct adjustments can be determined for caloric intake and expenditure recommendations.

Target Body Weight Formula

Fat mass = current body weight x (% body fat ÷ 100)

Fat-free mass (FFM) = current body weight - fat mass

$$\text{Target body weight} = \frac{FFM}{1 - \left\{\frac{\text{Desired \% BF}}{100}\right\}}$$

Example

A 30-year old male weights 185 lbs. and has a body fat percentage of 20%. His goal is to reach 15% body fat. What is his target bodyweight at 15% body fat?

Fat mass = 185 x .20 = 37 lbs

FFM = 185 lbs. - 37 lbs. = 148 lbs

$$\text{Target body weight} = \frac{148}{1 - \frac{(15)}{100}} = 174 \text{ lbs}$$

Male	<3%	5%	10%	15%	18%	22%	25%	30%
	Essential		*Lean*		*Early risk*	*Obesity*		*Morbidly Obese*
Female	<11%	14%	16%	22%	26%	28%	32%	40%

Using the previous example for a 155 lb. person, to change from 20% body fat to 15% he would have to lose approximately 9 lbs. Taking into account that 3,500 calories equals one pound of fat energy, this individual must create a negative caloric balance of 31,500 kcal to lose the 9 lbs. If the goal is one pound of weight loss per week, the client would have to create a negative caloric balance of 500 kcal everyday for nine weeks. Five hundred calories equates to about five miles of running, probably an unrealistic goal for a client to accomplish everyday. Instead, diet and exercise management can be used together to make sure each day ends with a 500 kcal negative balance. Realistic goals are the foundation of exercise adherence. This and other weight loss strategies will be covered in Chapter 11.

Key Terms

Skinfold Measurements- The most widely used body composition testing method to assess body fat percentage. This body composition technique involves the use of calipers to determine levels of subcutaneous fat.

Cellulite- A fatty deposit causing a dimpled or uneven surface.

Bioelectrical Impedance Analysis (BIA)- A body composition technique using the electrical impedance of body tissues, which provides an estimate of total body water (TBW). TBW can be used to estimate fat-free body mass and body fat.

Near-infrared (NIR) Light Interactance- A relatively new method in assessing body fat in which infrared light is emitted into a tissue and the amount reflected back is measured as fat absorbs, and lean mass reflects, the infrared light in determining overall percentage.

Target Body Weight Formula- A formula used to assist in setting short- and long-term weight loss goals.

Chapter Ten References

1. **Abate N and Garg A.** Heterogeneity in adipose tissue metabolism: causes, implications and management of regional adiposity. *Prog Lipid Res* 34: 53-70, 1995.

2. **Abernathy RP and Black DR.** Healthy body weights: an alternative perspective. *Am J Clin Nutr* 63: 448S-451S, 1996.

3. **Ammerman A, Leung MM and Cavallo D.** Addressing disparities in the obesity epidemic. *N C Med J* 67: 301-304, 2006.

4. **Ammerman A, Leung MM and Cavallo D.** Addressing disparities in the obesity epidemic. *N C Med J* 67: 301-304, 2006.

5. **Armellini F, Zamboni M and Bosello O.** Hormones and body composition in humans: clinical studies. *Int J Obes Relat Metab Disord* 24 Suppl 2: S18-S21, 2000.

6. **Armellini F, Zamboni M and Bosello O.** Hormones and body composition in humans: clinical studies. *Int J Obes Relat Metab Disord* 24 Suppl 2: S18-S21, 2000.

7. **Arner P.** Impact of exercise on adipose tissue metabolism in humans. *Int J Obes Relat Metab Disord* 19 Suppl 4: S18-S21, 1995.

8. **Arner P.** Impact of exercise on adipose tissue metabolism in humans. *Int J Obes Relat Metab Disord* 19 Suppl 4: S18-S21, 1995.

9. **Arner P, Engfeldt P and Lithell H.** Site differences in the basal metabolism of subcutaneous fat in obese women. *J Clin Endocrinol Metab* 53: 948-952, 1981.

10. **Ashwell M, Chinn S, Stalley S and Garrow JS.** Female fat distribution--a photographic and cellularity study. *Int J Obes* 2: 289-302, 1978.

11. **Basdevant A, Raison J and Guy-Grand B.** [Influence of the distribution of body fat on vascular risk]. *Presse Med* 16: 167-170, 1987.

12. **Basdevant A, Raison J and Guy-Grand B.** [Influence of the distribution of body fat on vascular risk]. *Presse Med* 16: 167-170, 1987.

13. **Bjorntorp P.** The regulation of adipose tissue distribution in humans. *Int J Obes Relat Metab Disord* 20: 291-302, 1996.

14. **Bjorntorp P.** The regulation of adipose tissue distribution in humans. *Int J Obes Relat Metab Disord* 20: 291-302, 1996.

15. **Blaak E.** Gender differences in fat metabolism. *Curr Opin Clin Nutr Metab Care* 4: 499-502, 2001.

16. **Blaak E.** Gender differences in fat metabolism. *Curr Opin Clin Nutr Metab Care* 4: 499-502, 2001.

17. **Blaak E.** Gender differences in fat metabolism. *Curr Opin Clin Nutr Metab Care* 4: 499-502, 2001.

18. **Blaak E.** Gender differences in fat metabolism. *Curr Opin Clin Nutr Metab Care* 4: 499-502, 2001.

19. **Bradley DW.** The epidemic of overweight and obesity: a challenge to medicine, public health and public policy. *N C Med J* 67: 268-272, 2006.

20. **Bradley DW.** The epidemic of overweight and obesity: a challenge to medicine, public health and public policy. *N C Med J* 67: 268-272, 2006.

21. **Brodie DA.** Techniques of measurement of body composition. Part I. *Sports Med* 5: 11-40, 1988.

22. **Busetto L, Baggio MB, Zurlo F, Carraro R, Digito M and Enzi G.** Assessment of abdominal fat distribution in obese patients: anthropometry versus computerized tomography. *Int J Obes Relat Metab Disord* 16: 731-736, 1992.

23. **Chan GM.** Performance of dual-energy x-ray absorptiometry in evaluating bone, lean body mass, and fat in pediatric subjects. *J Bone Miner Res* 7: 369-374, 1992.

24. **Collins MA, Millard-Stafford ML, Sparling PB, Snow TK, Rosskopf LB, Webb SA and Omer J.** Evaluation of the BOD POD for assessing body fat in collegiate football players. *Med Sci Sports Exerc* 31: 1350-1356, 1999.

25. **Conway JM, Norris KH and Bodwell CE.** A new approach for the estimation of body composition: infrared interactance. *Am J Clin Nutr* 40: 1123-1130, 1984.

26. **Fogelholm M and van Marken LW.** Comparison of body composition methods: a literature analysis. *Eur J Clin Nutr* 51: 495-503, 1997.

27. **Garcia AL, Wagner K, Hothorn T, Koebnick C, Zunft HJ and Trippo U.** Improved prediction of body fat by measuring skinfold thickness, circumferences, and bone breadths. *Obes Res* 13: 626-634, 2005.

28. **Gause-Nilsson I and Dey DK.** Percent body fat estimation from skin fold thickness in the elderly. Development of a population-based prediction equation and comparison with published equations in 75-year-olds. *J Nutr Health Aging* 9: 19-24, 2005.

29. **Goran MI, Toth MJ and Poehlman ET.** Cross-validation of anthropometric and bioelectrical resistance prediction equations for body composition in older people using the 4-compartment model as a criterion method. *J Am Geriatr Soc* 45: 837-843, 1997.

30. **Haffner SM.** Relationship of metabolic risk factors and development of cardiovascular disease and diabetes. *Obesity (Silver Spring)* 14 Suppl 3: 121S-127S, 2006.

31. **He Q, Horlick M, Thornton J, Wang J, Pierson RN, Jr., Heshka S and Gallagher D.** Sex and race differences in fat distribution among Asian, African-American, and Caucasian prepubertal children. *J Clin Endocrinol Metab* 87: 2164-2170, 2002.

32. **Heyward VH, Cook KL, Hicks VL, Jenkins KA, Quatrochi JA and Wilson WL.** Predictive accuracy of three field methods for estimating relative body fatness of nonobese and obese women. *Int J Sport Nutr* 2: 75-86, 1992.

33. **Hortobagyi T, Israel RG, Houmard JA, McCammon MR and O'Brien KF.** Comparison of body composition assessment by hydrodensitometry, skinfolds, and multiple site near-infrared spectrophotometry. *Eur J Clin Nutr* 46: 205-211, 1992.

34. **Ivanov Z and Ivanov M**. [Relation between body fat mass and lipid status in the obese working population]. *Srp Arh Celok Lek* 130: 361-366, 2002.

35. **Jones V**. The "diabesity" epidemic: let's rehabilitate America. *MedGenMed* 8: 34, 2006.

36. **Jurimae T, Jagomagi G and Lepp T**. Body composition of university students by hydrostatic weighing and skinfold measurement. *J Sports Med Phys Fitness* 32: 387-393, 1992.

37. **Kosti RI and Panagiotakos DB**. The epidemic of obesity in children and adolescents in the world. *Cent Eur J Public Health* 14: 151-159, 2006.

38. **Krotkiewski M**. Can body fat patterning be changed? *Acta Med Scand Suppl* 723: 213-223, 1988.

39. **Ley CJ, Lees B and Stevenson JC**. Sex- and menopause-associated changes in body-fat distribution. *Am J Clin Nutr* 55: 950-954, 1992.

40. **Lockner DW, Heyward VH, Griffin SE, Marques MB, Stolarczyk LM and Wagner DR**. Cross-validation of modified fatness-specific bioelectrical impedance equations. *Int J Sport Nutr* 9: 48-59, 1999.

41. **Lukaski HC and Siders WA**. Validity and accuracy of regional bioelectrical impedance devices to determine whole-body fatness. *Nutrition* 19: 851-857, 2003.

42. **Lukaski HC and Siders W**A. Validity and accuracy of regional bioelectrical impedance devices to determine whole-body fatness. *Nutrition* 19: 851-857, 2003.

43. **Lukaski HC and Siders WA**. Validity and accuracy of regional bioelectrical impedance devices to determine whole-body fatness. *Nutrition* 19: 851-857, 2003.

44. **McLean KP and Skinner JS**. Validity of Futrex-5000 for body composition determination. *Med Sci Sports Exerc* 24: 253-258, 1992.

45. **McTernan PG, Anderson LA, Anwar AJ, Eggo MC, Crocker J, Barnett AH, Stewart PM and Kumar S**. Glucocorticoid regulation of p450 aromatase activity in human adipose tissue: gender and site differences. *J Clin Endocrinol Metab* 87: 1327-1336, 2002.

46. **Mueller WH and Joos SK**. Android (centralized) obesity and somatotypes in men: association with mesomorphy. *Ann Hum Biol* 12: 377-381, 1985.

47. **Muralidhara DV and Bhat MR**. Body fat and lean body mass assessment in human subjects--a comparison of two different techniques. *Indian J Physiol Pharmacol* 42: 139-143, 1998.

48. **Nemeth A, Bodzsar EB and Eiben OG**. Comparisons of fatness indicators in Budapest children. *Anthropol Anz* 57: 325-337, 1999.

49. **Neovius M, Hemmingsson E, Freyschuss B and Udden J**. Bioelectrical impedance underestimates total and truncal fatness in abdominally obese women. *Obesity (Silver Spring)* 14: 1731-1738, 2006.

50. **Oppliger RA, Clark RR and Nielsen DH**. New equations improve NIR prediction of body fat among high school wrestlers. *J Orthop Sports Phys Ther* 30: 536-543, 2000.

51. **ORPIN MJ and SCOTT PJ**. ESTIMATION OF TOTAL BODY FAT USING SKIN FOLD CALIPER MEASUREMENTS. *N Z Med J* 63: 501-507, 1964.

52. **Paijmans IJ, Wilmore KM and Wilmore JH**. Use of skinfolds and bioelectrical impedance for body composition assessment after weight reduction. *J Am Coll Nutr* 11: 145-151, 1992.

53. **Pollock ML and Jackson AS**. Research progress in validation of clinical methods of assessing body composition. *Med Sci Sports Exerc* 16: 606-615, 1984.

54. **Pollock ML and Jackson AS**. Research progress in validation of clinical methods of assessing body composition. *Med Sci Sports Exerc* 16: 606-615, 1984.

55. **Pollock ML and Jackson AS**. Research progress in validation of clinical methods of assessing body composition. *Med Sci Sports Exerc* 16: 606-615, 1984.

56. **Pollock ML and Jackson AS**. Research progress in validation of clinical methods of assessing body composition. *Med Sci Sports Exerc* 16: 606-615, 1984.

57. **Pollock ML and Jackson AS**. Research progress in validation of clinical methods of assessing body composition. *Med Sci Sports Exerc* 16: 606-615, 1984.

58. **Pollock ML and Jackson AS**. Research progress in validation of clinical methods of assessing body composition. *Med Sci Sports Exerc* 16: 606-615, 1984.

59. **Pollock ML and Jackson AS**. Research progress in validation of clinical methods of assessing body composition. *Med Sci Sports Exerc* 16: 606-615, 1984.

60. **Price GM, Uauy R, Breeze E, Bulpitt CJ and Fletcher AE**. Weight, shape, and mortality risk in older persons:

elevated waist-hip ratio, not high body mass index, is associated with a greater risk of death. *Am J Clin Nutr* 84: 449-460, 2006.

61. **Prior BM, Cureton KJ, Modlesky CM, Evans EM, Sloniger MA, Saunders M and Lewis RD**. In vivo validation of whole body composition estimates from dual-energy X-ray absorptiometry. *J Appl Physiol* 83: 623-630, 1997.

62. **Prior BM, Cureton KJ, Modlesky CM, Evans EM, Sloniger MA, Saunders M and Lewis RD**. In vivo validation of whole body composition estimates from dual-energy X-ray absorptiometry. *J Appl Physiol* 83: 623-630, 1997.

63. **Rippe JM and Hess S**. The role of physical activity in the prevention and management of obesity. *J Am Diet Assoc* 98: S31-S38, 1998.

64. **Scott EC and Johnston FE**. Critical fat, menarche, and the maintenance of menstrual cycles: a critical review. *J Adolesc Health Care* 2: 249-260, 1982.

65. **Shah B, Sucher K and Hollenbeck CB**. Comparison of ideal body weight equations and published height-weight tables with body mass index tables for healthy adults in the United States. *Nutr Clin Pract* 21: 312-319, 2006.

66. **Shah B, Sucher K and Hollenbeck CB**. Comparison of ideal body weight equations and published height-weight tables with body mass index tables for healthy adults in the United States. *Nutr Clin Pract* 21: 312-319, 2006.

67. **Shake CL, Schlichting C, Mooney LW, Callahan AB and Cohen ME**. Predicting percent body fat from circumference measurements. *Mil Med* 158: 26-31, 1993.

68. **Smith DB, Johnson GO, Stout JR, Housh TJ, Housh DJ and Evetovich TK**. Validity of near-infrared interactance for estimating relative body fat in female high school gymnasts. *Int J Sports Med* 18: 531-537, 1997.

69. **Smith DB, Johnson GO, Stout JR, Housh TJ, Housh DJ and Evetovich TK**. Validity of near-infrared interactance for estimating relative body fat in female high school gymnasts. *Int J Sports Med* 18: 531-537, 1997.

70. **Smith SC, Jr. and Haslam D**. Abdominal obesity, waist circumference and cardio-metabolic risk: awareness among primary care physicians, the general population and patients at risk--the Shape of the Nations survey. *Curr Med Res Opin* 23: 29-47, 2007.

71. **Smith SC, Jr. and Haslam D**. Abdominal obesity, waist circumference and cardio-metabolic risk: awareness among primary care physicians, the general population and patients at risk--the Shape of the Nations survey. *Curr Med Res Opin* 23: 29-47, 2007.

72. **Stern JS, Hirsch J, Blair SN, Foreyt JP, Frank A, Kumanyika SK, Madans JH, Marlatt GA, St Jeor ST and Stunkard AJ**. Weighing the options: criteria for evaluating weight-management programs. The Committee to Develop Criteria for Evaluating the Outcomes of Approaches to Prevent and Treat Obesity. *Obes Res* 3: 591-604, 1995.

73. **Stolarczyk LM, Heyward VH, Hicks VL and Baumgartner RN**. Predictive accuracy of bioelectrical impedance in estimating body composition of Native American women. *Am J Clin Nutr* 59: 964-970, 1994.

74. **Tchernof A, Belanger C, Morisset AS, Richard C, Mailloux J, Laberge P and Dupont P**. Regional differences in adipose tissue metabolism in women: minor effect of obesity and body fat distribution. *Diabetes* 55: 1353-1360, 2006.

75. **Terry RB, Page WF and Haskell WL**. Waist/hip ratio, body mass index and premature cardiovascular disease mortality in US Army veterans during a twenty-three year follow-up study. *Int J Obes Relat Metab Disord* 16: 417-423, 1992.

76. **Votruba SB and Jensen MD**. Sex differences in abdominal, gluteal, and thigh LPL activity. *Am J Physiol Endocrinol Metab* 2007.

77. **Votruba SB and Jensen MD**. Sex differences in abdominal, gluteal, and thigh LPL activity. *Am J Physiol Endocrinol Metab* 2007.

78. **Votruba SB and Jensen MD**. Sex differences in abdominal, gluteal, and thigh LPL activity. *Am J Physiol Endocrinol Metab* 2007.

79. **Votruba SB and Jensen MD**. Sex differences in abdominal, gluteal, and thigh LPL activity. *Am J Physiol Endocrinol Metab* 2007.

80. **Votruba SB and Jensen MD**. Sex differences in abdominal, gluteal, and thigh LPL activity. *Am J Physiol Endocrinol Metab* 2007.

81. **Votruba SB and Jensen MD**. Sex differences in abdominal, gluteal, and thigh LPL activity. *Am J Physiol Endocrinol Metab* 2007.

82. **Wake DJ, Strand M, Rask E, Westerbacka J, Livingstone DE, Soderberg S, Andrew R, Yki-Jarvinen H, Olsson T and Walker BR**. Intra-adipose sex steroid

metabolism and body fat distribution in idiopathic human obesity. *Clin Endocrinol (Oxf)* 66: 440-446, 2007.

83. **Walton C, Lees B, Crook D, Worthington M, Godsland IF and Stevenson JC**. Body fat distribution, rather than overall adiposity, influences serum lipids and lipoproteins in healthy men independently of age. *Am J Med* 99: 459-464, 1995.

84. **Wang J, Thornton JC, Kolesnik S and Pierson RN, Jr**. Anthropometry in body composition. An overview. *Ann N Y Acad Sci* 904: 317-326, 2000.

85. **Wang J, Thornton JC, Kolesnik S and Pierson RN, Jr**. Anthropometry in body composition. An overview. *Ann N Y Acad Sci* 904: 317-326, 2000.

86. **Weltman A, Levine S, Seip RL and Tran ZV**. Accurate assessment of body composition in obese females. *Am J Clin Nutr* 48: 1179-1183, 1988.

87. **Weltman A, Levine S, Seip RL and Tran ZV**. Accurate assessment of body composition in obese females. *Am J Clin Nutr* 48: 1179-1183, 1988.

88. **Wilmore KM, McBride PJ and Wilmore JH**. Comparison of bioelectric impedance and near-infrared interactance for body composition assessment in a population of self-perceived overweight adults. *Int J Obes Relat Metab Disord* 18: 375-381, 1994.

89. **Wysocki M, Krotkiewski M, Braide M and Bagge U**. Hemorheological disturbances, metabolic parameters and blood pressure in different types of obesity. *Atherosclerosis* 88: 21-28, 1991.

Chapter 11

Weight Management

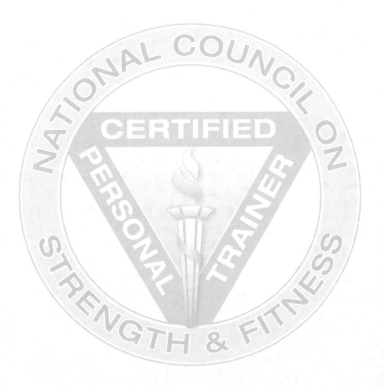

In This Chapter

Social, Economic, Physiological Factors

Energy Balance

Yo-Yo Dieting

Food Recalls and Logs

Metabolism

Weight Management Strategies

Social Behaviors and Weight Management

Weight Gain

Eating Disorders

Introduction

Rising obesity increasingly threatens the United States in terms of health risk to the overall population (17; 77). The current rate of weight gain and the medical costs associated with it have caused the government to create a formal initiative to combat the alarmingly steady rise in obesity (62). Estimates indicate that an obese individual costs six times more money in managed health care than a non-obese person (32). The obesity rate is climbing by 1% a year, and the World Health Organization predicts that America will reach a 70% obesity rate within the population by 2030 (75). This state of affairs could be economically catastrophic if it occurs (50).

The prevalence of overweight and obesity in America has pushed weight management to the forefront of personal trainers' job responsibilities. Most clients who hire personal trainers do so to look and feel better. Although the desire to lose weight is often vanity driven, the health outcomes associated with attaining a healthy weight are far more important. Weight loss is a relatively easy task to accomplish, in theory, because it is simply a reduction of energy consumed and an increase in energy expended. In reality though, most people find it very difficult to lose weight due to the number of factors associated with successful weight loss. Social, economic, physiological, psychological, and emotional factors can each play a part in creating barriers to adherence and success in a weight management program (28; 42; 57; 74). Addressing one factor alone may be ineffective due to the fact that the other factors may potentially create obstacles independent of the controlled variable, or the factors may compound, increasing the effort needed to comply with the original weight loss strategy. Therefore, an understanding of how each factor interacts with energy balance can assist in successfully managing a client's weight.

Social Factors

Social factors that effect weight stem from many different aspects of American tradition, behaviors, and lifestyle activities (59). Traditionally, food and drink have long been associated with celebrations, family gatherings, special events, and social environments. Linked with sensations of pleasure, the tendency for many people to indulge themselves with more calories than the body needs often occurs when eating during social activities. High calorie beverages, appetizers, large meals, and desserts are all part of normal eating patterns at weddings, holidays, get-togethers, and family events. Likewise, weekend activities often cause variations in eating habits and calorie intake compared to the more structured work week. Visits to restaurants,

social clubs, and gatherings with friends routinely dismantle efforts made during the week, as calories burned from exercise and conscious dietary restraint are easily replaced in a short period of time.

To contend with the additional caloric consumption associated with social events, weight management strategies should identify the specific problems and seek remedies to prevent or decrease the negative actions. Assessing the client's behaviors via interview can help identify common problem areas that warrant intervention or education. Some common habits that present obstacles to weight loss include:

Obstacles to Weight Loss

1. Over-consumption of food in attempts to try all the food dishes presented.

2. Eating large portions by loading the plate at a buffet or self-serve bar.

3. Consuming food and drink in response to boredom or social nervousness.

4. Location eating: close proximity to food increases likelihood of consumption.

5. Pressures to try dishes to acknowledge preparation effort by the party host.

6. Ordering multiple dishes or very large portions based on appetite at restaurants.

7. Not realizing the caloric density of foods prepared by others.

8. Throwing out restrictive habits due to the environment.

9. Allowing alcohol to skew judgment.

10. Eating or drinking in response to peer pressure.

There may be many contributing environmental factors that cause people to over eat when in social settings. Acknowledging the risks and obstacles in each environment helps clients to be conscious of the possible errors that can be made and the consequent limitations they place on goal attainment. Strategies to avoid these pitfalls should be discussed and documented as an ongoing part of the weight management program.

Economic Factors

Certain economic factors serve as obstacles to weight management as well (60). Recent identification of the impact of some of these factors has led to criticism of corporate and government practices (7; 30; 66). High calorie, low-cost foods have become a staple of many American diets, particularly for those in the lower socioeconomic income bracket (49). Fast food restaurants offer convenience, low price, and an abundance of calories. For individuals living within budgetary restraints, fast food has become an important dietary option. Higher quality food is often more expensive and harder to keep fresh than inexpensive alternatives. Fruits and vegetables, fish, lean meats, and whole grain products require a larger food budget for daily consumption, and they frequently have a shorter shelf-life. If shopping on a budget, boxed processed foods and lower quality foods high in fats and preservatives are a more cost-effective alternative. Sugar, for instance is an excellent preservative. Americans from the low socioeconomic brackets have less opportunity to eat healthy because their selections are limited to what they can afford (18).

The level of nutrition education and knowledge has also been linked to socioeconomic status (13; 44). Less affluent Americans have limited access to education resources compared to wealthier classes. Consequently, relative familiarity with nutrient value, caloric density, and healthy dietary practices are often lower in poorer communities, and the information availability is more limited. For instance, the **USDA** provides quality education and applications on the internet, but without a computer, this information is difficult to access. Risk for obesity has been linked to socioeconomic status, and the behaviors learned early in life tend to stay with an individual into adulthood. Those with less opportunity during the years of their youth may be more susceptible to weight gain as adults, regardless of their later economic status (43).

Physiological Factors

Hunger is the primary physiological determinant of eating behaviors. Stimulated by the **hypothalamus**, hunger is defined as the physiological sensation that leads to the urge to eat (6). It is a subjective feeling and therefore, does not discriminate the exact caloric intake needed. Response to hunger and subsequent satiety, or feeling of fullness, is multi-faceted, and as a result, variations in eating response often occur. Satiation is experienced when the body has consumed adequate food to satisfy its need, thereby shutting off the hunger response. Due to the large number of variables affecting the body's regulatory system for food intake, it is not a very concise mechanism (15; 29). The sensation of fullness may be attributed to the type of calories consumed, the amount of food in the stomach, or the extent food intake satisfies the demand created by the brain. Due to the variability in the regulatory response, a person may over-consume food before the mechanism to turn off eating occurs (21; 41).

Peripheral mechanisms are used to regulate food consumption via chemoreceptors and hormones (23; 33). The efficiency of these mechanisms is not always consistent, which is one reason why variations in eating patterns exist (24). One problem is that it is possible to consume calories at a rate faster than the food intake information can be processed. Likewise, different foods affect the speed and magnitude of satiation (27). Certain foods trigger peripheral mechanisms more efficiently than others. According to the University of Sydney's satiation index, over a two hour period, fish, fruits such as apples and oranges, and potatoes yield more efficient and effective satiety than croissants, cakes, donuts, peanuts, candy bars, and yogurt (38). Fibrous foods have also been linked with sensations of fullness due to the bulk they add in the diet. The duration of fullness seems to be tied to gastric emptying time (how long food remains in the stomach), fluid content, and overall bulk (54). According to laboratory results, the less water ingested and the longer the digestive process, the more hunger is staved off. In addition, biochemical evidence exists that suggests fat and protein content effects satiety as well.

When hunger is not addressed in a reasonable period of time the perception of the food needed by the body will often increase. Regularly consuming food throughout the day reduces the hunger mechanism, and therefore, may reduce total caloric intake. Selecting foods that quickly increase satiation, like apples and oranges, can help to regulate eating patterns when used as snacks. The inconsistencies in hunger satisfaction rates also suggest that foods should be consumed at slower rates and with adequate fluid to allow the body to recognize the nutrients and use the information to better regulate the chemical shut off valve in the hypothalamus.

Regulatory Center for Hunger

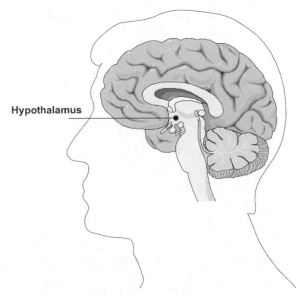

Hypothalamus

Psychological Factors

Appetite differs from hunger in that appetite is the primary psychological mechanism controlling eating, though it is often associated with the level of hunger experienced by the body (22). It represents a desire to eat based on the thought of food in the presence of hunger, but it can also occur without a physiological mediator. A person's appetite may be for a type of food, particular nutrient, or craving from environmental sights, smells, or thoughts. Planning to order a particular meal before getting to a favorite restaurant or craving a hot dog at a ball park are common examples. Appetite is often blamed for over consumption because it is linked with the psychological perception of satisfaction from food. Many people order a large entrée at a restaurant, but after consuming the appetizer, table breads, and their drink, actual hunger has subsided. When the additional food is delivered the pleasurable sights and smells stimulate appetite again, which often consequently help to motivate the person to further indulge in calories they probably do not need.

The psychological pleasure of eating contributes greatly to high calorie diets. Sensations associated with favorite foods cause chemicals to be released, driving people to eat (25). People find pleasure in tastes, textures, and sensations associated with certain foods or the environments where the food is consumed. This association causes people to desire the foods even when they are not hungry or to over consume the foods after they are full. High calorie foods rich in fats and sugar are often the foods with the most desirable tastes, and therefore present problems in a diet aimed at weight loss (26).

Psychological considerations also include behavior patterns, environmental cues, learned eating behaviors, and the psychological assignment of dollar value. Behavior eating patterns are commonly related to an association between locations, times, and events. A common example of this behavior is eating chips or popcorn while watching television or a movie. Events trigger eating responses as well: the Sunday football game, a trip to the fair, or even an ice cream stop while shopping at the mall has food-event associations. Familiar sites and sounds can trigger appetite without any presence of hunger (67).

Learned eating behaviors also contribute to psychological factors that surround consumption. Eating everything on the plate is a lesson taught early in life that sticks with people into adulthood. In some cases, these behaviors stem from cultural norms that instigate particular eating patterns or food choices. Families that

The Satiety Index

Each of the following foods are rated by how much food people consumed in order to satisfy their hunger
All are compared to white bread, ranked as "100"

Bakery Products		Snacks and Confectionary		Breakfast Cereals with Milk		Carbohydrate-Rich Foods		Protein-Rich Foods		Fruits	
Croissant	47%	Mars candy bar	70%	Mueslix	100%	White bread	100%	Lentils	133%	Bananas	118%
Cake	65%	Peanuts	84%	Sustain	112%	French fries	116%	Cheese	146%	Grapes	162%
Doughnuts	68%	Yogurt	88%	Special K	116%	White pasta	119%	Eggs	150%	Apples	197%
Cookies	120%	Crisps	91%	Cornflakes	118%	Brown rice	132%	Baked beans	168%	Oranges	202%
Crackers	127%	Ice cream	96%	Honeysmacks	132%	White rice	138%	Beef	176%		
		Jellybeans	118%	All-Bran	151%	Grain bread	154%	Ling fish	225%		
		Popcorn	154%	Oatmeal	209%	Wholemeal bread	157%				
						Brown pasta	188%				
						Potatoes, boiled	323%				

Adapted from S.H.A. Holt, J.C. Brand Miller, P. Petocz, and E. Farmakalidis, "A Satiety Index of Common Foods,"*European Journal of Clinical Nutrition, Sept 1995*

Disclaimer: The formula does not account for all known contributing factors for satiety. The formula is derived from a small data set. The data set is based on subjectively reported, rather than directly measured, criteria.

center their relationships on food and togetherness encourage large portions and longer time periods spent eating. There may be expectations to eat as a sign of affection and appreciation among the family members. Providing extra food to a son, daughter, or spouse is viewed as showing care for that person, as is eating all the food presented to acknowledge the appreciation for the offering.

In some cases over eating occurs to avoid wasting the food. The psychological and tangible value assigned to food can drive people to eat portions that they do not want or need. Commonly, people consume all the food presented at a restaurant because they paid for it, even though their hunger is satisfied before the meal was completely consumed. People routinely eat the last portions left in the serving containers to avoid having to deal with the leftovers. When food in the refrigerator reaches its termination date, it is often pushed for consumption, so it does not get thrown out and wasted.

Certain emotions or mental states can also drive people to consume food when they are not hungry (51). When people are in a state of boredom, eating provides a diversion. Without an alternate distraction, people often look through the kitchen and eat to pass the time. Likewise, particular emotions can drive people to eat (69). Depression, low self-worth, or sadness can cause people to find comfort in food because it provides pleasure (40). In other situations, people may eat as a reward for accomplishing something or because they have been good. Emotionally-driven food consumption may occur with or without hunger. The food choices selected are commonly associated with pleasure and often lead to indiscriminate eating. Personal trainers should identify these causes to help clients realize and recognize emotionally triggered eating patterns.

Energy Balance

When food is routinely consumed without the presence of hunger or above the caloric requirements of the body, the energy balance can become uneven. Energy balance is simply a comparison of the calories consumed versus the calories expended. Due to the fact that energy can neither be created nor destroyed, it must transfer into some appreciable form when it enters the body. If body energy is not used for enzymatic reactions or converted into heat and released into the air, it will likely be stored in cells or become a component of tissue. When the number of calories consumed is higher than the number of calories metabolized, the body experiences a positive caloric balance. Positive caloric balance leads to weight gain because the abundance of energy remains within the body. When the calories consumed match the calories expended, the body is isocaloric, or in a neutral

caloric balance, and consequently, weight should remain unchanged. When the calories expended by the body exceed the number of calories consumed, the body is in negative balance. Negative caloric balance is necessary for the reduction of body weight and body fat.

Concerns of Significant Caloric Restriction

Significant caloric restriction causes weight loss. However, much of this weight loss is accounted for by water and lean mass reduction (72). Defense mechanisms are in place so that when the body does not consume enough energy, it becomes catabolic. This is likely attributed to survival needs by early humans, who could not eat as regularly as we do today. When food was not available, their bodies reduced metabolic activity by reducing the tissue that required the most calories (i.e. muscle). Today, the same phenomenon occurs. Significantly cutting calories often leads to a reduction in metabolism due to lean mass diminution (71).

Some physicians prescribe **very low calorie diets (VLCD)** for severely obese clients even though the caloric intakes are below the recommended minimums. Diets containing only 800-1200 calories are prescribed and closely monitored for appropriate nutrients (53). These diets are completely inappropriate for individuals not suffering from life-threatening ailments or risk attributed to their weight (1). The diets are used in conjunction with metabolic, blood, and vital sign monitoring in hospital-based settings to prevent any significant negative health consequences from occurring. When individuals attempt to duplicate the VLCD plan by utilizing starvation type diets they risk damaging their metabolism and placing their organs under considerable stress (2). The minimum recommended caloric intake to maintain adequate nutrient composition is 1200 kcal/day. For many people, this value is still insufficient and can lead to negative outcomes if individual nutrient requirements are not met.

Yo-Yo Dieting

Physiological detriment has also been observed in people who routinely follow low calorie "fad" diets. The Yo-Yo dieting effect may be linked with reduced metabolism and increased body fat with age (11; 12; 65). The "10 lbs. off, 10 lbs. back on" trend commonly occurs in American dietary practices. People lose the weight in two months and gain it back in the four to six months following the diet's conclusion. Due to the restrictive nature of dieting, particularly without exercise, a loss of muscle may occur every time a new diet is employed. Lean mass is one of the primary

Effects of Yo - Yo Dieting

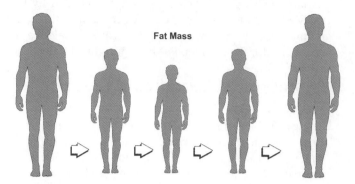

Fat Mass

Weight loss through diet   Weight gain when diet ends

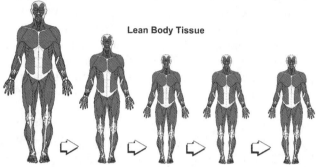

Lean Body Tissue

contributors to an individual's metabolic rate. The reduction in lean mass associated with dietary practices solely emphasizing caloric restriction increases the susceptibility of subsequent weight gain as a person ages.

Food Recalls and Logs

To appropriately manage weight, the correct balance between caloric expenditure and caloric intake must be attained on a routine basis. The resultant difference needs to be appropriate for the desired incremental changes to take place. To accomplish successful weight loss or weight gain, the values which contribute to the balance must be identified and managed correctly. To determine the caloric intake of an individual, a personal trainer can perform a dietary energy assessment. There are several protocols designed to identify or estimate the actual number of calories being consumed in a typical day. They are divided into food logs and food recall assessments. Food recalls are easily implemented and require minimal effort. The assessment requires a client to recall all of the food and drink consumed over a selected period of time. In most cases a 24-hour recall is used so that the information is still fresh in the mind of the client. The client is asked to record every calorie containing food or beverage by the serving or portion size consumed. It is important that the information be complete, recalled in detail, and measured as concisely as possible. To help enhance the accuracy of the information, personal trainers should use descriptions, household containers, or models to show clients what serving sizes and normal portions or food quantities are, as well as the standard household measures. If the client is inaccurate with the quantity of the food or drink consumed, the data collected may be invalid and skew any subsequent recommendations.

Food logs use a similar assessment protocol, but differ in the fact that the client records the foods as they are consumed. This difference in the data collection methodology increases potential accuracy above the recall method because the recording is done at the time of the intake, thereby reducing forgetfulness or inaccurate recall. Food records can be done for a 24-hour period, but the preferred method is to use three days of dietary consumption. The purpose of using a multiple day log is to identify variations in eating patterns and identify changes that occur between days in the week. Generally the days used should represent the beginning, middle, and end of the week. Commonly Monday, Thursday, and Saturday are designated for review. Including one weekend day is helpful because of common differences in eating habits on weekends compared to weekdays. This strategy enhances typical representation because it reflects the dietary habits consistent with different eating locations and frames of mind when consuming the foods. It is prudent to have the client identify the location where they consumed the food or drink and their feelings at the time of the

Sample Food Log

Amount (Serving Size)	Food Description (Cooking Method, Brand Name)	Location (Place, People, Social Environment)	Feeling (Hunger, Anger, Joy)	Time of Day
1 Cup	Kellogg's Corn Flakes	Home Breakfast table	Hungry	8 am
1/2 Cup	Low Fat milk 2%	Home Breakfast table	Hungry	8 am
1 Cup	Decaf Coffee	Home Breakfast table	Hungry	8 am
1	Banana	Home Breakfast table	Hungry	8 am

Common Errors in Food Recall or Food Log Assessments

Incorrect serving size or portion

Limited familiarity with container sizes or measurements

Forgotten items

Falsifying quantities or purposely leaving items out

Temporarily changing eating habits

Limited knowledge of mixed food contents or restaurant prepared foods

Overlooking use of condiments

Guessing rather than recalling

Assessing a non-typical eating pattern

Steps to Improve Recall Accuracy

Recall the activities in sequence from when they woke up until they went to bed.

Demonstrate the quantity using a tangible measuring model.

Describe the eating experience to improve detail; use drawings to show exact sizes.

Identify what was added to the food, if anything.

Recall the beverages separately.

Recall snacks consumed outside of main meals.

Ask the client if they have recalled everything or if there is anything they are not sure of.

consumption. This may provide data related to behavioral patterns and help identify intervention strategies. Food records require the same attentiveness and client education as the 24-hour recall. Clients should be clearly instructed on the protocol and advised to be conscious of the common errors found with the assessment. Clients should be convinced that they are not being judged nor will their food intake reflect negatively upon them. It is important for goal attainment to have accurate information. Otherwise, it may be a costly waste of time and effort.

Food recall and log data can be analyzed using a number of different computer diet analysis programs or performed manually using food composition tables. The government offers a free user-friendly database of foods as part of the USDA Food Guide Pyramid (www.mypyramidtracker.gov). The analysis program provides a detailed breakdown of foods' energy and nutrient composition. It also compares the nutrient intakes with the current food guide pyramid and identifies possible deficiencies that may negatively influence health.

Basic Nutrients to Evaluate

Percentage of Calories
Carbohydrates
Sugar
Fats
Proteins
Saturated fat

Additional Nutrients
Cholesterol
Fiber
Sodium
Calcium
Iron
Water

Once the data is compiled, it needs interpreting for both quantifiable and non-quantifiable information. Quantifiable information includes the food source and nutrient contents. Location and size of meal, why it was selected, and the time it was consumed represents non-quantifiable information. Both types of data are useful in identifying intake and food-selection patterns or habits.

The data should be evaluated for energy content, energy nutrient distribution, quality food choices, variety, and nutrient balance. Although the total caloric intake will be used in determining energy balance, particular nutrient quantities should also be evaluated for health purposes.

These nutrients can paint a broader picture of the diet's value as it pertains to health and may provide details that are useful to subsequent weight management strategies and recommendations. A diet high in fat, sugar, and processed carbohydrates will likely contribute as much to dietary problems as excess calories.

Metabolism

Identifying caloric intake provides information for half of the energy balance equation. The next step in completing the evaluation involves determining the daily caloric expenditure. Daily caloric expenditure is calculated by adding an individual's resting metabolic rate and their voluntary metabolism created from daily activity participation. Voluntary metabolism represents those calories expended through activity. The sum of the two measures is referred to as an individual's daily need. Daily need reflects the number of calories required for a neutral balance and weight maintenance.

Components of Metabolism

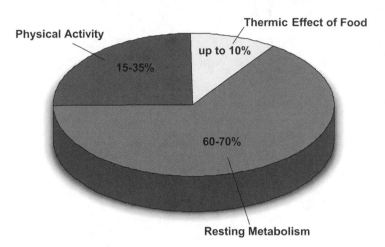

Physical Activity
15-35%

Thermic Effect of Food
up to 10%

60-70%

Resting Metabolism

Resting Metabolic Rate

Resting metabolic rate (RMR) generally represents between 60-70% of the total caloric expenditure in a given day (46). It is defined as the rate at which the body expends energy to support vital functions including heart contractions, digestion, and various cellular activities. Metabolic rates vary from person to person and are affected by several factors, including genetics, gender, age, height, weight, lean body mass, and hormone activity. In addition, certain conditions can cause increased metabolic activity at rest such as fever, stress, starvation, recovery from exertions, and malnutrition.

Several available methods can measure or predict metabolic rate in humans. Measurements are most commonly done in clinical environments using indirect calorimetry. Indirect calorimetry uses respiratory measurements of oxygen consumption and carbon dioxide production to calculate caloric expenditure. Although more accurate than predictive equations, the technique is not always practical for the personal trainer because the expensive equipment needed to perform the analysis and a complete understanding of the scientific protocol are not available. For logistical purposes, metabolic rate is more commonly predicted from equations. The use of equations to predict RMR allows

for close estimations based on known factors. The predictions are founded on the principles that 1) RMR is proportionate to body size, 2) RMR decreases with age, and 3) muscle is more metabolically active than fat. This relationship is reflected in all equations used to predict RMR. Two commonly used RMR equations are the **Cunningham Lean Mass Equation** and the **Revised Harris-Benedict Equations**.

The Lean Mass Equation is used to predict RMR when an individual's body composition has been accurately identified. It is not gender specific because it is calculated by the relative lean mass of an individual and therefore does not require adjustment for gender differences in fat storage. The value is useful for weight loss or weight gain programs because it focuses on the metabolically active lean mass. Identifying and using the quantity of lean mass in the calculation reduces the overestimation of RMR associated with the fat mass contribution to body weight found in other equations. One limiting factor to the calculation is that it does not account for age, which is known to affect metabolism independent of lean mass. Therefore, the predicted value will be more accurate for younger individuals.

The Revised Harris-Benedict Equations may be more appropriate when lean mass cannot be accurately determined. Unlike the lean mass equation, the Harris-

~Key Terms~

USDA- The United States Department of Agriculture.

Hypothalamus- The part of the brain that lies below the thalamus. The hypothalamus regulates bodily temperature, certain metabolic processes, and other autonomic activities.

Very Low Calorie Diet (VLCD)- A diet of 800 kilocalories a day or less.

Resting Metabolic Rate (RMR)- The rate at which the body expends energy to support vital functions including heart contractions, digestion, and various cellular activities.

Cunningham Lean Mass Equation- An equation used to predict resting metabolic rate (RMR) when an individual's body composition has been accurately identified.

Revised Harris-Benedict Equations- An equation used to predict resting metabolic rate (RMR) and may be more appropriate when lean mass cannot be accurately determined.

Lean Mass Equation

RMR = (21.6 x Fat Free Mass in Kilograms) + 370

Example

42 year old female weighing 142 lbs with 24% body fat

142 lbs x .24 = 34 lbs of fat mass

142 lbs - 34 lbs of fat mass = 108 lbs (fat free mass)

108 lbs ÷ 2.2 = 49 kg

RMR = (21.6 x 49 kg) + 370 = 1428 Calories

Benedict equations are multifactoral, utilizing gender, weight, height, and age to individualize the measurement and account for specific variations. Although it does not differentiate lean mass from fat mass, the equation does use weight and height based on predictive norms for body composition for a given age, and additionally, uses gender specific equations. It is important to note that the calculation of both equations uses the metric system.

Resting metabolic rate represents the largest portion of caloric need but does not completely cover the total daily need for calories. Physical activity generally accounts for 20-30% of a person's daily expenditure (47). This value contributes the most variability in total caloric need and therefore, has the most manipulability for increasing caloric expenditure. Predicting the average energy expenditure related to physical activity adds to the error of estimation unless it is measured using more direct means. Activity multiplier ranges have been developed to calculate daily need based on daily activity norms. When using the equations to predict daily need, estimates of calorie per kilogram of bodyweight have been established to enhance the accuracy of the prediction. Standard deviations of the RMR predictions are usually between 100-200 kcal, which may increase to 300-400 with inappropriate activity multiplier selection (31).

A third contributor to caloric expenditure is the thermic effect of food or dietary induced thermogenesis. It has been well documented that increasing caloric intake heightens metabolic functions related to digestion, transportation, and assimilation of nutrients. More complex foods or foods high in capsaicin like hot peppers, cause increases in metabolic rate above that of the normal American diet (19; 73). Lean proteins, vegetables, and whole grains are more difficult to breakdown and therefore, require more energy to digest. Depending on the contents of the diet, the thermic effect of food accounts for approximately 5-10% of caloric

expenditure (48). Certain dietary intakes can have more pronounced effects from both obligatory and facultative thermogenesis. The additional heat produced from the breakdown contributes as much as 12% of total caloric expenditure. Eating a lean diet high in complex carbohydrates, fruits, and vegetables helps contribute to weight loss through these mechanisms.

Subtracting caloric expenditure from caloric intake will predict the energy balance. This value is an important number, as it represents a predictable physiological outcome for the body. If a person consumes 2500 kcal in their diet and expends 2200 through **total energy expenditure (TEE)** the net gain is a positive 300 kcal. If this individual continually experiences a positive caloric balance, he or she is going to gain weight. It takes 3500 kcals to add a pound of fat and 2500 kcal for a pound of lean mass. Gains in lean mass occur with participation in fairly rigorous, high-volume resistance training. Any individual who experiences positive caloric balance without the addition of routine resistance exercise will likely gain fat mass at a rate consistent with their genetic predisposition. For a person prone to weight gain, every time the calories add up to a positive 3500 kcal, an additional pound of fat will potentially be added.

Most people will increase metabolism by over eating, partly in response to the thermic effect of the food. For the majority of people, this acute adjustment does not completely prevent the additions of fat mass. Additionally, individuals who do not dramatically over-eat, but routinely maintain a positive caloric balance of as little as 50-100 kcal per day can wind up gaining

Harris Benedict Equations

- **Males:**   66 + (5 x ht) + (13.8 x wt) – (6.8 x age)

- **Females:**   655 + (1.8 x ht) + (9.6 x wt) – (4.7 x age)

  - **RMR expressed in kilocalories per day**
  - **ht (height) expressed in centimeters**
  - **wt (weight) expressed in kilograms**
  - **age expressed in years**

  Example Conversions
  215 pound male subject
  215 ÷ 2.2 lb/kg = 97.7 kg

  Sample 6 ft. tall subject
  6 ft x 12 inches/ft = 72 inches
  72 inches x 2.54 cm/in = 182.9 cm

  Sample subject's RMR calculation

  RMR = 66 + (5 x ht) + (13.8 x wt) – (6.8 x age)
  RMR = 66 + (5 x 182.9) + (13.8 x 97.7) – (6.8 x 50)
  RMR = 1988 kcal per day

over 5 lbs. of weight in a single year. This gradual increase in weight from a positive caloric balance as a person ages is referred to as creeping obesity.

~Quick Insight~

Metabolism is based on how much oxygen the body needs each day. Therefore, the factors that affect the amount of oxygen used can be manipulated to increase a person's net caloric expenditure. RMR is primarily dependent upon a person's size or more importantly, their relative lean mass. Engaging in activities that promote lean mass maintenance or muscle hypertrophy can enhance metabolic expenditure. It is estimated that one pound of lean mass represents 11-15 calories of expenditure during rest per day. A two pound addition of lean mass can equate to more than a 5,000 kcal expenditure per year at resting levels. This number increases when that same tissue is put to work.

Physical activity can represent more than a third of caloric need when hard work is performed. Increasing the physical demands on the body through exercise or adding more activity throughout the day will increase metabolism. When vigorous exercise becomes routine, the post-exercise recovery demands also increase metabolic function. **Excess post-exercise oxygen consumption (EPOC)** can contribute positively to mean metabolic rate (64).

When prudent food choices are made in the diet this value again increases through thermic effects associated with the digestive processes. The combination of resistance training, routine high intensity exercise, and a healthy diet rich in complex foods can cause a person's mean metabolism to increase dramatically. Although resting metabolic rate is approximately 40% uncontrollable, 60% can be manipulated for improved metabolic fitness.

Weight Management Strategies

When weight management strategies are aimed at weight loss, the energy balance must be tipped to the negative side. Most people utilize dietary adjustment as a single means to create a caloric deficit. Dieting independent of other lifestyle changes has proven, in countless clinical trails, to be ineffective for long-term weight management. For fat weight to be reduced and

Daily Caloric Need

Resting Metabolism + Voluntary Metabolism =
Daily Caloric Need

Creeping Obesity

One Pound Fat Mass = 3,500 kcals

Daily Caloric Need = 2,200 kcals

Daily Caloric Expenditure = 2,100 kcals

Positive 100 kcal/day

100 kcal/day x 365 days/year = 36,500 kcals per year

36,500 kcals per year ÷ 3,500 kcals per lb of fat =

10.4 lbs of fat per year

remain under control, diet alone is not the answer. When additional factors that influence energy dynamics (i.e. exercise) are included in a weight loss strategy, the odds of success are increased proportionately.

Due to the inverse relationship that exists between a positive and negative energy balance, the factors that cause weight gain represent the same variables that must be controlled for successful weight loss. These variables can be categorized into three primary areas: energy output, energy input, and influential lifestyle behaviors. Each area alone serves as a contributing factor to weight loss, but when employed in a unified manner, they become far more effective than when applied independently. Energy output includes all actions that expend calories, including resting metabolic rate, diet-induced thermogenesis, daily activity, and structured physical activity or exercise. Energy input includes all energy that enters the body, the particular form the energy is in, and the specific quantities that are ingested at a given time. Influential behaviors represent all actions that affect the previous two categories.

Increasing physical activity in general relates importantly to total caloric output. Individuals who are sedentary except for the 30-40 minutes of exercise they perform three days a week may actually have a greater risk for weight gain than those who do not engage in any structured exercise but are physically active throughout most days of the week. This phenomenon occurs because the mean caloric output is higher with ongoing activity than it is with intermittent engagement of exercise combined with sedentary behaviors. This explains why a person who follows a structured exercise program may not lose weight, as energy balance is comprised of the sum of the total energy expended throughout the day. Combining structured exercise with regular physical activity improves caloric expenditure dramatically compared to exercise alone. Physical activity can be added into any lifestyle at varying dosages based upon the situation. Biking instead of driving, using the stairs instead of the elevator, and

Strategies for Weight Loss

Prepare food over eating out.

Prepare smaller quantities of food or enough to meet the caloric requirement of the meal.

Place small portions on the plate and wait two minutes before having additional servings.

Replace processed food with whole fruits and vegetables.

Carry healthy snacks to avoid feeling hungry.

Use smaller serving containers.

Avoid close proximity to snack trays and buffet tables.

Make eating additional portions more difficult.

Create obstacles to food availability by making small portions and putting ingredients away before sitting down to eat.

Eat slowly.

Avoid long periods between meals.

Be conscious of drink calories.

Shop from a specific grocery list.

Select low calorie or reduced fat sauces and dressings.

Serve whole fruits for dessert.

Offer low calorie appetizers at social events.

Do not be overly restrictive of foods - eat in moderation.

Let others know you are focusing on calorie control.

---

the same duration, resistance training burns more calories per minute of activity due to the higher intensity of the work.

To yield the greatest contribution to a negative caloric balance, an exercise plan should focus on performing the maximum amount of work in the allotted time. Different activities can be combined to form a complete exercise program that flows with only minimal transitional rest. Aerobic training, resistance training, and flexibility activities can be combined using various techniques to use the full amount of workout time. Resistance training can be performed in circuit formats, flexibility training can be made dynamic, and aerobic exercise can be employed at any time in the bout, consistent with the program structure. Maximizing the use of time available for structured activity is a key component of any exercise-related weight loss strategy.

Ideally, the actions and modalities used for exercise aimed at weight loss should include both resistance training and aerobic activities. The maintenance or addition of lean mass is an important consideration for TEE (5; 36). Equally important, aerobic activity should be employed to encourage additional caloric expenditure and improved fitness, so greater training intensities can be attained (20). Individuals who reach elevated levels of fitness are better able to burn additional calories during the exercise bout primarily due to an ability to handle higher exercise intensities. The contribution of post-exercise metabolism encouraged by high intensity training also warrants attention, as it enhances fat utilization throughout the body (10).

Quantity of Work

The quantity of physical activity is fundamental to the dietary strategies used to create the negative caloric balance. Lower intensity workouts require longer exercise duration to achieve the same caloric expenditure as higher intensity workouts. If one pound of weight loss is to be attained per week, the amount of physical activity and its intensity will determine the number of calories that will be removed from the diet. Low intensity activity participation requires a larger dietary deficit. An individual who burns 500 calories per week through exercise must eliminate 3000 kcal from their diet. This assumes they are currently maintaining a neutral energy balance. Personal trainers should encourage their clients to burn between 1,000 and 2,000 kcal

playing tennis instead of going to the movies are all examples of ways to infuse physical activity into an everyday lifestyle.

Structured exercise prescribed for weight loss should emphasize continuous activity aimed at maximal caloric expenditure. The body burns far fewer calories at rest than when active. For this reason, aerobic activity is often used for weight loss instead of weight training. The non-stop aerobic activity often burns more calories at a lower force output than the total calories accumulated through resistance training using high force outputs with intermittent rest periods. This occurs because the rest periods used between sets of resistance exercises are longer in duration than the time actual work is performed. In most 60 minute resistance training sessions, only about one-third of the time (20 min.) is actually used for activity. When total resistance training work is compared to aerobic training for

Caloric Balance

Positive Caloric Balance
Calories in are greater than calories out

Iso or Neutral Caloric Balance
Calories in equal calories out

Negative Caloric Balance
Calories in are less than calories out

Spot Reduction

Weight loss will occur at the body's discretion as determined by the severity of the caloric restriction, total energy expenditure, and the genetic predisposition of the individual. Exercise cannot dictate lipid metabolism in any particular area. Therefore, what is commonly referred to as "spot reduction" is not possible in humans. Emphasizing leg training will not ensure lower extremity body fat loss in the same way performing abdominal work will not increase lipid use around the trunk. In general, fat loss patterns are controlled via genetic predisposition rather than by the areas that are exercised. For example, running may cause one person to initially lose fat around the abdomen whereas a different person experiences the body fat changes in the lower body.

Gimmicks aimed at spot reduction include ab-isolation machines, low frequency electrode units, sweat suit devices, and cellulite creams. For fat loss to occur, the body must attain a negative caloric balance while maintaining adequate energy to prevent lean mass loss.

through physical activity per week. This reduces the emphasis of dietary change to between 200-300 kcal per day. When the dietary restriction is too significant, compliance is reduced and goal attainment becomes less likely. Caloric deficit requires daily changes to the diet. Overly aggressive caloric restriction programs do not work for most people. A 10-15% reduction of total caloric intake is reasonable, assuming the client can manage the physical activity requirements to create the appropriate total negative balance. When calories are removed from the diet, they should come from areas which are not nutritionally dense. Reducing fat, sugars, and processed carbohydrates are most desirable because the foods containing these nutrients are generally nutrient poor and are energy sources that often cause the most metabolic problems. Most people respond far better to incremental reductions in particular types of calories, compared to significant calorie restriction where the percentage of nutrient contents remain consistent. Studies show better compliance to significantly reduced fat in the diet compared to reduced calorie diets that include fat.

Providing proper distribution in meal frequency and size can be almost as important as the energy distribution itself. Large meals place heavy demands on the metabolic system and reduce the efficiency of nutrient utilization, thereby increasing risk for fat storage. High glycemic loads combined with long durations between feeding encourage lipogenic behavior. On the contrary, smaller meals consumed throughout the day reduce hunger, are utilized more efficiently without excess insulin, and encourage metabolic activity. Eating throughout the day also reduces the likelihood that hunger will lead to episodes of overeating.

The adjustments to the diet and physical activity are part of behavioral modification strategies, but they do not completely represent the full spectrum of behavioral considerations. Stress and social behaviors both affect weight management outcomes but through different means. Unregulated emotional or psychological stress causes cortisol to be released, increasing available energy to manage the fight or flight response. Derivatives of protein and fat storage are mobilized into the blood and sent to the liver for conversion to readily available fuel. This fuel is meant for the physical activity required for fight or flight. However, in modern times, stress exists without a need for physical action. The excess fuel is then stored proximal to the liver as visceral fat or stored in other areas of the body (56). Avoiding or better coping with stress reduces its detrimental effects on weight loss. To properly manage stress, one must know where the potential for stress exists. Creating viable strategies to avoid or alter the environment to reduce the severity or impact of the stress is part of a complete management approach.

Social Behaviors and Weight Management

Social behaviors do not affect weight management through hormonal means, but rather as obstacles to diet and physical activity adherence. As stated earlier, social activities often promote increased caloric consumption and are usually not physical in nature. This increases the likelihood that a positive energy balance will replace the potential negative contributions from the diet and impede weight loss.

Alcohol consumption is commonly used as part of social entertainment or to facilitate a feeling of relaxation for many Americans. At 7 kcal per gram, the caloric density of alcohol is almost as high as that of fat. Alcoholic beverages range between 100 kcal in a light beer to 450 kcal in some mixed drinks. Four or five alcohol containing beverages over a weekend can potentially add a large number of calories to one's diet. Likewise, the foods that are served in the presence of alcohol are also commonly high in calories. Foods consumed with alcohol have a greater propensity to be stored as lipids compared to when digested without the presence of alcohol (68). Alcohol is preferentially

Strategies to Avoid Poor Food Choices and Behaviors When in Social Environments

Never go out hungry; consume healthy low calorie foods before going out.

Drink water or low calorie beverages between alcohol containing beverages.

Avoid close proximity to high calorie snack foods.

Select healthy food choices before committing to bad food choice decisions.

Try to find social activities that include physical activity or a reduced emphasis on food and drink as the main form of entertainment.

Add ten minutes of cardiovascular activity for each alcoholic beverage consumed to negate the empty calories.

metabolized in the body with absorption starting in the stomach. This causes other foods to enter circulation without a demand for oxidation, leading to an increased likelihood of greater fat storage.

To reduce the consequential effects of social behavior on weight loss success, alternatives or compensatory actions should be considered. If high calorie consumption is a problem for a client, the personal trainer should plan for preventative action. Asking people to stop engaging in socially stimulating environments is inappropriate. Adding accountability and ways to avoid the pitfalls is warranted. Providing strategies to avoid poor food choices and behaviors when in social environments will help reduce the impact of social events.

Weight Gain

Not every person wants to lose weight. For some people, gaining weight is just as challenging as losing weight can be for others. Proper weight gain is accomplished in the same manner as proper weight loss, but instead of a negative caloric balance, the emphasis is on intelligently creating a positive energy balance. It would seem a positive caloric balance would be easily attained by simply eating high calorie food. Ideally however, weight gain should be from lean mass. Emphasizing a high caloric intake alone will likely increase fat mass and place the person at a higher risk for unhealthy blood lipid profiles.

Weight gain goals are often vanity or performance related. Healthy weight gain works on an incremental basis, inversely consistent with weight loss. If done

~Quick Insight~

Fad Diets

The popularity of fad diets has increased dramatically in recent years due to media promotion, elevations in body weight throughout the American population, and the misconception that weight can be reduced quickly with minimal effort. New books and remedies guaranteeing effective weight loss bombard consumers routinely and drive the message that there are alternatives to caloric restriction and exercise for weight management. It should be fairly obvious that singling out a particular energy nutrient or engaging in wholesale changes do not work. If any particular method did work only one diet book or diet strategy would be needed and everyone would gravitate towards it. Some common indications of unsound weight loss promotions include:

- Rapid or dramatic results
- A diet advertised as working without exercise
- Emphasis on short-term change
- Dramatic changes to normal patterns
- Celebrity, Athlete, or "Doctor" endorsed
- Claims of research such as "Independent studies prove"
- Claims to replace, or add to, metabolic or hormone function
- Emphasis on one nutrient or limited food choices
- Lack of emphasis on caloric reduction and behavior modification
- Assertion claiming to reduce cellulite or fat in specific locations

aggressively, both yield consequential results. Diets emphasizing excess calorie reduction frequently cause lean mass loss, while diets with excess calorie consumption cause fat mass gain. To avoid both scenarios, controlled changes in the diet and the activities engaged in will allow for the proper tissue to be affected. Weight gain attempts should emphasize resistance training combined with prudent caloric additions to the diet. An addition of 150-300 kcal per day with a focus on protein should be sufficient to encourage lean mass gain in conjunction with the adaptations associated with physical activity (3; 35). Some recommendations are more aggressive for individuals who find it extremely difficult to gain weight. Adding 500-750 kcals above caloric expenditure may be warranted for very lean clients who struggle with adding mass (63). Body composition should be tracked along with caloric intake to identify variations associated with excess or insufficient intakes.

Protein should represent the majority of the calories increased in the diet as long as the value stays below the 1.6-2.0 grams per kilogram of body weight upper limit. If additional calories are required, they should come from nutrient dense carbohydrates. High fat foods are not a good choice as they can lead to increased risk for negative blood lipid adjustments even though the foods are calorically dense. Feeding throughout the day may also positively contribute to the weight gain goals. For individuals who find it difficult to eat frequently, meal supplements may aid in fulfilling the calorie requirements. If protein supplements are used, whey protein is ideal for post-exercise consumption and casein protein can be used at night due to its slower absorption rate. Personal preferences will ultimately define the ideal dietary strategy.

Eating Disorders

Whenever clients attempt weight loss, personal trainers should consciously identify inappropriate behaviors. Disordered eating patterns are commonly associated with weight loss attempts, even in cases involving those educated about healthy strategies and weary of inappropriate behaviors. Two of the most common disordered eating patterns include restrained eating and binge eating behaviors. Although both behaviors characterize diagnosed eating disorders, individuals who engage in these behaviors are not necessarily suffering from a psychiatric disorder. Hoping to accelerate weight loss, individuals attempting to control calories often engage in episodes of severe restriction. This may be to compensate for over eating, to cause a negative caloric balance, or to prepare for an environment where the client knows they are likely to consume more calories than is appropriate for their

weight loss goals. Not uncommon, people intentionally do not eat all day, knowing they have an event that evening that will provide an abundance of food and drink.

Severe restriction is one of the worst habits to engage in because it changes the internal metabolic environment by promoting the loss of lean mass and increasing the likelihood of fat storage. Restriction is also likely to lead to binging: eating due to the psychological wear on the body from prolonged physiological signals of hunger. Binge eating occurs when people significantly surpass their caloric need. It commonly occurs due to the stress and fatigue of aggressive dieting or a temporary emotional lapse. For this reason, weight loss should be part of lifestyle changes that are not aggressively applied. Small changes do not cause significant stress on a person's normal behavior patterns and are thus, less likely to trigger an event.

When disordered eating patterns become routine, the behaviors may be psychologically motivated beyond the client's control. Eating disorders can start from attempts at weight modification that grow into damaging physiological patterns with roots in more significant underlying psychological pathology. Eating disorders are classified as psychological disorders by the American Psychological Association due to their potential for harm. They are complex, multi-faceted

Common Characteristics of Eating Disorders

Body dissatisfaction

Emphasis on bodyweight

Preoccupied with food and appearance

Avoid eating or noticeably overeat

Depression

Feelings of guilt, remorse, or self-loathing related to eating behavior

Body image distortion

Intense fear of being fat

Use of laxatives, appetite suppressants, purging or diuretics

Use of illegal drugs

Eating alone or avoiding eating in groups

Exercising excessively

Smoking cigarettes

~Key Terms~

Excess Post-exercise Oxygen Consumption (EPOC)- A measurably increased rate of oxygen intake following strenuous activity.

Total Energy Expenditure (TEE)- The overall amount of energy used throughout the day for activity and vital body functions: a combination of RMR plus voluntary metabolism and the thermic effect of food.

Anorexia Nervosa- A psychophysiological disorder, characterized by fear of becoming obese, distorted self image, persistent aversion to food, and severe weight loss.

Bulimia Nervosa- A psychiatric and medical condition which involves an individual engaging in episodes of binge eating, followed by various efforts to "purge" or expel the binged food.

Binge-eating disorder- A recurrent eating disorder characterized by the uncontrolled, excessive intake of any available food which often occurs following stressful events.

conditions that are presumed to stem from internal conflict and biochemical variations in the brain (34; 52). Unmet personal needs and issues of control are often linked to compensatory eating behaviors which attempt to cope with the emotional dysfunctions (8; 61).

The three most common eating disorders include **anorexia nervosa**, **bulimia nervosa**, and **binge-eating disorder**. Each has a specific diagnostic criteria listed in the Diagnostic and Statistical Manual of Mental Disorders of the American Psychological Association (16). A stereotypical physical characteristic does not exist for people with eating disorders except for severe, later-stage anorexia, where a person is visibly emaciated. A person may be of normal weight or even overweight and suffer from the afflictions of one of the disorders.

Anorexia Nervosa

Anorexia is probably the most well-known eating disorder. It is characterized by significant body image disorder, intense fear of becoming fat, and a preoccupation with weight (14). Although anorexia is most commonly diagnosed in females, nearly 10% of anorexics are male (37). Anorexia's most obvious symptoms include severe weight loss from caloric restriction, strict dietary practices, and heavy exercise participation (9). Although anorexics may engage in other compensatory activities, including vomiting and laxative use, caloric restriction is most common (45). Anorexia is a serious condition that results in death in

10% of the cases from suicide, cardiac arrest, or metabolic complications. Personal trainers who suspect an individual may suffer from the disorder should discuss it with their client and recommend counseling. Personal trainers should discuss the suspicions with the individual's designated emergency contact person in the case of clients under 18 years of age due to the severity of the disorder. Individuals suffering from anorexia will not be able to cure themselves and therefore, require psychological counseling or medical intervention (4).

Bulimia Nervosa

Bulimia Nervosa is more difficult to identify than anorexia because it is shadowed in secrecy; in fact, many bulimics are of normal weight or may be slightly overweight (39). Bulimia is often characterized by binge-eating and purging, seen in about 80% of the cases, or inappropriate compensatory actions, including heavy use of diet pills and laxatives (76). Weight changes may be limited in bulimics, so symptomatic identification is difficult. Estimates suggest that between 1-3% of the population is bulimic, with females showing a greater propensity for the disorder, representing 9 out of every 10 cases (37). Bulimics may experience episodes of severe compensatory behavior followed by periods of reduced symptomatic activity. Low self-esteem and body dissatisfaction are tied to weight, so body image often dictates the severity of the behavior (70). Fortunately most bulimics who seek counseling do so on their own to reduce their mental suffering.

Binge-Eating Disorder

Binge-eating disorder involves the consumption of large amounts of food followed by feelings of guilt, depression, and low self-worth (58). Binges may occur between 3-5 times per a week. Compensatory actions may be taken, but are done so on an irregular basis. It is estimated that binge-eating disorder affects up to 4% of the population (55). Binge eaters are more likely to be overweight or obese and experience feelings that they cannot control their eating (14). Most binge eaters have a long history of dieting or weight loss struggle and are not happy with their bodies (58). Caucasian women seem to represent the largest group of sufferers, but men and women of all races may suffer from the disorder.

Personal trainers should be knowledgeable as to the signs and symptoms of eating disorders. Individuals who are overly pre-occupied with exercise or feel the need to exercise every time they eat are candidates for these dysfunctions. Discussing concerns with clients may shed some light on the situation and help them identify negative behaviors.

CHAPTER ELEVEN REFERENCES

1. Position of the American Dietetic Association: very-low-calorie weight loss diets. *J Am Diet Assoc* 90: 722-726, 1990.

2. Position of the American Dietetic Association: very-low-calorie weight loss diets. *J Am Diet Assoc* 90: 722-726, 1990.

3. Promotion of healthy weight-control practices in young athletes. *Pediatrics* 116: 1557-1564, 2005.

4. Position of the American Dietetic Association: Nutrition intervention in the treatment of anorexia nervosa, bulimia nervosa, and other eating disorders. *J Am Diet Assoc* 106: 2073-2082, 2006.

5. **Ades PA, Savage PD, Brochu M, Tischler MD, Lee NM and Poehlman ET**. Resistance training increases total daily energy expenditure in disabled older women with coronary heart disease. *J Appl Physiol* 98: 1280-1285, 2005.

6. **Arora S and Anubhuti**. Role of neuropeptides in appetite regulation and obesity--a review. *Neuropeptides* 40: 375-401, 2006.

7. **Bagaric M and Erbacher S**. Fat and the law: who should take the blame? *J Law Med* 12: 323-339, 2005.

8. **Blinder BJ, Cumella EJ and Sanathara VA**. Psychiatric comorbidities of female inpatients with eating disorders. *Psychosom Med* 68: 454-462, 2006.

9. **Boris HN**. The problem of anorexia nervosa. *Int J Psychoanal* 65 (Pt 3): 315-322, 1984.

10. **Braun WA, Hawthorne WE and Markofski MM**. Acute EPOC response in women to circuit training and treadmill exercise of matched oxygen consumption. *Eur J Appl Physiol* 94: 500-504, 2005.

11. **Brownell KD, Greenwood MR, Stellar E and Shrager EE**. The effects of repeated cycles of weight loss and regain in rats. *Physiol Behav* 38: 459-464, 1986.

12. **Brownell KD, Greenwood MR, Stellar E and Shrager EE**. The effects of repeated cycles of weight loss and regain in rats. *Physiol Behav* 38: 459-464, 1986.

13. **Casey BR**. Kentucky's obesity epidemic. *J Ky Med Assoc* 104: 547-548, 2006.

14. **Cassin SE and von Ranson KM**. Personality and eating disorders: a decade in review. *Clin Psychol Rev* 25: 895-916, 2005.

15. **Chaudhri O, Small C and Bloom S**. Gastrointestinal hormones regulating appetite. *Philos Trans R Soc Lond B Biol Sci* 361: 1187-1209, 2006.

16. **Chizawsky LL and Newton MS**. Eating disorders: identification and treatment in obstetrical patients. *AWHONN Lifelines* 10: 482-488, 2006.

17. **Daniels J**. Obesity: America's epidemic. *Am J Nurs* 106: 40-9, quiz, 2006.

18. **Dastgiri S, Mahdavi R, TuTunchi H and Faramarzi E**. Prevalence of obesity, food choices and socio-economic status: a cross-sectional study in the north-west of Iran. *Public Health Nutr* 9: 996-1000, 2006.

19. **Diepvens K, Westerterp KR and Westerterp-Plantenga MS**. Obesity and thermogenesis related to the consumption of caffeine, ephedrine, capsaicin, and green tea. *Am J Physiol Regul Integr Comp Physiol* 292: R77-R85, 2007.

20. **Donnelly JE, Smith B, Jacobsen DJ, Kirk E, Dubose K, Hyder M, Bailey B and Washburn R**. The role of exercise for weight loss and maintenance. *Best Pract Res Clin Gastroenterol* 18: 1009-1029, 2004.

21. **Druce M and Bloom SR**. The regulation of appetite. *Arch Dis Child* 91: 183-187, 2006.

22. **Druce M and Bloom SR**. The regulation of appetite. *Arch Dis Child* 91: 183-187, 2006.

23. **Druce M and Bloom SR**. The regulation of appetite. *Arch Dis Child* 91: 183-187, 2006.

24. **Erlanson-Albertsson C**. How palatable food disrupts appetite regulation. *Basic Clin Pharmacol Toxicol* 97: 61-73, 2005.

25. **Erlanson-Albertsson C**. How palatable food disrupts appetite regulation. *Basic Clin Pharmacol Toxicol* 97: 61-73, 2005.

26. **Erlanson-Albertsson C**. How palatable food disrupts appetite regulation. *Basic Clin Pharmacol Toxicol* 97: 61-73, 2005.

27. **Erlanson-Albertsson C**. How palatable food disrupts appetite regulation. *Basic Clin Pharmacol Toxicol* 97: 61-73, 2005.

28. **Ewing R, Brownson RC and Berrigan D**. Relationship between urban sprawl and weight of United States youth. *Am J Prev Med* 31: 464-474, 2006.

29. **Flier JS**. Neuroscience. Regulating energy balance: the substrate strikes back. *Science* 312: 861-864, 2006.

30. **Forbes AL and Stephenson MG**. National Nutrition Monitoring System: implications for public health policy at FDA. *J Am Diet Assoc* 84: 1189-1193, 1984.

31. **Frankenfield DC, Rowe WA, Smith JS and Cooney RN**. Validation of several established equations for resting metabolic rate in obese and nonobese people. *J Am Diet Assoc* 103: 1152-1159, 2003.

32. **Golay A and Masciangelo ML**. [Burden of obesity: from epidemic to costs]. *Rev Med Suisse* 1: 807-10, 813, 2005.

33. **Goldstone AP**. The hypothalamus, hormones, and hunger: alterations in human obesity and illness. *Prog Brain Res* 153: 57-73, 2006.

34. **Gorwood P**. Eating disorders, serotonin transporter polymorphisms and potential treatment response. *Am J Pharmacogenomics* 4: 9-17, 2004.

35. **Grandjean A**. Nutritional requirements to increase lean mass. *Clin Sports Med* 18: 623-632, 1999.

36. **Hansen D, Dendale P, Berger J, van Loon LJ and Meeusen R**. The effects of exercise training on fat-mass loss in obese patients during energy intake restriction. *Sports Med* 37: 31-46, 2007.

37. **Hoek HW and van Hoeken D**. Review of the prevalence and incidence of eating disorders. *Int J Eat Disord* 34: 383-396, 2003.

38. **Holt SH, Miller JC, Petocz P and Farmakalidis E**. A satiety index of common foods. *Eur J Clin Nutr* 49: 675-690, 1995.

39. **Jenkins A**. Identifying eating disorders. *Br J Nurs* 14: 1034-6, 1038, 2005.

40. **Jirik-Babb P and Norring C**. Gender comparisons in psychological characteristics of obese, binge eaters. *Eat Weight Disord* 10: e101-e104, 2005.

41. **Jobst EE, Enriori PJ, Sinnayah P and Cowley MA**. Hypothalamic regulatory pathways and potential obesity treatment targets. *Endocrine* 29: 33-48, 2006.

42. **Johnson CA, Xie B, Liu C, Reynolds KD, Chou CP, Koprowski C, Gallaher P, Spruitj-Metz D, Guo Q, Sun P, Gong J and Palmer P**. Socio-demographic and cultural comparison of overweight and obesity risk and prevalence in adolescents in Southern California and Wuhan, China. *J Adolesc Health* 39: 925-928, 2006.

43. **Knol LL, Haughton B and Fitzhugh EC**. Dietary patterns of young, low-income US children. *J Am Diet Assoc* 105: 1765-1773, 2005.

44. **Loucks EB, Rehkopf DH, Thurston RC and Kawachi I**. Socioeconomic disparities in metabolic syndrome differ by gender: evidence from NHANES III. *Ann Epidemiol* 17: 19-26, 2007.

45. **Maddox RW and Long MA**. Eating disorders: current concepts. *J Am Pharm Assoc (Wash)* 39: 378-387, 1999.

46. **McCargar LJ**. Can Diet and ExerciseReally Change Metabolism? *Medscape Womens Health* 1: 5, 1996.

47. **McCargar LJ**. Can Diet and ExerciseReally Change Metabolism? *Medscape Womens Health* 1: 5, 1996.

48. **McCargar LJ**. Can Diet and ExerciseReally Change Metabolism? *Medscape Womens Health* 1: 5, 1996.

49. **Mello MM, Rimm EB and Studdert DM**. The McLawsuit: the fast-food industry and legal accountability for obesity. *Health Aff (Millwood)* 22: 207-216, 2003.

50. **Mensah GA and Brown DW**. An overview of cardiovascular disease burden in the United States. *Health Aff (Millwood)* 26: 38-48, 2007.

51. **Meyer C and Waller G**. The impact of emotion upon eating behavior: the role of subliminal visual processing of threat cues. *Int J Eat Disord* 25: 319-326, 1999.

52. **Monteleone P, Brambilla F, Bortolotti F and Maj M**. Serotonergic dysfunction across the eating disorders: relationship to eating behaviour, purging behaviour, nutritional status and general psychopathology. *Psychol Med* 30: 1099-1110, 2000.

53. **Moreno O, Meoro A, Martinez A, Rodriguez C, Pardo C, Aznar S, Lopez P, Serrano J, Boix E, Martin**

MD and Pico Alfonso AM. Comparison of two low-calorie diets: a prospective study of effectiveness and safety. *J Endocrinol Invest* 29: 633-640, 2006.

54. **Park MI, Camilleri M, O'Connor H, Oenning L, Burton D, Stephens D and Zinsmeister AR**. Effect of different macronutrients in excess on gastric sensory and motor functions and appetite in normal-weight, overweight, and obese humans. *Am J Clin Nutr* 85: 411-418, 2007.

55. **Patrick L**. Eating disorders: a review of the literature with emphasis on medical complications and clinical nutrition. *Altern Med Rev* 7: 184-202, 2002.

56. **Peeke PM and Chrousos GP**. Hypercortisolism and obesity. *Ann N Y Acad Sci* 771: 665-676, 1995.

57. **Pender JR and Pories WJ**. Epidemiology of obesity in the United States. *Gastroenterol Clin North Am* 34: 1-7, 2005.

58. **Pope HG, Jr., Lalonde JK, Pindyck LJ, Walsh T, Bulik CM, Crow SJ, McElroy SL, Rosenthal N and Hudson JI**. Binge eating disorder: a stable syndrome. *Am J Psychiatry* 163: 2181-2183, 2006.

59. **Pudel V and Ellrott T**. [Social and political aspects of adiposis]. *Chirurg* 76: 639-646, 2005.

60. **Ramsey PW and Glenn LL**. Obesity and health status in rural, urban, and suburban southern women. *South Med J* 95: 666-671, 2002.

61. **Sansone RA, Levitt JL and Sansone LA**. The prevalence of personality disorders among those with eating disorders. *Eat Disord* 13: 7-21, 2005.

62. **Shortt J**. Obesity--a public health dilemma. *AORN J* 80: 1069-1078, 2004.

63. **Smith NJ**. Gaining and losing weight in athletics. *JAMA* 236: 149-151, 1976.

64. **Speakman JR and Selman C**. Physical activity and resting metabolic rate. *Proc Nutr Soc* 62: 621-634, 2003.

65. **Steen SN, Oppliger RA and Brownell KD**. Metabolic effects of repeated weight loss and regain in adolescent wrestlers. *JAMA* 260: 47-50, 1988.

66. **Story M, Kaphingst KM and French S**. The role of schools in obesity prevention. *Future Child* 16: 109-142, 2006.

67. **Stubbs RJ**. Peripheral signals affecting food intake. *Nutrition* 15: 614-625, 1999.

68. **Suter PM**. Is alcohol consumption a risk factor for weight gain and obesity? *Crit Rev Clin Lab Sci* 42: 197-227, 2005.

69. **Toornvliet AC, Pijl H and Meinders AE**. Food and mood: a central connection. *Neth J Med* 41: 45-47, 1992.

70. **Tyrka AR, Waldron I, Graber JA and Brooks-Gunn J**. Prospective predictors of the onset of anorexic and bulimic syndromes. *Int J Eat Disord* 32: 282-290, 2002.

71. **Weiss EP, Racette SB, Villareal DT, Fontana L, Steger-May K, Schechtman KB, Klein S, Ehsani AA and Holloszy JO**. Lower extremity muscle size and strength and aerobic capacity decrease with caloric restriction but not with exercise-induced weight loss. *J Appl Physiol* 102: 634-640, 2007.

72. **Weiss EP, Racette SB, Villareal DT, Fontana L, Steger-May K, Schechtman KB, Klein S, Ehsani AA and Holloszy JO**. Lower extremity muscle size and strength and aerobic capacity decrease with caloric restriction but not with exercise-induced weight loss. *J Appl Physiol* 102: 634-640, 2007.

73. **Westerterp KR, Wilson SA and Rolland V**. Diet induced thermogenesis measured over 24h in a respiration chamber: effect of diet composition. *Int J Obes Relat Metab Disord* 23: 287-292, 1999.

74. **Wild S, Roglic G, Green A, Sicree R and King H**. Global prevalence of diabetes: estimates for the year 2000 and projections for 2030. *Diabetes Care* 27: 1047-1053, 2004.

75. **Wild S, Roglic G, Green A, Sicree R and King H**. Global prevalence of diabetes: estimates for the year 2000 and projections for 2030. *Diabetes Care* 27: 1047-1053, 2004.

76. **Yamanaka G and Kuboki T**. [Bulimia nervosa (BN)--epidemiology, etiology, clinical features, treatment, prognosis]. *Nippon Rinsho* 59: 540-543, 2001.

77. **Zarich SW**. Metabolic syndrome, diabetes and cardiovascular events: current controversies and recommendations. *Minerva Cardioangiol* 54: 195-214, 2006.

Chapter 12

Physical Fitness and Health

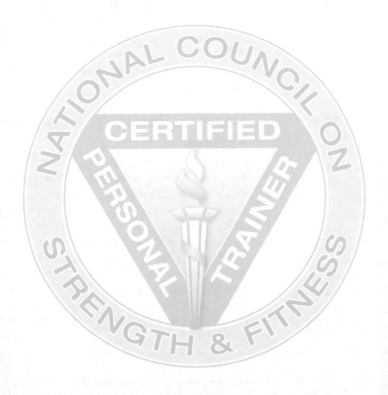

In This Chapter

Understanding Health & Wellness

The term "health" has been defined in many ways, and even today, not everyone agrees on a universally accepted meaning. Traditionally, the concept of health has applied to a person's susceptibility for disease. If a person did not have any diagnostic criteria for disease or present any known health problems, they were considered "healthy." Health professionals determined health status based on specific, quantifiable health measurements, such as blood pressure, and any self-reported problems. The problem with viewing health from this narrow diagnostic perspective is that, 1) it considers disease or symptomatic criteria, which may not be known to the individual, and 2) it does not consider the person's overall well-being as a defining characteristic. During the late seventies and early eighties, a broadened philosophy of health emerged that suggested viewing the person holistically, rather than by independent physiological measures. The term "wellness" evolved to reflect the combination of physical, mental, emotional, intellectual, social, and environmental health. The rationale was that each health-related component of wellness had potential implications for overall well-being. When individuals have control over these physiological and psychological areas, the negative impact each may have on health is reduced. For instance, good social health entails meaningful interrelationships and confident social interaction. Both are linked with reduced stress and a decreased risk for depression.

The concept of wellness is fairly mainstream among fitness professionals, but it is not a clearly understood term by the average population. Rarely will the term wellness be applied in conversation. Instead, people more often use the term healthy. Therefore, the term health is better understood as both the physical state of a person, and the assortment of lifestyle behaviors that affect that state, rather than simply being free from disease.

It is well-known and documented that health is affected by what enters the body, what the body is exposed to, and what the body is required to do each day. Therefore, lifestyle is the largest determinant to the outcome of these collectively-applied factors. Healthy lifestyle is defined as a group of actions and behaviors which positively affect a person's overall well-being. A person who lives a healthy lifestyle avoids stress, eats nutritionally appropriate foods, avoids behaviors that may negatively impact health, and engages in routine physical activity. The U.S. Department of Health and Human Services, Office of Disease Prevention and Health Promotion, has listed objectives to encourage healthy lifestyles by Americans in the *Healthy People*
2010 initiative. Through this initiative, Americans are being asked to take personal responsibility for their health through lifestyle management.

An important part of the plan to improve one's health is to routinely engage in physical activity. For most people, the term physical activity is synonymous with exercise. However, from a health standpoint, exercise and physical activity have two distinctly different meanings. Physical activity is defined as a period of time physical acts are performed. The definition is independent of the quantity of work, oxygen demand, and resultant energy expenditure. Examples of physical activity include gardening, walking the dog, and cleaning the house. Exercise, on the other hand, is defined as planned, structured, and repetitive bodily movement done to improve or maintain one or more components of physical fitness. Thus, exercise is physical activity, but physical activity may not be exercise. All types of physical activity can improve overall health, but exercise is physical activity with specific parameters that allow an individual to achieve defined outcomes when applied correctly.

Physical Fitness

Physical fitness is broken down into two categories: health-related physical fitness and performance-related physical fitness. The first category encompasses factors that quantifiably affect health, while the second category affects performance. The health-related components include **cardiorespiratory fitness**, muscular strength, muscular endurance, flexibility, and body composition. In some cases, metabolic fitness also qualifies as a health related component because it affects risk for metabolic disease including obesity and diabetes. The performance components of physical fitness include power, speed, **coordination**, balance, and **agility**. Each plays an important role in human performance and should be considered a secondary health component.

Health Related Components of Fitness

Health related components of fitness are fundamental to a person's overall well-being. They reflect quantifiable measures of efficiency and proper functionality of the movement systems of the body. Appropriate values or improvements in each of the respective components will promote positive health, while high score values in these categories of fitness will benefit the individual beyond that of basic health attainment. Although high rankings in some categories may be desirable for certain goal-related outcomes, it is important to maintain an acceptable level of fitness within each of the five areas.

~Quick Insight~

Health vs. Fitness

Many people believe that health and fitness are synonymous, but this may not always be the case. Health is a disease-free state of well-being that allows an individual to experience improved quality of life and independence. Fitness is a criterion-based measure of physical performance. A person does not have to be fit to be healthy, nor is a person guaranteed health because they are fit. Certainly, the two are interrelated, but distinct differences exist. An example of the differences can be seen in emotional, psychological, and physical assessment. A person who scores satisfactorily in the health-related components of fitness may be deemed fit by defined criteria, but experience high stress on the job, eat a diet high in saturated fats, and have hypertension and **hyperlipidemia**. The person is fit, but not necessarily healthy. On the other hand, a person may not score well on the assessments of physical fitness, but eat a very healthy diet, get enough physical activity to maintain functional performance levels, have low blood pressure, and a reasonable lipid profile. In this case, the person is classified as healthy but not physically fit.

In measures of skill or performance-related fitness, this difference can be even more significant. A person may show respectable scores in agility or on a vertical jump test but not be healthy by several categorical measures. Performance-related fitness is affected by genetics, exercise, and physical activity, but the activities that improve performance may not necessarily improve health. A weightlifter may exhibit high levels of power and low levels of cardiorespiratory fitness. Likewise, a person may have excellent balance and coordination, but be measured as obese. Skill measures are poor indicators of health, although people who score well on them often do so because they participate in sports and related physical activities.

When the level of physical activity is assessed in relation to health and fitness, there are two different criteria used to define acceptable values. Health simply requires routine physical activity of appropriate frequency and duration. Fitness requires a regimented program, designed to emphasize the specific components of health-related physical fitness. In general, moderate fitness may be attained from exercise performed 3 days a week at an intensity level of 60-70% of maximum. High level fitness however, often requires 4-6 days a week at 75-90% intensities.

Individuals who score very well in one or two components of fitness may be less healthy than a person who maintains a moderate level of fitness in all the health categories.

Cardiorespiratory Fitness

Cardiorespiratory fitness (CRF) includes several synonymous terms: aerobic fitness or endurance, cardiovascular efficiency or endurance, and cardiorespiratory efficiency. These all represent the same thing: the body's ability to consume and utilize oxygen. CRF is a factor of synergistic efficiency of the body's systems, as it includes the cardiopulmonary system, cardiovascular system, and the muscular system. CRF is the single most important health-related component of fitness because it links to risk for disease and death. Low measures of total-body oxygen efficiency are a risk factor for heart disease, diabetes, and obesity (198). On the contrary, high levels of CRF are associated with positive health, including improved self-reported quality of life (43).

Muscular Fitness

Muscular fitness is the body's ability to produce and sustain force output. It encompasses both muscular strength and muscular endurance. Muscular strength is

defined as the body's ability to exert a single maximal contractile force, whereas muscular endurance is the ability of muscle tissue to sustain force output or apply force for an extended period of time. Muscular fitness is essential for health because it determines movement capabilities, affects joint health, and is responsible for posture and stability. Low levels of muscular fitness are linked to functional decline and loss of independence (20). Beyond functional demands, the actual amount of strength and endurance needed by an individual is specific to the types of activities he or she participates in on a routine basis.

Key Terms

Hyperlipidemia – An excess of fats or lipids circulating in the blood.

Cardiorespiratory Fitness (CRF) - Refers to the ability and efficiency of the circulatory and respiratory systems to supply oxygen to working muscles during sustained activity.

Coordination - The harmonious adjustment or interaction of parts.

Agility - The ability of the body to change direction.

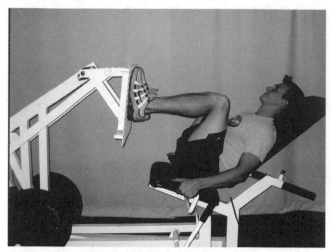

Muscular fitness is important for health because it determines movement capabilities, affects joint health, and is responsible for posture and stability.

Flexibility

Flexibility is probably the most undervalued and least-emphasized component of health-related fitness by most physically active adults. Anecdotally, this is likely due to three factors: 1) there is no vanity associated with improvements in flexibility; 2) high levels of flexibility are not needed to participate in most activities; and 3) the training is often viewed as time consuming, boring, and uncomfortable. This being said, flexibility is actually one of the most important components of physical fitness. Flexibility is tied into joint function, movement capabilities, risk for injury, and chronic pain. More importantly, it is associated with functional decline and is both a direct and indirect variable of health problems that can lead to disability in older adults (37; 160).

Body Composition

Body composition is defined as the ratio of fat mass to fat-free, or lean mass. Most people incorrectly view body composition as the amount of fat individuals maintain on their bodies. Although it is often expressed as a percentage of body fat, the important factor is the ratio. For example, a person measured at 20% body fat would see a decline in the percentage of fat by adding muscle. This occurs without actually changing the quantity of fat on the body because it is expressed as a percentage. However, individuals who lose muscle mass without changing body-fat mass will show an increase in fatness when expressed as a percentage. When analyzed for health risk, the percentile relationship is evaluated, not the actual pounds of fat on the body. Body composition is tightly linked with metabolic fitness and health (165; 218). The more lean mass a person maintains, the better their overall ability to manage caloric balance and the lower their respective

body composition will be when expressed as a fat percentage (175). Body composition directly correlates to risk for disease (197). Individuals who maintain high levels of body fat dramatically elevate their risk for disease and premature mortality.

Performance Related Fitness

Performance related fitness components have classically been the emphasis of sports-related conditioning for obvious reasons. Individuals looking to excel in competitive sports often train to improve nervous system function to enhance these particular components. In more recent years, an emphasis on the performance components has been placed on training for improved overall function. Power, speed, balance, coordination, and agility all have implications for health because they indirectly affect the health-related components. Without power, a person cannot rise from a chair; poor balance and coordination increases the risk of falls; gait speed decline correlates to functional decline (36; 159). Personal trainers should recognize the importance of integrating the performance components of fitness into exercise prescriptions for improved health, even in those clients who are not training for a particular sport. This is not to suggest training all clients with power cleans and high-speed pro agilities, but rather emphasizes utilizing activities that encourage improvements in neural contribution to these areas of human performance.

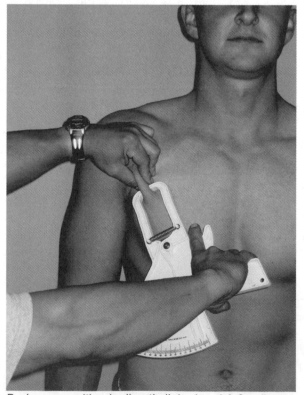

Body composition is directly linked to risk for disease.

Components of Health & Performance

Health Related Fitness	Performance Related Fitness
Cardiorespiratory Fitness	Power
Muscular Fitness	Speed
Flexibility	Balance
Body Composition	Coordination
	Agility

Power

Power is the speed at which work is performed. In performance enhancement, the focus is on acceleration. When power is emphasized in conditioning programs for athletes, the ability to move resistance at high speeds is fundamental. The **Olympic lifts**, **plyometrics**, and weighted throws all emphasize acceleration by calling on recruitment patterns which elicit the fastest development of force. This is necessary to improve jumping distance, forward drive, and speed. When power is viewed from a functional standpoint, it suggests the ability to generate adequate force velocity to allow body segments to effectively utilize momentum forces. For instance, getting up from a seated position requires powerful movements by the hip extensors to move the trunk anteriorly to assist in hip and knee extension. Individuals who lose this ability also increase risk of losing independence (35; 158). Many older adults find it difficult to get out of chairs or their car because of sarcopenic (muscular atrophy) decline. Thus, personal trainers should encourage power development in their exercise programs.

Speed

Speed is the ability to move the body or body parts (rate of positional change) over a distance in a period of time. Speed of movement also depends upon neural recruitment patterns and adequate muscle capabilities.

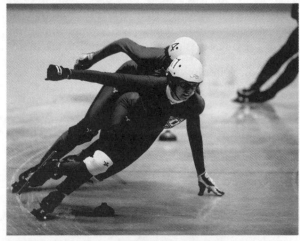

Speed of movement also depends upon neural recruitment patterns and adequate muscle capabilities.

Speed is crucial to successful athletic performance and is often considered to be the most valued performance measure in many sports. When speed capabilities are applied to the faculties of function, there is a noticeable age-related decline in older adults (206). The rate of decline is contingent on several health-related factors. Individuals who maintain higher levels of activity experience a slower rate of decline compared to their non-active counterparts. Movement speed should be appropriately addressed in activities designed for improved bodily function.

Balance

Balance can be described as the ability to manage forces which act to disrupt stability. Consistent with the other performance components, the nervous system plays the largest role in manipulating muscle tension to accommodate demand. Balance is needed in many occasions for sport and daily life activities in order to appropriately manage forces encountered in unstable environments and varying conditions. The stabilizing function of the muscles is used for efficient posture, movement, and body control during more dynamic applications. To improve balance, adequate strength, synergy of force and neural familiarity must be attained. When the body is appropriately challenged, the applied stress promotes improved neuromuscular coordination, which, in turn, enhances balance. Employing balance training across population segments encourages improved function and performance on several levels (11; 84). For the athlete, this means better management of force at higher speeds; for the general public, this suggests reduced risk of injury from falls or related accidents.

Coordination

Coordination is synonymous with neural efficiency. The better force is managed, the easier the body performs tasks. Webster's dictionary definition implies that coordination is the regulation of diverse elements into an integrated and harmonious operation. Coordination means integrating or linking together different parts of an organization to accomplish a collective set of tasks. For instance, hand-eye coordination suggests combining visual data with neuromuscular control. High levels of coordination associate with execution proficiency, which is intergral to sports performance. Adequate levels of coordination are needed to perform tasks safely and in a controlled manner. Although coordination is required for all physical activities, high levels are not necessary for health improvement.

Agility

Agility is the ability of the body to change direction and implies the quantifiable capability of being nimble. In object-based sports, agility allows the athlete to physically pursue the ball, puck, or other object that is constantly changing direction. Agility is often a defining quality in athletic pursuits and is necessary for effective contribution to success in many sports. The average person does not experience the same need for agility as a football running back or a point guard on a basketball team, but all people need to be able to manage direction change without losing balance, or to manage forces to avoid falls and injury from offsetting forces. Agility suggests quickness; therefore it applies most in situations where movement speeds are fast. Individuals who have low levels of agility have difficulty changing direction when faster movement velocities are present.

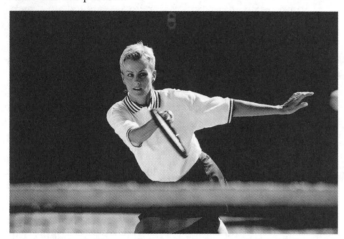

In object based sports, agility is important in tracking the ball, puck or other object that is constantly changing direction.

Factors that Affect Baseline Measures

Several factors affect a person's baseline measures on the fitness components. In untrained individuals, the strongest independent factor is genetic predisposition. Although genetics alone do not fully account for a person's physical fitness, they certainly cannot be overlooked. In addition to genetics, environmental factors, individual interest, and activity-related physical conditioning all contribute to the overall physical fitness of an individual.

Genetics, or heredity, contributes to the measurable components of physical fitness at any given time during a person's lifespan and determines the potential capabilities of the body. It is estimated that a person's genetics can determine up to 40% of uncontrolled factors that affect physical fitness (2; 78). With this being said, that leaves at least 60% of controllable or

somewhat-controllable factors that can be manipulated and improved. Almost everyone has the ability to improve his or her health or performance by engaging in activities and behaviors that act positively upon the body, regardless of genetic makeup.

The environmental factors that affect physical fitness are fairly numerous, and each primary factor carries a number of sub-factors. These factors may be social, such as the family one is born into and its respective values, personal attitudes, financial means, societal environments and opportunities, or physical, such as climate, altitude, or exposure to pollutants. Early learned behaviors yield very powerful influences on the lifestyles of adults. Individuals born into families that place little value on healthy behaviors, or are not educated to those behaviors, are less likely to ever engage in them. On the contrary, families that emphasize health through activity promotion, proper nutrition, and the avoidance of negative influences are more likely to transfer those values to their children and encourage the continuation of those behaviors into adulthood.

Interest also plays a key role in the types of behaviors in which people partake. Individual use of discretionary time is often connected with personal responsibility and feelings of enjoyment. Few people will voluntarily engage in activities that they find unpleasant. Fun activities are often preferably selected for participation over those that do not have a positive association to them. Exposure to a variety of activities during youth allows individuals to evaluate their interests and make decisions about adopting them into their lifestyle habits. In some cases, knowledge of the benefits from certain activities or behaviors influences participation, even when certain activities are viewed as less pleasurable. A sense of responsibility for one's health may cause people to exercise or eat right, even though they might prefer to make other decisions should consequences not exist. Education is an important factor in this decision making process. Individuals who understand that quality of life outcomes closely link to health are more

Controllable Versus Uncontrollable Factors Affecting Physical Fitness

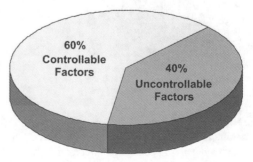

likely to participate in healthy behaviors. For example, a person looking to have an active retirement may emphasize healthy behaviors so as to be able to accomplish his or her retirement goals.

Physical Activity & Life Quality

The World Health Organization has acknowledged health-related quality of life (HRQL) as an important outcome from wellness behaviors. In 1982, Kaplan and Bush coined this multidimensional concept that acknowledges the influences that health status has on tangible and perceived measures of life quality. Clinical data has shown that physical activity has significant potential to positively influence a person's HRLQ (18; 39; 55; 82; 193). The areas that seem to be most directly affected include physical and psychological well-being, perceived physical function, and stress reduction (127). Additionally, a positive association exists between physical activity and self-esteem in people of all ages.

One important effect of physical activity is the perception of improved physical function in daily activities. Although most people can perform daily tasks, the ease or proficiency of accomplishing physical work seems to improve with regular activity. Individuals suffering from maladies, such as heart disease and arthritis, who participate in physical activity report the highest rate of perceived improvement in daily functional capabilities (4; 97; 164; 226). In clinical trials, self-reported outcomes identified improvements in physical function and health in subjects who engaged in physical activity (aerobic training) compared to controls (3). Again, the individuals who were diagnosed with disease presented the greatest magnitude of positive effects in both physical and psychological measures.

Physical Activity & Risk for Injury

Research clearly demonstrates that exercise can help most people improve quality of life (17; 39; 81; 192). This holds true for both apparently healthy individuals and those diagnosed with disease. Exercise, though, also offers the potential for negative outcomes. Individuals who increase physical activity should be familiar with the inherent risk of injury. Several types of common injuries are associated with exercise and sports participation. New exercisers are at particular risk for soft tissue strains, tears, and even bone fracture from inappropriately applied stress and repetitive motions. Progressing intensity too aggressively is associated with greater risk for multiple cause injury. Lower extremity injuries seem to be reported most commonly; in particular the articulation sites of the ankle, knee, and foot (62; 74; 156).

Metabolic abnormality is also a possibility with exercise participation. Although rare and mainly associated with prolonged duration, pre-existing exercise condition, or environmental influences, metabolic injury can be life threatening. Conditions such as **hyperthermia**, **hypothermia**, electrolyte imbalance, **hypoglycemia**, and **rhabdomyolysis** all may present acute emergency situations. Appropriate fluid consumption, acclimation to stress, and pre-exercise screening can help prevent incidence related to the aforementioned metabolic abnormalities.

Pre-Exercise Screening

Importantly, pre-exercise screening can also help reduce cardiac events during exercise. For some individuals suffering from cardiovascular pathology, exercise may cause more harm than good. Individuals may incite arrhythmia (abnormal heart rate or rhythm) triggers when exercising with compromised coronary circulation. Arrhythmias, acute angina, and myocardial infarction (heart attacks) may be precipitated by the combination of physical exertion and disease. Sudden death is not common but a definite possibility for high cardiac risk exercisers. It is important to recognize that the risk occurs not just during participation in the activity but also immediately following exercise. However, from a risk vs. benefit perspective, regular activity for medically cleared participants yields more protective effects from disease than the risk for injury from an exercise-related cardiovascular incident.

Other health concerns related to exercise may warrant attention as well. Overtraining increases risk for infection from immuno-suppression and can cause stress-related injuries (61). Likewise, pre-existing conditions, including asthma, musculoskeletal injury,

Common Activities & Injuries

Jogging/running	Torn cartilage, tendonitis, plantar faciitis, shin splints
Bicycling	Ulnar nerve palsies, ischial bursitis
Swimming	Shoulder pain
Aerobic dance	Shin splints, plantar fasciitis
Tennis	Epicondylitis, tendonitis

osteoporosis, and arthritis can lead to additional problems during exercise participation. Studies show that previous injury and existing conditions strongly predict subsequent injury related to physical activity (106; 229). Although a myriad of adverse events are associated with physical activity, the risk of participation is still outweighed by the problems associated with a sedentary lifestyle. Taking steps to identify risk factors and high risk environments and situations, screening participants, providing structured and appropriate acclimation to the physical stress, prescribing exercise within individual capabilities, avoiding activity when injury or risk is elevated, and having an emergency plan, all contribute to reduced risk and consequence of physical activity-related injury.

Key Terms

Olympic lifts – Clean, jerk, and snatch exercises.

Plyometrics – Exercises that use explosive movements to develop muscular power.

Genetics- The science of biological inheritance which contributes to the measurable components of physical fitness during a person's lifespan and also helps to determine the potential capabilities of the body.

Tendonitis- Inflammation of a tendon.

Plantar fasciitis- An inflammatory condition caused by excessive wear on the plantar fascia (bottom of the foot).

Ulnar nerve palsies- Paralysis caused by damage, compression, or trapping of the ulnar nerve.

Ischial bursitis- Inflammation of the bursa that separates the gluteus maximus from the underlying ischial tuberosity.

Epicondylitis- Inflammation of the muscles and soft tissues around an epicondyle.

Hyperthermia- Unusually high body temperature.

Hypothermia- Abnormally low body temperature.

Hypoglycemia- An abnormally low level of glucose in the blood.

Rhabdomyolysis- An acute, potentially fatal disease that destroys skeletal muscle and is often accompanied by the excretion of myoglobin in the urine.

Physical Activity & Risk for Disease

The rate of physical inactivity in the United States constitutes a societal health burden. The lack of participation in daily physical activity is, in part, blamed for elevated incidence of the Western Culture Diseases. The CDC estimates that the number of deaths associated with sedentary lifestyles is approximately 200,000 annually when viewed as an independent risk factor. Linked with poor diet, that estimate jumps to 300,000. It is likely that other risk factors associated with a sedentary lifestyle also contribute to these values, which speaks to the relevance of overall health accountability, rather than emphasis on any single factor (28; 53; 166). Simply removing a single factor may not reduce mortality risk when other negative factors exist.

Physical activity is associated with a reduction in risk of all-cause mortality, as well as mortality from all cardiovascular disease combined, coronary heart disease, hypertension, colon cancer, and non-insulin dependent diabetes mellitus (28; 45; 52; 167). Research presented in this chapter identifies the relationship of physical activity and cardiorespiratory fitness (CRF) to a variety of health consequences. Data collection results of epidemiological studies have identified the association of physical activity and health problems, the respective magnitude or strength of such relationships, and the biological mechanisms for the onset of the diseases in question.

Individuals regularly engaging in physical activity or those with high levels of CRF have a lower mortality rate than those classified as sedentary or those individuals who maintain low CRF (29; 45). The cited risk for dying from all cause mortality is 1.2- to 2-times higher for sedentary individuals and those with low CRF (46; 215). In addition to a reduction in death rates associated with activity participation, a correlation also exists between lifespan and the level of physical fitness (46). Individuals who engage in activities of longer duration and higher intensity tend to live longer regardless of the age that they begin participation (121; 169).

Studies show that changes from low-level fitness to moderate fitness yield the greatest impact on death rates (44; 120; 168). In other words, a sedentary individual who trains to modest levels of fitness condition will have a greater impact on his or her risk for disease than someone who already has a modest degree of CRF who attains a higher level. In longitudinal studies, improvement from low CRF to moderate levels caused a 44% lower death rate compared to those who remained at low fitness levels. After adjusting for other factors, that difference jumped to a 64% reduction in risk compared to those that remained sedentary (178). This information suggests that individuals who engage in physical activity reduce their risk for all-cause mortality. Regular physical activity is a strong indicator for overall mortality rates and shows a significant dose-response relationship (177). Adjusting lifestyle habits to include regular physical activity is an important part of taking control of one's health and risk for death. Further increasing the level of fitness through training at higher intensities and for longer durations adds to the marked effects on mortality risk (45).

Physical Activity & Cardiovascular Disease

The Center for Disease Control (CDC) identifies heart disease and stroke as the most common **cardiovascular diseases**, representing the first and third leading causes of death in the United States, respectively (27). Research suggests that these diseases account for 40% of all annual deaths, which equates to 1 death every 35 seconds from CVD (128). Although these largely preventable diseases are more common in older individuals, the risk of sudden death has increased in individuals less than 35 years of age (71; 222; 223). CVD in the form of coronary artery disease is also the leading cause of premature, permanent disability among United States workers (68). Additionally, over 1 million Americans are disabled from stroke alone. Collectively, CVD forces the hospitalization of over 6 million

Americans (54; 221). Estimates suggest that more than 70 million Americans currently live with some form of heart disease, and the cost associated with CVD is projected at $403 billion dollars in 2006 (224).

Physical activity has a dramatic effect on reducing risk for developing CVD (12). Several studies have shown that a dose-response gradient exists, further supporting the need for regular physical activity (191; 201; 219). As stated, lower CRF increases risk for mortality, which is consistent with its relationship with CVD-related death. Individuals with the highest levels of fitness show the greatest reduction of risk (139). The dose-response relationship suggests that benefits begin at moderate levels and increase consistently with activity intensity and duration. Therefore, physical activity strongly and inversely relates to CVD risk (138). Numerous studies have analyzed the impact of physical activity on risk for specific forms of CVD. The following text reviews the epidemiological literature related to the measured outcomes.

Coronary Heart Disease (CHD)

Earlier text acknowledged the transient risk of an acute coronary event with exercise participation by those with advanced coronary pathology. This being said, numerous studies have indicated a strong inverse relationship between physical activity and CHD (7; 42; 140; 196). In fact, active people have a significantly lower risk for coronary events compared to sedentary persons or those with low CRF (220). Participation in moderate to high intensity (60-80% VO_2) aerobic exercise has been shown to improve CRF and dramatically reduce the risk of CHD (141). Appropriate diet and lifestyle habits that reduce negative blood lipid profiles and stress enhances this benefit (100).

Although CHD is rare in children, enough evidence suggests that physical activity in childhood helps to prevent CHD in adulthood (182). The presence of CHD in adulthood is related to coronary plaque, and data shows atherosclerosis begins during childhood (173). Of particular relevance is that childhood behaviors linked to the initial development of coronary plaque persist into adulthood. Likewise, physical inactivity is linked to contributing factors for heart disease, including obesity, diabetes, hypertension, and hyperlipidemia (199).

The reduction in risk for CHD associated with aerobic activity and CRF is likely attained through several physiological mechanisms. Aerobic exercise demonstrates a positive effect on several factors that influence risk for CVD. These include reductions in

Coronary Heart Disease (CHD)

Clean Coronary Artery

Coronary Artery with Fatty Deposits

body fat, blood pressure, **myocardial ischemia**, blood clotting (thrombosis), and heart rhythm disturbances (cardiac arrhythmias), as well as improvements in plasma lipid profile (16; 41; 92; 142).

CHD is caused by occlusion of the coronary arteries due to vascular wall damage, which leads to atherosclerosis. Coronary plaque or atherosclerosis occurs when the arterial walls are injured from turbulent blood flow and high vascular pressure. Resultant lesions on the vessel wall cause fatty deposits in the lining of the artery. Circulating low density lipoproteins deliver cholesterol into the artery wall at the area of the initial insult. An inflammatory reaction then occurs, attracting macrophages, or immune cells, to accumulate in the cell wall, where they ingest the fatty deposits. These macrophages cause a proliferation of smooth muscle cells around the area, which are eventually replaced with collagen. A protective fibrous cap then forms between the fatty deposits and the artery lining. This process is commonly referred to as hardening of the arteries. At this point the lumen of the artery is not narrowed. However, over the course of years the plaque can form an aneurism (an abnormal dilation) of the vessel inner wall, which can rupture. When a plaque ruptures in the wall, a clot can form, which can narrow or even occlude the artery so that little to no blood passes through. The inner wall damage is subject to additional build-up of fatty deposits, platelets, and other circulatory elements. With this decrease in blood flow through the artery, the tissue being fed by the vessel becomes ischemic and can die from lack of oxygen.

Exercise & Atherosclerosis

Exercise and physical activity reduce the risk of atherosclerosis by lowering blood pressure, as well as circulating LDL cholesterol, a prime instigator in plaque formation. Extensive review has shown that high density lipoprotein (HDL) increases via liver production in response to aerobic exercise (15; 91; 99). This lipid scavenger picks up circulating LDL cholesterol and transports it back to the liver, where it is reabsorbed and

Quick Facts on Cardiovascular Disease

Causes 40% of all annual deaths in the United States

One death every 35 seconds

Leading cause of premature/permanent work disability

Over one million Americans are disabled due to stroke annually

Over six million Americans are hospitalized annually for CVD

Estimated 403 billion dollars spent in associated health costs in 2006

Smokers' Risk

70% greater level of risk for heart disease.

Smoking two packs a day results in a 2 to 3-fold greater risk for CVD .

After 15 years of smoking abstinence, CVD risk approaches the non-smoker.

Smoking cessation reduces risk for heart attack or stroke by 50%.

the cholesterol is used for bile. A dose-response relationship has been shown between the amount of regular physical activity and plasma levels of HDL (6; 98). Endurance-trained athletes have demonstrated 20% to 30% more circulating HDL cholesterol than same-aged sedentary healthy subjects (174). Moderate intensity activity seems to yield the same benefits in HDL production as high intensity exercise as long as one reaches an appropriate weekly energy expenditure value (1200-1600 kcal/week) (79). In addition, regular exercise reduces triglycerides and increases lipoprotein lipase, the enzyme responsible for removing fatty acids and cholesterol from the blood (67). Complementing the reduction in hazardous circulatory lipids, exercise also reduces platelet adhesion by influencing the stress response. Stress can increase circulatory lipids and make particles in the blood "sticky."(217) Aerobic exercise offers a protective effect against this phenomenon.

Myocardial Ischemia

When the heart requires an amount of oxygen that cannot be met via functional mechanisms, it becomes ischemic. Oxygen supply does not meet demand. When this occurs repeatedly over time the condition becomes symptomatic. Exertion and consequential ischemia causes angina pectoris or chest pains and may cause irregularities in heart rhythm. Endurance activities have been shown to cause adaptations in coronary circulation that can reduce ischemia (129). Routine aerobic exercise leads to improved coronary blood flow and oxygen utilization by the cardiac tissue. Adaptations to exercise that account for the improved efficiency include improved blood flow dynamics, the promotion of oxygen transfer, and remodeling of the vascular structures that augment oxygen delivery. The vascular structures increase in diameter, allowing more blood to pass, while new capillaries and arterioles are formed to enhance the myocardial vascular network. Improved blood flow is further promoted by vascular reactivity and subsequent distribution in conjunction with increased vascular compliance. Together, these adaptations to training cause a relative reduction in peripheral resistance, thereby reducing the oxygen demand of the myocardium by lowering its workload.

Cardiac events related to coronary heart disease

Common Cardiovascular Disease Medications

Diuretics - Act on the kidney to prevent re-absorption of water.

Beta-Blockers - Reduce myocardial vigor by inhibiting the nerve impulse to the heart and blood vessels.

Angiostensin Converting Enzyme (ACE) Inhibitors - Cause blood vessels to relax by preventing the formation of the hormone angiotensin II, which causes constriction.

Angiostensin Antagonists - Block angiostensin II, resulting in the prevention of vasoconstriction.

Calcium Channel Blockers - Prevent calcium from entering the myocardium, reducing contraction.

Alpha-Blockers - Reduces the nerve impulses to the blood vessels, which allows the blood to pass more easily.

Nervous System Inhibitors - Relax blood vessels by controlling nerve impulses.

Vasodilators - Directly open the blood vessels by relaxing the muscle in the vessel walls.

are often triggered by heart arrhythmias or by thrombosis. **Arrhythmias** are heart rhythm disturbances that often occur in the presence of heart disease. Although they may occur in healthy individuals from artery spasm, electrolyte imbalances, responses to certain medications or drugs, and states of dehydration, they are more common in individuals with myocardial ischemia. The largest threat from arrhythmias occurs with ventricular fibrillation, where blockage causes the heart conduction system to malfunction. With ventricular fibrillation the heart's electrical activity becomes disordered. When this happens, the heart's lower chambers contract in a rapid, unsynchronized manner and the heart pumps little or no blood. If the heart is not defibrillated, the person will die from the phenomenon known as sudden death, due to heart attack. Exercise reduces the risk of cardiac arrhythmias by increasing blood flow to the tissue, thereby better satisfying the myocardial oxygen demand while suppressing sympathetic nervous system activity. This combined effect reduces the risk of sudden death in both healthy persons and those diagnosed with disease by mediating the two primary triggers, ischemia and neural stimulus.

Thrombosis

A **thrombus,** or blood clot, may also trigger a heart attack by occluding a coronary artery which, in turn, cuts off the oxygen supply to a portion of the heart. The initiation of an acute thrombotic event often starts with a disruption or rupture of an atherosclerotic plaque, tearing the inner wall of the vessel. Platelets accumulate at the injury site, causing the aforementioned process of obstruction. The formation of a clot, or thrombosis, around the injury site creates a major obstruction to blood flow. Even without full occlusion, the ischemic

catalyst can cause lethal disturbances in the heart rhythm, resulting in a heart attack.

This process does not occur as rapidly as it may sound. It generally follows the slow progression of atherosclerosis, but the thrombosis is the acute precipitating event that sets the course into action. This development of blockage is the transition between silent coronary artery disease, where the lumen of the vessel is not disrupted and often asymptomatic, to significant occlusion and onset of symptoms. At this point, the individual may experience recurring chest pains called unstable angina, cardiac arrhythmias, acute myocardial infarction, or sudden death. Aerobic training reduces the threat of thrombosis by enhancing the enzymatic activity at the site. The enzymes produced from endurance training break down the blood clots and decrease platelet adhesion and aggregation, helping to reduce and prevent clot formation.

Hypertension & Physical Activity

High blood pressure has been implicated as a major underlying cause of cardiovascular pathology. It is linked with cardiovascular complications and mortality. Currently, about one in every three persons in the United States is classifiably hypertensive.

Development of a Thrombosis

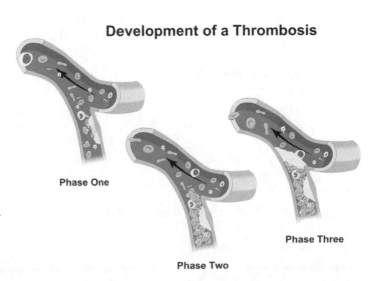

Phase One

Phase Two

Phase Three

Several large cohort studies have identified a relationship between physical activity and risk for hypertension (51). Physical activity, measured through sport and structured aerobic exercise, has shown an inverse relationship between hours per week of participation and risk for the development of high blood pressure (76; 208; 214). Epidemiological cohort studies have consistently demonstrated that sedentary, unfit persons have a 20% to 50% higher prospective risk of hypertension, as compared to exercising, physically fit persons (123). Following adjustments for age, sex, baseline blood pressure, and BMI, low cardiorespiratory fitness was identified as an independent risk factor for the development of hypertension. Low CRF was linked to a 52% higher risk of later development of the disease. Consistent with other studies, a dose-response relationship exists between the amount of activity and the degree of protection from hypertension (5; 170; 185). Individuals who are the least active were shown to have a 30% increase in risk compared to those who were highly active. It should be noted that none of these studies analyzed higher-risk minorities.

Conclusions of several meta-analyses suggest that aerobic exercise has a significant effect on both diastolic and systolic blood pressure response (49). Participation in aerobic training 30-60 minutes a day, 3-4 days per week, at intensity ranges of 60-70% VO_2 Max caused a consistent decrease of approximately 6-7 mmHg in both diastolic and systolic measures (213). Different studies, lasting between 10 and 36 weeks, analyzed the intensity of the aerobic training to determine the dose-response implications of the training (50; 207; 212). Interestingly, lower-intensity training yielded more positive results (184). In the low intensity groups (50%, 53% of maximum intensity), a mean decrease of 6 mmHg and 11-12 mmHg diastolic blood pressure were found, and systolic reductions between measures were 9 mmHg and 20 mmHg, respectively. The high intensity groups (73%, 75% of maximum intensity) did not fair as well with diastolic reductions of 11-12 mmHg and 5 mmHg and systolic reductions of

Blood Pressure Categories

	Systolic	Diastolic
Optimal Blood Pressure	≤ 115	≤ 75
Normal Blood Pressure	<120	<80
Prehypertension	120-139	80-89
Hypertension	≥ 140	≥ 90
Medical Referral	≥ 160	≥ 100

8 mmHg and 3 mmHg, respectively. Based on these studies and others, moderate intensity may offer an even more pronounced effect at lowering blood pressure than high intensity training (95). The reason for these findings is unclear and more data is needed to conclusively confirm these results.

Blood pressure is the product of cardiac output and peripheral resistance in the blood vessels. Exercise has been shown to present a relaxation effect on vascular wall resistance (48). Acute response by the body to a bout of aerobic exercise causes an immediate and temporary reduction effect on vascular resistance through peripheral blood vessel dilation. This response has been measured several hours following a session of exercise. With chronic and appropriate exercise stress, peripheral resistance lowers via attenuation of sympathetic nervous system activity. Routine aerobic exercise may cause a reduction in renin-angiotensin system activity (hormones secreted from the kidney to control blood pressure), arterial vasodilation, and baroreceptor (the brain's blood pressure monitoring system) adjustment (32). Additionally, the positive effect aerobic training has on circulating insulin levels contributes to a further enhancement in blood pressure reduction by decreasing insulin-mediated re-absorption of sodium by the kidneys (47).

Obesity & Physical Activity

Obesity is a major issue facing the American population. It is a risk factor for diabetes, heart disease, hypertension, osteoarthritis, high cholesterol, various cancers, and all-cause mortality (56; 232). Documented increases in bodyweight have occurred in all race and sex groups and have led to concerns of epidemic proportion. The combination of high-calorie diets and low levels of physical activity has created an energy balance disturbance (positive caloric balance), leading to progressive weight gain. This weight increase is most pronounced between the third and sixth decade of life (23; 94). Recently, childhood obesity has also become a major concern facing the United States. Reductions in activity and poor diets have made children fatter than ever before. Childhood obesity

Complications Related to Hypertension

Health Problems and Complications Related to Hypertension
Organ damage
Congestive heart failure
Hemorrhagic stroke
Aortic aneurysms and dissection
Renal failure
Retinopathy

Atherosclerosis Complications of Hypertension
Coronary heart disease
Ischemic stroke
Peripheral vascular disease

is directly linked to adult obesity, and overweight children present an elevated risk for adult diseases later in life, including hypertension, diabetes, and CVD (181).

A common theme that links many diseases and chronic illness is uncontrolled cellular inflammation. It is a factor in diseases including cardiovascular disease, diabetes, cancer, arthritis and many autoimmune-related conditions. Obesity has recently been added to this group of diseases as it is now known to present a low grade inflammatory response within many of the body's tissues, which cause deleterious effects, often leading to the development of cardiovascular and metabolic disease (115). It is well-known that being overweight is detrimental to one's health, but until recently the known mechanisms were limited. Scientists over the last decade have started to unravel the mystery of why obesity leads to premature death.

Inflammation is, by design, a protective response leading to the repair of tissue. When inflammation becomes chronic, as is the case with obesity, chemical mediators derived from different cellular activities change their dynamics causing a progressive deterioration. Fat cells are now considered a dynamic immune organ that secretes numerous immune modulating chemicals (72; 119). Visceral fat, in particular, is associated with the low-grade inflammation that seems to be a contributing pathologic feature for metabolic disease through insulin resistance and the promotion of atherosclerotic build-up in circulatory vessels (33). When high levels of visceral fat are combined with physical inactivity, over-nutrition, and advancement in age, the effect becomes more pronounced. Visceral fat is highly metabolic and contributes to cytokine (a chemical signal used between cells) hyperactivity (10). Adipokines secreted from fat tissue influence the metabolic process and contribute to proper function (86). The consequent low-grade inflammation associated with obesity causes disturbance in the secretion and function of adipokines. Research has identified changes in adiponectin, leptin, and resistin that exhibit harmful effects upon the body in obese individuals (149).

Adiponectin is an antiatherogenic agent, meaning it helps prevent the development of atherosclerotic plaque in blood vessels and slows the progression of atherosclerosis in coronary vessels. It does this by acting directly upon the vessel wall, inhibiting adhesive molecules from contributing to plaque formation and acts as a blocking agent to the formation of foam cells. In the skeletal muscle and the liver, adiponectin serves to promote insulin sensitivity and a positive blood lipid profile. Visceral adiposity reduces adiponectin concentrations (155). Lowering the adiponectin concentrations lessens the cardioprotective effect, leading to increased cardiovascular risk.

Leptin regulates energy metabolism and balance in conjunction with the brain's hypothalamus. Leptin is currently being touted as having cardioprotective benefits among its others roles in metabolism. Leptin concentrations adjust in response to obesity and contribute to insulin resistance (147). The changes in leptin concentration have also been recognized as a risk factor for coronary heart disease. Likewise, increased resistin concentrations correlate with obesity related inflammation and may be associated with the initiation and progression of atherosclerotic lesions (150). Resistin also promotes insulin resistance, although the actual mechanism is not known.

Insulin resistance due to adipokine dysfunction is further influenced by free fatty acids liberated directly into the liver from visceral fat tissue (112; 148). Visceral fat releases chemicals and fatty acids into the portal system, where they act on the connecting organs. The portal circulation system is a specialized network of blood vessels that connect the visceral organs to the liver. The excess fat in portal circulation has detrimental effects on insulin action, which is worsened by sympathetic hyperactivity in response to obesity. Sympathetic hyperactivity causes heightened lipolytic action resulting in excess free fatty acids in the blood. These actions combined with beta cell hypersecretion and reduced insulin clearance resulting in hyperinsulinemia, lead to early stage diabetes (111).

Interleukin-6 (IL-6) is possibly another factor associated with obesity-related inflammatory detriment within the portal system. High levels of IL-6 are a marker for inflammation and vascular pathology (118). Obese subjects demonstrated a 50% greater portal vein IL-6 concentration, demonstrating again the profound effect visceral fat has on pathogenic indicators. Portal vein IL-6 correlates with systemic C-reactive protein concentrations (154). C-reactive protein is associated with cardio- and peripheral vascular disease. C-reactive protein and oxidative stress are now presumed to interact in the early inflammatory processes of atherosclerosis. This is significant for young obese individuals. Although more research is necessary for conclusive association, C-reactive protein may be a new risk factor for CAD in individuals under 25 years of age (93).

The imbalance between increased inflammatory stimuli with a concurrent reduction in anti-inflammatory activity may be the foundation for the accelerated endothelial dysfunction and insulin resistance associated with obesity and the comorbid disorders of metabolic disease. More research is needed to clearly delineate the particular relationships, but it seems evident that the low-grade inflammation caused by obesity and visceral adiposity, lead to the premature development of disease. This, more so than ever before, identifies the importance of weight management during the developmental years and ongoing efforts to control weight throughout one's lifespan. For individuals who are currently obese, there is still hope. Weight loss is related to a reduction of oxidative stress and inflammation, and these beneficial effects likely translate into reduction of cardiovascular risk in obese individuals (9). Likewise, exercise and dietary management, along with pharmacologic intervention, can lead to atherosclerotic reversal in the earlier stages of CAD (8; 13).

Exercise may provide some protection against the onset of obesity related inflammation via heightened caloric expenditure and the attenuation of some of the side effects. It is assumed that individuals who engage in physical activity are more likely to be lean and experience a lower incidence of obesity than sedentary persons. These presumptions have not been conclusively backed by research. Physical activity has shown to be inversely related to risk of becoming overweight (83; 172). However, other research trials have not come to the same conclusion (40; 90). This suggests that an active lifestyle alone may not be enough to compensate for dietary intakes. Investigations comparing physical activity and childhood weight gain have shown higher activity levels in non-obese children and a reduction in BMI with increasing activity (14). However, inconsistent results have been seen in cross sectional studies examining physical activity and lower BMI and skinfold measures.

Studies examining the impact of exercise training on body weight and obesity have had more positive outcomes. Several reviews have concluded that exercise and physical activity positively affect weight by

Key Terms

Myocardial Ischemia – Lack of oxygen to the myocardium

Cardiovascular disease (CVD) - A general diagnostic category, consisting of several separate diseases of the heart and circulatory system.

Coronary heart disease (CHD) - Progressive reduction of blood supply to the heart due to narrowing or blocking of the coronary arteries.

Arrhythmia- An abnormal heart rhythm.

Thrombosis- Formation of a blood clot in the heart or blood vessel.

reducing fat mass and maintaining muscle. In addition, a dose-response gradient exists, based upon the frequency and duration of the activity (190). Most studies suggest that physical activity alone yields positive, but limited benefits for weight loss. When diet is factored in, the results become more favorable. The combination of caloric control and physical activity appears to be substantially more beneficial than either diet or physical activity alone. However, independently, physical activity seems to be an important factor in body fat distribution. Physical activity may favorably affect central storage through several measures to be discussed in the coming sections.

Weight gain is a factor of energy balance. When energy intake exceeds caloric expenditure, weight gain often results. Physical activity contributes most favorably to metabolic expenditure, and therefore is an important component in weight loss. Increasing physical activity contributes to greater caloric expenditure and consequently improves weight management. Exercise yields positive results for the maintenance of metabolic rate, whereas diet alone does not. Additionally, physical activity reduces the prevalence of central storage, which is important for lowering risk of metabolic disease.

It is suggested that decreases in physical activity may be a cause and consequence of weight gain. Adult weight gain has been linked with decreasing physical activity (189). As people reduce activity without appropriate adjustments in caloric intake, weight gain is likely to occur. When this occurs continuously over time risk for obesity increases significantly. To prevent creeping obesity, regular physical activity should be combined with caloric control.

Stroke & Physical Activity
Stroke stands as the third leading cause of death and is implicated as a major contributor to disability, making it

Body Mass Diagnostic Criteria

	Male	Female
Overfat Bodyfat	21-24%	28-31%
Obesity Bodyfat	≥25%	≥32%
Obesity BMI	≥30	≥30
Obesity Height-Weight	>20% mean	>20% mean
Morbid Obesity Bodyfat	≥30%	≥40%

a major problem in developed countries like the United States. A stroke is the sudden death of an area of brain cells caused by a lack of oxygen to the brain. The primary causes are vascular blockage, which impairs blood flow to the tissue (ischemic stroke) or an artery rupture (hemorrhagic stroke), causing bleeding within the brain. Ischemic stroke accounts for 80% of all stroke cases (134). In ischemic stroke, interruption of the blood supply to the brain results in tissue hypoperfusion, hypoxia, and eventual cell death. The main mechanisms involved in the development of ischemic stroke are associated with atherothrombotic and embolic disease.

In atherothrombotic disease, the pathophysiology resembles CAD in the heart (231). Lipid deposition leads to the formation of plaque, which narrows the vessel lumen and results in turbulent blood flow through the area of stenosis. The turbulence of the flow and the resultant alterations in flow velocities lead to vessel wall disruption or plaque rupture, both of which activate the clotting cascade. This process causes platelets to become activated and adhere to the plaque surface, where they eventually form a fibrin clot. As the lumen of the vessel becomes more occluded, ischemia develops distal to the obstruction and can eventually lead to infarction (death) of the tissue that relies on the parent vessel for oxygen delivery. Embolic stroke occurs when dislodged thrombi travel distally and

Stroke Facts

Stroke is the leading cause of serious long term disability.

25% of strokes occur in people under 65.

Stroke costs in 2005 :$57 billion in direct and indirect expense.

The southern United States has the highest rate of stroke-related death in the country.

occlude vessels downstream. One-half of all embolic strokes are caused by atrial fibrillation (an abnormal rhythm of the heart atria), while the rest are attributable to a variety of causes, including left ventricular dysfunction secondary to acute myocardial infarction or severe congestive heart failure, and atheroemboli. These latter emboli often arise from atherosclerotic lesions in the aortic arch, carotid arteries, and vertebral arteries, which break off and travel to the brain. Two of the most common risk factors for stroke include cigarette smoking and high blood pressure (75; 107; 108).

Hemorrhagic stroke, as indicated above, is caused by an intracerebral (within the brain) hemorrhage and results from the rupture of a vessel within the brain tissue. The primary cause of these ruptures is hypertension. Hypertension can cause an aneurism (an abnormal ballooning of a vessel) to form in a brain artery. This aneurysm can burst, which causes bleeding into the brain. Although limited data exists to support the benefits of physical activity on stroke risk, no conclusive evidence has directly linked reduced risk of either type of stroke to physical activity participation (137). The CDC reported that one study attempted to distinguish the difference between stroke pathophysiology and physical activity participation (114). It suggested that inactive men were more likely than active men to have hemorrhagic stroke, and ischemic stroke risk was reduced in smokers, but not non-smokers. More research is necessary to unequivocally support the association between physical activity and stroke, but physical activity has been shown to reduce risk for hypertension, a leading cause of stroke.

Diabetes & Physical Activity

Diabetes mellitus, commonly referred to as diabetes, is a chronic disease involving abnormalities in the body's ability to use sugar. In healthy individuals, the hormone insulin is secreted by the pancreas in response to carbohydrates absorbed into the blood stream, usually in the form of glucose, through normal digestion. Insulin signals muscle and other cells to take up glucose, thereby lowering the blood

Diagram of a Stroke

Affected area of brain

Unaffected area of brain

Hemorrhage disrupts blood flow to brain tissue

Blocked vessel cutting off blood supply

Diabetes Facts

Type I - 5-10% of diagnosed cases.

Type II accounts for 90-95% of diagnosed cases.

Highest risk: African American, Hispanic/Latino Americans, American Indians and Pacific Islanders.

Children born after the year 2000 have a 20-30% chance of developing type II diabetes.

Women who had gestational diabetes have a 20-50% chance of developing the disease in the next 5-10 years.

glucose level. The glucose taken up by cells is then used for normal metabolism, stored as glycogen, or converted into fat for later use. Diabetes is diagnosed when the body either has an inability to make insulin, or the cells have an inability to act in response to insulin (insulin insensitivity.)

Diabetes is one of the largest threats to the health of the United States population. According to the American Diabetes Association, individuals born after the year 2000 have a 24% (males) to 33% (females) chance of developing diabetes in their lifetime (131). Of the estimated 16 million Americans with diabetes, only 8 million have been diagnosed. Diabetes is the 7th leading cause of death from direct means, but this statistic greatly underestimates the role diabetes plays in premature death and disability. When diabetes is analyzed as a secondary cause (the disease that precipitated the event) the number of deaths associated with the disease doubles (34). Diabetes usually kills through cardiovascular disease, including stroke, CHD, peripheral vascular disease, and congestive heart failure (205). Diabetes-related illness or injury accounts for 1 out of 10 hospital visits. Predictions suggest that by age 65, approximately 40% of Americans will have glucose tolerance impairment (an inability of the body to appropriately handle digested carbohydrates) (130).

Diabetes is classified into groups based on the cause of the metabolic disease. **Insulin Dependent Diabetes Mellitus (IDDM)**, or type I as it is commonly known, is thought to be caused by a genetic autoimmune disorder that occurs in children. The beta cells in the pancreas responsible for the production of insulin are destroyed by the immune system, leading to a deficiency of circulating insulin. **Non-Insulin Dependent Diabetes Mellitus (NIDDM)**, or type II diabetes, results from insulin insensitivity of muscle cells, a reduction of insulin due to impaired secretion or a combination of both. Diabetes may also occur during pregnancy due to metabolic disruption that occurs during the fetal development process.

NIDDM is the most common form of diabetes, representing more than 90% of all diagnosed cases. Although the most prevalent form of diabetes, NIDDM is also the most preventable. Even though strong genetic factors exist, and the disease is more common in older age, the primary causes of NIDDM are all modifiable. Physical inactivity, obesity (particularly android), and poor diet lead to the development of insulin resistance, glucose intolerance, and hyperinsulinemia (excessive secretion of insulin). When circulating glucose is not managed and remains elevated, it damages large and small vessels of the vascular system. Diabetic damage to blood vessels causes chronic complications and accounts for the significant morbidity and mortality related to the disease. As indicated above, these can be divided into large vessel (macrovascular) disorders, including coronary artery disease, stroke, and peripheral vascular disease, which are the main causes of death, and small vessel (microvascular) disorders including retinopathy, nephropathy, erectile dysfunction, and neuropathy which are the main causes of morbidity (decreased quality of life and disability). Diabetic macrovascular disease is caused by the acceleration of atherogenesis. However, how hyperglycemia causes small vessel disease is not clearly understood. Two predominant theories are the advanced glycation endproduct theory and the reactive oxygen species theory. The advanced glycation endproduct theory is based on the fact that hyperglycemia causes increased glycation of proteins (the attachment of sugar molecules to protein molecules). A variety of extracellular and intracellular products of glycation have been termed advanced glycation endproducts (AGE). Extracellular AGE may alter protein function, and intracellular AGE may alter gene expression, the net result being abnormal cellular and vascular function. Inhibitors of AGE have been used in animal studies, but their efficacy was limited by toxicity in clinical trials. Diabetes-induced oxidative stress milieu is one of the oldest theories for hyperglycemia-induced microvascular damage. The oxidation of glucose releases free radicals, which may account for a number of cellular dysfunctions. Unfortunately, in recent human trials, the promise of antioxidants (such as vitamin C and vitamin E) in reducing diabetic complications has not materialized.

Inactive lifestyles are linked with the development of NIDDM. Considerable evidence exists which shows that sedentary lifestyle habits are a risk factor for NIDDM (30; 157; 230). Physical activity, to the contrary, has shown to both protect against and have a pronounced effect on NIDDM by reducing circulating

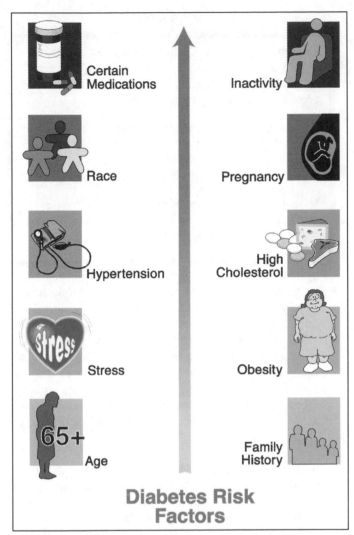

Diabetes Risk Factors

Labels: Certain Medications, Inactivity, Race, Pregnancy, Hypertension, High Cholesterol, Stress, Obesity, 65+ Age, Family History

Exercise has demonstrated an improvement in carbohydrate metabolism and glucose tolerance by enhancing the cellular uptake of sugar. Contracting muscle tissue likely causes a synergistic effect between insulin and cellular sensitivity, increasing glucose transport into the cell. Single prolonged bouts of exercise increase cellular permeability for 24 hours, enabling better glucose management as the cells replenish the lost glycogen stores. The increased sensitivity to insulin prevents hyperinsulinemia and improves glucose tolerance, providing a protective effect from the onset of the disease.

Both endurance and resistance training have been shown to provide benefits (176; 233). Endurance athletes have demonstrated greater insulin sensitivity, allowing for lower insulin levels at relative glucose concentrations compared to sedentary subjects. Likewise, it has been reported that resistance-trained individuals experience similar glucose insulin dynamics (183). Physical activity has been shown to improve glucose management through muscle cell changes and fat cell response. Physical activity also leads to indirect benefits, including weight management, reduced central fat storage, and metabolic efficiency.

The combination of diet and exercise is recommended to prevent and treat diabetes. Individuals with mild disease not taking medication seem to experience the most benefit from the therapy. Individuals with advanced NIDDM may experience complications with excessive physical activity, including ketosis, an abnormality of the body's metabolic process resulting in an increase of ketones in the blood, hyperglycemia (high blood sugar), and hypoglycemic (low blood sugar) response to vigorous exercise. Additionally, foot wounds, cardiovascular complications, and eye damage due to retinopathy are potential problems. Proper medical evaluation and screening can help identify individuals at greater risk and determine proper precautions.

glucose in a process that causes insulin re-sensitivity in the cells. Physically inactive women ages 55-69 were found to have twice the risk for NIDDM as their physically active counterparts (31). Prospective cohort studies identified that physical activity provides a protective effect and is inversely related to the incidence of the disease (126; 179; 180). The highest risks identified in the studies were high BMI and/or family history of hypertension or diabetes. It is suggested that for each additional 500 kcal of expenditure per week from physical activity, risk for NIDDM is reduced 6% (225). Additionally, more vigorous activities were associated with the greatest benefit. A study of 34-59 year old women who reported engaging in vigorous physical activity at least once a week experienced a reduction in risk by 16% compared to women who did not participate in vigorous activities (122).

Diagnosing Diabetes

Pre-diabetes
Impaired Fasting Glucose 100-125 mg/dl ,following over night fast

Impaired Glucose Tolerance 140-199 mg/dl, following 2-hour glucose test

Diabetes Diagnostic criteria
Fasting plasma glucose >126 mg/dl

Casual plasma glucose >200 mg/dl

Oral Glucose test >200 mg/dl

Osteoarthritis & Physical Activity

Osteoarthritis, the most common form of arthritis, is not a single disease but rather the end result of a variety of disorders leading to the structural or functional failure of one or more joints in the body. Osteoarthritis involves the entire joint, including the nearby muscles, underlying bone, ligaments, joint lining (synovium), and the joint cover (capsule). It is characterized by an advancing loss of cartilage. As the cartilage attempts to repair itself, the bone remodels, the underlying (subchondral) bone hardens, and bone cysts form. Age is a key risk factor for osteoarthritis, with the greatest prevalence in older adults. Osteoarthritis is credited with being the leading cause of activity limitation among many older adults. The actual cause of osteoarthritis is unknown. It seems to be more common in individuals who pursue competitive sports or engage in high-intensity activity (60). Competitive running, football, soccer, and weightlifting are all associated with increased risk for the development of the disease (116). The development of osteoarthritis seems to occur more frequently in joints used repetitively and excessively (24). In one study, a small sample of pitchers reported greater incidence in the shoulder and elbow of the throwing arm (200).

Osteoarthritis is linked with injury in sedentary and active persons alike. Researchers suggest that osteoarthritis may be more prevalent in athletes than non-athletes because of the high incidence of injury reported in competitive sports (59). Soccer players who did not experience injury during competition demonstrated no greater incident of arthritis than sedentary controls (171). It appears that physical activity is not the impetus for osteoarthritis but increases the risk of injury, which may be the underlying cause (26). Regular noncompetitive physical activity that is dose appropriate does not appear to be harmful to joints that have not been injured (101).

Key Terms

Insulin dependent diabetes mellitus (IDDM) - Type I diabetes, is an autoimmune disorder in which the body's own immune system attacks cells of the pancreas, sufficiently reducing insulin.

Non-insulin dependent diabetes mellitus (NIDDM)- Type II diabetes is a metabolic disorder characterized by insulin resistance, insulin deficiency, and hyperglycemia.

Osteoarthritis- A form of arthritis, occurring mainly in older individuals, that is characterized by chronic degradation of the cartilage in the joints.

Physical activity using non-impact resistance and aerobic modalities, when performed at moderate levels, can improve function, reduce joint swelling, and relieve symptoms with both osteo- and rheumatoid arthritis (145). Increased levels of activity have been demonstrated to improve status in physical, psychosocial, and functional measures (146). In addition, self reports by subjects with osteoarthritis suggest moderate intensity activity raises pain threshold, improves energy levels, and self-efficacy (203).

The benefits of moderate intensity exercise are likely related to the mechanisms that naturally keep joints healthy. Joints require movement to receive nourishment. Nutrients diffuse through the cartilage matrix via pressure gradients that cause fluid to flow when compressed. When the joints are appropriately loaded through normal functional range of motion, proteoglycan synthesis is increased by the chondrocytes, increasing the cushioning effect. On the contrary, high impact, high intensity loading performed repeatedly disrupts this process, inhibiting cartilage matrix function. Inactivity also affects the cartilage matrix by reducing proteoglycan synthesis and cartilage

Osteoarthritis

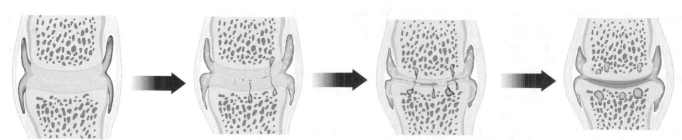

The gradual breakdown of articulating cartilage over time

integrity. Physical inactivity, particularly immobility, causes cartilage decline and makes the joint more susceptible to injury. Prolonged disuse associates with fibrous replacement and a loss of function. When comparing injured versus non-injured joints, running had a positive effect on healthy joint water content and proteoglycan synthesis but had negative outcomes on injured joints, ultimately leading to the development of osteoarthritis (25; 85).

Osteoporosis & Physical Activity

Osteoporosis is a progressive bone disease that occurs due to a loss of bone mass and structural deterioration of the bone tissue. The development of the disease is linked to three compounding factors: deficient level of peak bone mass, a reduction in bone mass after age thirty, and further loss of bone after age fifty. Osteoporosis causes the bone to become frail and brittle, increasing the risk for fracture. The vertebra, hip, and wrist experience the greatest risk of injury from the disease. Fractures in the vertebra are usually asymptomatic and lead to structural changes that often present as kyphotic disorders of the spine. Kyphosis, or hunchback, is associated with significant functional decline, gastrointestinal and abdominal problems, and chronic back pain. Injuries at the hip usually occur from falls. Hip fractures account for 16% of osteoporosis-related fractures each year (63; 228). Death or disabilities are expected outcomes from hip fractures related to osteoporosis, with 15-20% of sufferers dying within 12 months (227). Osteoporosis is more common in women than men due to lower peak bone mass, post-menopausal bone loss, and the fact that women live longer than men.

Physical activity is a vital part of bone health. Regular participation in physical activity increases peak bone mass during youth and maintains the mass into adulthood. Athletic young adults demonstrate greater bone mass than their sedentary counterparts. The strength of the attached musculature, amount and intensity of physical activity performed, and level of CRF correlate with the bone mineral density. This suggests that activities promoting the greatest bone stress have the largest magnitude of benefit for bone mass. Activities that encourage higher force outputs, such as resistance training, plyometrics, and weight bearing endurance events have the greatest impact on bone maintenance. All persons should engage in routine weight-bearing physical activity to maintain appropriate bone health. This is particularly true for postmenopausal women due to the resultant reduction of estrogen experienced during menopause. Some evidence suggests that osteoporotic women may be able to reduce bone loss and facilitate improved bone mineral density with exercise. Other studies have found no such evidence (143). It is likely that the degree of bone stress determines the outcome. Resistance exercise seems to have a more pronounced effect compared with endurance exercise, which may be due to more muscle mass used and greater bone stress, particularly in the axial skeleton. Estrogen levels in both men and women seem to be an important component to bone improvement as well. In postmenopausal women, greater improvements have been demonstrated with the use of estrogen replacement therapy (113).

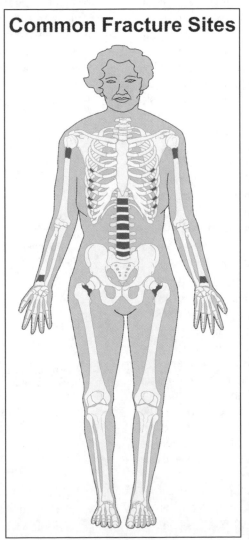

Common Fracture Sites

Bone stress from load-bearing activity is likely to be the most important factor in bone remodeling. Bone cell formation occurs in response to mechanical loading, which improves structural balance and density. The effects of the load placed upon the bone are mediated by glucose-6-phosphate, prostaglandins, and nitric oxide, all of which augment the adaptation response. Without appropriate stress, bone mass is compromised. In addition to mechanical factors, nutrition, medications, hormone concentrations, and age each have a relative contribution to bone health. Proper nutrition (in the form of calcium and vitamin D) and physical activity are necessary throughout a person's lifespan to reduce the risk of osteoporosis.

In addition to the improvements and maintenance of bone that protect against osteoporosis, physical activity also reduces risk of fractures from falls. As previously mentioned, osteoporotic hip fractures account for a higher risk for premature death and disability than all the other fractures combined. Studies analyzing physical activity and hip fracture

Osteoporosis

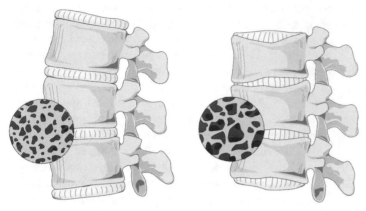

Healthy Bone   **Demineralized Bone**

occurrence found a lower risk among more active adults (19; 202). The magnitude of the benefit seems to be related to the level of activity, although even exercise walking showed protective effects. A person's risk for falls correlates to performance fitness scores and measures of functional task efficiency (132). Compromised gait, balance, reaction time, strength, range of motion, and impaired vision are all factors that affect fall risk. Exercise profoundly reduces risk by enhancing strength and balance. Additionally, improvements in functional capacity, gait efficiency, and speed and reaction time may positively impact risk. In measures of stair-climbing power, movement gait, and other functional tasks, frail elderly subjects suffering from chronic disease demonstrated improvements and reduced incidence of falls with weight training (77; 80). Individuals at high risk for falls should be encouraged to perform resistance training activities aimed at improving strength and balance to reduce risk of injury and hip fractures.

Cancer & Physical Activity

Cancer is reported to be the most feared of all diseases and is the second leading cause of death in the United States, accounting for one-fourth of all deaths (88). According to the American Cancer Society, the rate of new-case cancer is rising, with estimates of newly diagnosed cases well above one million per year (89). Cancer is actually several diseases, characterized by an abnormal and uncontrolled growth and spread of cells which have numerous forms and causes. Of all the cancers, colorectal cancer has been the most studied in relation to physical activity. Interestingly, there seem to be differences between the effects of physical activity on colon cancer and rectal cancer when viewed independently. Although two studies investigating colorectal adenomatous polyps (a pre-cancerous lesion) reported an inverse relationship between level of

physical activity and risk for adenomas, other studies have not found the same association (64; 66; 87; 110; 117; 216).

Colon cancer seems to show more promise for physical activity as a preventive measure than rectal cancer (102). Although job title was the only criteria for physical activity status, numerous studies showed consistency, reporting an inverse relationship between cancer risk and physical activity related to job responsibilities (163; 194; 211). Five out of ten studies using two categories of physical activity for investigating the dose-response relationship found statistical significance with an inverse dose gradient (103; 135; 186; 188). Additionally, two studies found the same relationship when using leisure time activity as the measure of physical work (162; 209).

When diet is added as a measured factor the relationship becomes stronger. Studies that controlled for dietary intake found significant inverse relationships with various types of physical activity (161; 187; 204). The research suggests that physical activity, whether leisure, structured, or related to job responsibility reduces risk for colon cancer. The risk for rectal cancer seems to remain unchanged with activity participation, but recent studies show a possible link.

Types of Colorectal Cancer

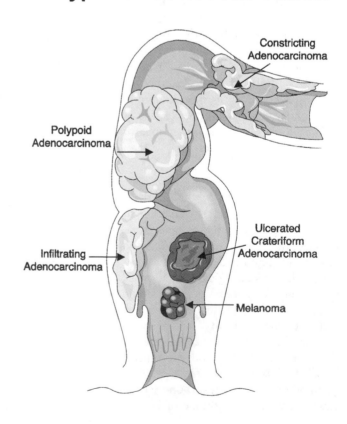

Constricting Adenocarcinoma

Polypoid Adenocarcinoma

Infiltrating Adenocarcinoma

Ulcerated Crateriform Adenocarcinoma

Melanoma

Breast cancer may also possibly be affected by regular participation in activity, but little data exists to support this possibility. Two of five studies found strong significance between physical activities during youth and later development of breast cancer, whereas only 20% of the epidemiologic studies analyzing physical activity and breast cancer risk demonstrated significance (104; 210). The inconsistencies may be related to confounding factors not accounted for in the research trials. The benefits of physical activity for breast cancer may exist through the possible benefits of exercise on weight control (96). According to the National Cancer Institute, risk for cancers of the colon, breast, endometrium, kidney, and esophagus are linked to obesity (65; 73; 105; 109). Therefore, activity that reduces risk for weight gain may also indirectly help reduce the risk of these cancers.

For all other cancers, too little information exists to make inferences related to the effect physical activity has on risk. The probable cause for the effect seen in colon cancer is the alteration of local prostaglandin synthesis. When activities are performed at higher intensities, prostaglandin (F2 alpha) synthesis increases and prostaglandin (E2) may become suppressed. This leads to increased intestinal motility, which in theory reduces contact time between carcinogens (toxins that cause cancer), co-carcinogens, and related promoters with the intestine mucosa. Although inconsistent results have been demonstrated in research trials, scientists believe mechanisms for enhanced motility will likely help reduce risk of colon cancer.

Mental Health & Physical Activity

Depression, anxiety disorders, and subjective feelings of self-worth affect psychological well-being. These disorders affect millions of people and are linked to suicide, currently the nation's ninth leading cause of death (136). Statistical reports suggest 1 out of 10 adults suffer from some type of depressive disorder, and approximately 15% of people experience anxiety disorders during any given year (125). One study found 25% of people ages 15-54 reported mental disorders during the previous year (1). Mental health and psychological well-being relate to mood, personality, cognition, and perception. Consequently, these factors are linked to physical health and perceived quality of life (153). Due to this relationship, it has been surmised that physical activity can improve mood, self-esteem, self-efficacy, and cognitive function.

Epidemiologic research demonstrates an association between physical activity and symptoms of depression, clinical depression, symptoms of anxiety, improvements in positive affect (disposition), and general well-being

(69; 152). These trials suggest that improvements associated with physical activity occur in persons with diagnosed disorders and in the general public, among persons reporting mood disturbances (124). Studies using aerobic training have demonstrated a temporary change in mental state based on a single episode of physical activity (144). Subjects reported reduced anxiety, reduced muscle tension, and improvements in transient mood, lasting 2-6 hours post-exercise. For exercise to affect trait measures, it is suggested that participation must be routine. It is not known if chronic participation causes actual trait adjustments or simply results in "carry-over effect" of the transient state changes associated with the exercise bout. Adults who engaged in routine physical activity from exercise or sport experienced reduced symptoms of depression and anxiety compared to individuals reporting no physical activity (151). In a cross sectional study involving over 46,000 individuals, physical activity was associated with improved mood and general well-being and fewer symptoms of anxiety and depression (70). On the contrary, studies analyzing the effects of physical inactivity on mental health found that individuals who engaged in little or no recreational physical activity had greater incidence of depressive symptoms.

The activity engaged in and frequency of participation may play a role in the mental shifts associated with physical activity (22). Women reported improvements in positive affect when the activity was recreational but did not show the same outcome when housework was a contributor to the physical activity measured by energy expenditure (21; 195). Men reported a 27% lower incidence of depression when engaged in activity 3 or more days per week (195). Additionally, individuals who expended 1,000-2,499 kcal per week showed a 17% reduction in risk, while those who exceeded 2500 kcal per week experienced a 28% reduction compared to those that expended less than 1,000 kcal in a one week period of time (38). In a similar study, an inverse dose-response relationship was found between energy expended and incidence of depression (58). Greater participation in activity seems to reduce risk for depression, consistent with the frequency and amount of work performed, up to a certain point. When individuals engage in strenuous or excessive activity, subjects reported negative mental health effects. No threshold of intensity or duration has been identified, nor has an optimal volume been demonstrated, but endurance athletes performing vigorous exercise have reported negative effects on mental health (57; 133). These included mood disturbances, increased fatigue, anxiety, and symptoms of depression. These negative effects are consistent with some of the symptoms identified in overtraining syndrome. It would seem that the deleterious effects from strenuous, high volume exercise are related to overtraining, as mood improved when excessive work was tapered back.

The suggested biological mechanism for improved mental state with exercise relates to the concentration of brain neurotransmitters (chemicals that transmit signals from one brain nerve to another) and neuroreceptors. Dopamine, norepinephrine, and serotonin, as well as endorphins, enkephalins, and dynorphins have been proposed components in mood adjustments associated with activity. Additionally, the temperature changes and physiological adaptations associated with increased core

temperature possibly explain the reduction in tension reported by subjects. It is also likely that some of the positive effects from exercise are psychosocial. Social interaction, healthy competitiveness, and social support that many people experience in environments associated with physical activity may be added factors to improved self-esteem, self-efficacy, and relief of daily stressors. No matter what the particular impetus for improvement in mental health and well-being, it seems physical activity performed at moderate levels throughout the week can improve mental health.

Chapter Twelve References

1. Self-reported frequent mental distress among adults-- United States, 1993-1996. *MMWR Morb Mortal Wkly Rep* 47: 326-331, 1998.

2. Nutrition and fitness: Diet, genes, physical activity and health. Proceedings of the 4th International Conference on Nutrition and Fitness. Athens, Greece, May 25-29, 2000. *World Rev Nutr Diet* 89: XI-191, 2001.

3. Physical activity programs and behavior counseling in older adult populations. *Med Sci Sports Exerc* 36: 1997-2003, 2004.

4. **Ades PA, Savage PD, Cress ME, Brochu M, Lee NM and Poehlman ET**. Resistance training on physical performance in disabled older female cardiac patients. *Med Sci Sports Exerc* 35: 1265-1270, 2003.

5. **Afghani A, Abbott AV, Wiswell RA, Jaque SV, Gleckner C, Schroeder ET and Johnson CA**. Central adiposity, aerobic fitness, and blood pressure in premenopausal Hispanic women. *Int J Sports Med* 25: 599-606, 2004.

6. **Afghani A, Abbott AV, Wiswell RA, Jaque SV, Gleckner C, Schroeder ET and Johnson CA**. Central adiposity, aerobic fitness, and blood pressure in premenopausal Hispanic women. *Int J Sports Med* 25: 599-606, 2004.

7. **Afghani A, Abbott AV, Wiswell RA, Jaque SV, Gleckner C, Schroeder ET and Johnson CA**. Central adiposity, aerobic fitness, and blood pressure in premenopausal Hispanic women. *Int J Sports Med* 25: 599-606, 2004.

8. **Aldhahi W and Hamdy O**. Adipokines, inflammation, and the endothelium in diabetes. *Curr Diab Rep* 3: 293-298, 2003.

9. **Aldhahi W and Hamdy O**. Adipokines, inflammation, and the endothelium in diabetes. *Curr Diab Rep* 3: 293-298, 2003.

10. **Aldhahi W and Hamdy O**. Adipokines, inflammation, and the endothelium in diabetes. *Curr Diab Rep* 3: 293-298, 2003.

11. **Alexander NB and Goldberg A**. Gait disorders: search for multiple causes. *Cleve Clin J Med* 72: 586, 589-4, 2005.

12. **Amundsen BH, Wisloff U and Slordahl SA**. [Exercise training for prevention, treatment and rehabilitation of cardiovascular disease]. *Tidsskr Nor Laegeforen* 127: 446-448, 2007.

13. **Bassuk SS and Manson JE**. Physical activity and the prevention of cardiovascular disease. *Curr Atheroscler Rep* 5: 299-307, 2003.

14. **Berkey CS, Rockett HR, Gillman MW and Colditz GA**. One-year changes in activity and in inactivity among 10- to 15-year-old boys and girls: relationship to change in body mass index. *Pediatrics* 111: 836-843, 2003.

15. **Bertoli A, Di Daniele N, Ceccobelli M, Ficara A, Girasoli C and De Lorenzo A**. Lipid profile, BMI, body fat distribution, and aerobic fitness in men with metabolic syndrome. *Acta Diabetol* 40 Suppl 1: S130-S133, 2003.

16. **Bertoli A, Di Daniele N, Ceccobelli M, Ficara A, Girasoli C and De Lorenzo A**. Lipid profile, BMI, body fat distribution, and aerobic fitness in men with metabolic syndrome. *Acta Diabetol* 40 Suppl 1: S130-S133, 2003.

17. **Bish CL, Michels BH, Maynard LM, Serdula MK, Thompson NJ and Kettel KL**. Health-related quality of life and weight loss among overweight and obese U.S. adults, 2001 to 2002. *Obesity (Silver Spring)* 14: 2042-2053, 2006.

18. **Bish CL, Michels BH, Maynard LM, Serdula MK, Thompson NJ and Kettel KL**. Health-related quality of life and weight loss among overweight and obese U.S. adults, 2001 to 2002. *Obesity (Silver Spring)* 14: 2042-2053, 2006.

19. **Borer KT**. Physical activity in the prevention and amelioration of osteoporosis in women : interaction of mechanical, hormonal and dietary factors. *Sports Med* 35: 779-830, 2005.

20. **Brill PA, Macera CA, Davis DR, Blair SN and Gordon N**. Muscular strength and physical function. *Med Sci Sports Exerc* 32: 412-416, 2000.

21. **Brooks AG, Withers RT, Gore CJ, Vogler AJ, Plummer J and Cormack J**. Measurement and prediction

of METs during household activities in 35- to 45-year-old females. *Eur J Appl Physiol* 91: 638-648, 2004.

22. **Brown DW, Brown DR, Heath GW, Balluz L, Giles WH, Ford ES and Mokdad AH**. Associations between physical activity dose and health-related quality of life. *Med Sci Sports Exerc* 36: 890-896, 2004.

23. **Bruunsgaard H and Pedersen BK**. Age-related inflammatory cytokines and disease. *Immunol Allergy Clin North Am* 23: 15-39, 2003.

24. **Buckwalter JA**. Sports, joint injury, and posttraumatic osteoarthritis. *J Orthop Sports Phys Ther* 33: 578-588, 2003.

25. **Buckwalter JA and Martin JA**. Sports and osteoarthritis. *Curr Opin Rheumatol* 16: 634-639, 2004.

26. **Buckwalter JA and Martin JA**. Sports and osteoarthritis. *Curr Opin Rheumatol* 16: 634-639, 2004.

27. **Callow AD**. Cardiovascular disease 2005--the global picture. *Vascul Pharmacol* 45: 302-307, 2006.

28. **Carlsson S, Andersson T, Wolk A and Ahlbom A**. Low physical activity and mortality in women: baseline lifestyle and health as alternative explanations. *Scand J Public Health* 34: 480-487, 2006.

29. **Castillo Garzon MJ, Ortega Porcel FB and Ruiz RJ**. [Improvement of physical fitness as anti-aging intervention]. *Med Clin (Barc)* 124: 146-155, 2005.

30. **Choi BC and Shi F**. Risk factors for diabetes mellitus by age and sex: results of the National Population Health Survey. *Diabetologia* 44: 1221-1231, 2001.

31. **Choi BC and Shi F**. Risk factors for diabetes mellitus by age and sex: results of the National Population Health Survey. *Diabetologia* 44: 1221-1231, 2001.

32. **Cornelissen VA and Fagard RH**. Effects of endurance training on blood pressure, blood pressure-regulating mechanisms, and cardiovascular risk factors. *Hypertension* 46: 667-675, 2005.

33. **Das UN**. Obesity, metabolic syndrome X, and inflammation. *Nutrition* 18: 430-432, 2002.

34. **Davidson JA**. Introductory remarks: diabetes care in America - "a sense of urgency". *Endocr Pract* 12 Suppl 1: 13-15, 2006.

35. **De Luca CR, Wood SJ, Anderson V, Buchanan JA, Proffitt TM, Mahony K and Pantelis C**. Normative data from the CANTAB. I: development of executive function over the lifespan. *J Clin Exp Neuropsychol* 25: 242-254, 2003.

36. **De Luca CR, Wood SJ, Anderson V, Buchanan JA, Proffitt TM, Mahony K and Pantelis C**. Normative data from the CANTAB. I: development of executive function over the lifespan. *J Clin Exp Neuropsychol* 25: 242-254, 2003.

37. **De Luca CR, Wood SJ, Anderson V, Buchanan JA, Proffitt TM, Mahony K and Pantelis** C. Normative data from the CANTAB. I: development of executive function

over the lifespan. *J Clin Exp Neuropsychol* 25: 242-254, 2003.

38. **De Moor MH, Beem AL, Stubbe JH, Boomsma DI and De Geus EJ**. Regular exercise, anxiety, depression and personality: a population-based study. *Prev Med* 42: 273-279, 2006.

39. **de Vreede PL, van Meeteren NL, Samson MM, Wittink HM, Duursma SA and Verhaar HJ**. The effect of functional tasks exercise and resistance exercise on health-related quality of life and physical activity. A randomised controlled trial. *Gerontology* 53: 12-20, 2007.

40. **Dekker MJ, Lee S, Hudson R, Kilpatrick K, Graham TE, Ross R and Robinson LE**. An exercise intervention without weight loss decreases circulating interleukin-6 in lean and obese men with and without type 2 diabetes mellitus. *Metabolism* 56: 332-338, 2007.

41. **Duncan GE, Perri MG, Anton SD, Limacher MC, Martin AD, Lowenthal DT, Arning E, Bottiglieri T and Stacpoole PW**. Effects of exercise on emerging and traditional cardiovascular risk factors. *Prev Med* 39: 894-902, 2004.

42. **Duncan GE, Perri MG, Anton SD, Limacher MC, Martin AD, Lowenthal DT, Arning E, Bottiglieri T and Stacpoole PW**. Effects of exercise on emerging and traditional cardiovascular risk factors. *Prev Med* 39: 894-902, 2004.

43. **Duscha BD, Slentz CA, Johnson JL, Houmard JA, Bensimhon DR, Knetzger KJ and Kraus WE**. Effects of exercise training amount and intensity on peak oxygen consumption in middle-age men and women at risk for cardiovascular disease. *Chest* 128: 2788-2793, 2005.

44. **Dvorak RV, Tchernof A, Starling RD, Ades PA, Dipietro L and Poehlman ET**. Respiratory fitness, free living physical activity, and cardiovascular disease risk in older individuals: a doubly labeled water study. *J Clin Endocrinol Metab* 85: 957-963, 2000.

45. **Erikssen G**. Physical fitness and changes in mortality: the survival of the fittest. *Sports Med* 31: 571-576, 2001.

46. **Erikssen G**. Physical fitness and changes in mortality: the survival of the fittest. *Sports Med* 31: 571-576, 2001.

47. **Evans EM, Racette SB, Peterson LR, Villareal DT, Greiwe JS and Holloszy JO**. Aerobic power and insulin action improve in response to endurance exercise training in healthy 77-87 yr olds. *J Appl Physiol* 98: 40-45, 2005.

48. **Fagard RH**. Exercise is good for your blood pressure: effects of endurance training and resistance training. *Clin Exp Pharmacol Physiol* 33: 853-856, 2006.

49. **Fagard RH**. Exercise is good for your blood pressure: effects of endurance training and resistance training. *Clin Exp Pharmacol Physiol* 33: 853-856, 2006.

50. **Fagard RH and Cornelissen VA**. Effect of exercise on blood pressure control in hypertensive patients. *Eur J Cardiovasc Prev Rehabil* 14: 12-17, 2007.

51. **Fagard RH and Cornelissen VA**. Effect of exercise on blood pressure control in hypertensive patients. *Eur J Cardiovasc Prev Rehabil* 14: 12-17, 2007.

52. **Fattirolli F, Cellai T and Burgisser C**. [Physical activity and cardiovascular health a close link]. *Monaldi Arch Chest Dis* 60: 73-78, 2003.

53. **Fattirolli F, Cellai T and Burgisser C**. [Physical activity and cardiovascular health a close link]. *Monaldi Arch Chest Dis* 60: 73-78, 2003.

54. **Fox CS, Evans JC, Larson MG, Kannel WB and Levy D**. Temporal trends in coronary heart disease mortality and sudden cardiac death from 1950 to 1999: the Framingham Heart Study. *Circulation* 110: 522-527, 2004.

55. **Fox KR, Stathi A, McKenna J and Davis MG**. Physical activity and mental well-being in older people participating in the Better Ageing Project. *Eur J Appl Physiol* 2007.

56. **Fulop T, Tessier D and Carpentier A**. The metabolic syndrome. *Pathol Biol (Paris)* 54: 375-386, 2006.

57. **Galper DI, Trivedi MH, Barlow CE, Dunn AL and Kampert JB**. Inverse association between physical inactivity and mental health in men and women. *Med Sci Sports Exerc* 38: 173-178, 2006.

58. **Galper DI, Trivedi MH, Barlow CE, Dunn AL and Kampert JB**. Inverse association between physical inactivity and mental health in men and women. *Med Sci Sports Exerc* 38: 173-178, 2006.

59. **Garrick JG and Requa RK**. Sports and fitness activities: the negative consequences. *J Am Acad Orthop Surg* 11: 439-443, 2003.

60. **Garrick JG and Requa RK**. Sports and fitness activities: the negative consequences. *J Am Acad Orthop Surg* 11: 439-443, 2003.

61. **Gerson LW and Stevens JA**. Recreational injuries among older Americans, 2001. *Inj Prev* 10: 134-138, 2004.

62. **Gerson LW and Stevens JA**. Recreational injuries among older Americans, 2001. *Inj Prev* 10: 134-138, 2004.

63. **Geusens P, Milisen K, Dejaeger E and Boonen S**. Falls and fractures in postmenopausal women: a review. *J Br Menopause Soc* 9: 101-106, 2003.

64. **Giacosa A, Franceschi S, La Vecchia C, Favero A, Frascio F and Andreatta R**. Overweight and colorectal cancer risk. *Minerva Gastroenterol Dietol* 47: 235-240, 2001.

65. **Giovannucci E, Ascherio A, Rimm EB, Colditz GA, Stampfer MJ and Willett WC**. Physical activity, obesity, and risk for colon cancer and adenoma in men. *Ann Intern Med* 122: 327-334, 1995.

66. **Giovannucci E, Ascherio A, Rimm EB, Colditz GA, Stampfer MJ and Willett WC**. Physical activity, obesity, and risk for colon cancer and adenoma in men. *Ann Intern Med* 122: 327-334, 1995.

67. **Glueck CJ**. Nonpharmacologic and pharmacologic alteration of high-density lipoprotein cholesterol: therapeutic approaches to prevention of atherosclerosis. *Am Heart J* 110: 1107-1115, 1985.

68. **Goldberg RJ, Glatfelter K, Burbank-Schmidt E, Lessard D and Gore JM**. Trends in community mortality due to coronary heart disease. *Am Heart J* 151: 501-507, 2006.

69. **Goodwin RD**. Association between physical activity and mental disorders among adults in the United States. *Prev Med* 36: 698-703, 2003.

70. **Goodwin RD**. Association between physical activity and mental disorders among adults in the United States. *Prev Med* 36: 698-703, 2003.

71. **Goraya TY, Jacobsen SJ, Kottke TE, Frye RL, Weston SA and Roger VL**. Coronary heart disease death and sudden cardiac death: a 20-year population-based study. *Am J Epidemiol* 157: 763-770, 2003.

72. **Greenberg AS and Obin MS**. Obesity and the role of adipose tissue in inflammation and metabolism. *Am J Clin Nutr* 83: 461S-465S, 2006.

73. **Greenwald P**. Cancer prevention clinical trials. *J Clin Oncol* 20: 14S-22S, 2002.

74. **Grimmer KA, Jones D and Williams J**. Prevalence of adolescent injury from recreational exercise: an Australian perspective. *J Adolesc Health* 27: 266-272, 2000.

75. **Guilmette TJ, Motta SI, Shadel WG, Mukand J and Niaura R**. Promoting smoking cessation in the rehabilitation setting. *Am J Phys Med Rehabil* 80: 560-562, 2001.

76. **Hagberg JM, Park JJ and Brown MD**. The role of exercise training in the treatment of hypertension: an update. *Sports Med* 30: 193-206, 2000.

77. **Harada A**. [Exercise for fall prevention and osteoporosis treatment]. *Nippon Rinsho* 64: 1687-1691, 2006.

78. **Harpending H and Cochran G**. Genetic diversity and genetic burden in humans. *Infect Genet Evol* 6: 154-162, 2006.

79. **Haskell WL**. Physical activity and health: need to define the required stimulus. *Am J Cardiol* 55: 4D-9D, 1985.

80. **Henderson NK, White CP and Eisman JA**. The roles of exercise and fall risk reduction in the prevention of osteoporosis. *Endocrinol Metab Clin North Am* 27: 369-387, 1998.

81. **Herrero F, Balmer J, San Juan AF, Foster C, Fleck SJ, Perez M, Canete S, Earnest CP and Lucia A**. Is cardiorespiratory fitness related to quality of life in survivors of breast cancer? *J Strength Cond Res* 20: 535-540, 2006.

82. **Herrero F, Balmer J, San Juan AF, Foster C, Fleck SJ, Perez M, Canete S, Earnest CP and Lucia A**. Is cardiorespiratory fitness related to quality of life in survivors of breast cancer? *J Strength Cond Res* 20: 535-540, 2006.

83. **Hill JO and Wyatt HR**. Role of physical activity in preventing and treating obesity. *J Appl Physiol* 99: 765-770, 2005.

84. **Hindmarsh JJ and Estes EH, Jr**. Falls in older persons. Causes and interventions. *Arch Intern Med* 149: 2217-2222, 1989.

85. **Hohmann E, Wortler K and Imhoff A**. [Osteoarthritis from long-distance running?]. *Sportverletz Sportschaden* 19: 89-93, 2005.

86. **Invitti C**. [Obesity and low-grade systemic inflammation]. *Minerva Endocrinol* 27: 209-214, 2002.

87. **Isomura K, Kono S, Moore MA, Toyomura K, Nagano J, Mizoue T, Mibu R, Tanaka M, Kakeji Y, Maehara Y, Okamura T, Ikejiri K, Futami K, Yasunami Y, Maekawa T, Takenaka K, Ichimiya H and Imaizumi N**. Physical activity and colorectal cancer: the Fukuoka Colorectal Cancer Study. *Cancer Sci* 97: 1099-1104, 2006.

88. **Jemal A, Siegel R, Ward E, Murray T, Xu J, Smigal C and Thun MJ**. Cancer statistics, 2006. *CA Cancer J Clin* 56: 106-130, 2006.

89. **Jemal A, Siegel R, Ward E, Murray T, Xu J and Thun MJ**. Cancer statistics, 2007. *CA Cancer J Clin* 57: 43-66, 2007.

90. **Kay SJ and Fiatarone Singh MA**. The influence of physical activity on abdominal fat: a systematic review of the literature. *Obes Rev* 7: 183-200, 2006.

91. **Kelley GA, Kelley KS and Tran ZV**. Aerobic exercise and lipids and lipoproteins in women: a meta-analysis of randomized controlled trials. *J Womens Health (Larchmt)* 13: 1148-1164, 2004.

92. **Kelley GA, Kelley KS and Tran ZV**. Aerobic exercise and lipids and lipoproteins in women: a meta-analysis of randomized controlled trials. *J Womens Health (Larchmt)* 13: 1148-1164, 2004.

93. **Kelly AS, Wetzsteon RJ, Kaiser DR, Steinberger J, Bank AJ and Dengel DR**. Inflammation, insulin, and endothelial function in overweight children and adolescents: the role of exercise. *J Pediatr* 145: 731-736, 2004.

94. **Kennedy RL, Chokkalingham K and Srinivasan R**. Obesity in the elderly: who should we be treating, and why, and how? *Curr Opin Clin Nutr Metab Care* 7: 3-9, 2004.

95. **Keul J, Lehmann M and Dickhuth HH**. [Hypertension, the heart and physical activity (sports)]. *Z Kardiol* 78 Suppl 7: 199-209, 1989.

96. **Key TJ, Schatzkin A, Willett WC, Allen NE, Spencer EA and Travis RC**. Diet, nutrition and the prevention of cancer. *Public Health Nutr* 7: 187-200, 2004.

97. **Knap B, Buturovic-Ponikvar J, Ponikvar R and Bren AF**. Regular exercise as a part of treatment for patients with end-stage renal disease. *Ther Apher Dial* 9: 211-213, 2005.

98. **Kokkinos PF and Fernhall B**. Physical activity and high density lipoprotein cholesterol levels: what is the relationship? *Sports Med* 28: 307-314, 1999.

99. **Kokkinos PF and Fernhall B**. Physical activity and high density lipoprotein cholesterol levels: what is the relationship? *Sports Med* 28: 307-314, 1999.

100. **Kokkinos PF and Fernhall B**. Physical activity and high density lipoprotein cholesterol levels: what is the relationship? *Sports Med* 28: 307-314, 1999.

101. **Kraus JF, D'Ambrosia RD, Smith EG, Van Meter J, Borhani NO, Franti CE and Lipscomb PR**. An epidemiological study of severe osteoarthritis. *Orthopedics* 1: 37-42, 1978.

102. **Kruk J and Aboul-Enein HY**. Physical activity in the prevention of cancer. *Asian Pac J Cancer Prev* 7: 11-21, 2006.

103. **Kruk J and Aboul-Enein HY**. Physical activity in the prevention of cancer. *Asian Pac J Cancer Prev* 7: 11-21, 2006.

104. **Kruk J and Aboul-Enein HY**. Physical activity in the prevention of cancer. *Asian Pac J Cancer Prev* 7: 11-21, 2006.

105. **Kruk J and Aboul-Enein HY**. Physical activity in the prevention of cancer. *Asian Pac J Cancer Prev* 7: 11-21, 2006.

106. **Kurowski K and Chandran S**. The preparticipation athletic evaluation. *Am Fam Physician* 61: 2683-2688, 2000.

107. **Kurth T, Kase CS, Berger K, Schaeffner ES, Buring JE and Gaziano JM**. Smoking and the risk of hemorrhagic stroke in men. *Stroke* 34: 1151-1155, 2003.

108. **Kurth T, Moore SC, Gaziano JM, Kase CS, Stampfer MJ, Berger K and Buring JE**. Healthy lifestyle and the risk of stroke in women. *Arch Intern Med* 166: 1403-1409, 2006.

109. **Lagra F, Karastergiou K, Delithanasis I, Koutsika E, Katsikas I and Papadopoulou-Zekeridou P**. Obesity and colorectal cancer. *Tech Coloproctol* 8 Suppl 1: s161-s163, 2004.

110. **Larsson SC, Rutegard J, Bergkvist L and Wolk A**. Physical activity, obesity, and risk of colon and rectal cancer in a cohort of Swedish men. *Eur J Cancer* 42: 2590-2597, 2006.

111. **Lazar MA**. How obesity causes diabetes: not a tall tale. *Science* 307: 373-375, 2005.

112. **Lazar MA**. How obesity causes diabetes: not a tall tale. *Science* 307: 373-375, 2005.

113. **Le Pen C, Maurel F, Breart G, Lopes P, Plouin PF, Allicar MP and Roux C**. The long-term effectiveness of preventive strategies for osteoporosis in postmenopausal women: a modeling approach. *Osteoporos Int* 11: 524-532, 2000.

114. **Lee IM, Hennekens CH, Berger K, Buring JE and Manson JE**. Exercise and risk of stroke in male physicians. *Stroke* 30: 1-6, 1999.

115. **Lender D and Sysko SK**. The metabolic syndrome and cardiometabolic risk: scope of the problem and current standard of care. *Pharmacotherapy* 26: 3S-12S, 2006.

116. **Lequesne MG, Dang N and Lane NE**. Sport practice and osteoarthritis of the limbs. *Osteoarthritis Cartilage* 5: 75-86, 1997.

117. **Little J, Logan RF, Hawtin PG, Hardcastle JD and Turner ID**. Colorectal adenomas and energy intake, body size and physical activity: a case-control study of subjects participating in the Nottingham faecal occult blood screening programme. *Br J Cancer* 67: 172-176, 1993.

118. **Lobner K and Fuchtenbusch M**. [Inflammation and diabetes]. *MMW Fortschr Med* 146: 32-36, 2004.

119. **Lyon CJ, Law RE and Hsueh WA**. Minireview: adiposity, inflammation, and atherogenesis. *Endocrinology* 144: 2195-2200, 2003.

120. **Manini TM, Everhart JE, Patel KV, Schoeller DA, Colbert LH, Visser M, Tylavsky F, Bauer DC, Goodpaster BH and Harris TB**. Daily activity energy expenditure and mortality among older adults. *JAMA* 296: 171-179, 2006.

121. **Manini TM, Everhart JE, Patel KV, Schoeller DA, Colbert LH, Visser M, Tylavsky F, Bauer DC, Goodpaster BH and Harris TB**. Daily activity energy expenditure and mortality among older adults. *JAMA* 296: 171-179, 2006.

122. **Manson JE, Rimm EB, Stampfer MJ, Colditz GA, Willett WC, Krolewski AS, Rosner B, Hennekens CH and Speizer FE**. Physical activity and incidence of non-insulin-dependent diabetes mellitus in women. *Lancet* 338: 774-778, 1991.

123. **Marti B**. [Physical activity and blood pressure. An epidemiological brief review of primary preventive effects of physical exercise activities]. *Schweiz Rundsch Med Prax* 81: 473-479, 1992.

124. **Martinsen EW**. [Physical activity for mental health]. *Tidsskr Nor Laegeforen* 120: 3054-3056, 2000.

125. **Martinsen EW**. [Physical activity for mental health]. *Tidsskr Nor Laegeforen* 120: 3054-3056, 2000.

126. **Martinson BC, O'Connor PJ and Pronk NP**. Physical inactivity and short-term all-cause mortality in adults with chronic disease. *Arch Intern Med* 161: 1173-1180, 2001.

127. **Mielenz T, Jackson E, Currey S, DeVellis R and Callahan LF**. Psychometric properties of the Centers for Disease Control and Prevention Health-Related Quality of Life (CDC HRQOL) items in adults with arthritis. *Health Qual Life Outcomes* 4: 66, 2006.

128. **Minino AM, Heron MP and Smith BL**. Deaths: preliminary data for 2004. *Natl Vital Stat Rep* 54: 1-49, 2006.

129. **Moe IT, Hoven H, Hetland EV, Rognmo O and Slordahl SA**. Endothelial function in highly endurance-trained and sedentary, healthy young women. *Vasc Med* 10: 97-102, 2005.

130. **Molitch ME, Fujimoto W, Hamman RF and Knowler WC**. The diabetes prevention program and its global implications. *J Am Soc Nephrol* 14: S103-S107, 2003.

131. **Molitch ME, Fujimoto W, Hamman RF and Knowler WC**. The diabetes prevention program and its global implications. *J Am Soc Nephrol* 14: S103-S107, 2003.

132. **Nakatsuka K, Kawakami H and Miki T**. [Exercise and physical therapy in osteoporosis]. *Nippon Rinsho* 52: 2360-2366, 1994.

133. **Netz Y, Wu MJ, Becker BJ and Tenenbaum G**. Physical activity and psychological well-being in advanced age: a meta-analysis of intervention studies. *Psychol Aging* 20: 272-284, 2005.

134. **Neu I and Schrader A**. [Clinical picture and therapy of cerebral apoplexy]. *Fortschr Med* 95: 904-908, 1977.

135. **Nieman DC**. Exercise immunology: practical applications. *Int J Sports Med* 18 Suppl 1: S91-100, 1997.

136. **Nock MK and Kessler RC**. Prevalence of and risk factors for suicide attempts versus suicide gestures: analysis of the National Comorbidity Survey. *J Abnorm Psychol* 115: 616-623, 2006.

137. **Oczkowski W**. Complexity of the relation between physical activity and stroke: a meta-analysis. *Clin J Sport Med* 15: 399, 2005.

138. **Oja P**. Dose response between total volume of physical activity and health and fitness. *Med Sci Sports Exerc* 33: S428-S437, 2001.

139. **Okura T, Nakata Y and Tanaka K**. Effects of exercise intensity on physical fitness and risk factors for coronary heart disease. *Obes Res* 11: 1131-1139, 2003.

140. **Okura T, Nakata Y and Tanaka K**. Effects of exercise intensity on physical fitness and risk factors for coronary heart disease. *Obes Res* 11: 1131-1139, 2003.

141. **Okura T, Nakata Y and Tanaka K**. Effects of exercise intensity on physical fitness and risk factors for coronary heart disease. *Obes Res* 11: 1131-1139, 2003.

142. **Okura T, Nakata Y and Tanaka K**. Effects of exercise intensity on physical fitness and risk factors for coronary heart disease. *Obes Res* 11: 1131-1139, 2003.

143. **Paganini-Hill A, Atchison KA, Gornbein JA, Nattiv A, Service SK and White SC**. Menstrual and reproductive factors and fracture risk: the Leisure World Cohort Study. *J Womens Health (Larchmt)* 14: 808-819, 2005.

144. **Paluska SA and Schwenk TL**. Physical activity and mental health: current concepts. *Sports Med* 29: 167-180, 2000.

145. **Panush RS and Brown DG**. Exercise and arthritis. *Sports Med* 4: 54-64, 1987.

146. **Panush RS and Lane NE**. Exercise and the musculoskeletal system. *Baillieres Clin Rheumatol* 8: 79-102, 1994.

147. **Paquot N and Tappy L**. [Adipocytokines: link between obesity, type 2 diabetes and atherosclerosis]. *Rev Med Liege* 60: 369-373, 2005.

148. **Paquot N and Tappy L**. [Adipocytokines: link between obesity, type 2 diabetes and atherosclerosis]. *Rev Med Liege* 60: 369-373, 2005.

149. **Paquot N and Tappy L**. [Adipocytokines: link between obesity, type 2 diabetes and atherosclerosis]. *Rev Med Liege* 60: 369-373, 2005.

150. **Paquot N and Tappy L**. [Adipocytokines: link between obesity, type 2 diabetes and atherosclerosis]. *Rev Med Liege* 60: 369-373, 2005.

151. **Penedo FJ and Dahn JR**. Exercise and well-being: a review of mental and physical health benefits associated with physical activity. *Curr Opin Psychiatry* 18: 189-193, 2005.

152. **Penedo FJ and Dahn JR**. Exercise and well-being: a review of mental and physical health benefits associated with physical activity. *Curr Opin Psychiatry* 18: 189-193, 2005.

153. **Penedo FJ and Dahn JR**. Exercise and well-being: a review of mental and physical health benefits associated with physical activity. *Curr Opin Psychiatry* 18: 189-193, 2005.

154. **Pihl E, Zilmer K, Kullisaar T, Kairane C, Magi A and Zilmer M**. Atherogenic inflammatory and oxidative stress markers in relation to overweight values in male former athletes. *Int J Obes (Lond)* 30: 141-146, 2006.

155. **Pihl E, Zilmer K, Kullisaar T, Kairane C, Magi A and Zilmer M**. Atherogenic inflammatory and oxidative stress markers in relation to overweight values in male former athletes. *Int J Obes (Lond)* 30: 141-146, 2006.

156. **Powell KE, Heath GW, Kresnow MJ, Sacks JJ and Branche CM**. Injury rates from walking, gardening, weightlifting, outdoor bicycling, and aerobics. *Med Sci Sports Exerc* 30: 1246-1249, 1998.

157. **Pradhan AD, Skerrett PJ and Manson JE**. Obesity, diabetes, and coronary risk in women. *J Cardiovasc Risk* 9: 323-330, 2002.

158. **Puggaard L**. Effects of training on functional performance in 65, 75 and 85 year-old women: experiences deriving from community based studies in Odense, Denmark. *Scand J Med Sci Sports* 13: 70-76, 2003.

159. **Puggaard L**. Effects of training on functional performance in 65, 75 and 85 year-old women: experiences deriving from community based studies in Odense, Denmark. *Scand J Med Sci Sports* 13: 70-76, 2003.

160. **Puggaard L**. Effects of training on functional performance in 65, 75 and 85 year-old women: experiences deriving from community based studies in Odense, Denmark. *Scand J Med Sci Sports* 13: 70-76, 2003.

161. **Quadrilatero J and Hoffman-Goetz L**. Physical activity and colon cancer. A systematic review of potential mechanisms. *J Sports Med Phys Fitness* 43: 121-138, 2003.

162. **Quadrilatero J and Hoffman-Goetz L**. Physical activity and colon cancer. A systematic review of potential mechanisms. *J Sports Med Phys Fitness* 43: 121-138, 2003.

163. **Quadrilatero J and Hoffman-Goetz L**. Physical activity and colon cancer. A systematic review of potential mechanisms. *J Sports Med Phys Fitness* 43: 121-138, 2003.

164. **Quist M, Rorth M, Zacho M, Andersen C, Moeller T, Midtgaard J and Adamsen L**. High-intensity resistance and cardiovascular training improve physical capacity in cancer patients undergoing chemotherapy. *Scand J Med Sci Sports* 16: 349-357, 2006.

165. **Reaven G**. Syndrome X. *Curr Treat Options Cardiovasc Med* 3: 323-332, 2001.

166. **Richardson CR, Kriska AM, Lantz PM and Hayward RA**. Physical activity and mortality across cardiovascular disease risk groups. *Med Sci Sports Exerc* 36: 1923-1929, 2004.

167. **Richardson CR, Kriska AM, Lantz PM and Hayward RA**. Physical activity and mortality across cardiovascular disease risk groups. *Med Sci Sports Exerc* 36: 1923-1929, 2004.

168. **Rognmo O, Hetland E, Helgerud J, Hoff J and Slordahl SA**. High intensity aerobic interval exercise is superior to moderate intensity exercise for increasing aerobic capacity in patients with coronary artery disease. *Eur J Cardiovasc Prev Rehabil* 11: 216-222, 2004.

169. **Rognmo O, Hetland E, Helgerud J, Hoff J and Slordahl SA**. High intensity aerobic interval exercise is superior to moderate intensity exercise for increasing aerobic capacity in patients with coronary artery disease. *Eur J Cardiovasc Prev Rehabil* 11: 216-222, 2004.

170. **Rognmo O, Hetland E, Helgerud J, Hoff J and Slordahl SA**. High intensity aerobic interval exercise is superior to moderate intensity exercise for increasing aerobic capacity in patients with coronary artery disease. *Eur J Cardiovasc Prev Rehabil* 11: 216-222, 2004.

171. **Roos H**. [Increased risk of knee and hip arthrosis among elite athletes. Lower level exercise and sports seem to be "harmless"]. *Lakartidningen* 95: 4606-4610, 1998.

172. **Ross R and Janssen I**. Physical activity, total and regional obesity: dose-response considerations. *Med Sci Sports Exerc* 33: S521-S527, 2001.

173. **Saakslahti A, Numminen P, Varstala V, Helenius H, Tammi A, Viikari J and Valimaki I**. Physical activity as a preventive measure for coronary heart disease risk factors in early childhood. *Scand J Med Sci Sports* 14: 143-149, 2004.

174. **Sagiv M and Goldbourt U**. Influence of physical work on high density lipoprotein cholesterol: implications for the

risk of coronary heart disease. *Int J Sports Med* 15: 261-266, 1994.

175. **Saltin B and Pilegaard H**. [Metabolic fitness: physical activity and health]. *Ugeskr Laeger* 164: 2156-2162, 2002.

176. **Saltin B and Pilegaard H**. [Metabolic fitness: physical activity and health]. *Ugeskr Laeger* 164: 2156-2162, 2002.

177. **Samitz G**. [Physical activity for decreasing cardiovascular mortality and total mortality. A public health perspective]. *Wien Klin Wochenschr* 110: 589-596, 1998.

178. **Samitz G**. [Physical activity for decreasing cardiovascular mortality and total mortality. A public health perspective]. *Wien Klin Wochenschr* 110: 589-596, 1998.

179. **Sawada S, Muto T and Tanaka H**. [Epidemiologic study on physical activity and type 2 diabetes]. *Nippon Rinsho* 58 Suppl: 379-384, 2000.

180. **Sawada S, Muto T and Tanaka H**. [Epidemiologic study on physical activity and type 2 diabetes]. *Nippon Rinsho* 58 Suppl: 379-384, 2000.

181. **Schwarzenberg SJ and Sinaiko AR.** Obesity and inflammation in children. *Paediatr Respir Rev* 7: 239-246, 2006.

182. **Scrutinio D, Bellotto F, Lagioia R and Passantino A**. Physical activity for coronary heart disease: cardioprotective mechanisms and effects on prognosis. *Monaldi Arch Chest Dis* 64: 77-87, 2005.

183. **Shaibi GQ, Cruz ML, Ball GD, Weigensberg MJ, Salem GJ, Crespo NC and Goran MI**. Effects of resistance training on insulin sensitivity in overweight Latino adolescent males. *Med Sci Sports Exerc* 38: 1208-1215, 2006.

184. **Shephard RJ**. Absolute versus relative intensity of physical activity in a dose-response context. *Med Sci Sports Exerc* 33: S400-S418, 2001.

185. **Shephard RJ**. Absolute versus relative intensity of physical activity in a dose-response context. *Med Sci Sports Exerc* 33: S400-S418, 2001.

186. **Shephard RJ**. Absolute versus relative intensity of physical activity in a dose-response context. *Med Sci Sports Exerc* 33: S400-S418, 2001.

187. **Slattery ML**. Physical activity and colorectal cancer. *Sports Med* 34: 239-252, 2004.

188. **Slattery ML**, Edwards S, Curtin K, Ma K, Edwards R, Holubkov R and Schaffer D. Physical activity and colorectal cancer. *Am J Epidemiol* 158: 214-224, 2003.

189. **Slentz CA, Duscha BD, Johnson JL, Ketchum K, Aiken LB, Samsa GP, Houmard JA, Bales CW and Kraus WE**. Effects of the amount of exercise on body weight, body composition, and measures of central obesity: STRRIDE--a randomized controlled study. *Arch Intern Med* 164: 31-39, 2004.

190. **Slentz CA, Duscha BD, Johnson JL, Ketchum K, Aiken LB, Samsa GP, Houmard JA, Bales CW and Kraus WE**. Effects of the amount of exercise on body weight, body composition, and measures of central obesity: STRRIDE--a randomized controlled study. *Arch Intern Med* 164: 31-39, 2004.

191. **Smith JK, Dykes R, Douglas JE, Krishnaswamy G and Berk S**. Long-term exercise and atherogenic activity of blood mononuclear cells in persons at risk of developing ischemic heart disease. *JAMA* 281: 1722-1727, 1999.

192. **Sorensen JB, Kragstrup J, Kjaer K and Puggaard L**. Exercise on Prescription: Trial protocol and evaluation of outcomes. *BMC Health Serv Res* 7: 36, 2007.

193. **Sorensen JB, Kragstrup J, Kjaer K and Puggaard L**. Exercise on Prescription: Trial protocol and evaluation of outcomes. *BMC Health Serv Res* 7: 36, 2007.

194. **Steindorf K, Tobiasz-Adamczyk B, Popiela T, Jedrychowski W, Penar A, Matyja A and Wahrendorf J**. Combined risk assessment of physical activity and dietary habits on the development of colorectal cancer. A hospital-based case-control study in Poland. *Eur J Cancer Prev* 9: 309-316, 2000.

195. **Stephens T**. Physical activity and mental health in the United States and Canada: evidence from four population surveys. *Prev Med* 17: 35-47, 1988.

196. **Stewart KJ, Bacher AC, Turner K, Lim JG, Hees PS, Shapiro EP, Tayback M and Ouyang P**. Exercise and risk factors associated with metabolic syndrome in older adults. *Am J Prev Med* 28: 9-18, 2005.

197. **Stewart KJ, Bacher AC, Turner K, Lim JG, Hees PS, Shapiro EP, Tayback M and Ouyang P**. Exercise and risk factors associated with metabolic syndrome in older adults. *Am J Prev Med* 28: 9-18, 2005.

198. **Stewart KJ, Bacher AC, Turner K, Lim JG, Hees PS, Shapiro EP, Tayback M and Ouyang P**. Exercise and risk factors associated with metabolic syndrome in older adults. *Am J Prev Med* 28: 9-18, 2005.

199. **Strock GA, Cottrell ER, Abang AE, Buschbacher RM and Hannon TS**. Childhood obesity: a simple equation with complex variables. *J Long Term Eff Med Implants* 15: 15-32, 2005.

200. **Stulberg SD**. Sports injuries and arthritis. *Compr Ther* 6: 8-11, 1980.

201. **Sundberg CJ and Jansson E**. [Reduced morbidity and the risk of premature death. Regular physical exercise is beneficial for health at all ages]. *Lakartidningen* 95: 4062-4067, 1998.

202. **Suominen H**. Muscle training for bone strength. *Aging Clin Exp Res* 18: 85-93, 2006.

203. **Sutton AJ, Muir KR, Mockett S and Fentem P**. A case-control study to investigate the relation between low and moderate levels of physical activity and osteoarthritis of the knee using data collected as part of the Allied Dunbar National Fitness Survey. *Ann Rheum Dis* 60: 756-764, 2001.

204. **Tamakoshi K, Tokudome S, Kuriki K, Takekuma K and Toyoshima H**. [Epidemiology and primary prevention

of colorectal cancer]. *Gan To Kagaku Ryoho* 28: 146-150, 2001.

205. **Tanasescu M, Leitzmann MF, Rimm EB and Hu FB**. Physical activity in relation to cardiovascular disease and total mortality among men with type 2 diabetes. *Circulation* 107: 2435-2439, 2003.

206. **Teixeira-Salmela LF, Santiago L, Lima RC, Lana DM, Camargos FF and Cassiano JG**. Functional performance and quality of life related to training and detraining of community-dwelling elderly. *Disabil Rehabil* 27: 1007-1012, 2005.

207. **Thiele H, Pohlink C and Schuler G**. [Hypertension and exercise. Sports methods for the hypertensive patient]. *Herz* 29: 401-405, 2004.

208. **Thiele H, Pohlink C and Schuler G**. [Hypertension and exercise. Sports methods for the hypertensive patient]. *Herz* 29: 401-405, 2004.

209. **Thune I and Furberg AS**. Physical activity and cancer risk: dose-response and cancer, all sites and site-specific. *Med Sci Sports Exerc* 33: S530-S550, 2001.

210. **Thune I and Furberg AS**. Physical activity and cancer risk: dose-response and cancer, all sites and site-specific. *Med Sci Sports Exerc* 33: S530-S550, 2001.

211. **Thune I and Furberg AS**. Physical activity and cancer risk: dose-response and cancer, all sites and site-specific. *Med Sci Sports Exerc* 33: S530-S550, 2001.

212. **Tsai JC, Yang HY, Wang WH, Hsieh MH, Chen PT, Kao CC, Kao PF, Wang CH and Chan P**. The beneficial effect of regular endurance exercise training on blood pressure and quality of life in patients with hypertension. *Clin Exp Hypertens* 26: 255-265, 2004.

213. **Tsai JC, Yang HY, Wang WH, Hsieh MH, Chen PT, Kao CC, Kao PF, Wang CH and Chan P**. The beneficial effect of regular endurance exercise training on blood pressure and quality of life in patients with hypertension. *Clin Exp Hypertens* 26: 255-265, 2004.

214. **Tsai JC, Yang HY, Wang WH, Hsieh MH, Chen PT, Kao CC, Kao PF, Wang CH and Chan P**. The beneficial effect of regular endurance exercise training on blood pressure and quality of life in patients with hypertension. *Clin Exp Hypertens* 26: 255-265, 2004.

215. **Tuomainen P, Peuhkurinen K, Kettunen R and Rauramaa R**. Regular physical exercise, heart rate variability and turbulence in a 6-year randomized controlled trial in middle-aged men: the DNASCO study. *Life Sci* 77: 2723-2734, 2005.

216. **Vitetta L and Sali A**. Colorectal cancer and. *Aust Fam Physician* 35: 339, 2006.

217. **Vogel RA**. Coronary risk factors, endothelial function, and atherosclerosis: a review. *Clin Cardiol* 20: 426-432, 1997.

218. **Vsetulova E and Bunc V**. [Effect of body composition on physical fitness and functional capacity in obese women]. *Cas Lek Cesk* 143: 756-760, 2004.

219. **Wannamethee SG and Shaper AG**. Physical activity in the prevention of cardiovascular disease: an epidemiological perspective. *Sports Med* 31: 101-114, 2001.

220. **Wannamethee SG and Shaper AG**. Physical activity in the prevention of cardiovascular disease: an epidemiological perspective. *Sports Med* 31: 101-114, 2001.

221. **Watkins LO**. Epidemiology and burden of cardiovascular disease. *Clin Cardiol* 27: III2-III6, 2004.

222. **Watkins LO**. Epidemiology and burden of cardiovascular disease. *Clin Cardiol* 27: III2-III6, 2004.

223. **Watkins LO**. Epidemiology and burden of cardiovascular disease. *Clin Cardiol* 27: III2-III6, 2004.

224. **Watkins LO**. Epidemiology and burden of cardiovascular disease. *Clin Cardiol* 27: III2-III6, 2004.

225. **Wei M, Schwertner HA and Blair SN**. The association between physical activity, physical fitness, and type 2 diabetes mellitus. *Compr Ther* 26: 176-182, 2000.

226. **Westby MD, Wade JP, Rangno KK and Berkowitz J**. A randomized controlled trial to evaluate the effectiveness of an exercise program in women with rheumatoid arthritis taking low dose prednisone. *J Rheumatol* 27: 1674-1680, 2000.

227. **White SC, Atchison KA, Gornbein JA, Nattiv A, Paganini-Hill A and Service SK**. Risk factors for fractures in older men and women: The Leisure World Cohort Study. *Gend Med* 3: 110-123, 2006.

228. **White SC, Atchison KA, Gornbein JA, Nattiv A, Paganini-Hill A and Service SK**. Risk factors for fractures in older men and women: The Leisure World Cohort Study. *Gend Med* 3: 110-123, 2006.

229. **Woodfin BA**. Orthopaedic sports medicine and the adult male athlete: a review of common exercise-related injuries. *J Med Assoc Ga* 87: 17-21, 1998.

230. **Wylie-Rosett J, Mossavar-Rahmani Y and Gans K**. Recent dietary guidelines to prevent and treat cardiovascular disease, diabetes, and obesity. *Heart Dis* 4: 220-230, 2002.

231. **Wyndham CH**. The role of physical activity in the prevention of ischaemic heart disease. A review. *S Afr Med J* 56: 7-13, 1979.

232. **Xavier Pi-Sunyer F**. The relation of adipose tissue to cardiometabolic risk. *Clin Cornerstone* 8 Suppl 4: S14-S23, 2006.

233. **Yeater RA, Ullrich IH, Maxwell LP and Goetsch VL**. Coronary risk factors in type II diabetes: response to low-intensity aerobic exercise. *W V Med J* 86: 287-290, 1990.

Chapter 13

Pre-Exercise Screening & Test Considerations

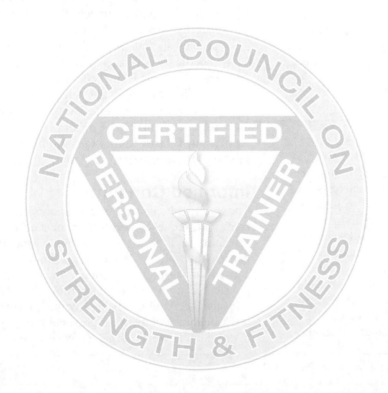

In This Chapter

Informed Consent

Par-Q

Health Status
Questionnaire

Behavior Questionnaire

Resting Battery of
Physical Tests

Assessing Heart Rate

Assessing Blood
Pressure

Physical Exam and
Lipid Screening

Medical Clearance Form

Pre-Exercise Screening

There is a significant quantity of evidence that encourages daily physical activity as a vital part to healthy aging. Data suggests that the absence of routine exercise is far more dangerous than the inherent risks of participating in physical activity (4; 13; 14). Although this may be true, cautious steps can and should be taken by personal trainers when encouraging exercise participation. Pre-exercise health screening is an important part of the health management services a personal trainer should provide. The primary purpose for screening a client before activity participation is to identify possible factors that may increase the risk of injury when performing exercise or a particular activity. Factors may include physical limitations, medical conditions, or behaviors that may put the client at risk for a negative outcome from exercise testing or physical activity participation. Failure to appropriately screen a client that leads to an untoward event can place significant liability on the personal trainer (15). Health screening is a necessary part of fulfilling the duty of care owed to a client paying for professional fitness services.

Exercise screening provides additional benefits beyond simply attempting to reduce risks for injury associated with participation. Secondary purposes for screening clients before activity are listed in the table below.

Benefits of Client Screening

1. Educating client about relative health risks associated with their lifestyle, behaviors, and history.

2. Identifying current health status compared to recommended ranges.

3. Providing data that will be used to create a needs analysis as the basis for the exercise prescription.

4. Establishing starting points and predictions of performance.

5. Identifying particular interests, aptitudes, or possible limitations.

Screening for exercise participation provides valuable information for creating an exercise prescription, as well as identifying client aptitude and interests in different types of activities. It is important to identify the data that is most relevant to the purpose and goal of the screening process so that the prescribed exercise program starts with a high likelihood for success and the client is able to participate with very low inherent risk. Exercise screening should not become an obstacle to participation nor be an unnecessary burden to initiating an exercise program. For these reasons, the screening protocols and depth of evaluation should

reflect the individual. In the recent past, criticisms have been made about requiring unnecessary testing and evaluation for clearance in an unrestricted exercise program (23; 26). Some stringent screening protocols required men ($\geq$45 years) and women ($\geq$55 years) to undergo cardiac stress tests, cardiopulmonary tests, and the completion of blood chemistry tests before being cleared for participation. The primary goal of this type of evaluation is to identify those individuals at risk of a cardiac event (i.e. myocardial infarct) during exercise participation. Although this type of screening generates a thorough evaluation, the requirements were viewed as excessive and costly for participating in activities aimed at improving health (6; 11).

Pre-exercise screening was originally designed to determine if a person could participate in vigorous exercise without risk of serious adverse effects. The reality is that most individuals who engage in activity do so at a moderate level and would not even be capable of vigorous activity until they were acclimated to the intensity over an extended period of time. In addition, most instruments used for the screening have significant limitations and are cost prohibitive for the majority of fitness facilities. Furthermore, cardiovascular events are fairly rare and unpredictable and cardiac stress tests and self-reported screening documents only effectively identify a small subset of individuals at risk (5; 8; 22; 23; 29). Screening should be practical, viable across multiple population segments, and effective at identifying those at risk.

The goals of screening are to help get people to safely participate in activity and identify those individuals who truly need appropriate medical evaluation and clearance. Personal trainers should identify health problems and risks for potential problems, and tailor the exercise based on the specific results and findings. Several documents can be used in conjunction with industry guidelines to help the screening process become more efficient and effective. Some common forms include: **Informed Consent, ParQ, Health Risk Appraisal, Health Status Questionnaire** and **Medical History Questionnaire**.

Informed Consent

The informed consent is not necessarily a screening form but requests permission or consent for health screening, fitness evaluations, and/or exercise participation. It is defined as a knowing and willful consent to testing procedures or to participation in physical activity after being properly advised of the relevant facts and the risks involved. Informed consent is a valuable document for personal training services, as it provides powerful legal defense against claims that suggest a client was not informed about the protocols and the inherent risks associated with the activities they were asked to engage in. By law, clients who are exposed to, or may be subject to, possible physical or psychological injury must give informed consent prior to participation in the described activities (7; 18; 25).

For the document to provide maximal value, it must be clearly explained and contain specific details related to the activities employed by the trainer and the associated risks. The informed consent should contain information that demonstrates the risks, benefits, rationale, and expectations of the program components. For optimal performance during litigation, the document should be administered and explained in easily understood terms, so the client fully understands the written language before signing it. Initials by each paragraph or section are useful in identifying that the client was properly informed of the information contained in the document. Additionally, in order to fulfill full disclosure and informed consent requirements, the reading level of the consent form must be comprehensible by the client, so they fully understand the described conditions, taking into account important differences based on the educational level of the individuals being serviced (10; 18).

The informed consent can serve, in part, as a waiver of liability when implemented properly using the appropriate language and signed in the presence of a witness. Because of its legal implications, it is important to use a document that has been reviewed and approved by a lawyer to ensure the document serves its intended role. It is important to realize that a signed informed consent does not prevent the client from having the right to take legal action. It does, however, provide legal defensibility when the procedures in question have been correctly performed by a qualified practitioner. The informed consent should be the first document completed and added to a client's file. It serves the permission to move ahead with the personal training services, as it suggests the client is privy to the described procedures and expected outcomes. Once completed, the screening protocols can be initiated.

Par-Q

Par-Q stands for physical activity readiness questionnaire. It was designed to be used with the Canadian Fitness Testing program, serving as an assessment of self-reported health information. Its primary objective is to identify those individuals at risk for a cardiac event. The Par-Q includes seven questions which serve as red flag indicators designed to identify individuals who require medical clearance before participating in any physical testing or starting an exercise program. Essentially, a "yes" answer to any of the questions dictates medical clearance requirements. This basic screening instrument is practical for large numbers of individuals and requires little time or expertise to implement.

Key Terms

Informed Consent – Consent from an exercise participant, given prior to engaging in any physical activity, that indicates they are fully aware of the risks, benefits, rationale, and expectations of the program's components.

Par-Q – The physical activity readiness questionnaire is a self-reported assessment of health information consisting of seven questions that serve as red flag indicators for individuals ages 15-69 who may require medical clearance before participating in any physical testing or exercise program.

Health Risk Appraisal - A health risk appraisal is a health promotional tool, consisting of a questionnaire, a formula for estimating health risks, an advice database, and a means to generate reports.

Medical History Questionnaire – A form that an individual should complete, prior to engaging in any activity, in order to answer any significant questions about their medical history that may restrict certain activities.

Health Status Questionnaire- A structured self-report questionnaire that generates subscale scores for physical functioning, role limitations due to physical problems, bodily pain, general health perceptions, vitality, social functioning, role-limitations due to emotional problems, and mental health.

Components of Informed Consent

Background and purpose

Assumed risks of participation

Reasonably expected benefits

Reasonable explanation of procedures

Normal physiological expectations

Opportunity for inquiry

Right of refusal

Right of confidentiality

INFORMED CONSENT

Purpose and Explanation of Service

I understand that the purpose of the exercise program is to develop and maintain cardiorespiratory fitness, body composition, flexibility, muscular strength and endurance. A specific exercise plan will be given to me, based on my needs and abilities. All exercise prescription components will comply with proper exercise program protocols. The programs include, but are not limited to aerobic exercise, flexibility training, and strength training. All programs are designed to place a gradually increasing workload on the body in order to improve overall fitness.

Risks

I understand, and have been informed, that there exists the possibility of adverse changes when engaging in a physical activity program. I have been informed that these changes could include abnormal blood pressure, fainting, disorders of heart rhythm, stroke and very rare instances of heart attack or even death. I have been told that every effort will be made to minimize these occurrences by proper screening and by precautions and observations taken during the exercise session. I understand that there is a risk of injury, heart attack, or even death as a result of my participation in an exercise program, but knowing those risks, it is my desire to partake in the recommended activities.

Benefits

I understand that participation in an exercise program has many health related benefits. These may include improvements in body composition, range of motion, musculoskeletal strength and endurance, and cardiorespiratory efficiency. Furthermore, regular exercise can improve blood pressure and lipid profile, metabolic function, and decrease the risk of cardiovascular disease.

Physiological Experience

I have been informed that during my participation in the exercise program I will be asked to complete physical activities that may elicit physiological responses/symptoms that include, but are not limited to, the following: elevated heart rate, elevated blood pressure, sweating, fatigue, increased respiration, muscle soreness, cramping, and nausea.

Confidentiality and Use of Information

I have been informed that the information obtained in this exercise program will be treated as privileged and confidential and will consequently not be released or revealed to any person without my express written consent. Any other information obtained, however, will be used only by the program staff to evaluate my exercise status as needed.

Inquiries and Freedom of Consent

I have been given an opportunity to ask questions about the exercise program. I further understand that there are also other remote health risks. Despite the fact that a complete accounting of all these remote risks has not been provided to me, I still desire to proceed with the exercise program. I acknowledge that I have read this document in its entirety or that it has been read to me if I was unable to read. I consent to the rendition of all services and procedures as explained herein by all program personnel.

_____

Date

_____

Participant's Signature

_____

Witness's Signature

_____

Trainer's signature

It is limited to evaluating risk for low to moderate exercise but should not be used as clearance for vigorous activities.

For the personal trainer, the Par-Q offers little value beyond medical referral identification and basic clearance for low to moderate client activity. Investigative instruments including the Health Status Questionnaire, Health Risk Appraisal, and Medical History Questionnaire can provide more significant data identifying individuals at risk of injury from a variety of possible events. Additionally, the screening tools help identify those clients requiring medical clearance and are useful for specific program participation and exercise decision making. The assessment of a person's overall health profile provides coronary risk analysis, disease risk classification, lifestyle and health evaluation, and general physical activity and behavior risk stratification. Additionally, the implementation process can help facilitate improved client-trainer rapport and help the client realize important health markers, while becoming more educated about his or her current condition.

Health Status Questionnaire

Traditionally, health status questionnaires are split into sections which include the following: general client information, current medical information, medical history, self-reported health and physical fitness status, and self-reported psychological considerations. Numerous questionnaires are available for pre-exercise screening, which vary by format, number of questions, degree of thoroughness, and the actual complexity level of each question.

Taking the time to orally administer the questionnaire is very effective for collecting the data. It helps initiate trust and confidence in the client-trainer relationship, enables the use of probing questions to expand on the questionnaire item and helps ensure that the client understands the question so that the response represents the best and most complete answer. Likewise, administering the questionnaires verbally, provides the opportunity for client education as the trainer can explain the relevance of the question's subject matter and explain why the information is valuable. Trainers should pay particular attention to key risk areas, including family history of cardiovascular and metabolic disease, smoking history, sedentary lifestyle, **obesity**, high blood pressure, undesirable blood lipid profiles, and impaired glucose tolerance. These areas are most likely associated with heightened disease risk, health complications, and risk of cardiovascular events.

~Quick Insight~

Pre-activity screening.
Although a complete screening assessment employs fitness testing and ECG evaluations, a pre-activity screen uses non-activity protocols. Personal trainers should employ pre-activity screening instruments before performing exercise testing. Failure to screen individuals prior to physical activity participation and testing may be viewed as negligent behavior, depending on the population being tested. Utilizing a pre-activity screen is important for program data decision making, better familiarizing yourself with the client, and making prudent decisions in their lifestyle behavior management.

Good health screening evaluations have a specific section for identifying diagnosed diseases, such as hypertension or diabetes, that warrant medical clearance, as well as a separate section for symptoms that may represent an undiagnosed disease that requires a medical evaluation prior to exercise participation. Examples of symptoms that are warning signs include any chronic pain, dizziness or breathlessness, **heart palpitations**, **edema**, unusual fatigue, frequent thirst, and/or frequent urination. It is important to understand that it is not the role of the personal trainer to diagnose disease within a client but only to identify those clients who require either medical referral or clearance prior to an exercise program initiation.

Behavior Questionnaire

In a comprehensive screening, the health status questionnaire should be followed by a behavior questionnaire. The behavior questionnaire provides details about routine lifestyle habits, common behavior trends, and dietary practices. It can also help identify personal preferences and learned behavior traits. The behavior questionnaire can be very useful for several reasons, including:

1. Identifying obstacles to the program goals and needed improvements in health status.

2. Identifying factors correlating to current health status.

3. Providing the opportunity to educate clients of how their behaviors impact their health.

4. Identifying appropriate behavior management strategies.

Unhealthy behaviors can have a significant impact on a person's physical and mental condition. If unaccounted for, these behaviors can cause barriers to program goal

HEALTH STATUS QUESTIONNAIRE

SECTION ONE - GENERAL INFORMATION

1. Date_____

2. Name_____

3. Mailing Address_____   Phone (H)_____

   _____   Phone (W)_____

   Email   _____

4. *EI* Personal Physician_____   Phone_____

       Physician Address_____   Fax_____

       _____

5. *EI* Person to contact in case of emergency_____   Phone_____

6. Gender (circle one):   Female   Male *RF*

7. *RF* Date of birth_____/_____/_____

8. Height _____   Weight _____

9. Number of hours worked per week: Less than 20   20-40   41-60   over 60

10. *SLA* More than 25% of the time at your job is spent (circle all that apply)

       Sitting at desk   Lifting loads   Standing   Walking   Driving

SECTION TWO - CURRENT MEDICAL INFORMATION

11. Date of last medical physical exam:_____

12. Circle all medicine taken or prescribed in last 6 months:

Blood thinner *MC*	Epilepsy medication *SEP*	Nitroglycerin *MC*
Diabetic *MC*	Heart rhythm medication *MC*	Other_____
Digitalis *MC*	High blood pressure medication *MC*	
Diuretic *MC*	Insulin *MC*	

13. Please list any orthopedic conditions. Include any injuries in the last six months.

_____

14. Any of the following health symptoms that occur frequently (two or more times/month) requires medical attention. Please check any that apply.

a. ___ Cough up blood *MC*		g. ___ Swollen joints *MC*
b. ___ Abdominal pain *MC*		h. ___ Feel faint *MC*
c. ___ Low-back pain *MC*		i. ___ Dizziness *MC*
d. ___ Leg pain *MC*		j. ___ Breathlessness with slight exertion *MC*
e. ___ Arm or shoulder pain *MC*		k. ___ Palpitation or fast heart beat *MC*
f. ___ Chest pain *RF MC*		l. ___ Unusual fatigue with normal activity *MC*

Other_____

SECTION THREE - MEDICAL HISTORY

15. Please circle any of the following for which you have been diagnosed or treated by a physician or health professional:

Alcoholism *SEP*	Diabetes *SEP*	Kidney problem *MC*
Anemia, sickle cell *SEP*	Emphysema *SEP*	Mental illness *SEP*
Anemia, other *SEP*	Epilepsy *SEP*	Neck strain *SLA*
Asthma *SEP*	Eye problems *SLA*	Obesity *RF*
Back strain *SLA*	Gout *SLA*	Phlebitis *MC*
Bleeding trait *SEP*	Hearing loss *SLA*	Rheumatoid arthritis *SLA*
Bronchitis, chronic *SEP*	Heart problems *MC*	Stress *RF*
Stroke *MC*	Cancer *SEP*	High blood pressure *MC*
Thyroid problem *SEP*	Cirrhosis *MC*	HIV *SEP*
Ulcer *SEP*	Concussion *MC*	Hypoglycemia *SEP*
Congenital defect *SEP*	Hyperlipidemia *RF*	Other_____

16. Circle any operations that you have had:

Back *SLA*   Heart *MC*   Kidney *SLA*   Eyes *SLA*   Joint *SLA*   Neck *SLA*

Ears *SLA*   Hernia *SLA*   Lung *SLA*   Other_____

17. *RF* Circle any who died of heart attack before age 55:

Grandfather   Father   Brother

18. *RF* Circle any who died of heart attack before age 65:

Grandmother   Mother   Sister

SECTION FOUR - HEALTH-RELATED BEHAVIORS

19. Have you ever smoked?   Yes   No

20. *RF* Do you now smoke?   Yes   No

21. *RF* If you are a smoker, indicate the number smoked per day:

Cigarettes: 40 or more   20-39   10-19   1-9

Cigars or pipes only: 5 or more or any inhaled less than 5

22. *RF* Do you exercise regularly?   Yes   No

23. Last physical fitness test:_____

How many days a week do you accumulate 30 minutes of moderate activity?

0   1   2   3   4   5   6   7   days per week

24. How many days per week do you normally spend engaging in at least 20 minutes in vigorous exercise?

0   1   2   3   4   5   6   7   days per week

What activities do you engage in a least 1x per week?

_____

25. Weight now:_____   One year ago:_____   Age 21:_____

SECTION FIVE - HEALTH-RELATED ATTITUDES

26. These are traits that have been associated with CAD-prone behavior. Circle the number that corresponds to how you feel toward the following statement:

I am an impatient, time-conscious, hard-driving individual.

Circle the number that best describes how you feel:

6= Strongly agree   3= Slightly disagree
5= Moderately agree   2= Moderately disagree
4= Slightly agree   1= Strongly disagree

27. How often do you experience "negative" stress from each of the following:

	Always	Usually	Frequently	Rarely	Never
Work:	_____	_____	_____	_____	_____
Home or family:	_____	_____	_____	_____	_____
Financial pressure:	_____	_____	_____	_____	_____
Social pressure:	_____	_____	_____	_____	_____
Personal health	_____	_____	_____	_____	_____

28. List everything not included on this questionnaire that may cause you problems in a fitness test or fitness program:

_____

_____

_____

_____

Action Codes

EI= Emergency Information- must be readily available

MC= Medical Clearance needed-do not allow exercise without physician's permission.

SEP= Special Emergency Procedures needed- do not let participant exercise alone; make sure the person's exercise partner knows what to do in case of an emergency

RF= Risk Factor of CHD (educational materials and workshops needed).

SLA= Special or Limited Activities may be needed- you may need to include or exclude specific exercises.

Other (not marked)= Personal information that may be helpful for files or research.

attainment, even with a properly constructed and implemented exercise prescription. Personal trainers usually have 2-3 hours per week of control over the client's environment and behaviors. The other 165 hours are at the client's discretion. If the client makes poor eating and drinking decisions, engages in sedentary living, or places him or herself in stress related environments, much of the work accomplished during the personal training sessions may be squandered. This is most relevant if the behaviors increase risk of exacerbating a current health condition. Individuals at risk for diabetes, **hypertension**, **dyslipidemia**, **CAD**, and obesity must comply with the recommendations for managing their condition. Of particular concern is unhealthy eating, smoking, and sedentary living, as these are clear markers for increased disease risk.

Compiling the Data

The health behavior questionnaire should complement the Health Status Questionnaire to correlate findings. For instance, if a client has been diagnosed with hypertension and their diet consists of high salt or fatty foods, it becomes evident that their lifestyle habits promote the disease, rather than work to prevent it. Additionally, if a client's weight measurements over time indicate a propensity for creeping obesity, and their normal lifestyle habits show a preference for nonphysical activities, it should be identified and explained that they are creating barriers to improved health and increasing their susceptibility to additional weight gain. Most behavior questionnaires provide supportive causes for the problems found on the HSQ. Rarely will someone live a very healthy lifestyle and suffer the consequences of Western culture diseases.

Upon review of the HSQ and behavior questionnaire, personal trainers should attempt to identify and list all the health problems and risks associated with the client. Once a list has been constructed, it should be ranked by order of health risk significance. Immediate and primary risks should be listed first. These risks can cause direct damage to a person's health and include smoking, physical inactivity, obesity, CVD, **metabolic disease**, and other major health problems like **asthma**, leg pain, chronic low back pain, and orthopedic injuries. The next group of risks should include those factors that worsen these conditions or increase the potential adverse effects of current conditions. Some examples are high fat diet, unmanaged stress, excessive alcohol consumption, and high sugar intake. These risks and any important information should be evaluated for relevance and used to correlate related factors. This model will allow for a more complete strategy to address the conditions. Jointly employed, the two forms can provide relevant

details for effective risk stratification and program decision making.

Resting Battery of Physical Tests

To further enhance the screening process, personal trainers should implement a resting battery of physical testing. These tests do not require physical activity and therefore can be used before participation status has been determined. The purpose of the resting battery is to use physical measures that predict potential risk. These measures include resting heart rate and blood pressure, body composition assessment, height and weight measures, waist girth, and BMI. In addition, it may be worthwhile to have a client's blood chemistry evaluated to aid in the needs analysis and subsequent program decision-making process. This collection of data provides physical information about the body's current condition at rest.

Key Terms

Obesity – An abnormal accumulation of body fat, usually 20% or more over an individual's ideal body weight.

Heart palpitations – A sensation in which a person is aware of an irregular, hard, or rapid heartbeat.

Edema – An excessive accumulation of fluid in tissue spaces or a body cavity.

Hypertension – Arterial disease in which high blood pressure is the primary symptom.

Dyslipedemia – An abnormality in the amount of lipids in the blood.

Coronary Artery Disease (CAD) – A narrowing or blockage of the arteries and vessels that provide oxygen and nutrients to the heart.

Metabolic Disease – Any disorder that involves an alteration in the normal metabolism of carbohydrates, lipids, proteins, water, and nucleic acids evidenced by various syndromes and diseases, such as hypertension, hyperlipidemia, obesity, and diabetes.

Asthma – A chronic respiratory disease, often arising from allergies, characterized by sudden recurring attacks of difficult breathing, chest constriction, and coughing.

BEHAVIOR QUESTIONNAIRE

1. How many servings of fruits and vegetables do you eat per day?

           0   1   2   3+

2. How many caffeinated drinks (coffee, tea, cocoa, soft drinks) do you drink per day?

           0   1-2   3-4   5+

3. How many glasses (8 ounces) of water do you drink per day?

           0-3   4-5   6-7   8+

4. How many meals do you consume per day?

           1-2   3-4   5-6   7+

5. I cook with and eat fats:

     ___Nearly always cook/eat high fat foods (fried foods, shortening, butter, creams)
     ___Cook/eat mostly high fat
     ___Cook/eat both high and low fat foods
     ___Cook/eat mostly low fat
     ___Cook/eat only low fat

6. My bread/grain eating habit is:

     ___Nearly always eat refined (white bread, grains, rolls, crackers, cereal)
     ___Eat mostly refined grain products
     ___Eat a mixture of refined and whole grain products
     ___Eat primarily whole grain products
     ___Eat only whole grain products

7. How often do you eat out:

     ___I eat out nearly every day
     ___I eat out several times each week
     ___I eat out a few times each month
     ___I seldom or never eat out

8. My salty food habit is: (check all that apply)

     ___I rarely eat salty foods (chips, pickles, soups, added salt)
     ___Occasionally I eat salty foods
     ___I regularly eat salty food
     ___I add salt to the foods I eat

9. During the past 30 days, did you diet to lose weight or to keep from gaining weight?

           Yes   No

     If Yes, Explain:_____

10. My high fat snack eating habit is:

     ___I eat high fat snack foods (potato chips) 3 or more times daily
     ___I eat high fat snacks once or twice daily
     ___I eat high fat snacks a few times each week
     ___I rarely or never eat high fat snacks

11. How often do you eat red meat:
       ___I eat red meat nearly every day
       ___I eat red meat several times each week
       ___I eat red meat a few times each month
       ___I seldom or never eat red meat

12. How often do you eat cookies, cakes, sweets:
       ___I eat cookies, cakes, sweets nearly every day
       ___I eat cookies, cakes, sweets several times each week
       ___I eat cookies, cakes, sweets a few times each month
       ___I seldom or never eat cookies, cakes, sweets

13. How many alcoholic beverages do you consume per week?
                    0-3   4-5   6-7   8+

14. On average, I sleep _____ hours a night.
                    3-4   5-6   7-8   8+

15. Outside of work, what physical and/or social activities do you engage in?

Resting Heart Rate

Resting heart rate indicates the functional efficiency of the heart under non-stressed conditions. Due to the fact that the resting heart rate increases based upon stress factors, it indicates internal dynamics that the heart must contend with on a daily basis. The efficiency of the heart is the first variable. When the heart expels appropriate amounts of blood and the tissues can easily extract the oxygen, the resting heart rate remains low. To run a healthy, lean body, the heart requires a rate of about 30 beats per minute, as evidenced by marathon runners. The combination of high stroke volume with efficient oxygen extraction capabilities and low body mass causes the heart to run optimally. When the heart is detrained, it is not efficient and works harder to pump blood. Low stroke volumes, poor oxygen extraction capabilities, added fat mass, lower hemoglobin levels, and unregulated stress hormones cause resting heart rates to elevate. Deconditioned individuals often have heart rates in the eighties. Interestingly, factors that cause an elevated resting heart rate eventually lead to its dysfunction. By contrast, aerobic exercise, weight management, and physical activity reduce resting measures and consequently lead to a healthier heart. Chapter 12 identified that mortality was related to oxygen efficiency, with the heart playing a key role in this effect.

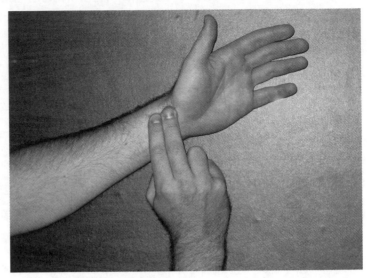

An illustration of proper technique when measuring the radial pulse.

Assessing the Radial Pulse

1. Assessing resting heart rates requires a calm and relaxed physiological environment. Any stimulus, perceived stress, or anxiety will cause the heart rate to accelerate beyond its resting requirements.

2. Personal trainers should instruct clients to avoid stimulants, such as caffeine and tobacco products, prior to assessing the pulse.

3. During the assessment, the client should not talk, as this can also elevate the heart rate. Have clients sit or lie down and place the arm to be assessed on a supportive structure. Have them maintain the position for two to five minutes to ease the postural shift and talk to them to reduce the anxiety of being tested.

4. Next, identify the site for measurement. Keep the arm supported at approximately heart height and palpate the radial pulse using the index and middle fingers.

5. For resting heart rate, the assessment should be for 60 seconds. Exercise heart rate can use a 15 second pulse count multiplied by four. Multiple recordings on subsequent visits will help predict an average waking resting heart rate.

6. If the value is consistently above 100 beats $\cdot$ min^{-1} the client should be referred to a physician before engaging in any physical testing or activity above walking.

Resting Heart Rate in Men and Women (beats/min)

%	MEN					WOMEN				
	20-29 y	30-39 y	40-49 y	50-59 y	60+ y	20-29 y	30-39 y	40-49 y	50-59 y	60+ y
90	50	50	50	50	52	55	55	55	55	52
80	54	55	54	55	55	59	58	60	60	57
70	58	58	58	58	58	60	62	62	61	60
60	60	60	60	60	60	63	65	64	64	62
50	63	63	62	63	62	65	68	66	67	64
40	66	65	65	65	65	70	70	70	69	66
30	70	68	69	68	68	72	74	72	72	72
20	72	72	72	72	72	75	76	76	75	74
10	80	77	78	77	77	84	82	80	83	79

Data from the US Department of Health and Human Services

Blood Pressure

Blood pressure is another cardiovascular measure that illustrates the internal environmental condition of the body during resting metabolism. It has been well documented that high blood pressure leads to numerous deleterious consequences for the body (9; 17). Vascular damage, **stroke**, kidney damage, and congestive heart failure all can occur in the presence of high blood pressure. The latest recommendations are to maintain a resting blood pressure at or below 115/75 mg/dl (24). Diagnostic criteria for hypertension include a diastolic value of 90 mmHg and systolic value of 140 mmHg. Pre-hypertension values include diastolic ranges between 80 and 89 mmHg and systolic ranges between 120 and 139 mmHg. High normal ranges are those that occur between 85 and 89 mmHg for diastolic measures, and 130 and 139 mmHg for systolic measures. These values have gained attention recently, as they are considered predictors for the later development of hypertension (1; 9). Blood pressure measurements above acceptable levels should be taken seriously and addressed as a key component in the exercise prescription and as part of the behavior management strategy. It is important to inform clients of the threat blood pressure presents because its development and the damage it causes occur without pain or discomfort. According to the US Department of Health and Human Services between 50 to 60 million Americans are hypertensive, which represents a large sample of the population hiring personal trainers.

Assessing Blood Pressure

1. Have the subject sit in a chair with feet flat on the floor and arm supported by a desk or table.

2. Place the appropriate sized cuff around the right arm so that the bottom of the cuff is two fingers from the flexion crease of the elbow.

3. The arm used for the assessment should be at the same elevation as the heart. If using an electronic device, be sure the sensor is over the brachial artery.

4. A cuff that is too small will falsely increase the reading, whereas a cuff that is too large will have the opposite effect.

5. Inflate the cuff to 165 mmHg for females and 185 mmHg for males or 20 mmHg above the previous systolic reading. Let the client know you will take the measurement twice to validate the initial measure. This will prevent anxiety if the client suspects the second measure is being taken because something was wrong with the first reading.

Note

Hypertension cannot be diagnosed by a personal trainer even though it seems obvious given elevated measures on 3 different days. Clients with blood pressure above 140/90 mmHg should be referred to their physician for proper diagnosis. If the measures are above 100 mmHg diastolic or 160 mmHg systolic, medical referral should be required before any activity participation.

Classification of Blood Pressure for Adults

Blood Pressure Classification	Systolic Blood Pressure (mmHg)	Diastolic Blood Pressure (mmHg)
Normal	<120	And <80
Prehypertension	120-139	Or 80-89
Stage 1 hypertension	140-159	Or 90-99
Stage 2 hypertension	≥160	≥100

Body Composition and Anthropometrics

Obesity is well known to be a comorbid disorder. As defined previously, comorbidity consists of one or more disorders or diseases in addition to a primary disease or disorder. Individuals who become obese dramatically increase their risk for other diseases and orthopedic problems (27; 28). Measuring relative body fat is important, as body fat compositions above specific values associate with higher rates of other diseases. Individuals with body fat compositions that are measured above 25% (males) and 32% (females) are at an elevated risk for having or developing diseases, including hypertension, diabetes, hyperlipidemia, CAD, and some cancers. Individuals who reach measures of 30% (males) and 40% (females) are considered morbidly obese and require a physician's referral before exercise testing can be performed. For visibly obese clients, skinfold assessments are not recommended. Instead select girth measures or a similar non-invasive technique. The reason for this choice is that skinfold measures are much less accurate when performed on individuals with excessive subcutaneous fat mass, and the experience unsettles the client.

Height and weight measurements should also be included in the resting battery, as the data is needed for BMI calculation, body fat and lean mass weight determination, and resting metabolic rate predictions. As previously stated, height and weight measures may also serve some purpose in mortality prediction, but generally serve as raw data and are not major criteria for exclusion in program participation. BMI is more commonly used by health care professionals than height and weight charts for prediction of disease and related consequences. A BMI value above 27 is considered high risk, while a calculated value of 30 is considered a predictor of obesity and a very high risk indicator. Keep in mind that BMI risk predictions are less meaningful in muscular clients, in which case, body composition is a better predictor of risk.

Waist circumference also strongly predicts risk of developing metabolic disease and CVD. Waist girth helps identify both central storage of subcutaneous and visceral fat. Individuals with high BMI values and large centralized girth are at a notably elevated risk, compared to someone who has low measures in both (3; 19-21). Males who exceed 40 inches and females who exceed 35 inches in circumference are considered to be at high risk. When both values are high, personal trainers should recommend the client see a physician for blood lipid profiling and fasting glucose measures to ensure they do not already suffer from pre-diabetes and/or hyperlipidemia.

Physical Exams and Lipid Screening

Only a qualified health care professional can perform a blood chemistry profile. Information gained from a complete blood analysis helps in making program and behavior modification decisions. Fasting blood glucose and blood lipid profiles are of particular importance due to their use in identifying certain diseases (2). Medical clearance is recommended for clients who present with the following values:

Blood Lipid Profiles for Medical Referral	
LDL-C	>135 mg/dl
HDL-C	<40 mg/dl
Total Cholesterol	>240 mg/dl
Cholesterol Ratio	>5
Triglycerides	>200 mg/dl
Blood Glucose (fasting)	>110 mg/dl

Regular exercise participation will result in positive adaptations for these blood elements. Therefore, elevated measured values should not be viewed as an impediment to participation in aerobic exercise, but as a risk factor that warrants physician review. For adults over 20 years of age, the National Cholesterol Education Program recommends that blood lipid profiles be evaluated every five years. Additionally, other risk factors compound the detriment these blood metabolites may cause, so tracking risk factors becomes even more important for individuals with multi-factorial risk.

Physical examinations by a physician are not required for the majority of clients prior to exercise participation, but personal trainers should encourage their clients to visit their physician for an annual physical and check-

Physiological Markers for Medical Referral

SBP > 160 mmHg
DBP > 100 mmHg
RHR > 100 beats · min^{-1}

Body Fat
Males   >30%
Females   >40%

up. When physiological problems are identified early, it makes them much easier to manage, and in most cases the consequential effects can be minimized. Individuals who go long periods of time without any physical assessment may place themselves at an unnecessarily high risk for disease or related complications. Pre-disease states respond much more positively to intervention compared to when they reach diagnostic criteria levels.

Exercise Participation Clearance

The findings from the resting battery should be added to the needs analysis and thoroughly reviewed for added risk for activity participation. The quantity of data collected using the aforementioned screening tools should provide a fairly clear picture as to someone's risk for potential adverse problems from engagement in physical activity. At this point, activity participation status must be determined before exercise testing can occur. Individuals who do not present any significant risk are cleared for unrestricted activity and tested for physical fitness. Individuals who possess a concerning level of risk factors or any signs and symptoms of disease should be medically cleared before exercise. A personal trainer may be acting negligently if they identify criteria that necessitate a medical referral but allow the client to engage in activities that place them at possible risk. In some cases, findings by a physician may require a medically supervised program, but these cases are rare among the general population.

No one wants medical clearance to be a barrier to participation, particularly when the participation is likely to improve the client's condition. However, sticking with generally accepted protocol does reduce liability. If the client has been to the physician in the past year, the standard method for efficiently clearing a client for exercise is to attain a physician contact form and have the client fax it to their general practitioner for clearance. The form indicates that the client willingly requests to engage in activity and allows the physician to make recommendations and restrictions for participation. The advantage to this process is that the client can simply fax the document to his or her

Signs and Symptoms of Disease

Cardiovascular
High blood pressure
Hypotension
High resting heart rate
Leg pain
High lipid profile
Chest or left arm pain
Dyspnea* on exertion
Edema
Heart palpitations

Metabolic
Increased thirst
Increased urination
Glucose intolerance
Obesity
High or low blood glucose
Increased or unexplained fatigue
Unexplained weight loss
Ammenorhea
Blurred vision
Insomnia
Jaundice (yellow colorization of skin and eyes)
Delayed wound healing

Pulmonary
Labored breathing
Breathlessness (mild exertion)
Nocturnal dypsnea
Frequent or chronic cough
Exercise induced asthma
Hemoptysis (coughing up blood)
Wheezing

*Dyspnea or shortness of breath (SOB) is perceived difficulty breathing or pain on breathing.

MEDICAL CLEARANCE FORM

Name of Patient_____ Date _____

Your patient wishes to take part in an exercise program and/or fitness assessment at or with _____ . After initial screening it has been determined that this individual requires physician consent prior to engaging in the exercise program and/or fitness assessments due to _____.

The participant will engage in the following exercise programming and/or fitness assessments:

Exercise Programming	**Fitness Assessments**
___Muscular Strength	___Muscular Strength
___Flexibility	___Muscular Endurance
___Muscular Endurance	___Flexibility
___Cardiorespiratory Fitness	___Body Composition
___Other*	___Cardiorespiratory Fitness

*Explain: _____

_____

Physician's Recommendations
Please indicate below for which of the following your patient is cleared to participate

Muscular Strength & Endurance Training and Assessment

___Yes, with no limitations   ___Yes, with limitations below   ___No, cannot participate

Limitations/recommendations: _____

_____

Cardiorespiratory Fitness and Assessment

___Yes, with no limitations   ___Yes, with limitations below   ___No, cannot participate

Limitations/recommendations: _____

_____

Flexibility Training and Assessment

___Yes, with no limitations   ___Yes, with limitations below   ___No, cannot participate

Limitations/recommendations: _____

_____

_____   _____
Signature of Physician/Primary Care Provider   Date

_____   **Please return this form to:**
Printed Name of Physician/Medical Group

_____
Street Address

_____
City   State   Zip

Disease Risk Classifications

Low risk - asymptomatic with one or fewer risk factors.

Moderate risk - asymptomatic with two or more risk factors.

High risk - multiple risk factors and/or signs and symptoms of disease.

---

physician and attain clearance without going through the process of a complete physical examination. Trainers should comply with any recommendations or restrictions, and in some cases, a physician may require a face-to-face visit. Due to the transfer of liability attained from the medical clearance document, trainers must adhere to any requirements outlined by the physician.

If the client needs to see his or her physician for clearance, the personal trainer should provide the client with the appropriate documents. A person acknowledging clearance without written documentation does not count as sufficient means for reducing trainer liability. Personal trainers must keep a written history of all activities and clearance documentation for proper risk management. In addition, this information assists in the development of an exercise prescription and the subsequent tracking of health changes.

Creating a client file should be a part of the first step to providing appropriate client services. Throughout the screening process, all documentation should be recorded and filed appropriately. Documents that are recommended for effective risk management include the informed consent, health status and behavior questionnaires, documentation of any resting battery assessments, any medical referral documents, physical testing records and all subsequent program documents. Trainers should implement an organized filing and tracking system to ensure a consistent and ongoing paper trail of the client's history while receiving personal training services. Although this adds responsibilities to the requirements of the job, it is beneficial for successful business activity. Taking the time to document and track services allows for insight into what is working and what may require modification within the program or behavior management strategies, while simultaneously reducing the risk of liability. Additionally, tracking and reviewing files can help to identify compliance with recommendations and ascertain obstacles to goal attainment.

Exercise Testing

One of the purposes for screening clients is to ensure a client will not be injured or suffer from a cardiovascular event during fitness testing. Fitness testing is a fundamental part of designing an exercise prescription. Results and findings from physical fitness tests allow personal trainers to create a health-fitness profile of each client and make educated decisions for addressing his or her current condition.

The rationale for testing is well justified and fairly extensive; however, each individual test should have a specific purpose. Test selection decision making is not arbitrary. Quite a bit of thought should go into test selecting to ensure its validity, reliability, and appropriateness for the client. The tests need to be chosen, based on specific criteria.

Test Rationale	Test Selection Criteria
Identifying baseline data of physical measures	What is the purpose of the test?
Identifying strengths and weaknesses	Is the test valid, reliable, and objective?
Assessing capabilities	What does the data provide and how will it be used?
Identifying starting points	How will improvements in subsequent test measures affect the goals of the training?
Determining readiness for training activities	
Establishing program and progress tracking criteria	What does it predict?
Determining goal setting data	Does it match the goals of the training?
Evaluating psychological considerations	Is it consistent with important program components?
Educating clients	Is it appropriate for the specific individual being tested?
Establishing program activities and evaluating their effectiveness	Will the client be able to effectively perform the test?
	Is it safe for the client?
	Does the test present psychological barriers or anxiety?
	Is the client comfortable performing the test?

Answering these questions will help to individualize the battery of tests for the client. Individualizing the test selection for the client maximizes the effectiveness and experience of the testing, and ensures the best outcome for his or her well-being. Recognizing the client's experience, capabilities, training status, age, and gender will be relevant for deciding on the most appropriate tests and selecting the assessments that will provide the best data. Personal trainers must remain conscious of any health risks or safety issues when selecting tests to avoid a negative experience or outcome associated with the testing protocol or testing environment.

When deciding on the test or protocol to be used for a particular client, it is important to evaluate each test's validity, reliability, and objectivity. A test is considered valid when it accurately measures what it is designed to measure. The goal is to identify assessment protocols that have been proven valid through appropriate research methodology and will best match the client's particular characteristics. When tests are validated by clinical trials and are appropriate for the population being tested, the personal trainer has an excellent opportunity to collect valid data by performing the protocols consistent with the intended methodology. This suggests understanding the assessment protocol and being proficient at implementing it in the correct environment. It is easy to illustrate how validity can be gained or lost by considering the following scenarios:

Scenario 1. A personal trainer asks a previously sedentary 37-year old female to run a mile on a high school track. The trainer assumes that the track distance is 1,320 ft because when he ran the mile in High School, four laps was a mile. The test takes place on the third meeting, but the trainer did not inform the client what exercises or tests she would be performing that day. The client has worn designer athletic shoes, but they are not ideal for running. In addition, the environment is somewhat hot and humid because the client trains at lunch time, and the season of the year is summer.

Scenario 2. A personal trainer researches the distance of an indoor track before deciding to use it with her 28-year old male client. He has routinely jogged between 6-9 miles per week for the past six months to stay fit. She asks him to bring his running shoes with him for the training session because she wants to test his performance in a maximal one mile run. In the previous two meetings, she used the track for some cardio interval training with the client, and he is familiar with the surface and running distance. She instructs him not to run any significant distance the two days before the test and gives him a pretest checklist to follow.

After reviewing the two scenarios, it should be evident that the second situation would provide a much better experience for the client and would likely have a much higher validity of testing for cardiorespiratory fitness. The trainer has provided the client with a test consistent with his capabilities and experience, provided exposure to the specific factors of the test, assessed the distance for accuracy, accounted for environmental factors, and properly planned the event. Conversely, scenario one may actually place the client at risk. The trainer did not match the test to the client, did not mentally prepare her for the event, failed to account for environmental influences, and did not provide pretest information that would increase the accuracy of the assessment. It is the personal trainer's job to account for all the factors that may invalidate a test and ensure that they have been removed before implementing a test for physical fitness.

Validity is also affected if the methodology deviates in any way from the proper protocol. This is commonly seen when subjects incorrectly perform the techniques used in the assessment. Incorrect body position, poor biomechanics, and using momentum or other compensatory action for improved scoring all serve to invalidate the assessment. Validity may also be compromised when the testing equipment or the evaluation instrument performs poorly. This can occur from using inferior equipment, not calibrating the equipment before employing it, or having depleted batteries in the device. Poor assessment instrument performance wastes everyone's time and effort.

When the proper steps have been taken to ensure only minimal error exists, the measure can provide high test validity. A personal trainer should document the testing environment and the specific details related to the client preparation and protocol implementation. In doing so, he or she can increase the opportunity for effective reliability in follow-up testing. Reliability suggests reproducibility, or a test's ability to provide valid measures in subsequent re-testing. Any change in the testing activities or environment may decrease predictive reliability and invalidate the data for comparative purposes. Consistency is the key to reliability. With subsequent testing, everything should be the same in order to maximize the accuracy of the data for comparison to previous trials. This means using the same methods, instruments, testing environment and pretest protocols for each subsequent retest. Reproducibility affects retest validity, but the two are not synonymous. Something can be invalid and reproducible. For instance, the sit-and-reach test has been used for years and has demonstrated consistent reproducible measures but investigations have shown the test is not necessarily valid due to the large number of variables that can affect it (12; 16).

Validity and reliability errors may be impossible to completely remove because test participants are human and subject to an innumerable amount of physiological and psychological variables which may affect a test's outcome. The one person who can enhance the validity and reliability of the testing is the test administrator. Objectivity is the same as inter-tester reliability. When personal trainers are highly trained and well versed in the testing protocols, they add to the validity and reliability of the tests. Applying meticulous detail to all the test factors adds to the success of the program.

Testing Environment

The testing environment can either add to, or detract from, validity and reliability. Obvious environmental factors include ambient air temperature, altitude, humidity, and pollution, including gases, noise, and toxins. However, most variables that affect the testing environment are not as obvious. Recalling that the human factor is the hardest to account for, it must also be the one emphasized for control. If the testing environment is around, or in the sight of others, it is likely the client will be distracted and possibly self-conscious, thereby affecting the testing. For this reason, private testing may help the client to focus on the task, rather than experience test-related anxiety due to the environment. Safety is another factor that should be thoroughly accounted for when creating the test environment. Making sure the client has a safe area in which to work, the equipment has been tested and deemed safe, and the client has the appropriate clothing and footwear, are all key factors to assess before testing should begin.

Test Administration

Test administration is a crucial factor in the outcome of the client assessments. Properly organized and administered testing procedures provide quality data for the exercise program. Acquiring the technical skills and mastering the test protocols is vital to being a successful personal trainer. A test administrator's proficiency in implementing and managing the assessment is easily enhanced by gaining expertise and experience in the protocols being employed. Performing the tests and practicing the protocols on others helps to identify problems and circumstances that may reduce the accuracy of client testing. Test invalidation due to administrator error or incompetence, related to the procedure can be avoided by practice and using a premeditated, organized plan. Making a checklist and complying with it can be a valuable step in efficient test management.

Test Economy

Another variable, test economy often compromises test validity. Test economy describes the proficiency of the subject in performing the test and his or her compliance with the test instructions. When personal trainers do not properly instruct their clients in the test techniques or fail to point out pitfalls and common errors, the test is likely to provide poor data. Personal trainers should have clients practice the testing techniques and allow for adequate skill acquisition before implementing the protocol. When the client is proficient at the techniques required of the test the validity increases dramatically. By practicing the skills required by a specific test prior to the actual test implementation, the client's confidence increases and the exposure to the test reduces the anxiety that often comes from testing and new experiences.

The psychological component of testing should not be underestimated. In addition to the physical requirements asked of a client, some psychological aspect to testing is always present. People experience different levels of test anxiety. In some cases, the anxiety stems from the pressure to perform well, internal questioning of one's capability to perform the test, or concerns that they may perform poorly on the tests and become embarrassed. In other

---

Increasing Validity and Reliability of Tests

Validity

- Make sure the protocol is valid.
- Make sure the tester is skillful and experienced in the test protocols.
- Make sure the client is proficient in the test action.
- Use strict discrimination in measurement.
- Psychologically prepare the client for the event and properly motivate them.
- Make sure the environment is safe and ideal for the test.
- Make sure all the equipment functions properly and is calibrated.
- Make sure the client has met pretest instructions.
- Make sure no variable has entered the equation such as illness or high stress.
- Clearly defined scoring system.

Reliability

- Duplicate the conditions (time, environment, location, recovery).
- Strict adherence to the protocol.
- Consistent pretest factors: warm-up and motivation.
- Consistency with scoring system.
- Emphasize tester consistency.
- Use the same assessment instrument.

cases, they may have had a negative experience or have not performed well on similar tests in the past. These feelings are often brought to the forefront of consciousness when individuals are faced with a similar situation.

Test preparation checklists and practice work well to help contend with many of these factors. There are two types of pretest checklists: one for the administrator and one for the client. For the test administrator, the checklist should include factors that will ensure the test is performed safely and efficiently. It will contain items such as having the right equipment, ensuring it is calibrated and functioning properly, having the appropriate forms and using a properly prepared environment. The client's pretest instructions will include test day preparations such as appropriate clothing, adequate rest and hydration, and the avoidance of stimulants or other ingested items that may affect the outcome of the test. The best test administrators are organized and detail oriented. When everything is properly accounted for, the likelihood of success is very high. On the other hand, with a lack of preparation, the chance for error increases significantly.

Testing Format

When more than one test is to be administered on a given day, it is necessary to establish a well organized test format. The two primary components to the format decisions are time and validation. Some tests take more time than others to set up and administer. Others have minimal time requirements but can invalidate subsequent tests by causing fatigue. Identifying an appropriate sequence can help ensure the test session's efficiency and accuracy. Attempting to perform all the tests in one day may be better from a time perspective, but if this process dilutes the data, then the time saved was of little value.

Knowledge is the key to proper decision making when determining the test sequence or what tests should be administered together. Tests that are demanding of the nervous system and/or the immediate energy system should be performed first in a sequence of testing. Tests that produce fatigue should be placed later in the test sequence. When deciding on a logical progression, the following guidelines can assist in the sequencing decision.

Test Order

1. Resting test or test of minimal fatigue: body composition, flexibility, balance and coordination.

2. Strength and power tests: maximal repetition tests, anaerobic power tests.

3. Endurance tests: push-ups, curl-ups.

4. Anaerobic capacity tests: one minute squat, 400m run.

5. Aerobic tests: 12-min run, step tests.

For maximum effectiveness, tests should be split up and implemented on different days. Aerobic tests, anaerobic capacity tests, and strength tests are generally most valid when performed independently of other tests. If several tests are being performed on a single day, non-fatigue tests may occur between tests of more intense activity to provide a rest period for the client. Specific decisions will be relative to the tests employed, the capabilities of the client, and other relevant factors. A good strategy is to implement a particular test and then practice the other physical fitness tests to be performed on subsequent test days.

Pretest Checklists

Client Pretest Instructions
____ I have read and understand any pretest procedures.
____ I am familiar with the tests I will perform.
____ I have acquired adequate rest the night before testing.
____ I have consumed adequate fluid.
____ I have consumed a moderate dietary intake.
____ I have abstained from tobacco, stimulants, and nonprescription medications.
____ I have the proper clothing and footwear for the activity.
____ I am not ill or injured.

Administrator Checklist for Testing
____ Client has been screened and signed informed consent.
____ Equipment is available, in working condition, and calibrated.
____ All records and scoring sheets are prepared.
____ Protocol is clearly understood.
____ Subject has practiced the test.
____ Subject has been properly instructed for the test.
____ Testing environment has been defined and is prepared.
____ External conditions are appropriate for testing.
____ Test termination criteria.
____ Warm-up and cool-down procedures defined.

Health and Safety Considerations

Safety must be a fundamental concern in the delivery of services by personal trainers. As with any trainer-supervised environment, the testing conditions must be controlled and managed in a way that will ensure the best possible outcome for the client. Using the aforementioned strategies will certainly assist in helping to prevent any incidents from occurring, but a premeditated safety and emergency plan should always be in place. Even though clients have gone through a proper screening process before being cleared for exercise testing, problems may still arise, as injury is an inherent element of physical activity. In addition to establishing a safe environment and implementing a pretest checklist, trainers should also explain stop test protocols, communicate methods to help reduce injury during testing, visually survey the area before and during the test for external hazards, and ensure the client is adequately prepared in mind and body for the assessment. Likewise, trainers should have the emergency plan in order to efficiently address any situation that may arise. Some prudent considerations include having ice available (bagged in a portable cooler) in case of a musculoskeletal injury, having juice or sugar-based fluids to address a hypoglycemic reaction, and an EMS action plan in the event of a more serious situation.

Test Interpretation

Once the data has been collected from exercise testing, it needs to be analyzed and interpreted for the client. Clients are often very interested in how they perform compared to others in their population group. To help clients understand their level of fitness, it is necessary to compare the test scores to established age and gender norms. In some cases, the scoring system uses ranges that the client's scores will fall into for the purposes of identifying the current fitness level. Other test norms use percentile ranking to classify how the client performed on a given test. Explaining scores and the respective classification in understandable terms and context helps clients recognize where they fall on the fitness continuum. A goal of an effective personal training service is to always maintain a positive outlook on the situation. Some clients may fall into categories that define their current fitness level as low. This can often lead to feelings of embarrassment and worthlessness. These feelings must be avoided. Poor results should be explained in positive terms. Personal trainers should emphasize that these are starting points and the training program is designed specifically to enhance the scores attained during assessment. Avoid using negative terms, such as "poor" or "low," by applying action words that will be viewed as something possible to accomplish. Letting the client know that the deficient area can be improved upon and that it will be emphasized during the exercise program is often helpful. Additionally, help them realize that many of their peers fall into these categories and that improvement in fitness is the reason that they are there in the first place.

It is also helpful to focus on the end result, rather than on current deficiencies. Let the client know that, in a reasonable period of time, his or her scores can improve to the level they would like to attain. This is also an appropriate time to initiate motivational strategies. Focus on the steps to success and reinforce your confidence in their ability to reach those goals. Let them know that their progress will be tracked, and if they comply with the program recommendations, they will see improvement by the next evaluation.

When interpreting the scores for program decision making purposes, personal trainers should evaluate each area of fitness and decide on the greatest areas of need. For individuals with low scores in most or all the categories of fitness, cardiorespiratory fitness (CRF) should be the initial emphasis, due to its role in health and disease prevention. This does not suggest that the other areas should be overlooked, but low CRF is the most detrimental on health of the fitness measures. All of the values ascertained from fitness testing should be added to the needs list so they can be appropriately emphasized in the exercise program. Each area will warrant appropriate attention, which will help to define the program matrix.

Needs Analysis

The long list of data collected will have relevant findings that will dictate the appropriate response from the exercise prescription. Reviewing the information and identifying the specific issues to address in the exercise program is referred to as the needs analysis. This process requires personal trainers to determine the goals of the exercise prescription, based on the data collected and the relationship of the findings to positive and negative health outcomes. The initial review should single out negative factors as they present the greatest consequence and may be barriers to improvements in the health status of the client. The negative factors should be evaluated and addressed in an attempt to come up with plausible solutions to the problems they present. For instance, if flexibility scores are low, the personal trainer should identify effective solutions that will improve upon the identified limitations. Using the listing system, the identified needs will each reflect a suitable remedy. The remedies will provide the trainer with appropriate options to use within the exercise program. The combination of the need and remedy can then be used to determine short- and long-term goals and the daily objectives that will lead to successful attainment of the goals.

Goal Setting

Nearly all new personal trainers find goal setting initially difficult. It is an area where common errors frequently occur. Most individuals set goals that are too difficult to attain in the designated period of time, which sets the client up for failure. When goals are not attained, clients lose momentum, and this failure negatively affects their motivation and compliance to the program due to feelings of inadequacy and apathy. When goals are set appropriately they are reinforcing, and increase adherence, compliance, and effort, further accelerating improvements. The two most common errors made when defining goals are setting unrealistic goals and not creating an appropriate system of objectives and short-term goals to attain the requirements of the long-term goal.

To effectively set goals, personal trainers should analyze the capabilities of the client, the time defined to reach the goals, and the effort necessary to attain them. Effective goal setting starts with understanding the characteristics that separate quality goals from those that may be unrealistic or ineffective. Goals should reflect controllable behaviors, be specific and measurable, and be challenging but realistic; meaningful and rewarding to the client. They should have a designated time frame that matches the client's individual characteristics, motivations, and capabilities.

Goal setting is essentially outlining an action plan. In most cases, a reverse approach is most effective in defining the planned items that will make up the measurable components within the goal continuum. The first step is defining a timeline in which reasonable adaptations will occur. Long-term goals in personal training should be split into two categories: 1) the ultimate goal to be achieved by the program, and 2) a goal that is of lesser degree that can be accomplished in three to six months. Losing thirty pounds for instance, would reflect an ultimate long-term goal, whereas losing twelve pounds would reflect a long-term goal that falls within a 12-week training cycle. Defining the term is ultimately going to be on a case-by-case basis due to relative differences among individual clients. A person new to exercise who is fairly deconditioned and previously sedentary may

Needs Analysis Examples

Identified Need	Remedies	Long-term goal
Risk Factors		
Physical inactivity	Increase daily physical work	200 kcal increase in energy expenditure per day
High stress	Identify stressors and environments	Reduce perception Increase coping skills
Low back pain	Abdominal strength Hip flexor/ext. flexibility Improve postural stability	Reduce daily occurrence
Resting Battery		
RBP: 138/88 mmHg	Increase aerobic activity Decrease body weight Modify diet	Reduce to 120/80 mmHg
RHR: 82 bpm	Improve stroke volume	Reduce to 75bpm
Body fat: 23%	Increase caloric expenditure Increase metabolism Caloric restriction Reduce sugar & fat intake	Reduce to 18%
Waist girth: 39 inches	Increase exercise output Same as above	34 inches
Exercise Testing Flexibility:		
Tight hip extensors Poor spinal extension Poor spinal rotation	Dynamic & static stretching	Improve ROM
Upper body strength: average	Resistance training	Above average measures
Lower body strength: average	Resistance training	Above average measures
Cardiovascular fitness: fair	Aerobic training	Improve to average

require more time to accomplish a goal than a well-conditioned client.

The long-term goal helps to establish the short-term goals. In the same example, a weight loss of twelve pounds in a twelve week period suggests that the short-term goal would be one pound of weight loss a week or four pounds of weight loss per month. Short-term goals are generally accomplishable in less than a month and can be broken down further into weekly goals. The short-term goals must be attainable because they are a valuable asset in motivation. The weekly short-term goals can further be broken down into daily objectives. If the long-term goal is twelve pounds in three months and the short-term goal is a pound a week of weight loss, than the daily objective would be defined as a negative caloric balance of 500 calories. If a client focuses on the daily effort of caloric restriction and physical activity in an attempt to expend 500 calories and is able to meet the objective, then the short-term goal will be reached at the end of the week and the long-term goal will be reached at the end of the training cycle. Keeping the focus on daily objectives is conceptually the same as taking one step at a time. The inability to attain goals is most often traced back to unrealistic expectations. Behavior change and adaptations are fairly slow, progressive elements. Therefore, attempting to force the rate of change beyond the typical human process will most often result in failure.

Key Terms

Stroke – The sudden death of brain cells in a localized area due to inadequate blood flow.

Hypotension – Abnormally low blood pressure.

Dyspnea – Difficulty in breathing, often associated with lung or heart disease, resulting in shortness of breath.

Hemoptysis – The coughing up of blood or bloody sputum from the lungs or airway.

Amenorrhea – A menstrual irregularity, seen especially in women who are involved in regular, high-intensity exercise.

Insomnia – Chronic inability to fall asleep or remain asleep for an adequate length of time.

Emergency Medical Service (EMS) – Responsible for providing pre-hospital care by paramedics, emergency medical technicians, and medical first responders.

Chapter Thirteen References

1. **Bakx JC, Deunk L, van Gerwen WH, van Aalst M, van den Hoogen HJ and van den Bosch WJ**. [Relationship between te general practice guidelines for the diagnosis of hypertension and the indication for treatment and practice in the Nijmegen region, the Netherlands, 1983-2001]. *Ned Tijdschr Geneeskd* 147: 612-615, 2003.

2. **Ballantyne C, Arroll B and Shepherd J**. Lipids and CVD management: towards a global consensus. *Eur Heart J* 26: 2224-2231, 2005.

3. **Bergman RN, Kim SP, Hsu IR, Catalano KJ, Chiu JD, Kabir M, Richey JM and Ader M**. Abdominal obesity: role in the pathophysiology of metabolic disease and cardiovascular risk. *Am J Med* 120: S3-S8, 2007.

4. **Chinn DJ, White M, Howel D, Harland JO and Drinkwater CK**. Factors associated with non-participation in physical activity promotion trial. *Public Health* 120: 309-319, 2006.

5. **Corrado D, Basso C, Schiavon M and Thiene G**. Does sports activity enhance the risk of sudden cardiac death? *J Cardiovasc Med (Hagerstown)* 7: 228-233, 2006.

6. **Cournot M, Taraszkiewicz D, Galinier M, Chamontin B, Boccalon H, Hanaire-Broutin H, Puel J and Ferrieres J**. Is exercise testing useful to improve the prediction of coronary events in asymptomatic subjects? *Eur J Cardiovasc Prev Rehabil* 13: 37-44, 2006.

7. **Dickens BM and Cook RJ**. Dimensions of informed consent to treatment. *Int J Gynaecol Obstet* 85: 309-314, 2004.

8. **Erbs S, Linke A and Hambrecht R**. Effects of exercise training on mortality in patients with coronary heart disease. *Coron Artery Dis* 17: 219-225, 2006.

9. **Fattirolli F, Cellai T and Burgisser C**. [Physical activity and cardiovascular health a close link]. *Monaldi Arch Chest Dis* 60: 73-78, 2003.

10. **Geller G, Tambor ES, Bernhardt BA, Fraser G and Wissow LS**. Informed consent for enrolling minors in genetic susceptibility research: a qualitative study of at-risk children's and parents' views about children's role in decision-making. *J Adolesc Health* 32: 260-271, 2003.

11. **Hecht HS**. Recommendations for preparticipation screening and the assessment of cardiovascular disease in masters athletes. *Circulation* 104: E58, 2001.

12. **Hui SS and Yuen PY**. Validity of the modified back-saver sit-and-reach test: a comparison with other protocols. *Med Sci Sports Exerc* 32: 1655-1659, 2000.

13. **Kappagoda CT, Ma A, Cort DA, Paumer L, Lucus D, Burns J and Amsterdam E**. Cardiac event rate in a lifestyle modification program for patients with chronic coronary artery disease. *Clin Cardiol* 29: 317-321, 2006.

14. **Kappagoda CT, Ma A, Cort DA, Paumer L, Lucus D, Burns J and Amsterdam E**. Cardiac event rate in a lifestyle modification program for patients with chronic coronary artery disease. *Clin Cardiol* 29: 317-321, 2006.

15. **Ladimer I**. Professional liability in exercise testing for cardiac performance. *Am J Cardiol* 30: 753-756, 1972.

16. **Lemmink KA, Kemper HC, de Greef MH, Rispens P and Stevens M**. The validity of the sit-and-reach test and the modified sit-and-reach test in middle-aged to older men and women. *Res Q Exerc Sport* 74: 331-336, 2003.

17. **Lloyd-Jones DM, Dyer AR, Wang R, Daviglus ML and Greenland P**. Risk factor burden in middle age and lifetime risks for cardiovascular and non-cardiovascular death (chicago heart association detection project in industry). *Am J Cardiol* 99: 535-540, 2007.

18. **Mozes T, Tyano S, Mano I and Mester R**. Informed consent: myth or reality. *Med Law* 21: 473-483, 2002.

19. **Ofei F**. Obesity - a preventable disease. *Ghana Med J* 39: 98-101, 2005.

20. **Onat A, Hergenc G, Turkmen S, Yazici M, Sari I and Can G**. Discordance between insulin resistance and metabolic syndrome: features and associated cardiovascular risk in adults with normal glucose regulation. *Metabolism* 55: 445-452, 2006.

21. **Onat A, Uyarel H, Hergenc G, Karabulut A, Albayrak S and Can G**. Determinants and definition of abdominal obesity as related to risk of diabetes, metabolic syndrome and coronary disease in Turkish men: A prospective cohort study. *Atherosclerosis* 191: 182-190, 2007.

22. **Peteiro JC, Monserrat L, Bouzas A, Pinon P, Marinas J, Bouzas B and Castro-Beiras A**. Risk stratification by treadmill exercise echocardiography. *J Am Soc Echocardiogr* 19: 894-901, 2006.

23. **Seto CK**. Preparticipation cardiovascular screening. *Clin Sports Med* 22: 23-35, 2003.

24. **Sever P**. New hypertension guidelines from the National Institute for Health and Clinical Excellence and the British Hypertension Society. *J Renin Angiotensin Aldosterone Syst* 7: 61-63, 2006.

25. **Shephard RJ**. Ethics in exercise science research. *Sports Med* 32: 169-183, 2002.

26. **Smith DM, Lombardo JA and Robinson JB**. The preparticipation evaluation. *Prim Care* 18: 777-807, 1991.

27. **Smith SC, Jr. and Haslam D**. Abdominal obesity, waist circumference and cardio-metabolic risk: awareness among primary care physicians, the general population and patients at risk--the Shape of the Nations survey. *Curr Med Res Opin* 23: 29-47, 2007.

28. **Stavropoulos-Kalinoglou A, Metsios GS, Koutedakis Y, Nevill AM, Douglas KM, Jamurtas A, Veldhuijzen van Zanten JJ, Labib M and Kitas GD**. Redefining overweight and obesity in rheumatoid arthritis patients. *Ann Rheum Dis* 2007.

29. **Whang W, Manson JE, Hu FB, Chae CU, Rexrode KM, Willett WC, Stampfer MJ and Albert CM**. Physical exertion, exercise, and sudden cardiac death in women. *JAMA* 295: 1399-1403, 200

Chapter 14

Assessment of Physical Fitness

In This Chapter

Submaximal VO₂ Testing

Predicting Maximal Values

Testing for Muscular Fitness

Testing Error

Anaerobic Power Capacity

Flexibility

Body Composition

Common Field Assessments

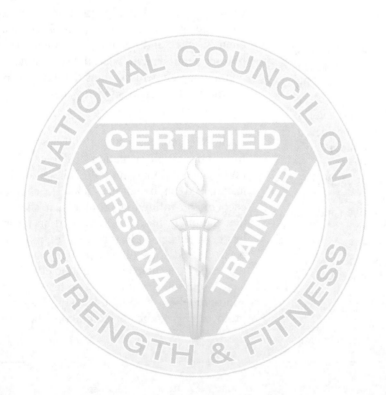

Introduction

Cardiorespiratory fitness (CRF) is probably the single most important measure of health-related fitness due to its role in physiological function and its relationship to disease and lifespan (1; 2; 7; 16). Participation in cardiovascular activities positively affects the other health related components of fitness, making it a key component to any exercise program. Physical fitness evaluations should include a cardiorespiratory assessment to ensure appropriate levels of aerobic fitness are maintained throughout a person's life.

When CRF tests are administered, they are intended to identify a person's **VO₂max,** or maximum oxygen uptake. VO₂max reflects the body's ability to intake, transport, and utilize oxygen. It is a measure of the efficiency with which the lungs, heart, and blood supply oxygen to the muscles, and the muscles' ability to extract and use the oxygen for energy metabolism during exercise. Tests to measure oxygen consumption may be maximal, where an individual is required to perform an all-out effort at 100% intensity, or submaximal, where heart rate is measured at lower intensities and extrapolated to predict the maximal oxygen uptake. Additionally, VO₂max can be determined by estimating oxygen demand, as determined by measured distance and time, and calculated using predictive equations. In most cases, submaximal efforts are preferred and are implemented via a variety of test protocols and modalities that employ large muscle action for a sustained period of time. The measured heart rates or test specific data are entered into predictive equations or graphed for predictive value.

Submaximal VO₂ Testing

Personal trainers rarely employ maximal testing protocols due to the risk of possible injury, the technical skills required for safe implementation, and the complexity of administering the assessment, as well as the lack of justification for placing the required level of stress upon the population being considered. Submaximal testing on the other hand, is often fairly easy to employ, presents limited risk for injury or cardiovascular incident, and is tolerable by most people. These tests include walking and running protocols, stationary bike tests, step tests, and may even include swim tests if warranted by the test population.

The majority of the submaximal assessments require subjects to perform activities at a set pace with a protocol-specified level of difficulty, though some utilize gradually increasing submaximal workloads. The tests are either performed for a designated period of time, until a particular distance is reached, or steady state heart rates have been attained at a particular intensity level. The specific test protocol determines the measuring system and termination criteria to be used. Once the test data has been collected, it will be entered into a protocol specific calculation or graph to identify a predictive score or value. Note that submaximal protocols differ from maximal protocols in that they generate a prediction of an individual's VO₂max and they are, to some extent, less accurate, whereas maximal protocols are a direct measurement.

Predicting Maximal Values

Predictive equations convert the measured performance unit into an expression of oxygen utilization. The predictive quantity of oxygen utilization is expressed in absolute terms, milliliters or liters of oxygen used per minute of activity (ml · min⁻¹ or L · min⁻¹), or in relative terms, milliliters of oxygen used per kilogram of body weight per minute of activity (ml · kg · min⁻¹). The absolute terms represent the total quantity of oxygen consumed by the body per minute, whereas the relative expression represents the oxygen used by the subject's body mass per minute. If a large person and small person both have the same absolute measure of oxygen usage, the smaller person is identified as possessing a better ability to utilize oxygen per pound or kilogram of their respective weight. For this reason, relative expressions are more commonly used so that the measures display the subjects' individualized efficiency levels and are therefore more useful for comparisons among individuals.

The predicted measure of oxygen utilization identified by the test will mean very little to the client. The findings should be explained in easy to understand language and compared to norms consistent with the client's age and gender. Personal trainers should become familiar with what the scores mean for different population segments so that the exercise prescription is appropriately constructed to help meet the client's defined goals.

Each CRF submaximal test will have specific protocols for proper implementation. Chapter 13 discussed the importance of matching the client to the appropriate test, based on his or her specific characteristics. For each of the following protocols, it should be assumed that the client has already signed an informed consent, has been successfully screened for risk factors, and has been cleared for exercise participation consistent with the level of testing being conducted. He or she should have complied with the pretest checklist and be appropriately prepared for testing. Additionally, each protocol has indicators to abort the test (Stop Test

Indicators) that should be strictly adhered to, along with an emergency plan in the unlikely event of a problem.

Indications for Test Termination

- Subject no longer feels comfortable doing the test.
- Subject's skin becomes pale.
- Subject fails to keep cadence for 20 seconds or more.
- Subject has an inability to focus attention.
- Subject experiences faintness, dizziness, or lightheadedness.
- Subject experiences upset stomach or vomiting symptoms.
- Subject experiences dysfunction in breathing.
- Subject experiences chest pain.
- Subject experiences side stitch, cramp, strain, fatigue.

Testing for Muscular Fitness

Testing for muscular fitness includes assessing a client's capacity for both **muscular strength** and **endurance**. Traditionally, these components of fitness have used specialized equipment such as hand grip dynamometers, cable tensiometers, and isokinetic machines to predict body strength and endurance in clinical settings, or 1RM dynamic resistance exercises for use with athletic populations. A problem with strength and endurance testing is that each individual muscle and joint action may vary in their ability to produce and sustain force. When only one or two measures are used to assess the body's force production capabilities or the ability of the body to sustain force output, the outcome may not be valid for movements or exercises other than the ones used for the testing. For instance, a person may perform well on a bench press test but not have the strength to perform a pull-up, or he or she may be able to leg press a respectable quantity of weight but not have adequate muscle strength/balance in his or her leg flexors, placing him or her at an increased risk for muscle strains due to muscle imbalances. For this reason, trainers should use a minimum of three different strength and endurance assessments; one each for the upper body, lower body, and trunk.

Adequate strength and endurance in all muscles of the body is a central goal for health. When measures such as the bench press or leg press are emphasized, the criteria for retest performance only apply to the muscle groups employed. A person may, in fact, perform well on those tests and receive a high ranking for muscle strength categorically, but this should not be viewed as a true representation of the whole body. In the ideal

situation, personal trainers would be able to ascertain the strength and fitness of all the major muscle groups to identify deficiencies and imbalances. Normalized data can be used for traditional assessments where population norms have been established, while multi-repetition max assessments and one repetition predictive calculations can help provide information regarding movements that do not currently have defined comparable data.

As previously alluded to, a balance of muscular strength between agonist and antagonist muscle groups aids proper joint stability and reduces risk of injury due to uneven force coupling, a problem which often leads to joint dysfunction. Each major muscle group has an opposing relationship with the muscle group responsible for moving the body segment in the opposite direction. Depending on the articulation, the strength relationship between the two groups requires a specific ratio to keep the joint functioning properly. Attaining the appropriate ratio for each group should be a primary goal of any exercise program.

Muscle Balance Ratio Goals

Trunk Flexors:Extensors	1:1
Hip Flexors:Extensors	1:1
Shoulder Flexors:Extensors	2:3
Knee Flexors:Extensors	2:3
Shoulder Int. Rotators:Ext. rotators	3:2
Elbow Extensors:Flexors	1:1
Ankle Plantar Flexor:DorsiFlexor	3:1

Muscular Strength Assessments

Strength assessments possess a level of risk for musculoskeletal injury due to strain, particularly in deconditioned clients. To reduce this risk, clients should be well versed in the movements and appropriately familiarized with the exercise being performed. Likewise, selecting higher repetition (5-10RM) tests over 1RM or 3RM is recommended for the average healthy population. Although it is possible to perform low repetition maximal tests safely with healthy populations, and these tests provide more accurate data, there are inherent problems with their inclusion. Some of these problems include the obvious risk associated with the testing, the difficulty in identifying the maximal load to be lifted, changes to the movement mechanics due to the load and stability requirements, and the dramatic increases in pressure associated with the lifts. Outside of the healthy, athletic population, low repetition, maximal strength tests are generally not recommended.

There are many variations of the type of resistance used for strength testing. Some tests employ static resistance, others use variable resistance or constant resistance machines, while others utilize free weight modalities. Although the decision for any test will be client specific, free weight assessments are often preferred over exercise machines. In addition to assessing strength, free weight tests can also identify relative joint stability during the performance of the movement. Machine tests only measure linear or angular force and will not identify weakness associated with an instable joint, as the machines use fixed movement arms. Humans require balance, coordination, and increased stability during real world applications of force production, so it is logical to employ these factors when testing.

Muscular Endurance Assessments

Endurance tests require the client to sustain an isometric contraction for an extended period of time, perform a maximal number of repetitions in a designated time frame, or perform a particular movement to failure. Chin hangs are one example of static contractile force assessed by time. Paced abdominal curl-ups represent a test in which the exerciser stays in cadence for an extended period of time and test termination occurs when the subject can no longer maintain the pace. Maximal repetition tests may have a time limitation, as seen with the one-minute body squat test, or allow the exerciser to reach failure, as is the case with the push-up test. No matter what the particular test criteria, the goal is to ascertain the decline in force production of a muscle over a period of time. The abdominal curl-up is likely the most common single assessment used for overall prediction because it focuses on the endurance capabilities of postural muscles. This assumes that postural muscle endurance reflects muscular endurance of other muscles, which is not always accurate. Local muscle endurance is, more often than not, dependent upon the activity status of the individual and the movements or actions they perform on a routine basis. A person who rides a bike most days of the week will likely have better endurance in the muscles used for that activity than others. Although trunk postural muscle endurance is important, trunk muscles are not the only ones in the body that have endurance requirements.

Much like strength testing, it is appropriate to perform endurance movements that do not have population norms for comparative scoring for assessment purposes. Although normative data is not available for comparison, the number of correctly performed movements with a certain resistance will provide details regarding the muscle's endurance and can be repeated for retesting purposes. This will allow the personal trainer to track changes within an individual muscle group. Additionally, identification of deficiencies that may present obstacles or increase risk for injury is necessary for effective program enactment.

One key consideration for endurance testing is that adequate strength is required for successful completion. A person who performs three push-ups or one pull-up is not being assessed for endurance. Rather, the tests actually identify strength measures. For local muscular endurance to be appropriately assessed, the number of repetitions should ideally reach double digits and emphasize the anaerobic glycolytic pathways. If a client cannot perform at least ten repetitions for a given assessment, then a different test should be selected. Modifications to the test can be made by reducing the resistance applied during the movement. Modified push-ups and pull-ups can be used as an alternative to traditional tests, even though there may not be appropriate gender norms for scoring. Having comparative norms is helpful, but the focus of the data should be for exercise program generation and retesting that individual. If a person performs poorly in all strength and endurance tests, resistance training should be encouraged, with repetition ranges between 12 and 15. This will provide for client acclimation to resisted movements and still encourage both strength and endurance adaptations.

Testing Error

Estimation error is very common in the tests used for muscular fitness. The error is most commonly attributed to four key measurement factors, which include:

1. Poor explanation of the test procedures and the performance criteria used for scoring.

2. Lack of client neuromuscular proficiency or familiarity in the tested movement.

3. Loose scoring guidelines used by the tester.

4. Lack of experience with the resistance loads used for the test.

Strategies to reduce the risk of error require identifying and accounting for the likely pitfalls. Following the guidelines outlined in Chapter 13 will aid in reducing organization and administration error and can also limit client-related error. Employing strict protocol in all testing procedures and scoring, ensuring the client is proficient in the movement and comfortable with the resistance used, and practicing the test so the client knows the scoring criteria before the assessment takes place, are all characteristics of quality testing procedures and will enhance test validity.

When strength tests are used for evaluating older adults, some additional considerations should be made to ensure their safety and successful outcomes. Standard strength protocols are inappropriate for most older adults. A battery of functional tests has been created to predict independence and the ability to successfully complete **activities of daily living (ADLs)**. ADLs include tasks such as cooking and cleaning, getting in and out of vehicles, climbing stairs, dressing, and bathing. The most common tests are the single arm-curl, 30-second chair stand, and the 8-foot up-and-go. These practical tests are easy to implement and provide valid, reliable, normalized data for individuals between the ages of 60 and 94. Classifications of scores should be viewed along a continuum of function. Difficulty or failure to perform these tests correlates with disability and a loss of independence.

Assessment of Anaerobic Power & Capacity

Muscular strength and endurance can contribute to a functional measure of anaerobic power and capacity. Note that neither strength and power nor endurance and anaerobic capacity are synonymous. Each is reflected in some degree within the other, but specific physiological factors distinguish each. Rather than analyzing neurophysiological contractile factors such as recruitment, synchronicity, and firing rate, anaerobic power and capacity emphasizes biochemical measures, including energy system efficiency, fatigue rate, and the resultant total work.

Power is the amount of work performed in a given time and is often associated with athletic performance in sports. Personal trainers should realize that power is not only a performance related component of fitness for athletes but also a key component to functional health performance. Individuals who do not possess adequate power will have difficulty rising from bed, getting out of a chair, and often suffer significant gait speed decline. Low levels of power correlate to disability and loss of independence.

Low power measures require special attention in the exercise prescription, with an emphasis on improving movement rate and body segment velocity to prevent functional attrition. The functional chair stand test is actually a power exercise for older adults with a goal of increasing rate of speed. Healthy individuals are more commonly tested by vertical jump or anaerobic power stepping.

Anaerobic capacity simply measures power-rate decline. In other words, it is the length of time that a muscle can perform an activity utilizing the anaerobic glycolytic pathway to regenerate ATP until fatigue. For an individual, anaerobic capacity is the ability to perform sustained work at elevated intensity levels for extended periods of time. Most capacity tests last 15, 30, 60, or 90 seconds, depending on what component of capacity is being emphasized. The two components of anaerobic capacity are either the body's ability to sustain high intensity levels for a short duration of time or the ability to perform moderate intensity levels until fatigue. Performances lasting less than 30 seconds gauge the duration of time maximal output can be sustained. Tests lasting 60 to 90 seconds analyze the power-rate of decline. Some tests can be used to identify both anaerobic power and capacity, including the Wingate bike test and anaerobic power step test, because their protocols use measures during different time segments throughout the test. A measure is done at 5 or 15 seconds and then again at 30 or 60 seconds. Each value is placed in a predictive equation to calculate watts or joules (units of power). Anaerobic capacity tests are probably better predictors of functional capability than strength tests due to the number of physiological factors involved, but they may also be associated with a degree of risk when employed with the wrong population. Clients should be categorized as healthy and maintain appropriate fitness before engaging in these tests.

~Key Terms~

VO$_2$ max - The highest rate at which oxygen can be taken up and utilized by an individual during exercise.

Muscular strength – The ability of a person to exert a maximal quantifiable force against an object.

Muscular endurance – The ability of a person to sustain a continual muscular exertion over a given period of time.

Activities of daily living (ADLs) – Activities that require a baseline functional ability and are completed every day such as sitting, standing, dressing, bathing, etc.

Anaerobic capacity – The length of time that a muscle can perform an activity utilizing the anaerobic glycolytic pathway to generate ATP until fatigue.

Flexibility Assessments

Flexibility testing is often overlooked or undervalued in many fitness evaluations. This is also true within the exercise prescription. Either due to lack of knowledge, or the fact that flexibility activities do not provide tangible changes in the body, flexibility is the least employed health-related component of fitness. Interestingly, flexibility directly relates to functional independence in the elderly and is a key factor in activity decline with age. A negative, self-perpetuating loop exists in which flexibility declines with reduced physical activity, and as flexibility declines, subsequent physical activity status declines due to reduced movement capacity. This further reduces individual flexibility and leads to significant decline in physical activity throughout later stages of life. A lack of flexibility is associated with acute and chronic lower back pain and musculoskeletal injuries. Personal trainers should emphasize flexibility in exercise programming and use a battery of tests to ensure adequate levels are maintained throughout a person's lifespan. In addition, it should be understood that flexibility contributes to specific sports related performance. Flexibility exercises should be further emphasized for those clients looking to increase performance in particular events above that required for normal function.

In traditional health and fitness testing batteries, flexibility testing has used the sit-and-reach as the staple evaluation protocol. However, since flexibility is joint specific, over the last decade, health professionals have recognized the limitations of the sit-and-reach test as a suitable assessment for total body flexibility. Additionally, the validity of the test has come under scrutiny and has been determined by many to be a poor measure of flexibility in the low back, as it was originally designed (3; 4; 8-12). The test requires a subject to sit with legs extended and feet flat against a measurement box, while reaching forward with outstretched arms using hip and trunk flexion. Limb length discrepancies, sacral angle, and spinal segment variability reduce the validity of the assessment when comparing individuals against normalized standard values. For these reasons the modified sit-and-reach may be a better indicator of hamstring flexibility compared to its predecessor, but limitations still exist in its use as a predictor of total body flexibility (5).

As indicated above, flexibility, like strength, is specific to a particular joint movement. This suggests that a number of assessments should be used to identify the range of motion in all movement capabilities of the body. The need for multiple measures is further supported by common differences between bilateral joints. For lateralized joints like the shoulder, it is important to assess both the right and left sides, as discrepancies often exist based on the actions an individual performs. For example, a tennis player who holds the racquet in his or her right hand may have excellent right shoulder flexibility, but limited left shoulder flexibility due to the difference in usage. Additionally, as seen with strength considerations, a similar agonist-antagonist relationship exists at each joint. Range of motion deficiencies on one side of a joint can lead to structural adjustments as the tight side places an uneven pull on the components of the articulation. Identifying areas of concern before they manifest into serious limitations or injuries should be a goal of any exercise program.

The difficulty with most flexibility assessments lies in the scoring method. The ideal situation is to utilize a **goniometer**, which measures the angle of a given joint during full attainable range of motion. The device works like a mathematical protractor. The pivot point, or axis of rotation, is placed over the joint, and the arms of the instrument are aligned with the bones of the joint to determine the angle. **Electronic inclinometers** and other specialized devices may also be used for accurate assessment but require a level of expertise and are often cost prohibitive. Limited normative data exists for all flexibility tests, but again, the primary goal of the assessment is to identify baseline measures for exercise prescriptions and retesting of an individual client.

Another group of measuring devices used for quantifiable data are alignment mats. These floor or wall mats use 360 degree or linear line patterns to identify the client's range of motion angle. They are relatively inexpensive, easy to use, and provide quality data for range determination and retest analysis. Any movement can be performed on, or in front of, the mat to assess the degree of range.

If a measuring device is not used, visual assessments can still be useful. Predetermined angles related to function can be fairly well identified and used in the evaluation process. Taking still photographs of the end range of motion on a digital camera can provide excellent data for retest comparisons. Additionally, observed biomechanical adjustments that occur during the assessment should be recorded for analysis, and any pain associated with the movements should be documented. Keeping detailed and organized records helps streamline the program and positively aids in the decision-making process.

Body Composition Assessments

Chapter 10 covered the relative importance of body fat testing, as well as the commonly used protocols. This section focuses on reinforcing some key elements of the testing rationale and common areas for testing error. Consistent with other fitness tests, the client is the central factor in the test selection for body composition analysis. Each specific type of assessment used for body composition has advantages and disadvantages related to the test, and some have population limitations. The four biggest factors related to the decision of using one testing method over another are: 1) validity of the test, 2) the client population, 3) the tester's skill set, and 4) the psychological impact on the client. Creating a value system for test selection may help in the decision to select one test over another.

Increasing accuracy related to these four factors can be gained by increasing understanding and proficiency in the test protocols. Test validity can easily be ascertained by reviewing the documented research that supports the test and identifying the populations the tests were designed for (see chapter 10). Matching the client population with tests that were devised for their characteristics will also help with validity. Testing accuracy is based on the tester's proficiency but also the standard estimation of error inherent to the test. In general, acceptable estimation error should not be higher than 4% because it may change the client's fitness profile and affect appropriate decisions made for the program. The last factor to consider is the psychological impact the testing will have on the client. Most people are embarrassed about their fat level and possess at least some level of body image distress. Non-invasive techniques like girth measurements or bioelectrical impedance should be selected for individuals with obviously higher levels of body fatness.

As a rule of thumb, use skinfold assessments on leaner individuals and girth measurements on everyone else. This limits the need for multi-protocol proficiency and caters to the advantages and disadvantages of both tests. Additionally, the standard estimation of error is about the same for both tests when competently administered and used for the appropriate population. If it is deemed necessary to have a more accurate measurement of body composition, then the client should be tested clinically using **hydrostatic weighing**, **air displacement plethysmography**, or dual-energy x-ray absorptiometry (DEXA). It should be noted that, in most cases, this will not be necessary.

Measurements related to body composition may also be used to identify risk related to disease. BMI measures above 27 are considered a high risk factor for disease and a value of 30 or greater places the individual into the obese category, even if other non-direct measures of body fat have been taken (6; 15; 17). Waist circumference and waist-to-hip ratio may also be used to predict risk for disease based on the charted findings. The identification of high levels of central adiposity correlates to elevated risk for disease (13; 14).

When personal trainers explain findings from body composition tests, many clients will be surprised and often convey feelings of disbelief. In general, most individuals underestimate their amount of body fat. Dealing with body fat results often requires a level of professional decorum and discretion so that the relevance of the information remains intact without causing the client to experience self-defeating emotions, such as acute depression and lack of self-worth. Emphasizing attainable change and adding a positive spin to the situation will help to keep the client focused on the important factors and prevent feelings of apathy. Additionally, body composition changes take some time to alter; therefore, the trainer should avoid testing too frequently, as this may decrease motivation.

~Key Terms~

Goniometer – An instrument used for measuring specific joint angles with full attainable range of motion.

Electronic inclinometers – An electronic device that helps accurately measure specific joint angles, when used correctly by trained individuals.

Hydrostatic weighing – A clinically analyzed method of determining an individual's body composition in which the individual is weighed in air and subsequently weighed in water of known density. The volume of the individual is equal to the loss of weight in the water, divided by the density of the water.

Air displacement plethysmography – Tested in an apparatus called the 'Bod Pod', this method of measuring an individual's body composition uses air displacement to measure body volume.

Fitness Test Preparation Checklist

Subject Preparation

1. Subject has completed the informed consent. ____

2. Subject has been screened and cleared for participation. ____

3. Subject has read and understands the test procedures. ____

4. Subject understands the starting and stopping procedures. ____

5. Subject knows the stop test indicators. ____

6. Subject understands what is expected for each stage of the test. ____

7. Subject has complied with all pre-test instructions concerning:

    A. Rest. ____

    B. Food. ____

    C. Beverage and hydration status. ____

    D. Drugs – including prescription, stimulants, depressants, alcohol, and tobacco. ____

    E. Appropriate attire. ____

8. Subject does not have illness or injury. ____

9. Subject is not fatigued, stressed, or anxious. ____

10. Subject is not on any medication (prescription or non-prescription). ____

11. Subject has participated in the proper warm-up procedure. ____

Tester Preparation

1. Test to be administered has been determined. ____

2. The protocols for administration are understood. ____

3. Equipment has been tested, calibrated, and is in good working order. ____

4. All necessary equipment, supplies, and recording sheets are ready. ____

5. The test environment is within acceptable limits for:

    A. Cleanliness. ____

    B. Temperature. ____

    C. Humidity. ____

    D. Noise. ____

6. The timing and sequence of testing are set. ____

7. The starting and stopping instructions are clear. ____

8. The subject has been prepared appropriately and meets all guidelines for testing. ____

9. The test atmosphere and environment are controlled. ____

10. Post test activities and responsibilities are set. ____

11. Emergency procedures are determined and understood. ____

Common Field Assessments

Field Test	Population	Type	Method of Scoring
Cardiorespiratory Tests			
1 mile walk	Healthy adult	Submax	Prediction equation
12 minute run	Healthy adult	Submax	Prediction equation
1.5 mile steady state	Healthy adult	Submax	Prediction equation
Forestry step test	Healthy teen/adult	Submax	Prediction equation
YMCA Bike Test	Healthy adult	Submax	Multistage equation
Muscular Strength Tests			
YMCA Bench press	Healthy adult	Max	Measured
Multi-rep Bench press	Athlete	Max	Prediction equation
5 RM Squat	Athlete	Max	Prediction equation
10 RM Leg press	Healthy Adult	Max	Prediction equation
Pull-up	Healthy Adult	Max	Measured
Muscular Endurance Tests			
Push-up	Healthy Adult	Max	Measured
Modified pull-up	Healthy Adult	Max	Measured
Curl-up	Healthy Adult	Max	Timed/measured
Muscular Power Tests			
Vertical jump	Athlete	Max	Measured
Chair stand	Older Adult	Max	Measured
Anaerobic power step	Healthy Adult	Max	Prediction equation
Body Composition Tests			
Skinfold	Non-obese		Prediction equation
Girth measurements	Non-muscular		Prediction equation
Flexibility Tests			
Back scratch	All		Measured
Thomas test	All		Measured
Trunk extension	All		Measured
Hip flexion	All		Measured
Bilateral knee flexion	All		Measured

Cardiorespiratory Test: 1 Mile Walk Test

Equipment

1 mile course
Stopwatch

Directions

1) **Test Preparation**: Client should comply with any pretest checklist requirements.

2) **Test Start**: Have client ready him or herself behind the beginning mark of the measured mile. Trainer initiates the test, stating "Ready, Go" and starts the watch as the client begins walking, as fast as possible, the measured mile or course.

3) **Test Finish**: At the end of the measured mile (4 laps on standard track), the trainer identifies the client's time as they cross the measured mile marker and record the number below.

Time to Completion _____

4) **Recording**: Immediately following the test, palpate and assess the client's heart rate for 10 seconds. Record the client's 10-second heart rate, and calculate the client's 60-second heart rate by multiplying by 6.

5) **Cool Down**: Have the client perform an adequate cool down following the assessment.

6) **Organize Data**: To calculate the client's fitness level you will need to have client data such as: age, current body weight, and gender (this information should have already been gathered prior to any physical activity assessments). In addition, your recording sheet should have the client's 1-mile walk time and 60-second pulse count from Steps 3 and 4.

7) **Calculating Fitness Level**: The following formula is used to calculate VO2max (ml · kg⁻¹ · min⁻¹) for the 1-mile walk test from the recorded information. Using the equation template below, calculate the estimated VO_2max.

$$VO_2max \ (ml \cdot kg^{-1} \cdot min^{-1}) = 132.853 - 0.0769 \ (weight) - 0.3877 \ (age) + 6.315 \ (gender) - 3.2649 \ (time) - 0.1565 \ (HR)$$

- Weight is in pounds
- Age is in years
- Gender = 0 for females and 1 for males
- Time is in minutes and hundredths of a minute (ex. 13.06)
- Heart rate is in beats per minute

Aerobic Fitness Classification (ml · kg · min⁻¹)					
MEN					
	20-29 Y	**30-39 Y**	**40-49 Y**	**50-59 Y**	**60+ Y**
Above Average	≥46.8	≥44.6	≥41.8	≥38.5	≥35.3
Average	42.5-46.7	41.0-44.5	38.1-41.7	35.2-38.4	31.8-35.2
Below Average	<42.4	<40.9	<38	<35.1	<31.7

Aerobic Fitness Classification (ml · kg · min⁻¹)					
WOMEN					
	20-29 Y	**30-39 Y**	**40-49 Y**	**50-59 Y**	**60+ Y**
Above Average	≥38.1	≥36.7	≥33.8	≥30.9	≥29.4
Average	35.2-38	33.9-36.6	30.9-33.7	28.3-30.8	25.9-29.3
Below Average	<35.1	<33.8	<30.8	<28.2	<25.8

Cardiorespiratory Test: 12 Minute Run Test

Equipment
Measured track
Stopwatch

Directions

1) **Test Preparation**: Client is checked for compliance with the pretest checklist and instructed in a proper warm-up activity.

2) **Test Start**: When ready to begin the test, the client will line up at the starting line of the pre-measured track. The trainer will say "Ready, Go" and the client will begin the test.

3) The client will run, jog, and/or walk for the designated time period (12 min) at the fastest tolerable pace.

4) The trainer should supply motivational support and shout out the duration of time remaining following each lap.

5) **Test Finish**: At the end of the 12 minutes, the trainer should place themselves in close proximity to the client to identify the specific location of the client on the track at the end of the allotted time and estimate the distance to the closest 10 yards.

6) Have the client perform a cool down activity.

7) **Calculating Fitness Level**: The fitness level of the client is determined by consulting the table below.

Fitness Level vs. 12-min Distance for Men and Women Ages 13-59 years

Fitness Level	Age (Years)	13-19	20-29	30-39	40-49	50-59
		12 – Minute Distance (Miles)				
Very Poor	Men	<1.30	<1.22	<1.18	<1.14	<1.03
	Women	<1.0	<0.96	<0.94	<0.88	<0.84
Poor	Men	1.30-1.37	1.22-1.31	1.18-1.30	1.14-1.24	1.03-1.16
	Women	1.00-1.18	0.96-1.11	0.95-1.05	0.88-0.98	0.84-0.93
Fair	Men	1.38-1.56	1.32-1.49	1.31-1.45	1.25-1.39	1.17-1.30
	Women	1.19-1.29	1.12-1.22	1.06-1.18	0.99-1.11	0.94-1.05
Good	Men	1.57-1.72	1.50-1.64	1.46-1.56	1.40-1.53	1.31-1.44
	Women	1.30-1.43	1.23-1.34	1.19-1.29	1.12-1.24	1.06-1.18
Excellent	Men	1.73-1.86	1.65-1.76	1.57-1.69	1.54-1.65	1.45-1.58
	Women	1.44-1.51	1.35-1.45	1.30-1.39	1.25-1.34	1.19-1.30
Superior	Men	>1.87	>1.77	>1.70	>1.66	>1.59
	Women	>1.52	>1.46	>1.40	>1.35	>1.31

Maximal Oxygen Consumption (VO₂max) vs. 12-Minute Distance

12-Min Distance (miles)	VO₂max (mL · kg⁻¹ · min⁻¹)
<1.0	<25.0
1.0-1.24	25.0-33.7
1.25-1.49	33.8-42.5
1.50-1.74	42.6-51.5
1.75-2.0	51.6-60.2
>2.0	>60.2

Cardiorespiratory Test: 1.5 Mile Steady State

Equipment
Measured track
Stopwatch

Directions

1) **Test Preparation**: Check that the client has complied with pretest checklist and have them perform an appropriate warm-up activity.

2) **Test Start**: Have client ready him or herself behind the beginning mark of the measured 1.5 miles. Trainer initiates the test, stating "Ready, Go" and starts the watch as the client begins running the 1.5 mile distance (6 laps on a standard track).

3) **Monitor**: As the client passes the start/stop line the trainer informs the client of the lap number they are on and the time. The trainer should also look for signs of physical distress.

4) **Test Finish**: At the completion of lap 6, or 1.5 miles, the trainer records the client's time and has them perform a cool down activity.

5) **Review of Formula**: Calculating the fitness level (estimated VO₂max) from the client's 1.5-mile run time involves the use of the following formula:

$$VO2 = \text{horizontal velocity m·min}^{-1} \times \frac{0.2 \text{ ml · kg}^{-1} \cdot \text{min}^{-1}}{\text{m · min}^{-1}} + 3.5 \text{ ml · kg}^{-1} \cdot \text{min}^{-1}$$

6) **Finding horizontal running velocity (m · min⁻¹)**: The first factor that must be calculated is the average horizontal running velocity of the client in meters per minute. To do this you must convert the distance run into meters and divide it by the number of minutes the client took to complete the run.

Example Meter Conversion
1.5 miles = 2,413.8 meters

2,413.8 must then be divided by the time it took to complete the run in minutes (use whole numbers)

Example (m · min⁻¹) conversion
If it took 12:00 minutes to complete the run, divide the 2,413 meters by 12 minutes.
2,413.8 m ÷ 12 min = 201.15 m · min⁻¹ (horizontal velocity)

If it took 12:13 to complete the run then the divisor would be 12.21

$$\{12 \text{ min} + (13 \text{ sec} \div 60 \text{ sec})\}$$

Perform your conversion below:

2,413.8 meters ÷ _____ minutes = _____ $m \cdot min^{-1}$ (horizontal velocity)

7) **VO$_2$max conversion:** The last calculation that must be performed is the one that will provide you with the client's estimated VO2max. Consider the above example:

$$VO_2 \text{ max} = \text{horizontal velocity } m{\cdot}min^{-1} \text{ x } \frac{0.2 \text{ ml} \cdot kg^{-1} \cdot min^{-1}}{m \cdot min^{-1}} + 3.5 \text{ ml} \cdot kg^{-1} \cdot min^{-1}$$

$$VO_2 max = 201 \, \cancel{m{\cdot}min^{-1}} \text{ x } \frac{0.2 \text{ ml} \cdot kg^{-1} \cdot min^{-1}}{\cancel{m \cdot min^{-1}}} + 3.5 \text{ ml} \cdot kg^{-1} \cdot min^{-1}$$

$$VO_2 max = 43.7 \text{ ml} \cdot kg^{-1} \cdot min^{-1}$$

The following chart can also be used as a quick reference

1.5 Mile Time min:s	VO$_2$max ml · kg^{-1} · min^{-1}	1.5 Mile Time min:s	VO$_2$max ml · kg^{-1} · min^{-1}
<7:31	75	12:31-13:00	39
7:31-8:00	72	13:01-13:30	37
8:01-8:30	67	13:31-14:00	36
8:31-9:00	62	14:01-14:30	34
9:01-9:30	58	14:31-15:00	33
9:31-10:00	55	15:01-15:30	31
10:01-10:30	52	15:31-16:00	30
10:31-11:00	49	16:01-16:30	28
11:01-11:30	46	16:31-17:00	27
11:31-12:00	44	17:01-17:30	26
12:01-12:30	41	17:31-18:00	25

Cardiorespiratory Test: Forestry Step Test

Equipment
Step or Box (15.75 inches or 13 inches)
Metronome
Stopwatch

Directions

1) **Test Preparation**: Ensure the client has complied with the pretest checklist. Using a 40 cm (15.75 in) box or step for men and 33 cm (13.0 in) box or step for women, have client stand facing toward the box.

2) **Practice stepping**: A metronome is set at 90 tones per minute and the client should practice stepping up and then down using a four-count cadence.
"Up-one" Foot #1 goes to the top of the step
"Up-two" The other foot (#2) follows to the top of the step
"Down-one" Foot #1 descends to the floor
"Down-two" Foot #2 descends to the floor
The client should practice until they can establish cadence.
Once proficiency has been demonstrated, allow the client a rest period for the duration of time it takes to return the pulse back to a resting state.

3) **Begin Assessment**: Following the rest interval, re-establish the metronome's pace, 90 tones per minute, and ask the client to take the starting position (facing the box). When they feel ready, they can begin stepping. As soon as the client takes the first step the trainer should begin timing the assessment.

4) **Test Performance**: Have the client continue stepping on and off the box, keeping with the cadence, for 5 minutes.

5) **RPE**: The trainer should maintain visual assessment of the client throughout the duration of the test. This is for proper identification of any signs and symptoms listed on the Stop Test Indicator check list. They should also periodically ask the client how they are feeling based on their RPE. The RPE for this type of submaximal assessment should not exceed 7 on a 1 to 10 scale, or 16 on a 1 to 20 scale.

6) **Palpation Preparation**: When the stopwatch reaches 5:00 have the client stop stepping. Be sure to keep the watch running as it will be used to assess the recovery heart rate of the subject. Immediately locate the client's radial pulse as the clock continues to run. Marking the site before beginning the test may aid in rapid identification.

7) **Recovery Heart Rate Palpation**: Once the stopwatch reads 5:15 the trainer begins counting the client's recovery heart rate through the palpation of the radial artery.

8) Monitoring/counting of the client's heart rate should start at the 5:15 mark and end at the 5:30 mark. This will provide the client's heart rate in 15 seconds.

9) Record 15-second recovery heart rate. Then have client perform a cool down.

   Recovery heart rate (15 seconds) _____ beats min^{-1}

Procedures for Estimating VO$_2$max:

10) **Calculate Fitness Level Score**: Using the 15-second recovery heart rate recorded in step #9, find the client's non-age adjusted fitness score on Table A. To do this, you must refer to the correct gender table (Table A). Follow the left-hand column down until you find the number that represents the client's 15-second recovery heart rate from step #9. Follow the row over to the right to intersect with the subject's weight listed at the bottom of the table. This number will provide you the subject's non-age adjusted fitness score.

    Enter score here _____ non-age-adjusted fitness score (ml · kg^{-1} · min^{-1})

11) **Calculate age-adjusted estimated VO$_2$max**: To find the age-adjusted fitness score you will need the value from above. Find the client's fitness score on the top column of the table labeled Age-Adjusted Fitness Score (Table B). Intersect this score with the closest age value listed down the left side column and you will have found the client's age-adjusted fitness level or VO$_2$max (ml · kg^{-1} · min^{-1}).

    Enter score here _____ age-adjusted fitness score (ml · kg^{-1} · min^{-1})

12) **Evaluating the Results**: To find out what fitness category the client falls into refer to the table titled Aerobic Fitness Categories in Men and Women (Table C). Intersect the client's age in the left-hand column with the client's age-adjusted fitness score from Table B. The fitness classification is listed across the top of the chart.

    Enter classification here _____

Table A - Non-Adjusted Aerobic Fitness (ml • kg^{-1} • min^{-1}) for MEN

Pulse Count	Max Oxygen Consumption												
45	33	33	33	33	33	32	32	32	32	32	32	32	32
44	34	34	34	34	33	33	33	33	33	33	33	33	33
43	35	35	35	34	34	34	34	34	34	34	34	34	34
42	36	35	35	35	35	35	35	35	35	35	35	34	34
41	36	36	36	36	36	36	36	36	36	36	35	35	35
40	37	37	37	37	37	37	37	37	37	37	36	35	35
39	38	38	38	38	38	38	38	38	38	38	38	37	37
38	39	39	39	39	39	39	39	39	39	39	39	38	38
37	41	40	40	40	40	40	40	40	40	40	40	39	39
36	42	42	41	41	41	41	41	41	41	41	41	40	40
35	43	43	42	42	42	42	42	42	42	42	42	42	41
34	44	44	43	43	43	43	43	43	43	43	43	43	43
33	46	45	45	45	45	45	44	44	44	44	44	44	44
32	47	47	46	46	46	46	46	46	46	46	46	46	46
31	48	48	48	47	47	47	47	47	47	47	47	47	47
30	50	49	49	49	48	48	48	48	48	48	48	48	48
29	52	51	51	51	50	50	59	50	50	50	50	50	50
28	53	53	53	53	52	52	52	52	51	51	51	51	51
27	55	55	55	54	54	54	54	54	54	53	53	53	52
26	57	57	56	56	56	56	56	56	56	55	55	54	54
25	59	59	58	58	58	58	58	58	58	56	56	55	55
24	60	60	60	60	60	60	60	59	59	58	58	57	
23	62	62	61	61	61	61	61	60	60	60	59		
22	64	64	63	63	63	63	62	62	61	61			
21	66	66	65	65	65	64	64	64	62				
20	68	68	67	67	67	67	66	66	65				
WT	120	130	140	150	160	170	180	190	200	210	220	230	240

Table A – Non-Adjusted Aerobic Fitness (ml • kg^{-1} • min^{-1}) for WOMEN

Pulse Count	Max Oxygen Consumption											
45										29	29	29
44								30	30	30	30	30
43							31	31	31	31	31	31
42			32	32	32	32	32	32	32	32	32	32
41			33	33	33	33	33	33	33	33	33	33
40			34	34	34	34	34	34	34	34	34	34
39			35	35	35	35	35	35	35	35	35	35
38			36	36	36	36	36	36	36	36	36	36
37			37	37	37	37	37	37	37	37	37	37
36		37	38	38	38	38	38	38	38	38	38	38
35	38	38	39	39	39	39	39	39	39	39	39	39
34	39	39	40	40	40	40	40	40	40	40	40	40
33	40	40	41	41	41	41	41	41	41	41	41	41
32	41	41	42	42	42	42	42	42	42	42	42	42
31	42	42	43	43	43	43	43	43	43	43	43	43
30	43	43	44	44	44	44	44	44	44	44	44	44
29	44	44	45	45	45	45	45	45	45	45	45	45
28	45	45	46	46	46	47	47	47	47	47	47	47
27	46	46	47	48	48	49	49	49	49	49		
26	47	48	49	50	50	51	51	51	51			
25	49	50	51	52	52	53	53					
24	51	52	53	54	54	55						
23	53	54	55	56	56	57						
WT	80	90	100	110	120	130	140	150	160	170	180	190

Table B – Age-Adjusted Fitness Score

Fitness Score From Table A																					
	30	31	32	33	34	35	36	37	38	39	40	41	42	43	44	45	46	47	48	49	50
AGE	Age-Adjusted score (ml • kg^{-1} • min^{-1})																				
15	32	33	34	35	36	37	38	39	40	41	42	43	44	45	46	47	48	49	50	51	53
20	31	32	33	34	35	36	37	38	39	40	41	42	43	44	45	46	47	48	49	50	51
25	30	31	32	33	34	35	36	37	38	39	40	41	42	43	44	45	46	47	48	49	50
30	29	30	31	32	33	34	35	36	37	38	39	40	41	42	43	44	45	46	47	48	49
35	27	28	29	31	32	33	34	35	36	37	38	39	40	41	42	43	44	45	46	47	48
40	26	27	28	30	31	32	33	34	35	36	37	38	39	40	41	42	43	44	45	46	47
45	25	26	27	29	30	31	32	33	34	35	36	37	38	39	40	41	42	43	44	45	46
50	24	25	26	28	29	30	31	32	33	34	35	36	37	38	39	40	41	42	43	44	45
55	23	24	25	27	28	29	30	31	32	33	34	35	36	37	38	39	40	40	41	42	43
60	22	23	24	25	26	27	28	30	31	32	33	34	35	36	37	37	38	39	40	41	42
65	21	22	23	24	25	26	27	28	29	30	31	32	33	34	35	36	37	38	38	39	40

Table B – Age-Adjusted Fitness Score

Fitness Score From Table A																				
51	52	53	54	55	56	57	58	59	60	61	62	63	64	65	66	67	68	69	70	71

AGE	Age-Adjusted score (ml · kg^{-1} · min^{-1})																			
15	54	55	56	57	58	59	60	61	62	63	64	65	66	67	68	69	70	71	72	74	75
20	52	53	54	55	56	57	58	59	60	61	62	63	64	65	66	67	68	69	70	71	73
25	51	52	53	54	55	56	57	58	59	60	61	62	63	64	65	66	67	68	69	70	72
30	50	51	52	53	54	55	56	57	58	59	60	61	62	63	64	65	66	67	68	69	71
35	49	50	51	52	53	54	55	56	57	58	59	60	60	61	62	63	64	65	66	67	69
40	48	49	50	51	52	53	54	55	55	56	57	58	59	60	61	62	63	64	65	66	68
45	47	48	49	50	51	52	52	53	54	55	56	57	58	59	60	61	62	63	64	65	66
50	45	46	47	48	49	50	51	52	53	53	54	55	56	57	58	58	59	61	61	62	64
55	44	45	46	46	47	48	49	50	51	52	53	53	54	55	56	57	58	59	59	60	62
60	42	43	44	45	46	46	47	48	49	50	51	51	52	53	54	55	56	57	57	58	60
65	41	42	42	43	44	45	46	46	47	48	49	50	50	51	52	53	54	54	55	56	58

Table C - Aerobic fitness categories for men and women for The Forestry Step Test

Age	Sex	Superior	Excellent	Very Good	Good	Fair	Poor	Very Poor
15	M	57+	56-52	51-47	46-42	41-37	36-32	<32
	F	54+	53-49	48-44	43-39	38-34	33-29	<29
20	M	56+	55-51	50-46	45-41	40-36	35-31	<31
	F	53+	52-48	47-43	42-38	37-33	32-28	<28
25	M	55+	54-50	49-45	44-40	39-35	34-30	<30
	F	52+	51-47	46-42	41-37	36-32	31-27	<27
30	M	54+	53-49	48-44	43-39	38-34	33-29	<29
	F	51+	50-46	45-41	40-36	35-31	30-26	<26
35	M	53+	52-48	47-43	42-38	37-33	32-28	<28
	F	50+	49-45	44-40	39-35	34-30	29-25	<25
40	M	52+	51-47	46-42	41-37	36-32	31-27	<27
	F	49+	48-44	43-39	38-34	33-29	28-24	<24
45	M	51+	50-46	45-41	40-36	35-31	30-26	<26
	F	48+	47-43	42-38	37-33	32-28	27-33	<23
50	M	50+	49-45	44-40	39-35	34-30	29-25	<25
	F	47+	46-42	41-37	36-32	31-27	26-22	<22
55	M	49+	48-44	43-39	38-34	33-29	28-24	<24
	F	46+	45-41	40-36	35-31	30-26	25-21	<21
60	M	48+	47-43	42-38	37-33	32-28	27-23	<23
	F	45+	44-40	39-35	34-30	29-25	24-20	<20
65	M	47+	48-42	41-37	36-32	31-27	26-22	<22
	F	44+	43-39	38-34	33-29	28-24	23-20	<20

Cardiorespiratory Test: YMCA Bike Test

Equipment
Cycle ergometer (Monark)
Blood pressure cuff
RPE chart
Stopwatch

Directions

1) **Test Preparation**: Ensure the client has complied with the pretest checklist.

2) **Start Test**: With a metronome set at the required cadence (100 beats · min^{-1}), start the timer as soon as the client begins pedaling at the required 50 rev · min^{-1} and required first stage work rate of 150 kgm · min^{-1} (.5 kp).

3) **Monitor Blood Pressure**: At 1:30 take and record client's blood pressure.

4) **Monitor Heart Rate**: At 2:00 take and record HR.

5) **Assess RPE**: Ask participant how they are doing and record subject's RPE.

6) **Monitor Heart Rate Response to Determine Subsequent Workload**: At 3:00 take and record HR. If the client's HR is less than 85% of max, blood pressure is responding normally, and the client is performing satisfactory, increase the resistance to the next stage.

7) Refer to the table below to find out the correct workload for the next stage. The subsequent workloads are based on the heart rate response at the end of the first stage.

8) Repeat steps 1-5, increasing workload by the correct increments until a steady-state HR of over 110 beats · min^{-1} is attained.

9) The client should then continue one more stage after a HR of 110 beats · min^{-1} is reached. For example, if during stage 2 the client's 2nd minute HR is 113 beats · min^{-1} and 3rd minute HR is 115 beats · min^{-1} then they have reached steady-state and also have reached the desired 110 beats per minute for the test. The trainer should then have the client proceed with one more 3 minute stage following the outlined workload protocols below and record all designated physiological values on a provided chart.

10) The trainer should plot the results from each stage on the graph on the following page.

11) After plotting the heart rate values at the completion of the 2 (or 3) workloads, extrapolate the line outward to the subject's age-predicted maximum heart rate. Then draw a line downward toward the x-axis. Where the line bisects the x-axis is the subject's predicted VO$_2$max.

12) Record the predicted VO$_2$ max value _____ L · min^{-1}

13) Convert to relative VO$_2$max _____ ml · kg^{-1} · min^{-1}

Time	Stage	Heart Rate Response and Corresponding Workload			
0:00-3:00	First	150 kgm · min^{-1}			
3:00-6:00	Second	HR <80 750 kgm·min^{-1} 2.5kp	HR 80-89 600 kgm·min^{-1} 2.0kp	HR 90-100 450 kgm·min^{-1} 1.5kp	HR >100 300 kgm·min^{-1} 1.0kp
6:00-9:00	Third	HR <80 900 kgm·min^{-1} 3.0kp	HR 80-89 750 kgm·min^{-1} 2.5kp	HR 90-100 600 kgm·min^{-1} 2.0kp	HR >100 450 kgm·min^{-1} 1.5kp
9:00-12:00	Fourth	HR <80 1050 kgm·min^{-1} 3.5kp	HR 80-89 900 kgm·min^{-1} 3.0kp	HR 90-100 750 kgm·min^{-1} 2.5kp	HR >100 600 kgm·min^{-1} 2.0kp

YMCA Data Recording Sheet

Name:	Sex:	Age:	Weight:	Max HR:	85% HR:
Stage 1 Work Rate	150 kgm · min⁻¹ (.5 kp)	150 kgm · min⁻¹ (.5 kp)	150 kgm · min⁻¹ (.5 kp)	150 kgm · min⁻¹ (.5 kp)	150 kgm · min⁻¹ (.5 kp)
0:00-3:00	2ⁿᵈ min HR	3ʳᵈ min HR	Steady State HR?	1:30 BP mmHg	RPE:1-10
			Y or N		
Stage 2 Work Rate	_____ kgm · min⁻¹	_____ kgm · min⁻¹	_____ kgm · min⁻¹	_____ kgm · min⁻¹	_____ kgm · min⁻¹
3:00-6:00	2ⁿᵈ min HR	3ʳᵈ min HR	Steady State HR?	1:30 BP mmHg	RPE:1-10
			Y or N		
Stage 3 Work Rate	_____ kgm · min⁻¹	_____ kgm · min⁻¹	_____ kgm · min⁻¹	_____ kgm · min⁻¹	_____ kgm · min⁻¹
6:00-9:00	2ⁿᵈ min HR	3ʳᵈ min HR	Steady State HR?	1:30 BP mmHg	RPE:1-10
			Y or N		
Stage 4 Work Rate	_____ kgm · min⁻¹	_____ kgm · min⁻¹	_____ kgm · min⁻¹	_____ kgm · min⁻¹	_____ kgm · min⁻¹
9:00-12:00	2ⁿᵈ min HR	3ʳᵈ min HR	Steady State HR?	1:30 BP mmHg	RPE:1-10
			Y or N		

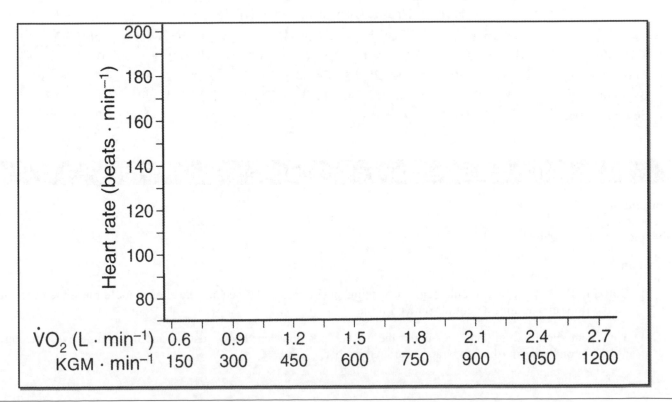

Muscular Strength Test: YMCA Bench Press

Equipment
Flat Bench
Olympic bar and weights
Metronome

Directions

1) **Set-up**: The trainer should set up the bar with the appropriate resistance: men use 80 lbs. (36 kg); women use 35 lbs. (16 kg).

2) The trainer then sets the metronome at a cadence of 60 beats · min^{-1}.

3) **Starting Position**: The client lies in a supine position on a bench with knees bent and feet flat on the floor.

4) Client grips bar using a pronated, shoulder width hand position.

5) The trainer asks the client to count to 3 when they are ready to begin, and the trainer provides a lift off of the bar.

6) The client presses on pace with the metronome by moving the bar upward until the arms are fully extended, but not locked, before returning to the chest – completing one repetition.

7) **Breathing**: Encourage the client to exhale during the concentric contraction and inhale at the top of the lift to initiate the eccentric movement. The client should also be instructed not to strain during the test.

8) The trainer should stop the test when the client no longer keeps pace with the metronome or technique is compromised.

9) **Recording**: The trainer should then record the successful number of repetitions.

Scoring: Identify the score and relative fitness value using the chart below.

Bench Press Classification Table									
	18-25 Y		**26-35 Y**		**36-45 Y**		**46-55 Y**		**56-65 Y**	
Classification	**M**	**F**	**M**	**F**	**M**	**F**	**M**	**F**	**M**	**F**
Above Average	30-42	28-40	26-40	25-40	24-34	21-32	20-28	21-30	14-24	16-30
Average	22-29	20-27	20-25	17-24	17-23	13-20	12-19	12-20	8-13	9-15
Below Average	<21	<19	<19	<16	<16	<12	<11	<11	<7	<8

Muscular Strength Test: Multi-rep Bench Press

Equipment
Flat bench
Olympic bar and weights

Directions

1) **Starting Position**: Client should begin in a supine position on a flat bench. The client should place their feet flat on the floor and assume a neutral spine position.

2) The client should align their eyes under the bar and position their hands just outside of shoulder width using a closed, pronated grip (thumps wrapped around the bar).

3) The client should then lift the bar off the rack with assistance from the trainer and position it over their chest with arms fully extended.

4) **Downward Movement Phase**: The client should begin lowering the bar in a slow and controlled movement down toward their chest. As the descent is made, the body should remain fixed on the bench with no extraneous body movement.

5) The bar should descend in a slow and controlled manner until it makes contact with the midline of the chest. The descent phase should last approximately 2 seconds.

6) **Upward Movement Phase**: Once bar contact has been made with the client's chest, the client presses the bar upward in the same plane of motion as used during the descent phase.

7) The bar is pressed upward until the arms are fully extended. The ascent phase should also last approximately 2 seconds, maintaining the controlled speed throughout the movement to avoid momentum forces.

8) **Spotting**: The trainer should lift the bar off the rack to the start position. This will reduce stress on the glenohumeral joint during the lift off.

9) As the bar is lowered during the eccentric phase, the trainer should spot the bar without contact, cueing controlled deceleration to the chest. Upon the concentric contraction, the trainer should monitor the upward movement phase with hands supinated under the bar inside the client's grip position.

10) When re-racking the bar it should be placed securely in the rack. If the rack has low rack arms, the trainer should be sure the bar does not exceed the height of the rack. This is of particular concern for individuals with long limbs and during close grip lifts.

11) The predicted maximum can be calculated using the following formula:

3% Formula

[(0.03 x Reps _____) + 1.0] x weight used _____ lb.

[_____ + 1.0] x _____ lb.

Bench Press Score = _____ lb.

12) *Interpret Results*. The table below illustrates Relative Bench Press Strength Norms based on body weight in both males and females. To find your subject's strength classification, divide the subject's calculated 1RM by current body weight.

Weight lifted ÷ body weight = Upper Body Strength Rating

Upper Body Strength Rating _____

Classification	20-29 Y		30-39 Y		40-49 Y		50-59 Y		60 +	
	M	F	M	F	M	F	M	F	M	F
Above Average	>1.17	>.72	>1.01	>.62	>.91	>.57	>.81	>.51	>.74	>.51
Average	.97-1.16	.59-.71	.86-1.00	.53-.61	.78-.90	.48-.56	.70-.80	.43-.50	.63-.73	.41-.50
Below Average	<.96	<.58	<.85	<.52	<.77	<.47	<.69	<.42	<.62	<.40

Muscular Strength Test: 5 RM Squat

Equipment
Squat rack
Olympic bar and weights

Directions

1) **Starting Position**: Prior to the performance of the exercise, the correct bar height must be set so that the client can safely position the bar on the trapezius and step clear of the bar holder (rack). To do this, the bar height should be set at approximately the height of the lifter's upper chest.

2) Once the bar is set at the correct height, the client faces the bar and grasps it with a closed, pronated grip. The hands should be placed slightly wider than shoulder width apart.

3) The client then steps under the bar and positions it across the superior aspect of the scapula – on top of the trapezius. *DO NOT place the bar across the cervical spine. The scapula should be retracted to help provide rigidity to the upper spine.

4) To attain the correct starting position, the client must extend the knees to lift the bar off the rack. Once the weight is suspended and the client has established control under load, they must slowly step backward (one to two foot clearance) to avoid coming in contact with the rack during the execution phase of the lift.

5) Once clear of the rack, the client again places the feet shoulder width apart and positions the feet so that they are pointing forward and slightly outward. The degree of outward rotation will be consistent with the natural standing gait of the client and is often dictated by hip complex anatomy.

6) **Downward Movement Phase:** The client initiates the downward movement by simultaneously flexing the hips and knees, pushing the glutes backward. The transversospinalis (erector spinae) group remains isometrically contracted, the head remains forward, and the chest elevated as the client further flexes the hips and knees to continue the descent.

7) The ideal end-point ROM is when the top of the thigh is parallel with the floor. However, this will be client specific. Never descend beyond functional ROM or compromise ROM to increase weight. Additionally, the knees should not break the plane of the toes during the entire downward movement phase. The descent phase should last approximately 2 to 3 seconds.

8) **Upward Movement Phase:** Once end-point ROM has been reached the client extends the knees and hips.

9) As the weight ascends, the spinal position is maintained through the isometric contraction of the transversospinalis group. The legs should not adduct or abduct during any phase of the execution process.

10) The client should return to the starting position but not lock their knees an athletic stance position should be maintained during the upright starting position. Once the 5RM has been completed, re-rack the bar, checking to be sure the bar is resting safely on the rack. The ascent phase should last approximately 2 to 3 seconds.

11) **Spotting**: Spotting the squat should utilize an upper trunk hand placement technique. The hands of the trainer/spotter should be placed on the outside of the rib cage, just under the chest with the trainer standing behind the lifter. Assume the position right at the lift off of the rack and walk the client to the starting position.

12) The trainer should mirror the lifter's form and speed. This allows the hips to extend and move the client safely into an upright position.

13) If breast contact on a female is a concern, the trainer can use slightly lateral hand position on the rib cage.

14) When the lift is complete the trainer should walk the client back to the rack and watch the bar to make sure it is racked correctly.

15) Calculate the predicted 1RM using the following formula.

Step One: 1.15 x _____ weight used = _____ predicted 1RM

Step Two: _____predicted 1RM / _____body weight

Classification of Relative Squat Strength (1 RM/body mass)									
	20-29 Y		30-39 Y		40-49 Y		50-59 Y		60+ Y	
Classification	**M**	**F**	**M**	**F**	**M**	**F**	**M**	**F**	**M**	**F**
Above Average	>1.84	>1.36	>1.64	>1.21	>1.57	>1.13	>1.47	>1.08	>1.37	>1.00
Average	1.63-1.84	1.26-1.36	1.55-1.64	1.13-1.21	1.50-1.57	1.06-1.13	1.40-1.47	.86-1.08	1.31-1.37	.85-1.00
Below Average	<1.63	<1.26	<1.55	<1.13	<1.50	<1.06	<1.40	<.86	<1.31	<.85

Muscular Strength Test: 10 RM Leg Press

Equipment
Leg press
Adequate weight

Directions

1) **Starting Position:** The client assumes a seated position in the leg press machine.

2) The back is pressed flat against the back pad and feet are placed flat on the footplate, approximately shoulder width apart.

3) The lumbar spine should be pressed firmly into the pad and the knees should be slightly flexed prior to disengaging the load from the machine.

4) **Downward Movement Phase:** The client extends the legs slowly and disengages the weight (usually by a rotating handle). With the back pressed firmly against the back pad, the weight is descended slowly toward the client, causing the knees to flex in front of the client's chest. As the weight descends, the lumbar spine and glutes **must** stay in contact with the back support pad.

5) The weight is lowered until full, functional ROM has been reached. This will vary from person to person. Individual flexibility limitations of the glutes, low back, and hamstrings will dictate specific endpoint ROM. At no point should the glutes rise off the back pad due to the engagement of a posterior pelvic tilt.

6) Consistent with all compound leg movements, the client's knees should not be flexed more than 90°, and at no point should the knees break the plane of the toes. The descent phase should last approximately 2 to 3 seconds.

7) **Upward Movement Phase:** Once full, functional ROM has been attained or the knees have reached 90° of flexion, the client applies additional force through the heels into the footplate and extends the legs.

8) The ascent is continued to a point just before full knee extension occurs. The knees are never placed into full extension or a "locked" position at any point during the execution. The ascent phase should last approximately 2 to 3 seconds.

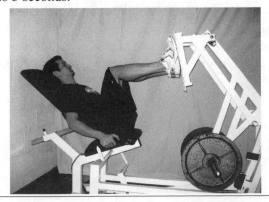 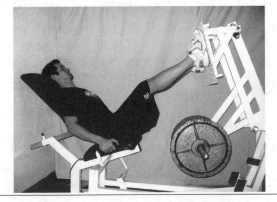

9) **Spotting**: Spotting the leg press requires the trainer to stand on the side of the machine. The trainer should provide support to the movement plate at the lift off and be sure the client is ready and supporting the weight.

10) Trainers should have client's perform the repetitions watching for controlled deceleration and smooth acceleration. If assistance is needed, the trainer should supply force to the footplate and hold it at the end point while the client locks the weight into place with the handles.

11) Use the following formula to calculate the predicted 1RM from a ten repetition performance.

Step One: 1.3 x _____ weight used = _____ predicted 1RM

Step Two: _____ predicted 1RM / _____ body weight

Classification of Relative Leg Press Strength (1 RM/body mass)

Classification	20-29 Y M	20-29 Y F	30-39 Y M	30-39 Y F	40-49 Y M	40-49 Y F	50-59 Y M	50-59 Y F	60+ Y M	60+ Y F
Above Average	>1.97	>1.42	>1.85	>1.47	>1.74	>1.35	>1.64	>1.24	>1.56	>1.18
Average	1.91-1.97	1.32-1.42	1.71-1.85	1.26-1.47	1.62-1.74	1.19-1.35	1.52-1.64	1.09-1.24	1.43-1.56	1.08-1.18
Below Average	<1.91	<1.32	<1.71	<1.26	<1.62	<1.19	<1.52	<1.09	<1.43	<1.08

Muscular Strength Test: Pull-up

Equipment
Pull-up bar

Directions

1) **Starting Position**: The client should start with hands in a pronated position and grasp a pull-up bar approximately shoulder width apart.

2) Extend the arms and slowly transfer the weight of the body to the extended arms. If the feet make contact with the ground, flex the knees so that no body to ground contact is possible at the lowest end range of motion during the test.

3) **Upward Movement Phase**: To initiate the upward phase of the movement, the client must flex the arms by contracting the biceps while simultaneously depressing and inwardly rotating the scapula. As the ascent progresses, the scapula will rotate further inward. The upward ascent should continue until the client's chin has passed the top of the bar.

4) **Downward Movement Phase**: After the chin has passed the top of the bar the client should begin initiating the downward phase of the movement by extending the arms.

5) As the descent progresses, the scapula should protract and outwardly rotate. The decent should be slow and controlled to a point of full arm extension. The descent phase should last approximately 2 to 3 seconds.

6) **Spotting**: The pull-up exercise is usually reserved for individuals who maintain a mid to high level of muscular strength. Trainers can effectively spot the exercise by providing assistance to the lower outside portion of the client's lats or upper torso. It is not recommended to spot the feet or legs due to changes in spinal alignment and grip failure concerns for the client. The exercise can be changed into a chin-up by narrowing the grip and using a supinated hand position.

Classification for Males (> 17 Y)				Classification for Females (> 17 Y)		
Below Average	Average	Above Average		Below Average	Average	Above Average
<7	8-10	≥11		0	1	>1

Muscular Endurance Test: Push-up

Equipment
Towel or foam roller
Stopwatch

Directions

1) **Starting Position**: Start with the client in a prone position on the floor with body extended. The client should place the hands approximately shoulder width apart with thumbs located directly under the shoulders. The feet should be or no more than 6" apart.

2) Have the client lift the body to a point where the arms are completely extended and the body is in proper alignment (Do not allow the body to engage in hip extension or hip flexion during any phase of the movement).

3) Place a towel (rolled up to a thickness of approximately 3" in width) or cut foam roll directly under the chest of the subject.

4) **Begin Assessment**: Once the towel is in place, the trainer should give the "Go" command and begin timing. The client should lower themselves in a rigid, straight position down to a point at which their elbows are at approximately 90° of flexion, a point which should have their chest making contact with the towel.

5) **Movement Repetition**: The client returns to the extended arm position by pushing upward until the elbows are fully extended.

6) This movement should be performed until failure or technique breakdown occurs. The trainer should count out loud each repetition the client completes correctly.

7) **Note:** During the execution of the test be sure that the client performs the movement through full ROM. It is not uncommon for a client to limit ROM to try and achieve a higher score. It is also important that the subject maintains rigid body position. At no time should the spine/torso be placed in a flexed or hyperextended position.

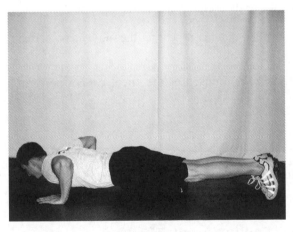 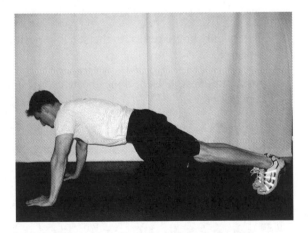

8) **Record**: The trainer should record the number of repetitions successfully performed in one minute on the Data Recording Sheet.

Number of Repetitions Completed _____

Classifications for Push-up Test

Men	15-19 Y	20-29 Y	30-39 Y	40-49 Y	50-59 Y	60-69 Y
Above Average	>28	>28	>21	>16	>12	>10
Average	22-28	21-28	17-21	13-16	10-12	8-10
Below Average	<22	<21	<17	<13	<10	<8
Women						
Above Average	>24	>20	>19	>14	>11	>10
Average	18-24	15-20	13-19	11-14	7-11	5-10
Below Average	<18	<15	<13	<11	<7	<5

Muscular Endurance Test: Modified Pull-up

Equipment
Smith machine or equivalent

Directions

1) **Start Position**: The client should stand with the Smith Machine bar at a point just below chest height (xyphoid process).

2) Using an overhand, pronated grip, the client should walk the feet forward until they have established a 45 degree floor to body position while hanging from the bar. Their body should be straight and their feet on the ground.

3) **Start the Test**: Once the position has been established, the client can initiate the pull and continue retracting the scapula and flexing the arms until the bar touches the chest or their chin is above the bar at a designated point.

4) The client should return to the starting position in a controlled manner repeating the movement as many times as possible.

5) **Stop the Test**: Discontinue the test once proper form is compromised or the client cannot perform any more repetitions.

6) **Record**: Document the results.

Number of Repetitions Completed _____

Classification for the Modified Pull-up (Adults 17+ Y)

	Male	Female
Above Average	≥22	≥9
Average	14-21	4-8
Below Average	<14	<4

Muscular Endurance Test: Abdominal Curl-up

Equipment
Mat
Metronome

Directions

1) **Starting Position**: Have the client assume the supine position with knees flexed and feet flat on the floor, approximately 12" apart.

2) The arms are extended with hands positioned palms down on the thighs with fingertips pointing at the knees.

3) **Begin Assessment**: Set a metronome for a cadence of 40 beats · min^{-1}.

4) On the "Go" command the trainer starts the metronome and the client curls-up in a controlled manner until the fingers reach the top of the knees as the cadence sounds.

5) Each beat represents a transitional change in the movement. The movements should be controlled and must remain on pace with the metronome.

6) **Movement Repetition**: The client then returns to the starting position (upper back contact with ground). The movements should not be jerky or use momentum. This should be repeated until the client cannot perform any more repetitions or completes 75 repetitions.

7) **Data Collection**: The trainer should count out loud each correct repetition.

8) **Stop the Test**: If the client performs 75 repetitions, stop the test and record the results.

9) Clients stopping before the terminal score should have their score recorded at the end of the test.

10) **Interpretation of Results**: The table below indicates the endurance ratings for trunk flexion for both males and females. It is based on the number of completed curl-ups for each   age category.

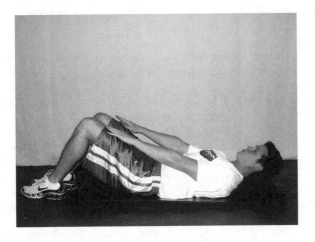 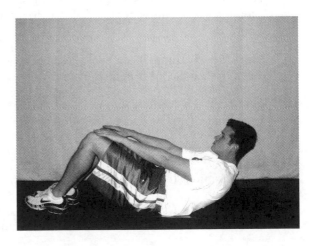

Number of Repetitions Completed _____

Classification for Abdominal Curl-up Test					
Men	**20-29 Y**	**30-39 Y**	**40-49 Y**	**50-59 Y**	**60-69 Y**
Above Average	$\geq$21	$\geq$18	$\geq$18	$\geq$17	$\geq$16
Average	16-20	15-17	13-17	11-16	11-15
Below Average	<16	<15	<13	<11	<11
Women					
Above Average	$\geq$18	$\geq$19	$\geq$19	$\geq$19	$\geq$17
Average	14-17	11-18	11-18	10-18	8-16
Below Average	<14	<11	<11	<10	<8

Muscular Power Tests: Non-Counter Movement Vertical Jump

Equipment
Tape measure
Chalk
Stopwatch

Directions

1) **Test Setup**: Secure a measuring tape against a sturdy surface at least 48 inches above the maximum reach point of the subject.

2) **Warm-up**: The client should perform a 5-10 minute warm-up consisting of activities designed to increase muscle temperature and to enhance nervous system excitation.

3) **Measure Reach**: The client should stand erect, with both feet flat on the floor with their dominant side facing the wall or measuring surface.

4) The client then extends the dominant arm straight up with the palm facing the measuring surface for a single arm maximum reach measurement. The highest point of the reach should be measured to the closest increment and recorded.

5) **Mark Reach Hand**: The client should chalk the tips of the fingers on the dominant hand (reach arm) prior to the initial trial so the measurement can be marked and maximum jump height assessed accurately.

6) **Test Prep**: The client then prepares to make the first attempt by getting in a comfortable jumping position. This entails having the feet shoulder width apart, knees flexed, and hips traveling in the sagittal plane.

7) Once the client has established jumping position their feet cannot move, nor may the client adjust body position. If the client uses any other preparatory action other than a single movement of the upper extremities and a single flexion of the legs (dip) prior to body extension, the jump should be avoided.

8) **Test**: The client should then make their first attempt by jumping and reaching as high as possible, placing a mark on the measurement surface with the chalked fingers.

9) The trainer should observe the reach mark and record its measurement value. Ideally, the trainer will be on an elevated surface to get a more accurate reading at eye level.

10) **Retest**: Three attempts should be performed (resting up to 90 sec. between trials), and the best trial should be used for statistical recording.

11) **Record and Calculate Data**: Record the subject's results.

12) Subtract the initial reach height from the recorded height on the tape to calculate vertical jump.

Recorded Height_____

Vertical Jump Classification (inches)				
	21-25 Y		26-30 Y	
	M	F	M	F
Above Average	≥25.7	≥16.6	≥25.2	≥16.4
Average	18.7-25.6	11.6-16.5	18.6-25.1	11.6-16.3
Below Average	<18.7	<11.6	<18.6	<11.6

Adapted from D. Patterson, D. Fred Peterson, 2004, "Vertical Jump and Leg Power Norms for Young Adults"
Measurement in Physical Education and Exercise Science

Muscular Power Test: 30-second Chair Stand

Equipment
Stable Chair
Stopwatch

Directions

1) For the chair stand test, select a stable chair that will not move during the test. The height of the chair should be at a level that allows for approximately 90 degrees of knee flexion at the starting position.

2) **Start Position**: The client should sit in the middle of the chair with back straight, knees flexed, and feet flat on the floor at shoulder width.

3) Arms should be crossed across the chest.

4) **Test Start**: Once the starting command is given by the trainer, the client should begin the movement and attempt to stand to an upright position and back down to the chair continually for 30 seconds.

5) **Test Stop**: At the end of the 30-second period the trainer should call "Stop." The number of correctly completed chair stands should be recorded by the trainer.

Number of Completed Chair Stands _____

30-Second Chair Stand (#. of Stands)													
	60-64 Y		65-69 Y		70-74 Y		75-79 Y		80-84 Y		85-89 Y		90-94 Y	
	M	F	M	F	M	F	M	F	M	F	M	F	M	F
Above Average	>19	>17	>18	>16	>17	>15	>17	>15	>15	>14	>14	>13	>12	>11
Average	14-19	12-17	12-18	11-16	12-17	10-15	11-17	10-15	10-15	9-14	8-14	8-13	7-12	4-11
Below Average	<14	<12	<12	<11	<12	<10	<11	<10	<10	<9	<8	<8	<7	<4

Anaerobic Capacity Test: Anaerobic Power Step

Equipment
Step or box
Stopwatch

Directions

1) **Start Position**: The client should stand alongside a box or bench. The height of the bench should allow the knee to be flexed at 90 degrees.

2) The client starts with the foot of their dominant leg (testing leg) centered on top of the box or bench. The step foot will remain in the same location throughout the duration of the test.

3) **Start Test**: On the "Go" command the trainer starts the timer and the client begins the step-up. On each step the client's legs and back should be straightened with the arms remaining at the sides used for balance only. The arms should not move for the purpose of momentum assistance.

4) The cadence for the test is a 1-2 count; the 1 count is up and the 2 count is down.

5) **Scoring**: A step is counted each time the client's step leg is straightened and then returned to the starting position. Steps are not counted if the client does not straighten the step leg or if the client's back is bent.

6) The trainer should call out the time remaining every 15 seconds. The total number of steps should be recorded for the sixty second trail.

7) Tests should not be paced, but performed at an all-out exertion for the entire duration (60 seconds).

8) **Stop Test**: At the end of the 60 second period the trainer should stop the test and record the number of steps following the completion of the test.

Number of Steps Completed _____

9) Have the client perform a cool down to prevent blood pooling in the action leg.

How to Calculate

Anaerobic Capacity (kgm · min^{-1}) = {_____ kg x [(0.4 m x _____ step score)/1]} x 1.33

= [_____ kg x (_____) m / 1] x 1.33

= _____ kg x _____ m · min^{-1} x 1.33

= _____ (kgm · min^{-1})

Watts = _____ (kgm · min^{-1}) ÷ 6.12 W/ kgm · m^{-1}

Example
A 100 kg (220 lb) male completed 60 steps for the entire one minute test duration.

Anaerobic Capacity (kgm · min^{-1}) = 100 x [(0.40 x 60)/1] x 1.33

= [100 x (24/1)] x1.33

= 100 x 24.0 x 1.33

= 3192 (kgm · min^{-1})

Conversion to Watts (6.12 kgm · min^{-1} = 1 W)

Watts = 3192 ÷ 6.12

= 521.6 W

Classification for Anaerobic Capacity		
	Male (W)	Female Power (W)
Above Average	≥507	≥339
Average	460-506	307-338
Below Average	<460	<307

Body Composition Test: Skinfold

Equipment
Skinfold calipers
Pen (to marking sites)

Directions

1) The trainers should locate the correct gender-specific anatomical location(s). The following chart and illustrations provide a detailed description of the 3-site Jackson-Pollock model. The trainer should refer to these when locating the correct gender-specific skinfold location. Once the site has been identified, the trainer should mark the site with an erasable marker so the trainer can return to the exact location for subsequent measurements. This will also allow the trainer to become more proficient at site identification and increase test reliability.

2) **Hand placement:** The trainer should place the calipers in the right hand with the index finger in a position to open the caliper. Slightly pronate the right hand so that the caliper can be easily read from above. Pronate the left hand to a point at which the thumb of the left hand is pointing downward.

3) **Pinching of skinfold:** Using a pinch width of approximately two inches, firmly pinch the skinfold between the thumb and the first two fingers, lifting the subcutaneous fat and skin from the underlying muscle tissue.

4) **Placement of the calipers:** Once the trainer has successfully separated the subcutaneous fat and skin from the underlying muscle belly, the calipers should be placed on the fold. The pinchers of the caliper should be placed across the long axis of the skinfold at the designated site.

5) Using a 1 cm separation between the trainer's fingers and the calipers should prevent the skinfold dimension from being affected by the pressure from the trainer's fingers. The depth of the caliper placement is about half the distance between the base of the normal skin perimeter and the top of the skinfold.

6) Place the jaws of the calipers perpendicular to the skinfold site.

7) **Reading of calipers:** Calipers have a compression tension of $10g \cdot mm^2$. In order to get an accurate reading and prevent compression of the fat by the caliper, the trainer must read the caliper to the closest half millimeter within 2 seconds of releasing the caliper jaws on the fold.

8) The measurements should be recorded and the test repeated two times allowing at least 15 seconds between subsequent measurements. If the measurements differ by more than 2 millimeters, a third measurement should be taken and an average of the three measurements used.

9) In non-obese individuals the skinfolds should not differ by more than two millimeters. The median values of the three trials are used for evaluation and prediction.

10) **Computation of results:** Once the data has been recorded, the trainer should add the three skinfolds together to obtain the sum of the skinfolds in millimeters.

11) The sum of the skinfolds is then charted, or used in a body density equation, to determine the estimated body fat of the individual. The following charts contain the estimated age-adjusted body composition computed by the Siri Equation. The trainer should find their client's estimated body fat by referencing the following gender specific table, and matching the sum of the skinfolds in the left hand column with the client's age across the top row.

Male Three Sites

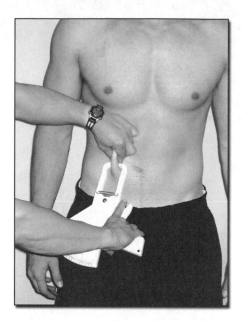

Abdominal Measurement:
Measure a vertical fold 2 cm from the midline of the umbilicus on the right side of the test subject. Be sure that neither the caliper nor the tester's fingers are in the umbilicus during the measurement.

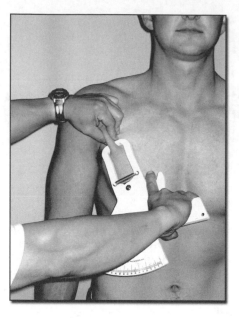

Chest Measurement:
The skinfold is a diagonal fold taken halfway between the anterior axillary line and the nipple. The right side is used for the pinch.

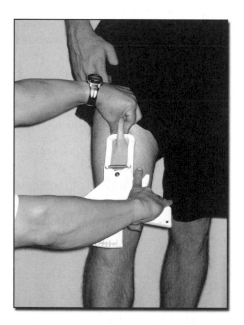

Thigh Measurement:
The measurement is a vertical fold taken over the quadricep muscles on the midline of the right thigh. The measurement should be located halfway between the inguinal crease and the top of the patella.

Female Three Sites

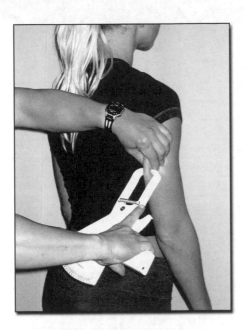

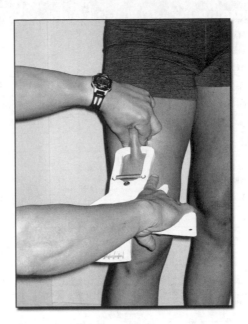

Tricep Measurement:

Measure the vertical fold over the belly of the tricep muscle. Be sure the test subject relaxes the arm. The specific site is located on the posterior midline of the right tricep, halfway between the acromion and olecranon process.

Thigh Measurement:

The measurement is a vertical fold taken over the quadricep muscles on the midline of the right thigh. The measurement should be located halfway between the inguinal crease and the top of the patella.

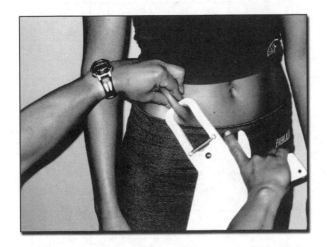

Suprailiac Measurement:

The skinfold is a diagonal fold measured in line with the natural angle of the iliac crest. The measurement should be taken along the anterior axillary line just above the iliac crest on the right side.

Percentage of Body Fat Estimation for *Women* From Age and Triceps, Suprailium, and Thigh Folds

Sum of skinfolds (mm)	Under 22	23 to 27	28 to 32	33 to 37	38 to 42	43 to 47	48 to 52	53 to 57	Over 57
23-25	9.7	9.9	10.2	10.4	10.7	10.9	11.2	11.4	11.7
26-28	11.0	11.2	11.5	11.7	12.0	12.3	12.5	12.7	13.0
29-31	12.3	12.5	12.8	13.0	13.3	13.5	13.8	14.0	14.3
32-34	13.6	13.8	14.0	14.3	14.5	14.8	15.0	15.3	15.5
35-37	14.8	15.0	15.3	15.5	15.8	16.0	16.3	16.5	16.8
38-40	16.0	16.3	16.5	16.7	17.0	17.2	17.5	17.7	18.0
41-43	17.2	17.4	17.7	17.9	18.2	18.4	18.7	18.9	19.2
44-46	18.3	18.6	18.8	19.1	19.3	19.6	19.8	20.1	20.3
47-49	19.5	19.7	20.0	20.2	20.5	20.7	21.0	21.2	21.5
50-52	20.6	20.8	21.1	21.3	21.6	21.8	22.1	22.3	22.6
53-55	21.7	21.9	22.1	22.4	22.6	22.9	23.1	23.4	23.6
56-58	22.7	23.0	23.2	23.4	23.7	23.9	24.2	24.4	24.7
59-61	23.7	24.0	24.2	24.5	24.7	25.0	25.2	25.5	25.7
62-64	24.7	25.0	25.2	25.5	25.7	26.0	26.2	26.4	26.7
65-67	25.7	25.9	26.2	26.4	26.7	26.9	27.2	27.4	27.7
68-70	26.6	26.9	27.1	27.4	27.6	27.9	28.1	28.4	28.6
71-73	27.5	27.8	28.0	28.3	28.5	28.8	29.0	29.3	29.5
74-76	28.4	28.7	28.9	29.2	29.4	29.7	29.9	30.2	30.4
77-79	29.3	29.5	29.8	30.0	30.3	30.5	30.8	31.0	31.3
80-82	30.1	30.4	30.6	30.9	31.1	31.4	31.6	31.9	32.1
83-85	30.9	31.2	31.4	31.7	31.9	32.2	32.4	32.7	32.9
86-88	31.7	32.0	32.2	32.5	32.7	32.9	33.2	33.4	33.7
89-91	32.5	32.7	33.0	33.2	33.5	33.7	33.9	34.2	34.4
92-94	33.2	33.4	33.7	33.9	34.2	34.4	34.7	34.9	35.2
95-97	33.9	34.1	34.4	34.6	34.9	35.1	35.4	35.6	35.9
98-100	34.6	34.8	35.1	35.3	35.5	35.8	36.0	36.3	36.5
101-103	35.3	35.4	35.7	35.9	36.2	36.4	36.7	36.9	37.2
104-106	35.8	36.1	36.3	36.6	36.8	37.1	37.3	37.5	37.8
107-109	36.4	36.7	36.9	37.1	37.4	37.6	37.9	38.1	38.4
110-112	37.0	37.2	37.5	37.7	38.0	38.2	38.5	38.7	38.9
113-115	37.5	37.8	38.1	38.2	38.5	38.7	39.0	39.2	39.5
116-118	38.0	38.3	38.5	38.8	39.0	39.3	39.5	39.7	40.0
119-121	38.5	38.7	39.0	39.2	39.5	39.7	40.0	40.2	40.5
122-124	39.0	39.2	39.4	39.7	39.9	40.2	40.4	40.7	40.9
125-127	39.4	39.6	39.9	40.1	40.4	40.6	40.9	41.1	41.4
128-130	39.8	40.0	40.3	40.5	40.8	41.0	41.3	41.5	41.8

Percentage of Body Fat Estimation for *Men* From Age and Chest, Abdominal, and Thigh Folds

Sum of Skinfold (mm)	Under 22	23 to27	28 to 32	33 to 37	38 to 42	43 to 47	48 to 52	53 to 57	Over 57
8-10	1.3	1.8	2.3	2.9	3.4	3.9	4.5	5.0	5.5
11-13	2.2	2.8	3.3	3.9	4.4	4.9	5.5	6.0	6.5
14-16	3.2	3.8	4.3	4.8	5.4	5.9	6.4	7.0	7.5
17-19	4.2	4.7	5.3	5.8	6.3	6.9	7.4	8.0	8.5
20-22	5.1	5.7	6.2	6.8	7.3	7.9	8.4	8.9	9.5
23-25	6.1	6.6	7.2	7.7	8.3	8.8	9.4	9.9	10.5
26-28	7.0	7.6	8.1	8.7	9.2	9.8	10.3	10.9	11.4
29-31	8.0	8.5	9.1	9.6	10.2	10.7	11.3	11.8	12.4
32-34	8.9	9.4	10.0	10.5	11.1	11.6	12.2	12.8	13.3
35-37	9.8	10.4	10.9	11.5	12.0	12.6	13.1	13.7	14.3
38-40	10.7	11.3	11.8	12.4	12.9	13.5	14.1	14.6	15.2
41-43	11.6	12.2	12.7	13.3	13.8	14.4	15.0	15.5	16.1
44-46	12.5	13.1	13.6	14.2	14.7	15.3	15.9	16.4	17.0
47-49	13.4	13.9	14.5	15.1	15.6	16.2	16.8	17.3	17.9
50-52	14.3	14.8	15.4	15.9	16.5	17.1	17.6	18.2	18.8
53-55	15.1	15.7	16.2	16.8	17.4	17.9	18.5	19.1	19.7
56-58	16.0	16.5	17.1	17.7	18.2	18.8	19.4	20.0	20.5
59-61	16.9	17.4	17.9	18.5	19.1	19.7	20.2	20.8	21.4
62-64	17.6	18.2	18.8	19.4	19.9	20.5	21.1	21.7	22.2
65-67	18.5	19.0	19.6	20.2	20.8	21.3	21.9	22.5	23.1
68-70	19.3	19.9	20.4	21.0	21.6	22.2	22.7	23.3	23.9
71-73	20.1	20.7	21.2	21.8	22.4	23.0	23.6	24.1	24.7
74-76	20.9	21.5	22.0	22.6	23.2	23.8	24.4	25.0	25.5
77-79	21.7	22.2	22.8	23.4	24.0	24.6	25.2	25.8	26.3
80-82	22.4	23.0	23.6	24.2	24.8	25.4	25.9	26.5	27.1
83-85	23.2	23.8	24.4	25.0	25.5	26.1	26.7	27.3	27.9
86-88	24.0	24.5	25.1	25.7	26.3	26.9	27.5	28.1	28.7
89-91	24.7	25.3	25.9	26.5	27.1	27.6	28.2	28.8	29.4
92-94	25.4	26.0	26.6	27.2	27.8	28.4	29.0	29.6	30.2
95-97	26.1	26.7	27.3	27.9	28.5	29.1	29.7	30.3	30.9
98-100	26.9	27.4	28.0	28.6	29.2	29.8	30.4	31.0	31.6
101-103	27.5	28.1	28.7	29.3	29.9	30.5	31.1	31.7	32.3
104-106	28.2	28.8	29.4	30.0	30.6	31.2	31.8	32.4	33.0
107-109	28.9	29.5	30.1	30.7	31.3	31.9	32.5	33.1	33.7
110-112	29.6	30.2	30.8	31.4	32.0	32.6	33.2	33.8	34.4
113-115	30.2	30.8	31.4	32.0	32.6	33.2	33.8	34.5	35.1
116-118	30.9	31.5	32.1	32.7	33.3	33.9	34.5	35.1	35.7
119-121	31.5	32.1	32.7	33.3	33.9	34.5	35.1	35.7	36.4
122-124	32.1	32.7	33.3	33.9	34.5	35.1	35.8	36.4	37.0

Body Composition Test: 2-3 Site Girth Measurements

Equipment
Tape measure

Directions

1) Identify the appropriate anatomical locations of the client by gender.

2) All circumference measurements should be taken over the client's skin where applicable.

3) Using a tape measure, assess each site so that the measuring tape lies parallel to the floor over the designated site location. The tape should lie flat against the skin. Each circumference measurement should be recorded in inches.

4) **For men**: Measure the body height to the closest half inch.

5) Abdominal girth - measure the circumference of the abdomen by aligning the tape so that it passes over the navel.

6) Neck girth - measure the circumference of the neck just inferior to the larynx (Adam's apple) with tape sloping slightly downward to the front.

7) **For Women**: Measure the body height to the closest half inch.

8) Upper abdominal girth - measure circumference at the level of minimal abdominal girth - about midway between the xiphoid process and the umbilicus.

9) Neck girth-Measure circumference just inferior to the larynx (Adam's apple) with tape sloping slightly downward to the front.

10) Hip girth-Measure circumference at the level of the greatest protrusion of the gluteal muscles.

11) **Calculate subject's derived circumference value**: From the data collected find the subject's estimated body fat using the gender specific charts.

12) Find the subject's derived circumference value by utilizing the following correct gender equation:

13) **Men**: Abdominal – Neck = Circumference value

    _____ - _____ = _____

14) **Women**: Upper abdominal + Hip – Neck = Circumference value

    _____ + _____ - _____ = _____

15) The following charts contain the estimated body fat percentages according to the 2-3 Site Girth model. To find the client's estimated body fat, the trainer must first refer to the correct gender table (Table A for men and Table B for women).

16) The trainer must then intersect the client's calculated circumference value with the client's height in inches. (The derived circumference values are located in the left hand column and the height values are located across the top of the table).

17) **Record the data.** _____

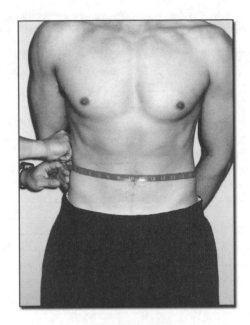

Abdominal
Across the umbilicus

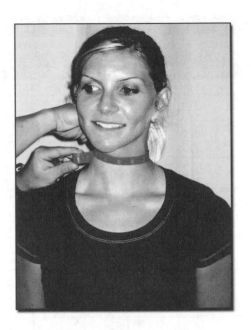

Neck
Across the center
of the neck

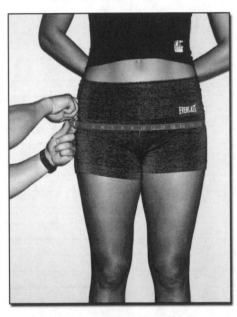

Hip
Across the thickest point
of the hip. Feet should be
inside the shoulders or
together

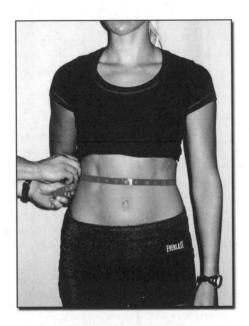

Upper Abdominal
½ way between the
umbilicus & xyphoid
process

Circumference value (in)	TABLE A Men's BF % 2-3 Girth									
	HEIGHT (IN)									
	60.0	60.5	61	61.5	62	62.5	63	63.5	64	64.5
11	3	2	2	2	2	1	1	1	1	1
11.5	4	4	4	3	3	3	3	2	2	2
12	6	5	5	5	5	4	4	4	4	3
12.5	7	7	6	6	6	6	6	5	5	5
13	8	8	8	8	7	7	7	7	6	6
13.5	10	9	9	9	9	8	8	8	8	8
14	11	11	10	10	10	10	10	9	9	9
14.5	12	12	12	11	11	11	11	11	10	10
15	13	13	13	13	12	12	12	12	12	11
15.5	15	14	14	14	14	13	13	13	13	12
16	16	15	15	15	15	15	14	14	14	14
16.5	17	17	16	16	16	16	15	15	15	15
17	18	18	17	17	17	17	16	16	16	16
17.5	19	19	19	18	18	18	18	17	17	17
18	20	20	20	19	19	19	19	18	18	18
18.5	21	21	21	20	20	20	20	19	19	19
19	22	22	22	21	21	21	21	20	20	20
19.5	23	23	23	22	22	22	22	21	21	21
20	24	24	23	23	23	23	22	22	22	22
20.5	25	25	24	24	24	24	23	23	23	23
21	26	26	25	25	25	25	24	24	24	24
21.5	27	26	26	26	26	25	25	25	25	24
22	28	27	27	27	27	26	26	26	26	25
22.5	28	28	28	28	27	27	27	27	26	26
23	29	29	29	29	28	28	28	28	27	27
23.5	30	30	30	29	29	29	29	28	28	28
24	31	31	30	30	30	30	29	29	29	29
24.5	32	31	31	31	31	30	30	30	30	29
25	33	32	32	32	31	31	31	31	30	30
25.5	33	33	33	33	32	32	32	31	31	31
26	34	34	34	33	33	33	32	32	32	32
26.5	35	35	34	34	34	33	33	33	33	32
27	36	35	35	35	34	34	34	34	33	33
27.5	36	36	36	35	35	35	35	34	34	34
28	37	37	36	36	36	36	35	35	35	35
28.5	38	37	37	37	37	36	36	36	36	35
29	38	38	38	38	37	37	37	37	36	36
29.5	39	39	39	38	38	38	37	37	37	37
30	40	39	39	39	39	38	38	38	38	37
30.5	-	-	40	40	39	39	39	39	38	38
31	-	-	-	-	40	40	39	39	39	39
31.5	-	-	-	-	-	-	-	40	40	39
32.0-35.0	-	-	-	-	-	-	-	-	-	40

	TABLE A Men's BF % 2-3 Girth									
	HEIGHT (IN)									
Circumference value (in)	65	65.5	66	66.5	67	67.5	68	68.5	69	69.5
11	0	0	-	-	-	-	-	-	-	-
11.5	2	2	1	1	1	1	1	0	0	-
12	3	3	3	3	2	2	2	2	2	1
12.5	5	4	4	4	4	4	3	3	3	3
13	6	6	6	5	5	5	5	5	4	4
13.5	7	7	7	7	6	6	6	6	6	5
14	9	8	8	8	8	8	7	7	7	7
14.5	10	10	9	9	9	9	9	8	8	8
15	11	11	11	10	10	10	10	10	9	9
15.5	12	12	12	12	11	11	11	11	11	10
16	13	13	13	13	12	12	12	12	12	11
16.5	14	14	14	14	14	13	13	13	13	13
17	16	15	15	15	15	14	14	14	14	14
17.5	17	16	16	16	16	16	15	15	15	15
18	18	17	17	17	17	17	16	16	16	16
18.5	19	18	18	18	18	18	17	17	17	17
19	20	19	19	19	19	19	18	18	18	18
19.5	21	20	20	20	20	19	19	19	19	19
20	22	21	21	21	21	20	20	20	20	20
20.5	22	22	22	22	22	21	21	21	21	20
21	23	23	23	23	22	22	22	22	22	21
21.5	24	24	24	24	23	23	23	23	22	22
22	25	25	25	24	24	24	24	24	23	23
22.5	26	26	25	25	25	25	25	24	24	24
23	27	27	26	26	26	26	25	25	25	25
23.5	28	27	27	27	27	26	26	26	26	26
24	28	28	28	28	27	27	27	27	27	26
24.5	29	29	29	29	28	28	28	28	27	27
25	30	30	30	29	29	29	29	28	28	28
25.5	31	31	30	30	30	30	29	29	29	29
26	32	31	31	31	31	30	30	30	30	29
26.5	32	32	32	32	31	31	31	31	30	30
27	33	33	32	32	32	32	32	31	31	31
27.5	34	33	33	33	33	33	32	32	32	32
28	34	34	34	34	33	33	33	33	33	32
28.5	35	35	35	34	34	34	34	33	33	33
29	36	36	35	35	35	35	34	34	34	34
29.5	36	36	36	36	35	35	35	35	35	34
30	37	37	37	36	36	36	36	35	35	35
30.5	38	38	37	37	37	37	36	36	36	36
31	38	38	38	38	37	37	37	37	37	36
31.5	39	39	39	38	38	38	38	37	37	37
32	40	39	39	39	39	38	38	38	38	38
32.5	-	-	40	40	39	39	39	39	38	38
33	-	-	-	-	40	40	39	39	39	39
33.5	-	-	-	-	-	-	-	40	40	39
34	-	-	-	-	-	-	-	-	-	40
34.5	-	-	-	-	-	-	-	-	-	-
35.0	-	-	-	-	-	-	-	-	-	-

TABLE A Men's BF % 2-3 Girth									
HEIGHT (IN)									
Circumference value (in)	70	70.5	71	71.5	72	72.5	73	73.5	74	74.5
11	-	-	-	-	-	-	-	-	-	-
11.5	-	-	-	-	-	-	-	-	-	-
12	1	1	1	1	0	0	0	-	-	-
12.5	3	2	2	2	2	2	1	1	1	1
13	4	4	4	3	3	3	3	3	2	2
13.5	5	5	5	5	4	4	4	4	4	4
14	7	6	6	6	6	6	5	5	5	5
14.5	8	8	7	7	7	7	7	6	6	6
15	9	9	9	8	8	8	8	8	7	7
15.5	10	10	10	9	9	9	9	9	9	8
16	11	11	11	11	10	10	10	10	10	9
16.5	12	12	12	12	12	11	11	11	11	11
17	13	13	13	13	13	12	12	12	12	12
17.5	14	14	14	14	14	13	13	13	13	13
18	15	15	15	15	15	14	14	14	14	14
18.5	16	16	16	16	16	15	15	15	15	15
19	17	17	17	17	17	16	16	16	16	16
19.5	18	18	18	18	18	17	17	17	17	17
20	19	19	19	19	18	18	18	18	18	17
20.5	20	20	20	20	19	19	19	19	19	18
21	21	21	21	20	20	20	20	20	19	19
21.5	22	22	22	21	21	21	21	21	20	20
22	23	23	22	22	22	22	22	21	21	21
22.5	24	23	23	23	23	23	22	22	22	22
23	25	24	24	24	24	23	23	23	23	23
23.5	25	25	25	25	24	24	24	24	24	23
24	26	26	26	25	25	25	25	25	24	24
24.5	27	27	26	26	26	26	26	25	25	25
25	28	27	27	27	27	27	26	26	26	26
25.5	28	28	28	28	28	27	27	27	27	27
26	29	29	29	29	28	28	28	28	27	27
26.5	30	30	29	29	29	29	29	28	28	28
27	31	30	30	30	30	30	29	29	29	29
27.5	31	31	31	31	30	30	30	30	30	29
28	32	32	32	31	31	31	31	31	30	30
28.5	33	33	32	32	32	32	31	31	31	31
29	33	33	33	33	33	32	32	32	32	31
29.5	34	34	34	33	33	33	33	33	32	32
30	35	35	34	34	34	34	33	33	33	33
30.5	35	35	35	35	35	34	34	34	34	33
31	36	36	36	35	35	35	35	34	34	34
31.5	37	36	36	36	36	36	35	35	35	35
32	37	37	37	37	36	36	36	36	36	35
32.5	38	38	37	37	37	37	37	36	36	36
33	39	38	38	38	38	37	37	37	37	37
33.5	39	39	39	38	38	38	38	38	37	37
34	40	39	39	39	39	39	38	38	38	38
34.5	-	-	40	40	39	39	39	39	39	38
35.0	-	-	-	-	40	40	40	39	39	39

TABLE A Men's BF % 2-3 Girth									
HEIGHT (IN)									
Circumference value (in)	75	75.5	76	76.5	77	77.5	78	78.5	79	79.5
11	-	-	-	-	-	-	-	-	-	-
11.5	-	-	-	-	-	-	-	-	-	-
12	-	-	-	-	-	-	-	-	-	-
12.5	1	1	0	0	-	-	-	-	-	-
13	2	2	2	1	1	1	1	1	1	0
13.5	3	3	3	3	3	2	2	2	2	2
14	5	4	4	4	4	4	3	3	3	3
14.5	6	6	5	5	5	5	5	5	4	4
15	7	7	7	6	6	6	6	6	6	5
15.5	8	8	8	8	7	7	7	7	7	6
16	9	9	9	9	8	8	8	8	8	8
16.5	10	10	10	10	10	9	9	9	9	9
17	11	11	11	11	11	10	10	10	10	10
17.5	12	12	12	12	12	11	11	11	11	11
18	13	13	13	13	13	12	12	12	12	12
18.5	14	14	14	14	14	13	13	13	13	13
19	15	15	15	15	15	14	14	14	14	14
19.5	16	16	16	16	16	15	15	15	15	15
20	17	17	17	17	16	16	16	16	16	16
20.5	18	18	18	18	17	17	17	17	17	16
21	19	19	19	18	18	18	18	18	18	17
21.5	20	20	20	19	19	19	19	19	18	18
22	21	21	20	20	20	20	20	19	19	19
22.5	22	21	21	21	21	21	20	20	20	20
23	22	22	22	22	22	21	21	21	21	21
23.5	23	23	23	23	22	22	22	22	22	21
24	24	24	24	23	23	23	23	23	22	22
24.5	25	25	24	24	24	24	24	23	23	23
25	26	25	25	25	25	25	24	24	24	24
25.5	26	26	26	26	26	25	25	25	25	25
26	27	27	27	26	26	26	26	26	25	25
26.5	28	28	27	27	27	27	27	26	26	26
27	28	28	28	28	28	27	27	27	27	27
27.5	29	29	29	29	28	28	28	28	28	27
28	30	30	29	29	29	29	29	28	28	28
28.5	31	30	30	30	30	30	29	29	29	29
29	31	31	31	31	30	30	30	30	30	29
29.5	32	32	31	31	31	31	31	30	30	30
30	33	32	32	32	32	32	31	31	31	31
30.5	33	33	33	33	32	32	32	32	32	31
31	34	34	33	33	33	33	33	32	32	32
31.5	34	34	34	34	34	33	33	33	33	33
32	35	35	35	34	34	34	34	34	33	33
32.5	36	35	35	35	35	35	34	34	34	34
33	36	36	36	36	35	35	35	35	35	34
33.5	37	37	36	36	36	36	36	35	35	35
34	37	37	37	37	37	36	36	36	36	36
34.5	38	38	38	37	37	37	37	37	36	36
35.0	39	38	38	38	38	38	37	37	37	37
35.5	39	39	39	39	38	38	38	38	38	37
36	40	40	39	39	39	39	39	38	38	38
36.5	-	-	40	40	39	39	39	39	39	38
37	-	-	-	-	-	40	40	39	39	39
37.5	-	-	-	-	-	-	-	40	40	40
38	-	-	-	-	-	-	-	-	-	-
38.5	-	-	-	-	-	-	-	-	-	-

TABLE B Women's BF % 2-3 Girth									
HEIGHT (IN)									
Circumference value (in)	58	58.5	59	59.5	60	60.5	61	61.5	62	62.5
34.5	1	0	-	-	-	-	-	-	-	-
35	2	1	1	1	0	-	-	-	-	-
35.5	3	2	2	2	1	1	0	0	-	-
36	4	3	3	3	2	2	1	1	1	0
36.5	5	4	4	4	3	3	2	2	2	1
37	6	5	5	4	4	4	3	3	3	2
37.5	7	6	6	5	5	5	4	4	4	3
38	7	7	7	6	6	6	5	5	5	4
38.5	8	8	8	7	7	7	6	6	5	5
39	9	9	9	8	8	7	7	7	6	6
39.5	10	10	9	9	9	8	8	8	7	7
40	11	11	10	10	10	9	9	8	8	8
40.5	12	12	11	11	10	10	10	9	9	9
41	13	12	12	12	11	11	11	10	10	10
41.5	14	13	13	13	12	12	11	11	11	10
42	14	14	14	13	13	13	12	12	12	11
42.5	15	15	15	14	14	13	13	13	12	12
43	16	16	15	15	15	14	14	14	13	13
43.5	17	17	16	16	15	15	15	14	14	14
44	18	17	17	17	16	16	16	15	15	14
44.5	19	18	18	17	17	17	16	16	16	15
45	19	19	19	18	18	17	17	17	16	16
45.5	20	20	19	19	19	18	18	18	17	17
46	21	20	20	20	19	19	19	18	18	18
46.5	22	21	21	20	20	20	19	19	19	18
47	22	22	22	21	21	20	20	20	19	19
47.5	23	23	22	22	22	21	21	21	20	20
48	24	23	23	23	22	22	22	21	21	21
48.5	25	24	24	23	23	23	22	22	22	21
49	25	25	25	24	24	23	23	23	22	22
49.5	26	26	25	25	24	24	24	23	23	23
50	27	26	26	26	25	25	24	24	24	23
50.5	27	27	27	26	26	26	25	25	24	24
51	28	28	27	27	27	26	26	25	25	25
51.5	29	28	28	28	27	27	27	26	26	25
52	29	29	29	28	28	28	27	27	27	26
52.5	30	30	29	29	29	28	28	28	27	27
53	31	30	30	30	29	29	29	28	28	27
53.5	31	31	31	30	30	30	29	29	28	28
54	32	32	31	31	31	30	30	30	29	29
54.5	33	32	32	32	31	31	31	30	30	29
55	33	33	33	32	32	32	31	31	30	30
55.5	34	34	33	33	33	32	32	31	31	31
56	35	34	34	33	33	33	32	32	32	31
56.5	35	35	34	34	34	33	33	33	32	32
57	36	35	35	35	34	34	34	33	33	33
57.5	36	36	36	35	35	35	34	34	34	33
58	37	37	36	36	36	35	35	35	34	34
58.5	38	37	37	37	36	36	35	35	35	34
59	38	38	38	37	37	36	36	36	35	35
59.5	39	38	38	38	37	37	37	36	36	36
60	39	39	39	38	38	38	37	37	37	36
60.5	40	40	39	39	39	38	38	37	37	37
61	41	40	40	39	39	39	38	38	38	37
61.5	41	41	40	40	40	39	39	39	38	38
62	42	41	41	41	40	40	40	39	39	38
62.5	42	42	42	41	41	40	40	40	39	39
63	43	42	42	42	41	41	41	40	40	40

	HEIGHT (IN)									
Circumference value (in)	63	63.5	64	64.5	65	65.5	66	66.5	67	67.5
34.5	-	-	-	-	-	-	-	-	-	-
35	-	-	-	-	-	-	-	-	-	-
35.5	-	-	-	-	-	-	-	-	-	-
36	0	-	-	-	-	-	-	-	-	-
36.5	1	1	0	-	-	-	-	-	-	-
37	2	2	1	1	1	0	-	-	-	-
37.5	3	3	2	2	2	1	1	1	0	-
38	4	3	3	3	2	2	2	1	1	1
38.5	5	4	4	4	3	3	3	2	2	2
39	6	5	5	5	4	4	4	3	3	3
39.5	7	6	6	6	5	5	5	4	4	4
40	7	7	7	6	6	6	5	5	5	4
40.5	8	8	8	7	7	7	6	6	6	5
41	9	9	8	8	8	7	7	7	6	6
41.5	10	10	9	9	9	8	8	8	7	7
42	11	10	10	10	9	9	9	8	8	8
42.5	12	11	11	11	10	10	10	9	9	9
43	12	12	12	11	11	11	10	10	10	9
43.5	13	13	13	12	12	12	11	11	11	10
44	14	14	13	13	13	12	12	12	11	11
44.5	15	15	14	14	14	13	13	13	12	12
45	16	15	15	15	14	14	14	13	13	13
45.5	16	16	16	15	15	15	14	14	14	13
46	17	17	17	16	16	16	15	15	15	14
46.5	18	18	17	17	17	16	16	16	15	15
47	19	18	18	18	17	17	17	16	16	16
47.5	19	19	19	18	18	18	17	17	17	16
48	20	20	20	19	19	18	18	18	18	17
48.5	21	21	20	20	20	19	19	19	18	18
49	22	21	21	21	20	20	20	19	19	19
49.5	22	22	22	21	21	21	20	20	20	19
50	23	23	22	22	22	21	21	21	20	20
50.5	24	23	23	23	22	22	22	21	21	21
51	24	24	24	23	23	23	22	22	22	21
51.5	25	25	24	24	24	23	23	23	22	22
52	26	25	25	25	24	24	24	23	23	23
52.5	26	26	26	25	25	25	24	24	24	23
53	27	27	26	26	26	25	25	25	24	24
53.5	28	27	27	27	26	26	26	25	25	25
54	28	28	28	27	27	27	26	26	26	25
54.5	29	29	28	28	28	27	27	27	26	26
55	30	29	29	29	28	28	28	27	27	27
55.5	30	30	30	29	29	29	28	28	28	27
56	31	31	30	30	30	29	29	29	28	28
56.5	32	31	31	31	30	30	30	29	29	29
57	32	32	32	31	31	31	30	30	30	29
57.5	33	32	32	32	31	31	31	30	30	30
58	33	33	33	32	32	32	31	31	31	30
58.5	34	34	33	33	33	32	32	32	31	31
59	35	34	34	34	33	33	33	32	32	32
59.5	35	35	35	34	34	34	33	33	33	32
60	36	35	35	35	34	34	34	33	33	33
60.5	36	36	36	35	35	35	34	34	34	33
61	37	37	36	36	36	35	35	35	34	34
61.5	38	37	37	37	36	36	36	35	35	35
62	38	38	37	37	37	36	36	36	35	35
62.5	39	38	38	38	37	37	37	36	36	36
63	39	39	39	38	38	38	37	37	37	36

TABLE B Women's BF % 2-3 Girth									
HEIGHT (IN)									
Circumference value (in)	63	63.5	64	64.5	65	65.5	66	66.5	67	67.5
64	40	40	40	39	39	39	38	38	38	37
64.5	41	41	40	40	40	39	39	39	38	38
65	41	41	41	40	40	40	39	39	39	38
65.5	42	42	41	41	41	40	40	40	39	39
66	43	42	42	41	41	41	40	40	40	39
66.5	43	43	42	42	42	41	41	41	40	40
67	44	43	43	43	42	42	41	41	41	41
67.5	44	44	43	43	43	42	42	42	41	41
68	45	44	44	44	43	43	43	42	42	42
68.5	-	45	44	44	44	43	43	43	42	42
69	-	-	45	45	44	44	44	43	43	43
69.5	-	-	-	-	45	44	44	44	43	43
70	-	-	-	-	-	45	45	44	44	44
70.5	-	-	-	-	-	-	-	45	44	44
71.0-75.5	-	-	-	-	-	-	-	-	45	45

TABLE B Women's BF % 2-3 Girth									
HEIGHT (IN)									
Circumference value (in)	68	68.5	69	69.5	70	70.5	71	71.5	72	72.5
34.5	-	-	-	-	-	-	-	-	-	-
35	-	-	-	-	-	-	-	-	-	-
35.5	-	-	-	-	-	-	-	-	-	-
36	-	-	-	-	-	-	-	-	-	-
36.5	-	-	-	-	-	-	-	-	-	-
37	-	-	-	-	-	-	-	-	-	-
37.5	-	-	-	-	-	-	-	-	-	-
38	0	0	-	-	-	-	-	-	-	-
38.5	1	1	1	0	0	-	-	-	-	-
39	2	2	2	1	1	1	0	0	-	-
39.5	3	3	3	2	2	2	1	1	1	0
40	4	4	3	3	3	3	2	2	2	1
40.5	5	5	4	4	4	3	3	3	2	2
41	6	5	5	5	5	4	4	4	3	3
41.5	7	6	6	6	5	5	5	4	4	4
42	8	7	7	7	6	6	6	5	5	5
42.5	8	8	8	7	7	7	6	6	6	6
43	9	9	9	8	8	8	7	7	7	6
43.5	10	10	10	9	9	8	8	8	7	7
44	11	10	11	10	9	9	9	9	8	8
44.5	12	11	12	11	10	10	10	9	9	9
45	12	12	12	11	11	11	10	10	10	10
45.5	13	13	13	12	12	12	11	11	11	10
46	14	14	14	13	13	12	12	12	11	11
46.5	15	14	15	14	13	13	13	12	12	12
47	15	15	15	14	14	14	13	13	13	13
47.5	16	16	16	15	15	15	14	14	14	13
48	17	17	17	16	16	15	15	15	14	14
48.5	18	17	18	17	16	16	16	15	15	15
49	18	18	18	17	17	17	16	16	16	15
49.5	19	19	19	18	18	17	17	17	17	16
50	20	19	20	19	18	18	18	18	17	17
50.5	20	20	20	19	19	19	19	18	18	18
51	21	21	21	20	20	20	19	19	19	18
51.5	22	21	22	21	21	20	20	20	19	19
52	22	22	22	22	21	21	21	20	20	20

TABLE B Women's BF % 2-3 Girth									
HEIGHT (IN)									
Circumference value (in)	68	68.5	69	69.5	70	70.5	71	71.5	72	72.5
52.5	23	23	23	22	22	22	21	21	21	20
53	24	23	24	23	23	22	22	22	21	21
53.5	24	24	24	23	23	23	23	22	22	22
54	25	25	25	24	24	24	23	23	23	22
54.5	26	25	26	25	24	24	24	24	23	23
55	26	26	26	25	25	25	24	24	24	24
55.5	27	27	27	26	26	25	25	25	25	24
56	28	27	28	27	26	26	26	25	25	25
56.5	28	28	28	27	27	27	26	26	26	25
57	29	29	29	28	28	27	27	27	26	26
57.5	30	29	29	29	28	28	28	27	27	27
58	30	30	30	29	29	29	28	28	28	27
58.5	31	30	31	30	29	29	29	29	28	28
59	31	31	31	30	30	30	29	29	29	28
59.5	32	32	32	31	31	30	30	30	29	29
60	32	32	32	32	31	31	31	30	30	30
60.5	33	33	33	32	32	31	31	31	31	30
61	34	33	33	33	32	32	32	31	31	31
61.5	34	34	34	33	33	33	32	32	32	31
62	35	34	34	34	34	33	33	33	32	32
62.5	35	35	35	34	34	34	33	33	33	33
63	36	36	35	35	35	34	34	34	33	33
63.5	36	36	36	35	35	35	35	34	34	34
64	37	37	36	36	36	35	35	35	35	34
64.5	38	37	37	37	36	36	36	35	35	35
65	38	38	37	37	37	37	36	36	36	35
65.5	39	38	38	38	37	37	37	36	36	36
66	39	39	39	38	38	38	37	37	37	36
66.5	40	39	39	39	38	38	38	37	37	37
67	40	40	40	39	39	39	38	38	38	37
67.5	41	40	40	40	39	39	39	39	38	38
68	41	41	41	40	40	40	39	39	39	38
68.5	42	41	41	41	40	40	40	40	39	39
69	42	42	42	41	41	41	40	40	40	39
69.5	43	42	42	42	42	41	41	41	40	40
70	43	43	43	42	42	42	41	41	41	40
70.5	44	43	43	43	43	42	42	42	41	41
71	44	44	44	43	43	43	42	42	42	41
71.5	45	44	44	44	43	43	43	43	42	42
72	-	45	45	44	44	44	43	43	43	42
72.5	-	-	-	45	44	44	44	44	43	43
73	-	-	-	-	45	45	44	44	44	43
735.5	-	-	-	-	-	-	45	44	44	44
74	-	-	-	-	-	-	-	45	45	44
74.5	-	-	-	-	-	-	-	-	-	45

TABLE B Women's BF % 2-3 Girth										
	HEIGHT (IN)									
Circumference value (in)	73	73.5	74	74.5	75	75.5	76	76.5	77	77.5
34.5-39.5	0	-	-	-	-	-	-	-	-	-
40	1	1	0	0	-	-	-	-	-	-
40.5	2	2	1	1	1	0	0	-	-	-
41	3	2	2	2	2	1	1	1	0	0
41.5	4	3	3	3	2	2	2	2	1	1
42	4	4	4	4	3	3	3	2	2	2
42.5	5	5	5	4	4	4	3	3	3	3
43	6	6	5	5	5	5	4	4	4	3
43.5	7	7	6	6	6	5	5	5	5	4
44	8	7	7	7	6	6	6	6	5	5
44.5	8	8	8	8	7	7	7	6	6	6
45	9	9	9	8	8	8	7	7	7	7
45.5	10	10	9	9	9	9	8	8	8	7
46	11	10	10	10	10	9	9	9	8	8
46.5	12	11	11	11	10	10	10	9	9	9
47	12	12	12	11	11	11	11	10	10	10
47.5	13	13	12	12	12	12	11	11	11	10
48	14	13	13	13	13	12	12	12	11	11
48.5	14	14	14	14	13	13	13	12	12	12
49	15	15	15	14	14	14	13	13	13	13
49.5	16	16	15	15	15	14	14	14	14	13
50	17	16	16	16	15	15	15	15	14	14
50.5	17	17	17	16	16	16	16	15	15	15
51	18	18	17	17	17	17	16	16	16	15
51.5	19	18	18	18	17	17	17	17	16	16
52	19	19	19	18	18	18	18	17	17	17
52.5	20	20	19	19	19	19	18	18	18	17
53	21	20	20	20	20	19	19	19	18	18
53.5	21	21	21	20	20	20	20	19	19	19
54	22	22	21	21	21	21	20	20	20	19
54.5	23	22	22	22	21	21	21	21	20	20
55	23	23	23	22	22	22	22	21	21	21
55.5	24	24	23	23	23	22	22	22	22	21
56	25	24	24	24	23	23	23	22	22	22
56.5	25	25	25	24	24	24	23	23	23	23
57	26	25	25	25	25	24	24	24	23	23
57.5	26	26	26	26	25	25	25	24	24	24
58	27	27	26	26	26	26	25	25	25	24
58.5	28	27	27	27	26	26	26	26	25	25
59	28	28	28	27	27	27	26	26	26	26
59.5	29	28	28	28	28	27	27	27	26	26
60	29	29	29	28	28	28	28	27	27	27
60.5	30	30	29	29	29	28	28	28	28	27
61	31	30	30	30	29	29	29	28	28	28
61.5	31	31	31	30	30	30	29	29	29	28
62	32	31	31	31	30	30	30	30	29	29
62.5	32	32	32	31	31	31	30	30	30	30
63	33	32	32	32	32	31	31	31	30	30
63.5	33	33	33	32	32	32	32	31	31	31
64	34	34	33	33	33	32	32	32	32	31
64.5	34	34	34	34	33	33	33	32	32	32
65	35	35	34	34	34	34	33	33	33	32
65.5	36	35	35	35	34	34	34	33	33	33
66	36	36	35	35	35	35	34	34	34	33
66.5	37	36	36	36	35	35	35	35	34	34
67	37	37	37	36	36	36	35	35	35	34
67.5	38	37	37	37	36	36	36	36	35	35
68	38	38	38	37	37	37	36	36	36	36

| TABLE B Women's BF % 2-3 Girth | | | | | | | | | | |
| HEIGHT (IN) | | | | | | | | | | |
Circumference value (in)	73	73.5	74	74.5	75	75.5	76	76.5	77	77.5
69	39	39	39	38	38	38	37	37	37	37
69.5	40	39	39	39	38	38	38	38	37	37
70	40	40	40	39	39	39	38	38	38	38
70.5	41	40	40	40	39	39	39	39	38	38
71	41	41	41	40	40	40	39	39	39	39
71.5	42	41	41	41	40	40	40	40	39	39
72	42	42	42	41	41	41	40	40	40	40
72.5	43	42	42	42	41	41	41	41	40	40
73	43	43	43	42	42	42	41	41	41	40
73.5	44	43	43	43	42	42	42	42	41	41
74	44	44	43	43	43	43	42	42	42	41
74.5	45	44	44	44	43	43	43	42	42	42
75	-	45	44	44	44	44	43	43	43	42
75.5	-	-	45	45	44	44	44	43	43	42

Adapted from Hodgdon and Beckett, 1984.

Flexibility Tests

Back Scratch Test/Shoulder rotators

Assessed Structures: Teres Major, Subscapularis, Infraspinatus, Teres Minor, Triceps, Latissimus Dorsi

Directions

1) Trainer should have the client stand or sit maintaining an upright posture.
2) Have the client place one arm behind their back; the other arm over their shoulder.
3) Trainers should instruct the client to try to touch their fingertips. Normal ROM is fingertip contact.
4) Trainers should then measure the distance between the tips of the middle fingers.
5) Be sure to repeat test with arms in the opposite positions.
6) Flexibility evaluation categorized as either: good, borderline, or needs work (could differ from left to right shoulder rotator).

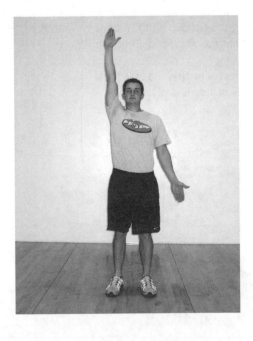
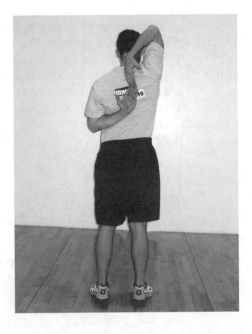

Hip Extension (Thomas Test)

Assessed Structures: Iliopsoas

Directions

1) With client lying in a supine position on a table or bench, the trainer should instruct them to pull both legs to their chest.
2) The trainer should then have the client release **one** leg, extending the released leg off the edge of the table.
3) The hamstring of the released leg should come to rest on the table for normal ROM.
4) Assess both hips.
5) To avoid excessive knee compression in the flexed leg, hand placement can anchor the leg from the hamstring.
6) Flexibility evaluation categorized as either: good, borderline, or needs work (could differ from left to right hip extensor).

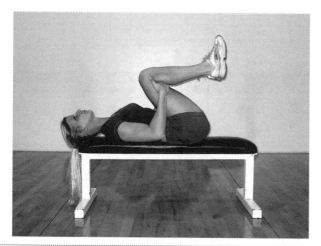 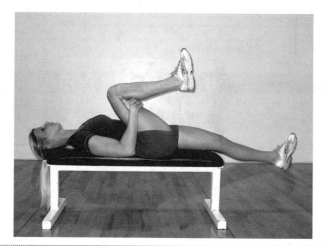

Trunk Extension

Assessed Structures: Hip Flexors, Abdominals

Directions

1) The trainer should have client lie in a prone position.
2) The client should place their hands directly under their shoulders.
3) The client should then fully extend their arms, while keeping the pelvis (hips) in contact with the mat or ground.
4) If the hips come off the ground, it indicates that the client has tight abdominals or hip flexors.
5) Women generally perform better on this test than men.
6) **If a client has a history of Low Back Pain (LBP) do not perform this assessment.**
7) Flexibility evaluation categorized as either: good, borderline, or needs work.

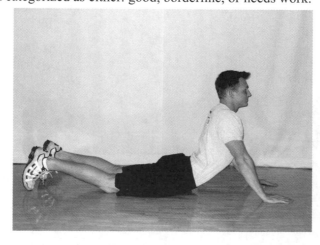

Trunk Flexion

Assessed Structures: Back Extensors

Directions

1) Have client sit on a chair or box.
2) Thighs should be parallel with the ground.
3) Legs should be abducted to 45°.
4) Have client reach down and backward between their legs.
5) Instruct the subject not to bounce while reaching as far as possible.
6) Normal ROM for this test is subject's shoulder joint in a parallel plane with the hip joint or the back parallel with the ground. Rounding of the back is acceptable for this test.

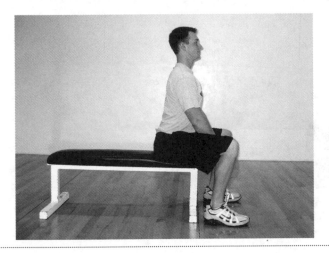 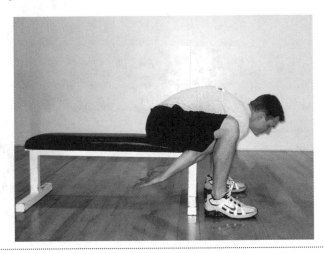

Bilateral Knee Flexion

Assessed Structures: Quadriceps

Directions

1) With client in a prone position and legs together, trainers should instruct them to bend one leg, bringing the heel to the gluteal of the same side.
2) Trainers should then have the client grasp their ankle and pull the leg as close as possible to the gluteal.
3) The heel should come within 2 inches of the gluteal for normal ROM.
4) Assess both quads.
5) Flexibility evaluation categorized as either: good, borderline, or needs work (could differ from left to right quadriceps).

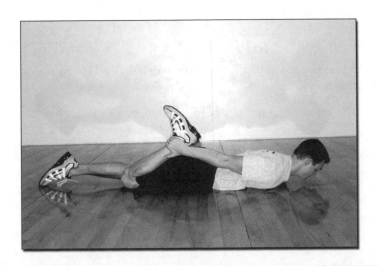

Knee Extension

Assessed Structures: Hamstrings

Directions

1) With client in a supine position, instruct them to bend one leg bringing the knee toward the chest.
2) Instruct the client to then extend the bent leg upwards.
3) Client should be able to hold the <u>fully extended</u> leg at 90° of flexion from the hip joint with the lower leg maintaining contact with the floor for normal ROM.
4) Assess both hamstrings.

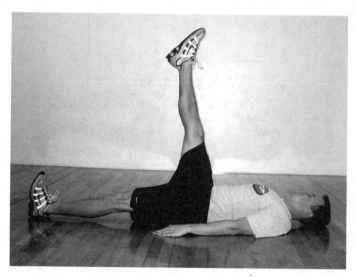

Agility Test: Pro Agility

Equipment
Measuring tape
Cones or equivalent
Stopwatch

Directions

1) **Test Preparation**: Using a measured area (10 yards in total length), place two markers on either end of the measured distance and one directly in the middle, separating the 10-yard distance into two, five-yard segments. The client should start in a lateral body position to the direction the linear movement will take place.

2) **Test Start**: The trainer signals "Ready, Go" and starts the stopwatch.

3) With a lateral start, the client runs 5 yards to the first marker from the starting point.

4) The client touches the line/ground at the first marker and makes a 180 degree change in direction (heading back toward the starting line).

5) The client then runs past the starting point to the second marker (5 yards past the starting marker in the opposite direction).

6) The client touches the line/ground at the second marker and makes a 180 degree change in direction.

7) **Test End**: Run 5 yards through the finish line (starting line). Timing ends when the client's body crosses the finish line.

8) **Record results**

Time to Completion _____ sec.

Pro Agility Test

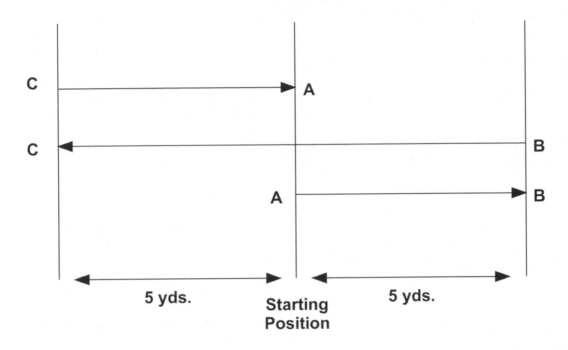

Speed Test: 40-yard Dash

Equipment
Measuring tape
Cones or equivalent
Stopwatch

Directions

1) **Test Preparation**: Measure a distance 40-yards from the designated starting line and form an end line using a marker.

2) The client should line up perpendicularly to the direction of movement at the starting line.

3) The client can assume a comfortable starting position at the start line.

4) **Test Start**: Timing begins when the client makes their first movement forward from the starting line.

5) **Test Stop**: Timing ends when any part of the clients' body crosses the 40 yard finish line.

6) **Record results**

Time to Completion _____ sec.

Chapter Fourteen References

1. **Al Khalili F, Janszky I, Andersson A, Svane B and Schenck-Gustafsson K**. Physical activity and exercise performance predict long-term prognosis in middle-aged women surviving acute coronary syndrome. *J Intern Med* 261: 178-187, 2007.

2. **Amundsen BH, Wisloff U and Slordahl SA**. [Exercise training for prevention, treatment and rehabilitation of cardiovascular disease.]. *Tidsskr Nor Laegeforen* 127: 446-448, 2007.

3. **Baltaci G, Un N, Tunay V, Besler A and Gerceker S**. Comparison of three different sit and reach tests for measurement of hamstring flexibility in female university students. *Br J Sports Med* 37: 59-61, 2003.

4. **Baltaci G, Un N, Tunay V, Besler A and Gerceker S**. Comparison of three different sit and reach tests for measurement of hamstring flexibility in female university students. *Br J Sports Med* 37: 59-61, 2003.

5. **Baltaci G, Un N, Tunay V, Besler A and Gerceker S**. Comparison of three different sit and reach tests for measurement of hamstring flexibility in female university students. *Br J Sports Med* 37: 59-61, 2003.

6. **Carey DG, Jenkins AB, Campbell LV, Freund J and Chisholm DJ**. Abdominal fat and insulin resistance in normal and overweight women: Direct measurements reveal a strong relationship in subjects at both low and high risk of NIDDM. *Diabetes* 45: 633-638, 1996.

7. **Ekelund U, Griffin SJ and Wareham NJ**. Physical activity and metabolic risk in individuals with a family history of type 2 diabetes. *Diabetes Care* 30: 337-342, 2007.

8. **Hoeger WW and Hopkins DR**. A comparison of the sit and reach and the modified sit and reach in the measurement of flexibility in women. *Res Q Exerc Sport* 63: 191-195, 1992.

9. **Hoeger WW and Hopkins DR**. A comparison of the sit and reach and the modified sit and reach in the measurement of flexibility in women. *Res Q Exerc Sport* 63: 191-195, 1992.

10. **Jackson A and Langford NJ**. The criterion-related validity of the sit and reach test: replication and extension of previous findings. *Res Q Exerc Sport* 60: 384-387, 1989.

11. **Minkler S and Patterson P**. The validity of the modified sit-and-reach test in college-age students. *Res Q Exerc Sport* 65: 189-192, 1994.

12. **Minkler S and Patterson P**. The validity of the modified sit-and-reach test in college-age students. *Res Q Exerc Sport* 65: 189-192, 1994.

13. **Panagiotakos DB, Pitsavos C, Yannakoulia M, Chrysohoou C and Stefanadis C**. The implication of obesity and central fat on markers of chronic inflammation: The ATTICA study. *Atherosclerosis* 183: 308-315, 2005.

14. **Shen W, Punyanitya M, Chen J, Gallagher D, Albu J, Pi-Sunyer X, Lewis CE, Grunfeld C, Heshka S and Heymsfield SB**. Waist circumference correlates with metabolic syndrome indicators better than percentage fat. *Obesity (Silver Spring)* 14: 727-736, 2006.

15. **Stranges S, Dorn JM, Muti P, Freudenheim JL, Farinaro E, Russell M, Nochajski TH and Trevisan M**. Body fat distribution, relative weight, and liver enzyme levels: a population-based study. *Hepatology* 39: 754-763, 2004.

16. **Turesson C and Matteson EL**. Cardiovascular risk factors, fitness and physical activity in rheumatic diseases. *Curr Opin Rheumatol* 19: 190-196, 2007.

17. **Van Pelt RE, Evans EM, Schechtman KB, Ehsani AA and Kohrt WM**. Waist circumference vs body mass index for prediction of disease risk in postmenopausal women. *Int J Obes Relat Metab Disord* 25: 1183-1188, 2001.

Chapter 15

Exercise Programming Components

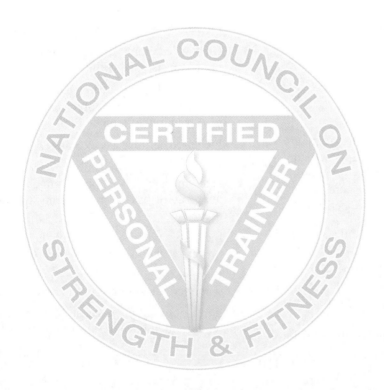

Introduction

When designing exercise programs, many factors and variables need to be considered before creating the actual exercise prescription matrix. The exercise prescription matrix is a compilation of prescribed individual exercise components and their interrelationships that collectively focus on achieving a client's program goals. The primary determinant for all client program decisions is the needs analysis created from the screening and assessment protocols. These findings will guide the exercise prescription, effectively addressing the key needs and goals of the client. That being considered, programming options for goal attainment present seemingly limitless possibilities, as the human body is capable of countless movement options and a variety of speeds at which these movements can be performed. The only constants are the principles of exercise program design. These principles are manipulated to reflect the desired adaptation response. They include the following:

Progressive Preparation – acclimating the body to harder work levels (warm-up).

Metabolic System – energy system used to fuel the work.

Exercise Selection – type of exercise or modality selected.

Exercise Order – sequence of exercises.

Training Frequency – number of exercise bouts per week.

Training Duration – length of time engaged in physical effort.

Training Intensity – level of effort performed.

Rest Periods – duration of time between each physical effort.

Training Volume – number of sets and repetitions.

Recovery Periods – duration of time between exercise sessions.

These training principles are also viewed as training variables, or components, and can be manipulated to attain the desired effect of the exercise program. Changes to one or more of these variables present a completely different outcome, so personal trainers must clearly recognize the independent characteristics of each variable and the effect altering any variable will have on the program. To take it a step further, the interrelationship among variables must also be known in order to appropriately create a coordinated and supportive program matrix, while concurrently preventing any conflict among variables. An easy way to view this program harmonization is to consider each program component as an ingredient in a recipe. In appropriate quantities, each ingredient complements the others to produce a predictable and desirable outcome. When imbalance or conflict among variables exists, the outcome may be neither completely predictable nor desirable when compared to the intended goal.

Warm-up

Based on the understanding of **kinetics**, mechanical objects function best when the resistive forces are reduced or controlled. When objects move under the duress of resistance caused by friction, tension, and other constraint mechanisms, they do not have the same abilities to accelerate. The human body works the same way. When body tissue is cold, it resists movement. Cold tissue is less pliable, cellular enzymes are less active, and neural conduction is less efficient (22; 31). For the body to function optimally during activity, it must be adequately warmed-up.

For most people, it is common knowledge that the performance of a warm-up should precede higher intensity physical activity; however, many individuals fail to understand the scientific rationale for this sequence. Warm-up is a generic term used to describe a preparation period prior to a designated physical activity. Its use has application prior to virtually any mode of physical movement, albeit recreational or competitive. As the name implies, warm-ups are designed to increase tissue temperature prior to engaging in elevated levels of physical work. The increase in body temperature assists the function of tissues through several proposed physiological mechanisms, (11; 14; 22; 28; 31) including:

- Increased speed of muscle action and relaxation.

- Greater economy of movement due to lowered viscous resistance within the active muscle.

- Increased delivery of oxygen to the muscles due to the fact that hemoglobin releases oxygen more readily at higher temperatures.

- Increased cellular gas exchange.

- Increased nerve transmission, enzymatic activity, and muscle metabolism due to the effect temperature has on accelerating the rate of bodily processes.

- Increased blood flow, which heightens metabolic processes and muscle temperature.

- Improved range of motion (ROM) capabilities seen with increases in muscle and core temperatures.

Scientific observation suggests that increasing muscle temperature facilitates the faster transfer of gases at the cellular level, increases blood flow through vasodilatation and the opening of dormant capillaries, lowers lactate levels, increases oxygen uptake and increases the energy metabolism within the muscle. (19) Arguments have been made as to whether or not these physiological changes actually reduce the risk of injury for individuals who employ them as a precursor to activity. However, most professionals will agree that that the performance of a warm-up will reduce activity-related injury risks (i.e., sprains, strains) (11; 28). This opinion is based on the fact that muscle tissue pliability increases as muscle temperature rises and the neural response time is accelerated, allowing for increased lengthening of the muscle-tendon unit and better neuromuscular control.

Further benefits of a warm-up performance are also seen, as the blood flow to the heart muscle mirrors the gradual intensity progression of the activity. Progressing from low to moderate to high intensity activity will help reduce stress on the cardiac muscle (smaller oxygen deficits in skeletal muscle and reduced lactate build up), which can help prevent spikes in systolic blood pressure and reduce the risk of abnormal electrical rhythms (cardiac arrhythmias).

Psychological enhancements accompany warm-up progressions as well. This preparation period can increase mental focus and arousal, which in turn can facilitate enhanced motor activity (11; 13; 28). Directing attention to specific movements, conditions, and environments can lead to improved performance. This combination of mental and physical preparation can make a warm-up effective in enhancing physical capabilities.

Types of Warm-ups

Warm-ups are usually designated into one of two categories: general or specific (27). Each holds particular merit for inclusion both before and during daily physical activity. The general warm-up is characterized by gross motor activation, designed to increase blood flow and temperature in the working musculature. General warm-ups often utilize basic movement patterns repeated continuously for a set period of time. Examples of this type of warm-up include walking, low speed jogging, jumping rope, **calisthenics**, and biking. Warm-ups usually last anywhere from three to ten minutes, depending on the client's physical fitness level and the activity that they are preparing to perform. Higher intensity activities require longer warm-up periods prior to their engagement. The actual duration of the warm-up is subject to the level of intensity at which the client will perform their training. Olympic athletes may use

gradual, progressive warm-ups lasting as long as thirty minutes for optimal physiological preparation.

Examples of General Warm-up Activities

Walking

Low-Speed Jogging

Jumping Rope

Calisthenics

Biking

Specific Warm-up

Specific warm-ups attempt to utilize actions and musculature which will be used during a particular activity and will often resemble, either in part or whole, the actual activity to be completed. They are effective in both warming up the muscles, as well as enhancing the specific neuromuscular pathways employed by the activity (27). Utilizing lighter weights for high repetitions on the bench press before heavier training sets are employed is a common example. Using specific sprint mechanics and slower speed sprinting before attempting full speed sprints is another. Both activities are event specific but still elicit all the aforementioned physiological and psychological responses. In either case, the goal is the same: increase performance, while reducing the likelihood of injury.

Examples of Specific Warm-ups

Activity	Specific warm-up
Bench Press	Light weight bench press
Sprinting	Low intensity sprints or form running
Squat	Light weight or body weight squats
Pitching (Baseball)	Low intensity throwing

Performance Warm-up

In addition to the traditional general and specific warm-ups, two hybrid models have gained popularity in various training environments. They include performance and functional warm-ups. Performance warm-ups combine general and specific warm-up modalities to enhance particular areas of performance fitness, while preparing for power and strength training. These activities combine large muscle continuous movement with gross sport-specific movements, completed through gradually increasing ranges of motion before becoming more specific to the speed and energy system used in the activity. The durations often reach 15-20 minutes before transitioning into the more intense work. An example would be jumping rope for 3 minutes before performing low level agility dot drills, then progressing to some agility ladder work and low intensity plyometrics such as skips, ankle pops, lateral shuffles, hops, medicine ball rebounds and passes. The intensity used is often 20-30% less than that employed for the actual training. The concept is to focus on skills and motor patterns that will improve the overall performance of the athlete.

Functional Warm-up

The fourth classification of warm-up has been termed the "functional warm-up." The functional training philosophy and its application are rooted in the physical rehabilitation setting. Allied health care professionals, such as occupational and physical therapists, have been using the "functional training" philosophy to complement other therapeutic modalities to improve movement capabilities after an injury has occurred. The premise behind functional training is to utilize integrated movement patterns that elicit increased joint stability through enhanced **proprioception** and improved transfer of energy across the kinetic chain. The goal is to create a more stable and functional joint for improved movement economy and improved function. Fitness professionals can, and have, applied this concept to fitness routines to help promote enhanced training responses and movement efficiency.

Applying the functional training concept to the warm-up component has several advantages. The most obvious is that the activities accomplish many of the same physiological and psychological benefits as the (traditional) general and specific warm-ups do, but with the added benefit of functional enhancement. Secondly, the functional warm-up addresses the ever-present injury prevention and core stabilization concerns of sound fitness programming. Although some of the activities employed within a functional warm-up may not fully present an integrated approach, they can be termed functional due to their injury prevention and core stabilization properties. Further clarification and exploration of integrated functional training techniques and the functional training paradigm will be covered

in the functional resistance training segment of Chapter 20.

To be classified as a warm-up activity, the actions should be directed at continuous movement. Walking on the treadmill for ten minutes is often inappropriately used as a complete warm-up before many training sessions. Walking is, in fact, continuous movement, but serves little purpose for a person seeking to improve his or her overall physical conditioning in a relatively short period of time. This becomes increasingly evident when the contact time a client and trainer have per week is usually between 120-180 minutes (2-3 sessions). For the average person hiring a personal trainer, the need for core strength and stability, improved movement proficiency, enhanced joint integrity, and improved musculoskeletal condition is a priority and should take precedent over a ten minute warm-up of walking or biking. With this in mind, 10 minutes on an aerobic machine should seem somewhat ineffective for the goals of the program. Rather than 10 minutes of low level movement by the muscles of the lower body in a single plane, it may better serve the needs of the client to use the warm-up period by combining total body activities in a continuous manner that will affect the conditions that require specific attention. This provides better use of the warm-up period and increases the amount of time designated for goal attainment.

Due to the fact that trainers are expected to show results for their client's time and money, activities directed at improving functional ability and range of motion are

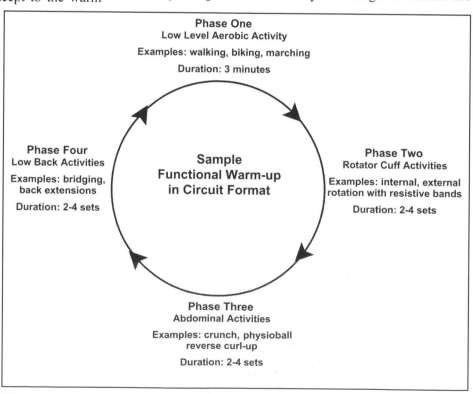

often passed over for actions that will elicit a visual change. Problems arise when the neglect of certain areas leads to some level of debilitation or deficiency. Back pain, shoulder problems, and similar ailments reduce training participation and effectiveness. To combat this scenario, the trainer should use the warm-up time to address preventative action, while keeping in mind the role of the warm-up in physiological preparation. Utilizing exercises in a circuit fashion enables multiple activities to function in a structured format of continuous movement, resulting in increased muscle temperature with the possible added benefits of injury prevention and improved functionality.

Designing Warm-ups

Any program component should be based on the client's personal profile and need. This is also true of warm-up activities. Deciding on the right warm-up for the client will be based on the intended goal, the training experience of the client, and their current physical capabilities. In some cases, the traditional general warm-up may be most appropriate as a client is introduced to exercise or for deconditioned individuals who are being gradually acclimated to routine exercise. In the case of a conditioned athlete, the warm-ups may be more aggressive than a new exerciser's entire workout. The movements and level of difficulty should mirror the capabilities of the client while still emphasizing the warm-up concept and purpose.

Likewise, the specific activities the trainer selects to incorporate into the warm-up depend on several factors that often stem from the activity being prepared for specific client needs. Warm-up modalities can range in difficulty and intensity. It is important that the trainer choose exercises that best meet their client's current fitness and ability levels.

The purpose of warming-up is to gradually increase temperature, range of motion, and intensity. Whether employing warm-ups aimed at performance preparation, functional movements, or traditional general preparation, the sequence of activities should be sensible. Large gross movements at a controlled pace will supercede faster, more specific actions. The selection of movements should logically support the subsequent activities and serve a desired purpose.

Deciding on the program components is the job of the personal trainer and should be based on the best interest of the client. Professional discretion will ultimately define the choices made for each aspect of the training regimen and will certainly be based on knowledge, personal philosophy, and experience. Gaining comprehension of different modalities and the particular benefits of each can enhance the program offerings and lead to more efficient goal attainment by the client. This concept can be implemented throughout the training session, starting with the warm-up.

Cool Downs

Warm-ups are used to progressively prepare the body for activity, whereas a cool down works in the opposite direction. The purpose of cooling down at the end of an exercise session is to bring the body back down to a pre-exercise state. The cool down should use low intensity, rhythmic, large muscle group exercise activities immediately following the exercise bout. The physiological rationale for the cool down includes the following (32; 33; 38):

1. Reduction of blood and muscle lactate.

2. Prevention of blood pooling.

3. Promotion of venous blood return, which positively effects cardiac output.

4. Reduced concentration of **catecholamines** in the blood.

5. Reduced risk of cardiac irregularities post-exercise.

Cool downs should be employed following both moderate to high intensity anaerobic and aerobic exercise. The actions promote a continued delivery of oxygen to the tissues that were placed under stress, which may aid in reducing delayed-onset muscle soreness related to cellular ischemia and tonic muscular spasm. Additionally, the prevention of blood pooling and the gradual decrease in activity enhances myocardial oxygen delivery and venous blood return to the heart, thereby promoting cardiac output (32; 34; 37). Although the primary activities should be of light aerobic nature, flexibility exercises can also be utilized at the end of the cool down to further promote a more relaxed state and take advantage of the warm tissue.

Key Terms

Kinetics – The mechanics concerned with the effects of force on the motion of a body.

Calisthenics – Exercises designed to develop muscular tone and promote physical fitness. Often used as a warm-up activity.

Proprioception – An unconscious perception of movement and spatial orientation in relation to functional training.

Catecholamine – Naturally occurring compounds in the body that serve as hormones or neurotransmitters in the sympathetic nervous system.

Metabolic System

As discussed in Chapter 4, the body utilizes different energy systems to create energy. Each system has specialized features that make it ideal for managing specific types of stress. Recall, the phosphagen system (ATP-CP) provided powerful burst energy when phosphate bonds were split. The fatigue rate is incredibly fast, but the force production output reached the maximum capabilities of the muscle. For this reason, power and absolute strength training requires use of this system in the training program. If the force is required for longer duration, the energy system is switched over to the glycolytic pathway. In the initial stages of the phosphagen energy system (<20 sec.), high force can still be produced if the movements are executed before lactic acid builds up in the tissue and blood. Training at near maximal or maximal levels for 8-10 repetitions will encourage some strength gain, but, perhaps more importantly, hypertrophy of the muscle tissue. When the activity duration extends even further (>30 sec.), the training enhances local muscular endurance and is used for "muscle tone" training. When extended from 60 to 90 seconds at near maximal levels, the exercise stress encourages improvements in anaerobic capacity. Exercise performed for longer than 90 seconds will cause a shift from the anaerobic energy system to aerobic metabolism. Aerobic metabolism accounts for prolonged work, but may be assisted by anaerobic metabolism for higher intensity portions of activities of a continuous nature. This leads to aerobic adaptations which include metabolic enzyme concentration changes, increased stroke volume, increased capillary density, and greater concentration of mitochondria in the muscle fibers (6; 12; 17; 20; 23).

Clearly, the metabolic system defines the capacity for work when expressed by time and **intensity**. Matching the energy system with the goals is fundamental to correct exercise prescription. Straying from the correct energy system or duration within that system can compromise results. For instance, lifting 15 repetitions maximum (RM) compared to a 6RM will have completely different results when applied over a training cycle, as reflected by the energy systems utilized. Knowing these systems is not only advantageous for exercise programming, but necessary for efficient goal attainment.

Exercise Selection

Exercise selection is equally important for proper prescription. Once the energy system for training has been identified, the modalities and specific exercises which maximize the system and best reflect the needs analysis can then be selected. Much like the options available for the exercise program, the specific exercises to be used have numerous variables for consideration. Aerobic training most frequently utilizes a single modality, performed for an extended period of time, such as jogging, biking, swimming, or stair climbing. This does not have to be the case. Creative prescription may employ any group of movements applied in a continuous fashion that results in

Metabolic System Continuum

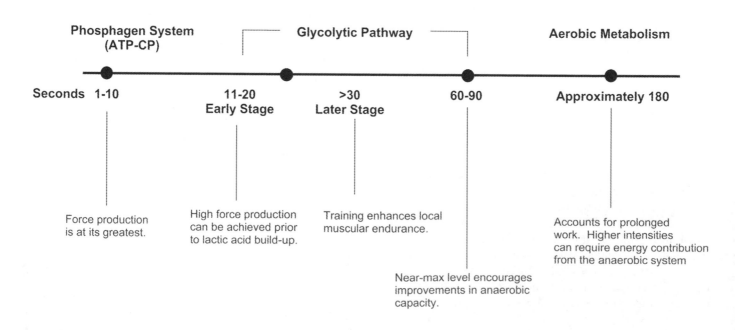

maintained elevated heart rates for the entire period of the performance. The exercise modality may change fifteen times during the specified exercise period, but as long as it is consistent with the aerobic energy system, it is acceptable. The main guidelines to consider are client-specific characteristics and sustained elevated heart rate for the designated time period. Cardiovascular **circuit training** is an excellent example of how many movements can be synergistically applied to form an aerobic workout, as long as the heart rate remains elevated for the duration.

Anaerobic training is far more complicated because it includes so many options and subcategories of those options. The needs analysis will once again provide the best guide for the exercise selection. Deficiency or a desire to improve in any particular area or movement will justify selecting from the group of exercises that specifically challenges the designated muscle or area for the desired adaptation, be it strength, power, speed, flexibility, or balance. Once the category of exercises has been identified, the client-specific criteria should be applied to the decision-making process. Utilizing this method, exercises may be identified as appropriate for consideration or left in reserve for a different time or different client. For instance, if a client has hamstring weakness and the knee extensor: flexor ratio is off balance, the decision to isolate the hamstring using a knee flexion exercise may be the most logical choice. On the other hand, if additional considerations, such as poor ROM in the hip extensors are determined, it may justify using a movement that may contribute to improved function like the Romanian Deadlift exercise. Each factor may define a particular exercise as advantageous or inappropriate depending on the goals of the training and the client's capabilities.

Although many more options in training are available to today's fitness professionals than in the past, researchers and practice-based exercise pioneers have helped to identify how each exercise challenges the body and what is most beneficial for the training program. These findings have been used to categorize exercises and modalities by their respective characteristics, including their usefulness and limitations. Reviewing the exercise usages, benefits, and disadvantages will help a trainer when deciding on the best solution to meet the client's need. Many of these findings will be reviewed in the following chapters and provide insight on the logical choices for each specific situation.

Exercise Order

When exercise selection causes different energy systems to be used in the same training bout, some

~Quick Insight~

Skill Acquisition and Movement Economy

The first step in implementing any exercise program or fitness activity is to teach the client to become proficient in the actions to be used within the training regimen. Although not a designated principle of programming, this work is a fundamental component in exercise instruction. Often referred to as the preparation phase of training, clients are taught how to properly execute each movement with correct biomechanical technique. Using physical and verbal cues, personal trainers can help clients become proficient at each exercise movement. Progressing a client toward more complex or resisted exercises before the techniques have been mastered often leads to a breakdown in form. Common consequences of poor form are repetitive **microtrauma**, which manifests into acute inflammatory syndrome at, or around, an articulation or joint, limiting results from the training (3; 18; 24; 29). Personal trainers should accept nothing less than perfect movement execution during each training bout. Trainers who allow clients to perform exercises incorrectly are being negligent in their job performance.

In sports, athletes routinely practice actions and movement sequences that they will perform on the field or court. They do this so they can become more efficient at managing the forces for precise execution during a competitive situation. By rehearsing the activity over and over again, the body learns to coordinate motor patterns via enhancements in neural efficiency. Once the pattern is learned, the nerves maintain a type of motor history, so every time the situation calls for the motor pattern, the body knows exactly what to do. This phenomenon explains why people do not forget how to ride a bike or throw a ball when they become adults, even though they may not have performed the actions routinely since they were age 10.

logical sequence considerations should be applied. The primary consideration relates to specific need. If a person has deficiencies or health risks that can be improved upon with training, they should be addressed first on the priority list of exercise order. Traditionally, aerobic exercise is performed after resistance training when the two are combined in a single training period. The reason for this order is that aerobic training will deplete muscle glycogen, and consequently reduce the client's ability to overload the muscle during the resistance training portion of the exercise session. However, if aerobic training tops the priority list based on the needs analysis, then it should precede anaerobic training in the exercise session. Hypertensive clients, those with low CRF, or those with risk factors for heart disease will benefit most from aerobic activities and warrant changing the traditional exercise order (1; 2; 9; 39). This may also be true for individuals competing at endurance events. In the latter example, the endurance stress is the most important part of the training bout based on the defined exercise goal; the resistance training is used as a complementary modality. Therefore, if the training bout employs both anaerobic and aerobic activities for an endurance athlete, the aerobic exercise should precede the anaerobic activities.

When aerobic and anaerobic activities are combined in a single bout for a healthy person with no underlying conditions, the order of exercises selected for the program will generally follow a preset consistent format. In most cases the order will be as follows:

1. Warm-up
2. Dynamic flexibility
3. Strength training
4. Hypertrophy training
5. Anaerobic endurance training
6. Aerobic training
7. Cool down
8. Static stretching

The type of anaerobic activities will vary by the client and may or may not include all the different training options in a single bout, but the energy systems and intensity used ultimately determine the order. Anaerobic exercise has additional characteristics that define the actual order used in the exercise session. Fast, compound, heavy, and complex movements are ordered first. Lighter, single-joint, isolated movements are used later in the session. Likewise, the size and number of muscle groups used also contribute to the order of operations. Larger muscle groups should take precedence over smaller groups in the exercise sequence. For instance, leg exercises precede arm exercises, and cross-joint hip movements precede cross-joint shoulder movements. This method ensures the physiologically most challenging activities are completed first in the exercise bout. These concepts will be further explored in the chapter devoted to anaerobic exercise prescription.

Training Frequency

The number of times a person engages in a particular activity per week defines the **frequency** of participation. Frequency is a relevant component to the exercise program because it plays a role in the rate and degree of adaptation response and serves as a preventative component for overtraining when properly manipulated. A common frequency choice in exercise programming for general health attainment is at least three times per week. Although it may be true that structured exercise performed three times per week will provide many health benefits, it would be ignorant to use this value to define the appropriate frequency for all exercise programs.

Generally speaking, the more frequent the exercise participation, the greater the rate and magnitude of the adaptations when all factors are properly considered. But before adopting the "more is better" philosophy, some key elements must be clarified. First, there is a tolerable upper limit to stress that the body can manage before reaching the exhaustion phase of Selye's General Adaptation Syndrome (10; 21; 30). This tolerable upper limit varies by the modality, intensity, and **duration** of the exercise, as well as by the individual. Jogging at a moderate level most days of the week will provide more health benefits than jogging two or three times per week (16; 26). On the contrary, high intensity running bouts at the maximal attainable distances most days of the week would cause a negative outcome due to overtraining effects. Even elite runners train at their maximal distances only a couple times per week, and then they complement the training with shorter running distances. This illustrates the need for balance between intensity, duration, and frequency. This scenario is also true of resistance training. Body builders train up to six days in a week, but they vary the muscles used so that each muscle has an appropriate opportunity to recover. Additionally, a less experienced exerciser who attempts a resistance workout at the same relative intensity and duration as an advanced body builder would likely have difficulty getting out of bed after the second or third day of training. This identifies that frequency is also a factor of training experience and physical condition.

Key Terms

Intensity – The magnitude, or level of degree, in which an activity is performed, often expressed as a percentage of maximum.

Circuit Training – A method of training or physical conditioning in which a person moves through different exercises/stations in a timed manner. The primary purpose is to maintain an elevated HR while resistance training.

Micro trauma – Relatively small injuries in the body, usually consisting of small tears in the muscle fibers.

Frequency – The number of times a person engages in a particular activity per given amount of time.

Duration – The period of time that an exercise session or training bout lasts.

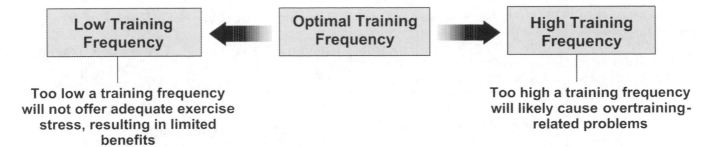

The stress stimulus is the basis for the physiological adaptation response, and frequency is a factor in the volume of stress to which the body is exposed. When the stress is excessive, the outcome is negative. On the other hand, when the stress is inadequate, the outcome is insignificant because the body resists adapting to stress when it is applied too infrequently. This being said, when the number of exercise bouts per week is considered, too high a frequency will likely cause overtraining-related problems, and conversely, if too low a training frequency is used, adequate exercise stress will not be experienced, resulting in limited benefits. Personal trainers must manage exercise frequency with other program components to ensure the adaptations are properly supported by the training stimulus. Guidelines exist that will help define frequency appropriateness, based on the client's capabilities and his or her respective goals.

Training Duration

The amount of time a person experiences training stress in a single bout of exercise is referred to as the duration of training. Training duration, like frequency, is specific to the exercise goals and the client's capabilities. Unlike frequency, however, duration is subject to a rate of fatigue. The faster an exerciser depletes his or her glycogen reserves, the earlier the bout will lose effectiveness. Fatigue most significantly defines the limit of the exercise session's duration. Second to fatigue is the duration of stress that is required to cause the intended adaptation response. For anaerobic adaptations, the duration a muscle is placed under stress can be relatively short. On the contrary, the duration of stress required for chronic aerobic adjustments is fairly lengthy by comparison. Duration differences even exist within the energy systems, depending on the intended goal. Strength training requires very heavy loads, applied for short periods of time. When the performed work is tallied, it may add up to a total of 12 minutes of actual resistance training for an hour long training session. Even though the exerciser remains in the gym for one hour, the body adapts mainly to the contact time with the resistance. When hypertrophy is the desired outcome, the duration of resistance training must increase over that necessary for strength gains. The

actual amount of weight lifted is slightly reduced, but the repetition ranges are increased to compensate for the difference. This places high levels of stress on the tissue for longer periods of time, a necessary element to increasing anabolic hormone response. Hypertrophy training duration may be two or three times that of strength training, even though both modalities utilize the anaerobic energy system.

A consistent relationship exists between duration and intensity. The more intense the work becomes the shorter the duration in which it can be performed. To the contrary, the lighter the work load, the longer the activity can be performed. Aerobic training performed at low intensity can last hours, but when the intensity is elevated, the duration of time to exhaustion is inversely affected. A balance between intensity and duration is necessary for effective exercise prescription. In addition, adequate fuel storage is also an important factor to consider for exercise performance duration. Writing an appropriate and effective exercise prescription will not be fully executable if the client presents low initial energy storage at the onset of the training bout.

Training Intensity

Training intensity often receives credit for being the key factor in exercise-induced adaptations. Although it can not truly exist independently in an exercise prescription, appropriate intensity is vital for physiological stress perception and hormonal response, as it denotes the level of effort exerted by the body. When added to exercise duration, the interrelationship becomes clearly evident, as previously discussed. Managing these two factors is fundamental to successful goal attainment. The specific intensity/duration values necessary for adaptations will be covered in Chapters 17 and 18 as they pertain to anaerobic and aerobic training, but some general guidelines do exist when viewed from a broad perspective of exercise prescription. Intensity has two relevant issues that determine the degree to which it is employed in an exercise regimen. The first issue is the physical aptitude and abilities of the client. Inherent to any exercise programming factor are safety and the relative capabilities of the client. Exercise that is too intense may cause injury or become a psychological barrier to exercise participation. The second key consideration in intensity planning is the energy system being utilized. Managing fatigue is a function of intensity and duration. Therefore, using incorrect workloads will throw off the body's adaptation to the stress. Intensity/energy system mismatches present an obstacle to successful program development for goal attainment.

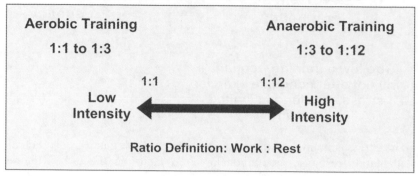

Rest Intervals

Rest intervals or rest periods are a crucial consideration for intensity prescription. Rest intervals are defined by the duration of time between each act of physical effort. High-intensity burst activities quickly use up the more powerful energy storage within the tissues. Once these energy stores deplete, or their metabolic byproduct accumulation becomes inhibitive, the action is stopped physiologically. To repeat the action, the body must rest while rephosphorylation occurs and lactate is removed (25; 36). Therefore, the rest intervals used for subsequent movement actions are secondary to the energy system consideration. The desired outcome and energy system replenishment cycles determine the rest interval length. In aerobic training, the rest interval may be between a 1:1 or 1:3 work to rest ratio, depending on the training system. In anaerobic bouts, that value jumps to 1:3 to 1:12 depending on the resistance used and the intended outcome. For example, between one mile run repeats that last seven minutes, the rest interval will be equivalent to the measured running times: in this case, seven minutes. In bouts of heavy resistance training such as a 5RM squat, the recovery may be over 2 minutes, even though the movement only takes 15 seconds to complete. Again, the duration of the energy replenishment cycle and the intensity used for the next action define these values.

Training Volume

Clearly, selected intensity and the other programming variables exist in an interdependent relationship. The exercise intensity level defines rest intervals, training duration, frequency, and the training volume used in the exercise bout and over the weekly training cycle. Training volume is the measure of total work performed. It combines sets, repetitions, and loads lifted. Training volume is calculated by multiplying the number of sets by the number of repetitions by the weight lifted per repetition. For instance, an individual who weighs 155 lbs. and completes four sets of body weight lunges for ten repetitions would have his or her training volume expressed as (4 x 10 x 155 lbs. body weight) = 6200 lbs. If the intensity is fairly consistent, then the total number of sets and repetitions can be used

to determine the volume instead. The goal is to approximate desired volumes per day or week consistent with intensity levels for recovery purposes. If volumes and intensities are high, the recovery demands will also be increased. Accounting for these variables will aid in the rate of adaptation and reduce the risk for over or under training.

Recovery Period

The recovery period is the duration of time between exercise bouts. It may reflect a four hour period of time between aerobic and anaerobic training in the same day, or a multiple day period between subsequent bouts of resistance training for a particular muscle group. Recovery periods replenish depleted energy sources (i.e. glycogen) and are necessary for cellular adaptations to occur from the stress experienced during the previous workout. It is important to recognize that adaptations to stress take place when the stress is eliminated. Simply stated, recovery periods are necessary for improvements. If the body is constantly stressed, it will become exhausted and break down. Injury, illness, and other negative side effects of overtraining can quickly occur with inadequate recovery.

Exercise Principles

The thoughtful arrangement of exercise prescription principles makes up a successful program matrix. In programming, the difficulty lies in creating balance in a complementary fashion so that the prescription is logical, client appropriate, goal-driven and outcome-based. To help ensure the program matrix makes sense for the client, personal trainers can make additional changes, which can enhance the program components. Program components should be evaluated for consistency with the principles of exercise. These principles add criteria, enhancing the ability of the prescription to effectively deliver the desired results. The principles of exercise include **specificity**, **overload**, and **progression**. Essentially, the three principles work together to ensure the exercise purpose reflects the goals of the client, the exercise provides adequate stress for the desired adaptation response, and the exercise is consistently applied in a progressive manner so that the body continues to improve. The exercise principles steer the program components to properly account for the necessary inclusion and quantity of exercise stress.

Principle of Specificity

The principle of specificity is very logical in its application. The principle states that, for a desired adaptation to occur in a physiological system, the stress demand must be appropriately and explicitly applied to that physiological system. Essentially, the adaptations are specific to the amount and type of applied physiological stress. If the proper amount of appropriate stress is placed on a system the system will respond by adapting to the stress. The principle of specificity guides the exercise selection and other components of programming to ensure the proper elements exist to enhance the desired function.

Principle of Overload

The principle of overload is defined as training stress which challenges a physiological system of the body above the level to which it is accustomed. Overload is applied by the manipulation of one or more of the training components, most commonly intensity, duration, or rest intervals, but possible adjustments are not limited to these three factors alone. The exercise selection, training volume, and frequency can also be modified to create a more physiologically stressful training experience. When overload is no longer perceived by the body, a fixed state is achieved and the adaptation response will discontinue. This phenomenon is

often referred to as staleness or hitting a plateau. Planned variations within the exercise program allow for the constant application of overload stress and continued improvement by the body's physiologic systems.

Principle of Progression

The planned, incremental increase in exercise stress is referred to as progressive overload and supports continued adaptations. The principle of progression suggests that the stress applied must continually be perceived as new for the physiological system to properly adjust to it. Progressions within an exercise program need to provide overload, but should not be excessive. Large increases in physical stress create a disparity between the rate of the adaptation process and the stress level increment. Rapid rates of progression lead to failure because the amount of overload is too great to manage and can potentially lead to injury. The actual quantity of the progression will be influenced by several factors, including:

1. The client's training experience
2. The client's physical condition
3. The client's genetic potential

Progressions are individual-specific and rates of change vary depending on previous exposure to the stress and the current physical state of the client. New clients with limited training experience often present a faster rate of improvement due to nervous system adaptations. On the contrary, individuals who have reached high levels of

Concept of Overload and Progressive Overload

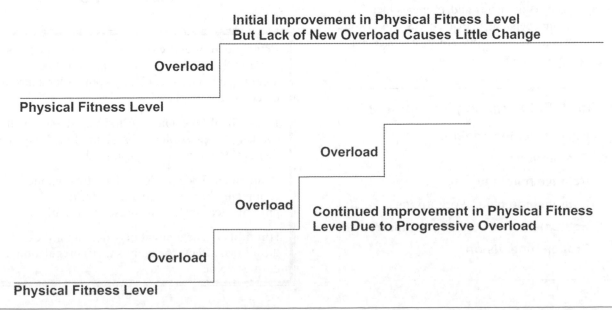

adaptation to a particular stress progress at a much slower rate relative to the percentage of change experienced. Another key factor in the application of the principle of progression is the person's level of fitness. Individuals who are in better physical condition can manage more stress, compared to less physically fit individuals. As a general rule of thumb, increases in exercise stress should be approximately 2-5% per week. Some more aggressive practitioners have suggested progressions as high as 10% per week, but the likelihood of sustaining a consistent adaptation rate of this magnitude is very unlikely.

Exercise Program Safety Factors

Several external factors need to be accounted for when implementing an exercise program safely and effectively. These are considered external factors because they do not necessarily play a direct role in the program components or the exercise principles themselves, but are necessary considerations for the proper execution of the program. Ensuring that these factors are appropriately managed will increase client safety and reduce the risk of liability associated with the training program.

Personal trainers must make sure the client is safe at all times when participating in physical activities under their guidance and supervision. It is well known that exercise comes with inherent risks for injury, but personal trainers can dramatically reduce the risk by accounting for many of the contributing factors that often lead to problems. Creating a safe environment is a key part of the trainer's job description. The concept of a safe environment spans across all aspects of the training area and conditions that affect the client. They include the client's acute condition, the ambient temperature and relative humidity, area safety hazards, the training space, equipment, and proper supervision. Each factor has independent relevance but can become compounded when other factors are also unaccounted for during the exercise session.

The client's acute condition is dependent on several daily variables, which may or may not contribute to concerns during training. Some acute considerations include mental distraction or lack of focus, acute illness, dehydration, drug or alcohol use, hypoglycemia, and excessive fatigue. Any one of these daily variables can lead to injury during the performance of physical activity, and they are therefore considered relative contraindications to exercise participation. If a personal trainer recognizes that a client is not functioning properly or experiencing an issue that may increase risk for injury, the activity should be discontinued and rescheduled for another day once the problem has subsided. Failure to do so constitutes poor professional judgment and can, in some cases, be considered negligent.

When the environmental conditions are analyzed for safety, temperature and relative **humidity** are often the first assessed. In some cases, pollution and altitude may also be factors, but they are less common agitators to exercise in most environments. High temperatures and humidity create physiological stress that increases the risk for dehydration and heat-related illnesses. Heat loss mechanisms can become relatively dysfunctional because heat loss from evaporation and convection can not properly occur (5; 15; 35). Training inside often alleviates any concerns related to temperature. However, if training is to be completed outside, temperature and humidity must be considered. Selecting the most appropriate time of the day is often the easiest and most controllable component involved in managing these conditions. Preplanning and having a contingency plan are necessary aspects to consider in dealing with environmental conditions.

Key Terms

Creating A Safe Training Environment

Client's acute condition

Temperature

Relative humidity

Establishing clear work space

Equipment's operating condition

Proper supervision

Principle of Specificity – For a desired adaptation to occur in the body, a stress demand must be appropriately and specifically applied for a desirable outcome to take place.

Principle of Overload – A training stress which challenges a physiological system of the body above the level to which it is accustomed.

Principle of Progression – The stress applied must continually be perceived as new for the physiological system to adjust accordingly.

Humidity – The amount of water vapor present in the air that affects the body's thermoregulation during exercise.

When the environmental conditions are controlled, a personal trainer's attention can be focused on other relevant program performance areas. The training space and the equipment used for the exercise performance must be evaluated for safety. Any time dynamic exercise is performed adequate space must be available to accommodate the movements. Before the exercise is performed, the work area should be evaluated to ensure it does not present any possible risks to the client. This includes establishing a clear work space, accounting for other people working in close proximity, and keeping an eye on concurrent activities within the environment.

The equipment being used constitutes another possible safety issue within the training area. All equipment should be evaluated for proper function, including making sure moving parts and cables are not damaged or excessively worn. If the equipment uses additional safety apparatus, such as clips, stoppers, and range-limiting devices, they should be employed during each performance to help reduce the risk in case the client

fails during the exercise. If a piece of equipment's ability to function properly is in question, avoid using it until it has received proper maintenance. Additionally, the client's capabilities should be evaluated before deciding on the equipment used within the program. For instance, hypertensive clients should avoid compression equipment like the leg press, and stability equipment may not be appropriate for clients not conditioned for less stable environments (4; 7; 8).

The personal trainer can further enhance the safety and effectiveness of the training environment by providing proper supervision. Spotting clients, evaluating their movements for poor mechanics and signs of fatigue, and providing instructional cues to enhance movement proficiency will all contribute to better training practices. Setting controls and providing assistance will improve the client's performance, while concurrently reducing safety-related issues. Trainers should be very active during the training session, observing the client and managing the environment for maximum safety.

Chapter Fifteen References

1.   **Banz WJ, Maher MA, Thompson WG, Bassett DR, Moore W, Ashraf M, Keefer DJ and Zemel MB**. Effects of resistance versus aerobic training on coronary artery disease risk factors. *Exp Biol Med (Maywood)* 228: 434-440, 2003.

2. **Belanger M and Boulay P**. Effect of an aerobic exercise training program on resting metabolic rate in chronically beta-adrenergic blocked hypertensive patients. *J Cardiopulm Rehabil* 25: 354-360, 2005.

3. **Blevins FT**. Rotator cuff pathology in athletes. *Sports Med* 24: 205-220, 1997.

4. **Braith RW and Stewart KJ**. Resistance exercise training: its role in the prevention of cardiovascular disease. *Circulation* 113: 2642-2650, 2006.

5. **Coris EE, Ramirez AM and Van Durme DJ**. Heat illness in athletes: the dangerous combination of heat, humidity and exercise. *Sports Med* 34: 9-16, 2004.

6. **Dickhuth HH, Rocker K, Mayer F, Konig D and Korsten-Reck** U. [Endurance training and cardial adaptation (athlete's heart)]. *Herz* 29: 373-380, 2004.

7. **Ewert R, Opitz CF, Wensel R, Winkler J, Halank M and Felix SB**. Continuous intravenous iloprost to revert treatment failure of first-line inhaled iloprost therapy in patients with idiopathic pulmonary arterial hypertension. *Clin Res Cardiol* 2007.

8. **Fagard RH and Cornelissen VA**. Effect of exercise on blood pressure control in hypertensive patients. *Eur J Cardiovasc Prev Rehabil* 14: 12-17, 2007.

9. **Fattirolli F, Cellai T and Burgisser C**. [Physical activity and cardiovascular health a close link]. *Monaldi Arch Chest Dis* 60: 73-78, 2003.

10. **Fry RW, Morton AR and Keast D**. Overtraining in athletes. An update. *Sports Med* 12: 32-65, 1991.

11. **Gamalei IA and Kaulin AB**. [Microscopic viscosity of muscle fibers. II. Temperature relations]. *Tsitologiia* 14: 1322-1327, 1972.

12. **Giada F, Bertaglia E, De Piccoli B, Franceschi M, Sartori F, Raviele A and Pascotto P**. Cardiovascular adaptations to endurance training and detraining in young and older athletes. *Int J Cardiol* 65: 149-155, 1998.

13. **Ingraham SJ**. The role of flexibility in injury prevention and athletic performance: have we stretched the truth? *Minn Med* 86: 58-61, 2003.

14. **Jacobson AL and Henderson J**. Temperature sensitivity of myosin and actomyosin. *Can J Biochem* 51: 71-86, 1973.

15. **Kamijo Y and Nose H**. Heat illness during working and preventive considerations from body fluid homeostasis. *Ind Health* 44: 345-358, 2006.

16. **Karacabey K**. Effect of regular exercise on health and disease. *Neuro Endocrinol Lett* 26: 617-623, 2005.

17. **Kemi OJ, Haram PM, Loennechen JP, Osnes JB, Skomedal T, Wisloff U and Ellingsen O**. Moderate vs. high exercise intensity: differential effects on aerobic fitness, cardiomyocyte contractility, and endothelial function. *Cardiovasc Res* 67: 161-172, 2005.

18. **Kiefhaber TR and Stern PJ**. Upper extremity tendinitis and overuse syndromes in the athlete. *Clin Sports Med* 11: 39-55, 1992.

19. **Kreuzer F**. Facilitated diffusion of oxygen and its possible significance; a review. *Respir Physiol* 9: 1-30, 1970.

20. **Lambert CP and Evans WJ**. Adaptations to aerobic and resistance exercise in the elderly. *Rev Endocr Metab Disord* 6: 137-143, 2005.

21. **McGowan CM, Golland LC, Evans DL, Hodgson DR and Rose RJ**. Effects of prolonged training, overtraining and detraining on skeletal muscle metabolites and enzymes. *Equine Vet J Suppl* 257-263, 2002.

22. **Mutungi G and Ranatunga KW**. Temperature-dependent changes in the viscoelasticity of intact resting mammalian (rat) fast- and slow-twitch muscle fibres. *J Physiol* 508 (Pt 1): 253-265, 1998.

23. **Pogliaghi S, Terziotti P, Cevese A, Balestreri F and Schena F**. Adaptations to endurance training in the healthy elderly: arm cranking versus leg cycling. *Eur J Appl Physiol* 97: 723-731, 2006.

24. **Renstrom P and Johnson RJ**. Overuse injuries in sports. A review. *Sports Med* 2: 316-333, 1985.

25. **Sesboue B and Guincestre JY**. Muscular fatigue. *Ann Readapt Med Phys* 49: 257-54, 2006.

26. **Sharman JE, Geraghty DP, Shing CM, Fraser DI and Coombes JS**. Endurance exercise, plasma oxidation and cardiovascular risk. *Acta Cardiol* 59: 636-642, 2004.

27. **Shellock FG and Prentice WE**. Warming-up and stretching for improved physical performance and prevention of sports-related injuries. *Sports Med* 2: 267-278, 1985.

28. **Shellock FG and Prentice WE**. Warming-up and stretching for improved physical performance and prevention of sports-related injuries. *Sports Med* 2: 267-278, 1985.

29. **Sheon RP**. Repetitive strain injury. 2. Diagnostic and treatment tips on six common problems. The Goff Group. *Postgrad Med* 102: 72-8, 81, 85, 1997.

30. **Shephard RJ**. Chronic fatigue syndrome. A brief review of functional disturbances and potential therapy. *J Sports Med Phys Fitness* 45: 381-392, 2005.

31. **Sidell BD**. Intracellular oxygen diffusion: the roles of myoglobin and lipid at cold body temperature. *J Exp Biol* 201: 1119-1128, 1998.

32. **Takahashi T, Okada A, Hayano J and Tamura T**. Influence of cool-down exercise on autonomic control of heart rate during recovery from dynamic exercise. *Front Med Biol Eng* 11: 249-259, 2002.

33. **van Mechelen W, Hlobil H, Kemper HC, Voorn WJ and de Jongh HR**. Prevention of running injuries by warm-up, cool-down, and stretching exercises. *Am J Sports Med* 21: 711-719, 1993.

34. **van Mechelen W, Hlobil H, Kemper HC, Voorn WJ and de Jongh HR**. Prevention of running injuries by warm-up, cool-down, and stretching exercises. *Am J Sports Med* 21: 711-719, 1993.

35. **Walsh NP and Whitham M**. Exercising in environmental extremes : a greater threat to immune function? *Sports Med* 36: 941-976, 2006.

36. **Westerblad H and Allen DG**. Cellular mechanisms of skeletal muscle fatigue. *Adv Exp Med Biol* 538: 563-570, 2003.

37. **Whitney JD, Stotts NA and Goodson WH, III**. Effects of dynamic exercise on subcutaneous oxygen tension and temperature. *Res Nurs Health* 18: 97-104, 1995.

38. **Whitney JD, Stotts NA and Goodson WH, III**. Effects of dynamic exercise on subcutaneous oxygen tension and temperature. *Res Nurs Health* 18: 97-104, 1995.

39. **Zanettini R, Bettega D, Agostoni O, Ballestra B, del Rosso G, di Michele R and Mannucci PM**. Exercise training in mild hypertension: effects on blood pressure, left ventricular mass and coagulation factor VII and fibrinogen. *Cardiology* 88: 468-473, 1997.

Chapter 16

Flexibility Assessment & Programming

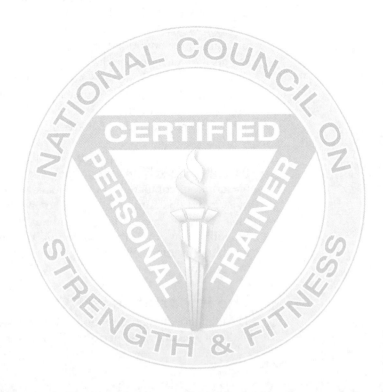

Introduction

Flexibility has numerous definitions that depend upon the point of reference from which it is being viewed. Webster's Dictionary defines it as "to bend, or having the ability to be bent." In fitness, flexibility is most often defined as the ability of a joint to move through a full range of motion. For the purposes of this book, **flexibility** and **range of motion (ROM)** will be used synonymously. This definition is more appropriate because flexibility is measured using an articulation site, a joint, as the reference point. In some cases, the measurement is quantified by angular units or degrees of movement. In others, the measurement is linear, often expressed as a distance covered in centimeters or inches. Regardless of how flexibility is quantified, it still reflects the ability of a joint to move around its axis.

Movement range at a particular joint is important because it defines the joint's functional capabilities. Each individual joint of the body is unique in its defined movement potential. The movement potential is determined by a joint's function in the **musculoskeletal** system. For example, both the hip joint and the shoulder joint are similar in structure; however, the hip joint has a limited ROM due to bony constraints. The hip must support the weight of the entire upper body, whereas the shoulder has a much greater ROM because it only has to support the weight of the arm, allowing greater functional range. In general, joints with less ROM

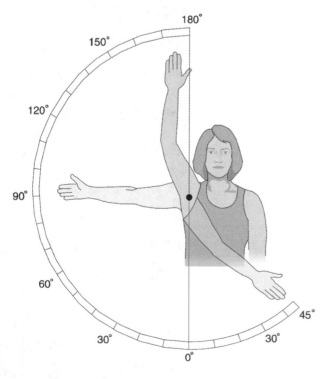

Example of ROM

potential offer greater stability, whereas joints with greater ROM potential are inherently less stable. This explains why shoulder dislocations are much more common than hip dislocations (44). Additionally, joint movement potentials may differ when comparing bilateral joints (i.e the right and left shoulder). Attainable movements in one shoulder may not be equaled in range by the joint of the opposite side. This suggests that measurement of one or more joint movements does not validly predict total body flexibility or possibly even bilateral flexibility. Differences between bilateral joint movement capabilities depend upon several variables, including genetic variations, activity participation, connective tissue discrepancy, and joint injury (36; 57). For example, a person performing right side dominant movement in his or her job will generally have greater ROM in the right shoulder compared to the left, secondary to the frequent placement of the right shoulder through its full ROM.

Flexibility is an inherent component of movement capabilities and therefore, plays a major role in human function and the ability to attain health through physical activity. Interestingly, although flexibility is a primary determinant in the body's ability to move, it receives very little attention in many exercise programs. From a health perspective, it is no less important than any other component of fitness, yet it only receives passive appreciation for what it actually offers. Most personal training clients expect visual changes in their physiques as a quantifiable measure of training effectiveness. Common goals of many programs are to lose body fat and improve muscle tone. Anecdotally speaking, there is a strong psychosocial association between exercise and improved vanity. The majority of individuals who exercise desire to look better for their efforts and take pleasure in the attention they receive when others notice the positive changes that have taken place. Flexibility is difficult to quantify upon visual observation and does little to improve a person's appearance. Due to this fact, much more attention is devoted to muscular enhancements and reduced body fat.

When markers of improvement are vanity-related, flexibility is likely to take a back seat in the exercise prescription, compared to other goals. Personal trainers must avoid this common mistake to appropriately serve their clients' needs. Understanding the benefits of flexibility can help in understanding the importance of including routine flexibility training in the exercise prescription.

The Importance of ROM

The attainable range of motion at a joint affects the way the joint functions and performs. Therefore, maintaining

Benefits of Flexibility

- Increased movement range
- Reduction in rate of functional decline
- Postural symmetry
- Stress reduction
- Reduced tension
- Muscle relaxation
- Reduced incidence of muscle cramps
- Reduced risk of injury
- Relief of muscle pain
- Improved quality of life

an optimal level of flexibility allows for efficient movement at various movement velocities and a high level of joint health. Likewise, proper functional range alleviates the consequences associated with poor range of motion. The maintenance of flexibility over the span of a lifetime associates with a decrease in functional decline and greater independence (26; 82). One of the most detrimental outcomes of range of motion decline is limitation in movement capabilities. As stated earlier in Chapter 15, the series of events that leads to reduced flexibility becomes problematic as rigidity reduces physical activity participation. This creates a negative feedback loop, as reduced physical activity further limits range of motion. As a result, the progressive downward spiral leads to chronic pain, dysfunction, and reduced quality of life (25; 81).

A lack of flexibility is implicated in a variety of musculoskeletal injuries. One key factor is postural symmetry. Tight muscles pull on bony structures, distorting the normal alignment. When the kinetic chain is compromised, soft tissues become stressed due to force variations that do not exist when the joint is properly aligned. This presents two problems that promote joint injury. The first problem is that the alignment change causes movement deviation, leading to undue stress on connecting structures (84). This is why a runner with a hip joint injury can develop a knee injury if he or she continues to train without allowing the hip to properly heal. The second problem is the body is subjected to ongoing forces that can lead to exhaustive strain. Some common examples of alignment alterations are an anterior shift of the shoulder, called upper cross syndrome and pelvic instability due to compromised tilt position. Both musculoskeletal misalignments can cause joint discomfort and may lead to chronic pain. Low back

pain, in particular, is often associated with lack of flexibility in the muscles that act on the hip and lower spine (37; 46; 58). Additionally, tight musculature is subject to injury when the joint is forcibly moved through a functionally unattainable movement range or at high velocities. Lack of flexibility related to musculoskeletal imbalances often lies at the root of muscle strains and connective tissue sprains in sports (21; 45).

Improved range of motion and participation in flexibility routines have been shown to positively affect stress. Reduced muscle tension through improved relaxation of the tissue is associated with improved self-reported stress reduction (8; 11; 75). Likewise, the activities employed to address range of motion, such as yoga, have shown to affect acute stress response (9; 11). The proposed mechanisms include the alleviation of tension, psychomotor distraction, and an overall state of relaxation. This information further supports the use of flexibility for improved health and well-being.

Properties of Soft Tissue

Soft tissue includes muscle, **fascia**, tendons, and ligaments. These tissues all possess some stretch quality or deformation potential. The property that allows stretched tissue to return to its original, or pre-stretched form, is referred to as the tissue's elasticity. A rubber band that is stretched can be significantly deformed from its starting position, but when the forces that pull the band into a stretched position are removed, the rubber band returns to its initial static position. The ability to return to its original form is based on the rubber band's elastic properties. The elastic properties of soft tissue work similarly and allow the tissue to be deformed beyond its resting state. The length attained is a factor of the relationship between the internal force

~Quick Insight~

Hypermobility

When a person can attain abnormal range of motion at a joint they are often said to be "double jointed" or to have extreme flexibility. In fact, neither concept is true. Flexibility refers to tissue extensibility or physiologically-controlled range of motion at a joint. Hypermobile joints are not as much a factor of tissue flexibility as they are a lack of stability. Laxity refers to a joint's stability. Therefore, the ability of an articulation to separate upon voluntary control is actually caused by excessive joint laxity. **Hypermobility** is undesirable due to the fact that the integrity of the joint system is compromised. Individuals with hypermobility at a joint should attempt to strengthen the attached musculature to increase the stability of the joint, thus preventing possible injury.

generated by the tissue, or resistive force, and the external force causing it to lengthen. When the resistive force is low within the tissue, and the external lengthening force rises above the tissue's internal force threshold, the tissue will lengthen to the magnitude of the external lengthening force.

Plasticity

Plasticity is the property of a tissue to become permanently deformed, or to attain a new length after being stretched. Appropriate levels of tissue-stretching-force applied routinely can cause the connective tissue to assume a chronic plastic state or new permanent length. This explains how tendons adapt to flexibility programs. Due to the limited elastic properties of tendons, they improve in range by permanently lengthening. If the external forces far exceed the resistive forces, the tissue may be lengthened beyond its elastic limit. When this occurs the tissue may become injured and become permanently deformed. An example of a negative consequence of plasticity is the permanent lengthening of spinal ligaments from the long-term application of stress due to poor seating posture (17; 32). When this occurs, the integrity of the system is compromised and injury is a likely outcome.

Viscosity

Another property that affects soft tissue is the variable fluid resistance, referred to as viscosity. This property is not as constant as elasticity or plasticity, but rather varies depending on acute tissue factors. When something is viscous, it adds to the tissue's resistance to change. When viscosity is reduced, so is the resistive force present in the tissue. This concept justifies warming up before stretching. Warming a tissue up before stretching will reduce the tissue's viscosity, consequently increasing its elastic response. Changes in viscosity are temporary and do not directly contribute to tissue adaptations to flexibility training (70; 83; 86). Decreased viscosity can indirectly cause a reduction in resistance, allowing for greater range during the performance of the flexibility program. Viscoelasticity describes the tissue's behavior related to external load and internal conditions and properties.

Factors Affecting Joint Range of Motion

Muscle Factors

Although the nervous system mediates tension within the muscle, myogenic mechanisms (mechanisms arising from within the muscle itself) also contribute to both an increase and decrease in range of motion. The variations in the range of motion are, in part, related to the

Key Terms

Flexibility – The ability of a joint to move through a full range of motion.

Range of motion (ROM) – The achievable distance between the flexed position and the extended position of a joint that can be measured.

Musculoskeletal – Relating to, or involving, the muscles and the skeleton.

Hypermobility – Describes joints that move further than a normal range of motion.

myofibrils within the muscle fibers. The number of **sarcomeres** and their ability to lengthen contributes to a muscle's range of motion. The ability of the sarcomeres to lengthen seems to be dependent on the elastic properties of the titin filaments (10; 18; 50). **Titin filaments** are the noncontractile protein filaments which make up the ends of the sarcomere (76). On the other hand, the contractile filaments, actin and myosin, do not change in length because they require extreme rigidity to produce force. These characteristics allow the contractile proteins to maintain their force generating qualities while still allowing the myofibril to reach greater lengths. If actin and myosin were to possess elastic properties, they would stretch under the application of stress, thereby reducing their force generating capabilities.

The sarcomeres also play a role in the passive length of the tissue. When muscle tissue is immobilized in a lengthened position using a cast, the result is an addition of sarcomeres along the myofibril at the end of the muscle toward the tendon (72; 73). The opposite effect occurs when a muscle is immobilized in a shortened length. The sarcomere numbers and length reduce, in compliance with the shortened position. Based on these findings, it can be surmised that muscle fiber elasticity is a factor of the number of sarcomeres along a myofibril and their respective ability to lengthen.

For the muscle to reach maximal length, the tissue must be in a relaxed state. Muscle relaxation is a passive act that occurs when the muscle no longer receives neural signals for tension. Most researchers agree that muscle relaxation is contingent upon the removal of calcium from troponin, causing disassociation of the contractile proteins (31). Muscles elongate as a result of external forces because the fibers do not have the ability to lengthen themselves. These forces may be due to a contraction of an antagonist muscle group, gravity, momentum force, or the force provided by a partner when stretching. The contractile component of the muscle can be elongated by up to 67% above the resting sarcomere length, which allows for a wide range of motion (42; 56). The ability of the muscle to relax when being stretched is a factor of its extensibility characteristics.

The amount of force necessary to lengthen a relaxed muscle is called passive tension. The greatest contributor to the lengthening resistance that exists in a relaxed muscle is related to the connective fascia within the tissue, including the **epimysium**, **perimysium**, and endomysium (48; 49). When muscle tissue is stretched in a relaxed state, the resistive properties become reduced. The acute response to a flexibility routine is a reduction in passive tension. This explains why participating in a flexibility program enables a person to attain a greater range than they were capable of before the flexibility exercises were performed. This is referred to as an elastic response. When the flexibility training is utilized on a routine basis, the elastic properties of the muscle increase, and in turn, the passive tension decreases, leading to an improved range of motion by way of a plastic response.

Connective Tissue Factors

Collagen represents approximately 33% of the protein structural component in the body. It presents limitations due to its inherent properties of high tensile strength and inextensibility. Collagen is the primary constituent of tendons and ligaments, as their functional roles warrant very limited extension capabilities. The more collagen in an area, the more resistant the tissue is to being elongated or deformed (29; 62). These properties contribute to the greatest limitation in joint range of motion. In fact, the connective tissue that comprises a joint's capsule provides almost 50% of the resistance to the joint's movement (28; 63).

Elastic fibers on the other hand provide for a greater magnitude of elongation. They are commonly located in close association with collagen fibers. When elastic fibers are found in greater quantity than collagen fibers in a particular tissue, the tissue will have greater extensibility characteristics. The elastic properties allow extended tissues to return to their prior state following a stretch.

Elastic tissue is present in different concentrations within the muscle connective tissue, or fascia, and plays a major role in determining the muscle's extensibility. Compared to tendons and ligaments, which are primarily composed of collagen, muscle connective tissue has higher quantities of elastic fibers. It is the elastic component that allows for the muscle's ability to

stretch. In addition, the elastic fibers in the tissue are responsible for several important functions, including conserving tone during muscle relaxation, enhancing coordination during rhythmic motion of the body, accommodating excessive force, and returning tissues to their original form, following deformation from force application.

Connective fascia makes up nearly one-third of the body's muscle mass. It serves several functions,

Contributors to Movement Resistance

Structure	Resistance
Joint Capsule	47%
Muscle Fascia	41%
Tendon	10%
Skin	2%

~Quick Insight~

Myofascial Release Technique

When muscle tissue is placed under significant stress, the myofascial alignment can be altered due to multidirectional restriction (27). These restrictions can cause the tissue to adopt a level of dysfunction and may manifest in pain. In some cases, the discomfort is localized. However, since fascia is continuous, restrictions to the tissue can affect other areas. In some cases, the pain is related to myofascial trigger points, which appear to be associated with the formation of pain circuits in the spinal cord in response to the disturbance of the nerve endings and abnormal contractile mechanisms at multiple dysfunctional sites (40). Myofascial restriction and trigger points can be managed or alleviated using different treatment methods, including stretching, manual massage, thermotherapy, and electrotherapy (2; 66). When myofascial restriction is significant, acupressure and myofascial release techniques, such as pressure rolling the affected area can return the compromised neurophysiological state of the tissue to its functional pathways (85). Foam rollers, rolling sticks, and related devices have gained popularity in addressing myofascial restriction, associated with physical activity and sport. The devices can provide self-massage, which has shown to be an effective means of soft tissue care. When the tissue alignment is not compromised by restriction and neural physiological mechanisms are functioning properly, the tissue will improve its performance.

including providing shape and a connective framework, fiber, blood vessel, and nerve alignment and even force transfer to the whole muscle. Under passive stretch, the muscle fascia provides the second greatest level of resistance to the movement.

Neural Factors

The three primary receptors used for neural management of the soft tissue related to range of motion are the muscle spindles, Golgi tendon organs, and the joint **mechanoreceptors**. The muscle spindles lie parallel to the muscle fibers in the belly of the muscle. They serve as the primary stretch receptor, identifying the length and velocity of the stretch. When a stretch is applied in a slow, controlled manner the muscle spindles remain dormant, allowing the tissue to extend. When the velocity of the stretch is increased, the muscle spindles activate to prevent the tissue from being overstretched by adding resistive tension. For this reason, high speed movements and **ballistic stretching** techniques do not allow the muscle tissue to relax due to counter tension development, which actually reduces the maximal attainable length (7; 61; 69). This is essentially the body's way of preventing injury. Muscle spindles activate before the tissue is stretched beyond the point where damage may occur.

The Golgi tendon organs are located in the musculotendinous junction. Although recent clinical attention has identified several roles of the receptors, an important function for tissue protection is the **autogenic inhibition** response to excessive force (47; 65). The receptors identify rapid changes in the muscle force and operate by inhibiting the muscle contraction to promote

tissue relaxation. This occurs to prevent forces that would damage the tissue during active stretching.

The articular mechanoreceptors are found in synovial articulations in four varieties. The receptors serve a variety of functions to sense joint changes. Some of the functions include:

1. Signals direction, amplitude, and velocity of the joint movements.
2. Regulates changes in joint pressure.
3. Contributes to postural and kinesthetic sensation.
4. Facilitates the CNS in regulating muscle tone.
5. Produces an inhibitory effect on pain.
6. Measures quick changes in the joint movement.
7. Produces reflex inhibition of muscles acting on the joint.
8. Signals pain reception within a joint.

These mechanisms contribute to the neural controls that protect a joint and help it to function efficiently. The combination of functions performed by the joint mechanoreceptors play a role in facilitating improved range of motion attainment when proper methods of stretching are employed.

Another neural factor that influences tissue elongation is a type of reflex inhibition called reciprocal innervation. When a muscle or muscle group contracts, the antagonist muscle or muscle group relaxes. Reciprocal innervation is what causes the hamstring muscles to relax during quadricep contraction. The purpose for this reflex is to prevent the agonist muscle group from having to overcome antagonistic tension in addition to the resistance it is accelerating against. Reciprocal innervation allows for coordinated muscle action. It has implications in flexibility because the excitatory impulses lead to greater relaxation in the stretched muscle if the reciprocating muscle contracts.

Age

Muscle, like other tissues in the body, experiences a functional decline with age. The actual age that this functional diminution occurs varies based on many factors, including genetics, health status, relative fitness level, and the quantity and type

Factors Limiting Range of Motion

Muscle Fascia
Tendon
Joint Capsule
Skin

Cross Section of Shoulder

Golgi Tendon Organ

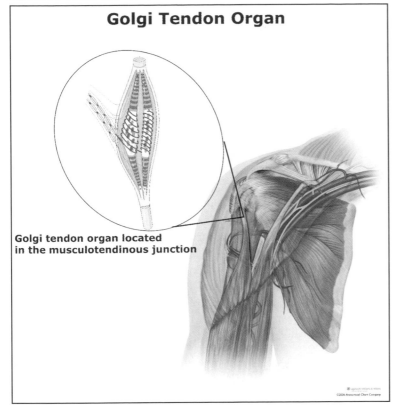

Golgi tendon organ located in the musculotendinous junction

physical fitness-related behaviors early in life increases the likelihood that health-related fitness will extend into the later years, and functional decline will be delayed. Flexibility training should be a valued part of all physical fitness programming, regardless of the age of the client.

Gender

It has been said that females are more flexible than males. Although supported by some clinical evidence, this statement is certainly lacking conclusiveness (39; 77). Simply selecting two random individuals on the street may quickly disprove this theory, as there are numerous factors which can easily invalidate the claim. In the defense of the researchers, some factors support the conclusion, as females are likely to display greater range of motion in some movements, compared to males. Although variations exist, upon observation, the female pelvis is noticeably broader at the top and narrower at the bottom. This marked gender difference allows for greater pelvic range of motion. Additionally, females show greater range

of physical activity performed (16; 67). The latter may have the greatest impact, as physically inactive individuals seem to experience a more rapid decline, which is further worsened by disease and injury. **Sarcopenia** is the term associated with the progressive atrophy of muscle mass, where the size and number of muscle fibers are reduced. The reduction in muscle mass negatively affects power, strength, endurance, speed, and flexibility.

The loss of flexibility with age is attributed to a reduction in sarcomeres along the muscle's length which are replaced with lipids and collagen fibers (20). In a process called fibrosis, the tissue loses its resiliency due to biochemical alterations in which connective tissue stiffness increases via an addition in the number of cross linkages (collagen). The tissue also experiences a series of mineralization processes, including calcification, further reducing the elasticity.

When a healthy level of flexibility is attained during youth, it is much easier to maintain over a lifespan, compared to initiating a flexibility program as an adult, particularly in the later years. Early research by Sermeev suggested that there is in fact an optimal time to begin flexibility training. Termed the "critical period" Sermeev observed the greatest improvements between the ages of 7 and 11 years of age with maximal values attained by 15 years of age (15; 33). This does not suggest that individuals above the age of 15 cannot benefit from flexibility training, but rather that adopting

Key Terms

Sarcomeres – A segment into which a fibril of striated muscle is divided.

Titin filaments – Non-contractile, structural protein filaments which make up the ends of the sarcomere.

Epimysium – The layer of connective tissue surrounding an entire muscle.

Perimysium – The layer of connective tissue enveloping bundles of muscle fibers.

Collagen – The fibrous protein constituent of bone, cartilage, tendon, and other connective tissue.

Mechanoreceptors – A specialized sensory end organ that responds to mechanical stimuli such as tension, pressure, or displacement.

Ballistic stretching – A form of passive or dynamic stretching, usually a bouncing motion, in which a limb or joint is forced into an extended range of motion when the muscle is not yet relaxed.

Autogenic inhibition – Caused by stimulating the GTO via an increase of tension, creating an inhibitory effect on the muscle spindles.

Sarcopenia – The degenerative loss of skeletal muscle mass and strength.

in elbow extension due to differences in the curvature of the olecranon process (the proximal end of the ulnar bone) and some show greater trunk flexibility attributed to shorter leg length and a lower center of gravity (68; 80). This being said, a person's gender will not ensure or prevent healthy flexibility.

Females may also experience range of motion adjustments due to the hormonal effects and physical changes related to pregnancy. It is well documented that peripheral joint laxity increases during pregnancy and it has been postulated that the hormone relaxin may be the cause, but evidence is not supportive of this claim. In fact, research suggests the changes in peripheral joint laxity do not seem to correlate well with maternal estradiol, progesterone, or relaxin levels (6; 12). Nonetheless, personal trainers should be aware of the orthopedic risks of joint laxity during and immediately following pregnancy and structure their programs appropriately.

Body Mass

It has been suggested that an increase in muscle mass reduces the tissue's range of motion. Taken at face value, this is not at all accurate. The limitations to flexibility have been discussed and have implicated several mechanisms by which flexibility may be reduced, none of which included the hypertrophy of a muscle fiber. The tissue possesses the same elastic properties, regardless of the diameter. It is likely this misconception is associated with some of the factors associated with hypertrophy training. When heavy resistance is moved through a limited range of motion, the muscle adapts to the environment. Routinely performing limited range movements may lead to a reduction in flexibility. Heavy bench pressing and bi-lateral rows have both been implicated in reduced range of motion in the upper back and shoulder. Individuals who perform resistance training with resistance appropriate for their strength capabilities, and move through a full range of motion, will not lose the lengthening qualities of the tissue. In fact, resistance training can aid in improving flexibility when performed correctly (19; 71). Unilateral activity seems to improve range of motion above bilateral movements due to the separation of the limbs and stabilization of attached structures more often influenced in bilateral movements.

The popularity of steroid use may also be a factor that leads people to believe resistance training and muscle mass make you less flexible. In addition to the aforementioned possibilities, individuals who use steroids often dramatically increase muscle mass beyond a normal attainable level. The excessive sizes reached by today's bodybuilders may create a limitation in movement range due to a muscle-bound phenomenon. Although these individuals would benefit from a flexibility routine, the excessiveness of their hypertrophy may become a physical obstacle to movement.

Muscle is not the only tissue that can present obstacles to movement range. Excessive fat mass stored in both visceral and subcutaneous areas can limit a person's ability to move. This is particularly true for central storage, as the midsection collides with other body segments when bending in a seated position. Obesity can have indirect effects as well. Obese individuals have a tendency to participate in less physical activity, move through more limited ranges, and experience musculoskeletal problems such as low back pain and orthopedic limitations. These factors further contribute to a reduction in range of motion and can manifest into significant limitations in movement capabilities if untreated.

Immobility

Immobility has detrimental effects on muscle tissue. Significant strength and flexibility loss can occur in a relatively short period of time (54; 79). Of particular concern is the loss of elasticity in the connective tissue elements. But the effects are not limited to the tissue structures. Chemical structure changes are also relevant, as they can result in reduced spacing between collagen fibers. When the fiber proximity is reduced to the point that contact occurs between the collagen fibers, cross linkages develop between fibers (3; 24; 41). This causes a reduction in extensibility and a consequent reduction in range of motion.

Immobility causes further detriment when the muscle is constricted in a shortened position. Evidence has shown that the reduced fiber length diminishes extensibility due to a loss of sarcomeres in series (4). Prolonged immobilization, particularly in a shortened muscle position, causes a notable decline in the functional range of motion of the tissue compared to the tissue's pre-immobilized state.

Pain

When stretching protocols are employed, discomfort and pain tolerance are factors in attainable range. The positions achieved when stretching to full ROM can cause different levels of discomfort, depending on pain inhibition which is modulated by receptors in the tissue. Individuals present variations in tolerance of discomfort, and therefore the tissue length reached may be limited by a person's relative pain threshold. Warming up tissue prior to stretching is fundamental to flexibility training but will also reduce resistance and discomfort at submaximal ranges.

Injury

Musculoskeletal injuries that result in loss of ROM usually are either the result of acute trauma or chronic overuse of a joint (60). Common injury-related ROM problems include **bursitis**, tendonitis, impingement syndromes, and **fasciitis** (43; 51; 74). Bursitis is the painful inflammation or irritation of the bursa. Bursa are soft, fluid-filled sacs that cushion the movement between the bones, tendons, and muscles near a joint. Bursitis usually occurs under the shoulder muscles, at the elbow (epitrochlear bursitis or "tennis elbow"), the hip socket (trochanteric bursitis), heel bone (retrocalcaneal bursitis), or the kneecap (called infrapatellar bursitis or "housemaid's knee"). Bursitis can be either acute or chronic.

When a joint is overused or when it stays under pressure or tension for extended periods of time, a nearby bursa can become inflamed. The bursa fills with excess fluid, causing pressure on the surrounding tissue and resulting in bursitis. Most commonly, bursitis is caused by trauma. Some specific factors possibly resulting in bursitis include overuse or injury to the joint areas, incorrect posture at work or rest, poor conditioning before exercise or sports participation, and an abnormal or poorly positioned joint or bone (such as leg length differences) that stresses soft tissue structures (23; 59). Movement pain associated with bursitis often leads to compensatory actions and limitations in range to avoid the pain.

Tendonitis describes inflammation, swelling, and irritation of a tendon. Tendonitis is a painful condition that is felt most at the tendon insertion site. Tendons are bands of fibrous material that attach muscle to bone. When these structures are irritated, they can swell and become inflamed, causing tendonitis. Tendonitis most commonly occurs in tendons associated with increased use. More common types of tendonitis include: Achilles tendonitis, Patellar tendonitis, and Elbow tendonitis (35).

Tendonitis can result from several different etiologies. However, overuse of the tendon during work or related to physical activity is the most common cause. Tennis and golf are two activities that commonly cause tendonitis of the elbow due to the repetitive motion at the elbow. Direct injury to the tendon can also result in tendonitis, as can various inflammatory conditions, such as rheumatoid arthritis (1; 22). Lastly, aging can make one more prone to developing tendonitis. As one ages, the tendons lose their elasticity, making them more susceptible to irritation and inflammation. Chronic tendonitis reduces activity and movement range, related to pain and discomfort.

Impingement syndromes are the painful entrapments of a tendon between the bony aspects of a joint. The most common example is shoulder impingement syndrome. With shoulder impingement syndrome, the **supraspinatus tendon**, **subacromial-subdeltoid bursa**, and/or the biceps tendon becomes entrapped between the humeral head and the **coracoacromial arch**. Shoulder impingement most often occurs in repetitive overhead activities such as swimming, serving a tennis ball, spiking a volleyball, or throwing a ball (22). Similar with the other injuries, pain becomes the limiting factor to attaining full range of motion.

Fasciitis is a condition in which the fascia that covers a surface of underlying tissue becomes inflamed. Though fasciitis can potentially occur with any fascia, the most prevalent is plantar fasciitis. Plantar fasciitis is a condition that occurs when the long, fibrous, plantar fascia ligament along the bottom of the foot develops tears in the tissue, resulting in pain and inflammation. The pain of plantar fasciitis is usually located close to where the fascia attaches to the calcaneous, or heel bone. The most common cause is an overload of physical activity or exercise. Excessive running, jumping, or other activities can easily place repetitive or excessive stress on the tissue and lead to tears and inflammation, resulting in moderate to severe pain that limits activity and movement range (14; 38).

Factors Affecting Flexibility

Knowledge of stretching techniques and stretches

Time availability

Identified deficiencies

Client's pain tolerance and interest

Imbalances

Injury

Orthopedic limitations

Disease

Disease

Several diseases can cause ROM limitations. The most common of these include osteoarthritis, **rheumatoid arthritis**, and **gout**. Osteoarthritis (OA) is a degenerative disorder of aging that can affect any joint, but is most commonly diagnosed in the hips, knees, toes, and the spine (13; 55; 85). Osteoarthritis increases water content and decreases protein makeup of cartilage. The cartilage begins to degenerate by becoming soft and flaking into the joints, losing its ability to cushion. This results in rubbing and friction between the joints. **Osteophytes** (outgrowth of new bone), commonly called "spurs" form at the edges of the joint surfaces, and the joint capsules and synovial membranes thicken. The joint spaces begin to narrow and lose their stability. All these changes lead to pain, inflammation, and limited mobility. A significant factor in addition to aging that may contribute to the development of OA is obesity. Other factors are repetitive stress to the joints, infection, or previous injury (13; 52; 55; 85).

Rheumatoid arthritis (RA) is an inflammatory disorder of unknown etiology. Its symptoms are generally caused by a person's immune system attacking his or her joints, resulting in inflammation. RA is characterized by symmetric, erosive synovitis (inflammation of the joint) and, in some cases, extra-articular involvement (involvement outside of the joint). Most people with RA experience a chronic, fluctuating course of disease that, despite therapeutic measures, may result in progressive joint destruction, deformity, disability, and premature death (5; 53; 64). The inflammation associated with RA damages the synovial joints of the wrists, shoulders, knees, ankles, and feet. Rheumatoid nodules that form close to the joints and other skin problems may be present in approximately 25% of RA patients and usually signal the most rapidly progressive form of the disease. Rheumatoid nodules usually develop in areas of the body where pressure is applied, including the **sacrum** and elbows. RA is debilitating and can significantly compromise movement capabilities associated with joint dysfunction.

Gout is a form of arthritis that primarily affects older males. It appears very quickly, often overnight, causing intense swelling and pain. The ball of the big toe is the most common site for gout. Gout is a condition in which uric acid, a by-product of metabolism, rises above normal levels. Uric acid is normally flushed out of the body in the urine. When a person has gout, the uric acid forms crystals which are deposited in the joints. These uric acid crystal deposits give rise to inflammation, in turn causing pain, swelling and redness which may limit attainable range of motion in the affected joint. Gout occurs more frequently in countries that have a high standard of living and is most likely diet related. The disease can usually be treated easily with medicine and prevented by changes in an individual's diet.

Testing Flexibility

The variability among joint range of motion requires a battery of flexibility assessments to determine range of motion deficiencies that may exist throughout the body. Ideally, each joint movement should be assessed using direct tests that assess rotational range in degrees of movement. Goniometer, inclinometer, and flexometer devices can be used to directly assess the joint range of motion with quantifiable data. If direct measurement is unattainable, indirect assessments can be performed to assess the functional range of motion in different joint movements. In some cases, indirect measures use assistive flexibility devices that provide data feedback such as the sit-and-reach box. In other cases, the movements are quantified using visual observation and/or tape measurement to determine range.

Key Terms

Bursitis – Inflammation of the bursa.

Fasciitis – Inflammation of the fascia.

Supraspinatus tendon – Runs along the top of the shoulder blade and inserts at the top of the humerus bone.

Subacromial-subdeltoid bursa – The fluid filled sac located between the coracoacromial arch and the rotator cuff.

Coracoacromial arch – A protective arch formed by the smooth inferior aspect of the acromion and coracoid process of the scapula.

Rheumatoid arthritis – A chronic autoimmune disease causing inflammation and deformity of the joints.

Gout – A disturbance of uric acid metabolism, usually occurring in males and often characterized by painful inflammation of the joints, typically in the feet and hands.

Osteophytes – Small, abnormal bony growths.

Sacrum – The triangular bone made up of five fused vertebrae and forming the posterior section of the pelvis.

Direct measurement using a goniometer is an effective means for assessing flexibility. The goniometer is a protractor-like device that uses a stationary arm fixed at zero degrees with a movable arm that is aligned with the bone of the movement limb or body segment. The goniometer's axis of rotation is aligned over the joint axis and the arms of the instrument are placed over bony landmarks along the longitudinal axis of body segments. The technique requires the body segment to move through its full range of motion and then to be held in a static position, at which time the goniometer is placed upon the respective bony landmarks and the degree of movement is measured and recorded. Norms exist for normal range of motion for each of the movements at each of the articulations. This assessment method provides quality data that can be used for evaluation of range and as a baseline measurement that can be used comparatively during later evaluations.

Similar to other administrator-reliant protocols, the validity and reliability is contingent upon strictness to protocol and technician expertise. The primary errors include improper alignment of rotational axis and boney landmarks. Some joints, particularly in the lower body present more difficulty in attaining true validity, compared to upper body measures. When compared to radiography, properly employed goniometer techniques show high levels of validity.

Indirect measurement methods are popular in non-clinical settings due to the relative ease of use, as well as limited technical skill and equipment requirements. In most cases, a linear measuring instrument, such as a cloth tape measure is used to quantify the range of motion attained in a select battery of field tests. The sit-and-reach and its successors including the V sit-and-reach, modified sit-and-reach, back saver sit-and-reach, and modified back saver sit-and-reach have been used as principal measures of flexibility in physical fitness assessments. These tests help assess low back and hamstring range of motion, often as a predictor of risk for low back pain (LBP). These tests have come under scrutiny for validity in measurement and predictability of incidence of LBP. For this reason, many professionals have gravitated away from these tests and migrated to other testing protocols.

Assessing ROM using Goniometric Measures

Average Range of Motion (ROM) Values for Healthy Adults

Joint	ROM (degrees)	Joint	ROM (degrees)
Shoulder		Hip	
Flexion	150-180	Flexion	100-120
Extension	50-60	Extension	30
Abduction	180	Abduction	40-45
Medial rotation	70-90	Adduction	20-30
Lateral rotation	90		
		Knee	
Elbow		Flexion	135-140
Flexion	140-150	Extension	0-10
Extension	0		
		Ankle	
Lumbar Spine		Dorsiflexion	20
Lateral Flexion	25-35	Plantar flexion	40-50
Rotation	30-45		

Data form the American Academy of Orthopedic Surgeons (Greene and Heckman 1994) and the American Medical Association (1988).

Procedure for Administering Goniometric Assessments

Joint	Body position	Axis of rotation	Stationary arm	Moving arm	Stabilization	Special considerations
Shoulder						
Extension	Prone	Acromion process	Midaxillary line	Lateral epicondyle of humerus	Scapula and thorax	Elbow is slightly flexed, and palm of hand faces body.
Flexion	Supine	Acromion process	Midaxillary line	Lateral epicondyle of humerus	Scapula and thorax	Palm of hand faces body.
Abduction	Supine	Anterior axis of acromion process	Midline of anterior aspect of sternum	Medial midline of humerus	Scapula and thorax	Palm of hand faces anteriorly: humerus is laterally rotated, elbow is extended.
Medial/lateral Rotation	Supine	Olecranon process	Perpendicular to floor	Styloid process of ulna	Distal end of humerus and scapula	Arm is abducted 90°; forearm is perpendicular to supporting surface in mid-pronated supinated position; humerus rests on pad so that it is level with acromion process.
Elbow						
Flexion (Triceps brachii)	Supine	Lateral epicondyle of humerus	Lateral midline of humerus	Lateral midline of radial head and styloid process	Distal end of humerus	Humerus is perpendicular to the floor, forearm is fully supinated
Extension (Biceps brachii)	Supine	Lateral epicondyle of humerus	Lateral midline of humerus	Lateral midline of radial head and styloid process	Distal end of humerus	Extend the elbow while holding the forearm in supination.
Hip						
Flexion / Extension	Supine / Prone	Lateral aspect of hip joint, using greater trochanter as reference	Lateral midline of pelvis	Lateral midline of femur, using lateral epicondyle for reference	Pelvis	Knee is allowed to flex as range of hip flexion is completed, knee is extended during hip extension

Procedure for Administering Goniometric Assessments Continued

Joint	Body position	Axis of rotation	Stationary arm	Moving arm	Stabilization	Special considerations
Knee						
Flexion (Quadricep)	Supine	Over the lateral epicondyle	Lateral midline of femur, using greater trochanter for reference	Lateral midline of fibula, using lateral malleolus and fibular head for reference	Femur to prevent rotation, abduction, and adduction	As knee flexes, the hip also flexes. Assesses quadricep muscle group minus the rectus femoris.
Flexion (Rectus femoris)	Prone	Over the lateral epicondyle	Lateral midline of femur, using greater trochanter for reference	Lateral midline of fibula, using lateral malleolus and fibular head for reference	Femur to prevent rotation, abduction, and adduction	Begin assessment with both feet off the end of the examination table.
Extension (Hamstring)	Supine	Over the lateral epicondyle of femur	Lateral midline of femur, using greater trochanter for reference	Lateral midline of fibula, using lateral malleolus and fibular head for reference	Femur to prevent rotation, abduction, and adduction	The end of the testing motion occurs when resistance is felt, and further knee extension causes the hip to move toward extension.
Ankle						
Dorsiflexion (Gastrocnemius)	Standing	Over the lateral aspect of lateral malleolus	Lateral midline of fibula, using head of fibula for reference	Parallel to lateral aspect of fifth metatarsal	Tibia and fibula	The subject maintains an extended knee and dorsiflexes the ankle by leaning the body forward. Endpoint reached when further dorsiflexion causes knee flexion.

Shoulder Extension

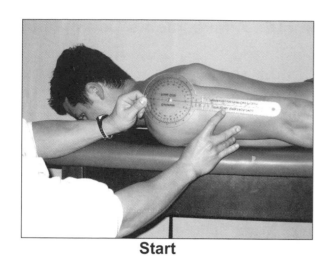 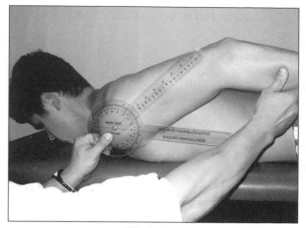

Start   **Finish**

Shoulder Flexion

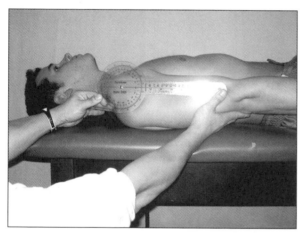 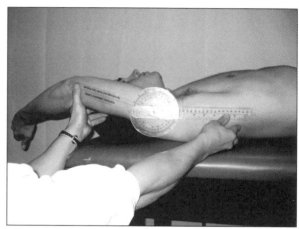

Start   **Finish**

Shoulder Abduction

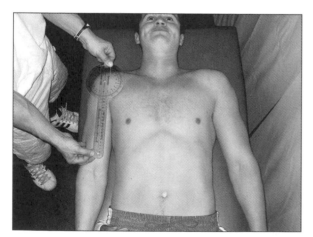 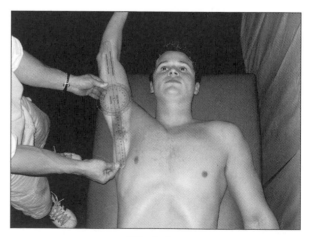

Start   **Finish**

Medial/Lateral Shoulder Rotation

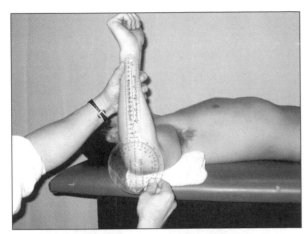

Start Lateral Rotation

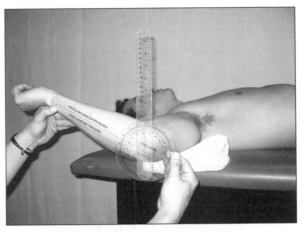

Finish Lateral Rotation

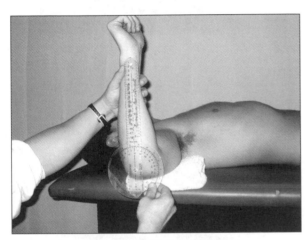

Start Medial Rotation

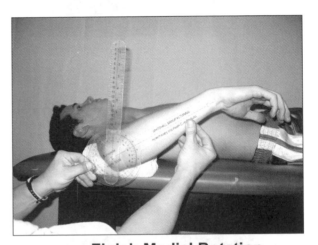

Finish Medial Rotation

Elbow Flexion (Triceps brachii)

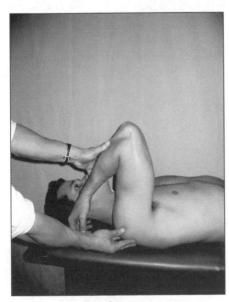

Start

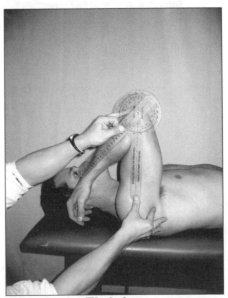

Finish

Elbow Extension (Biceps brachii)

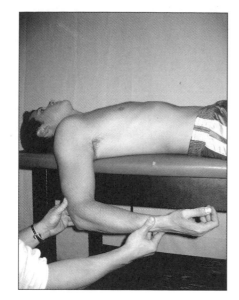

Start

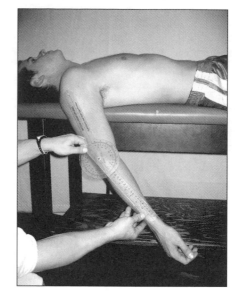

Finish

Hip Flexion

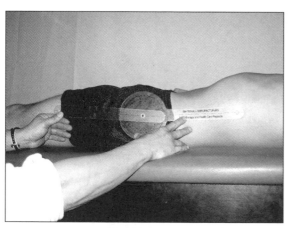

Start

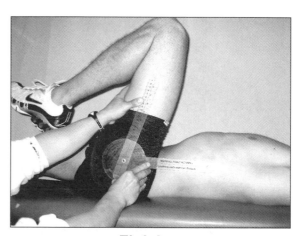

Finish

Hip Extension

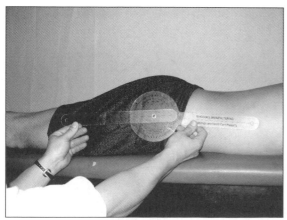

Start

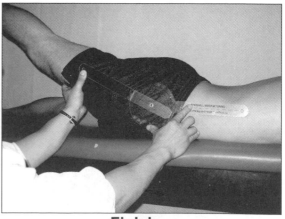

Finish

Knee Flexion (Quadricep)

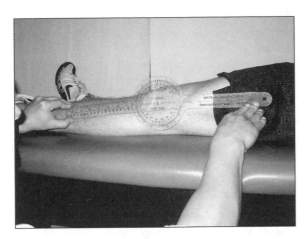

Start

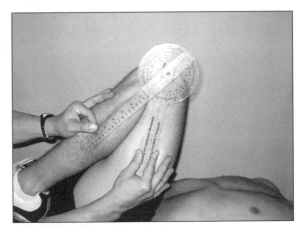

Finish

Knee Flexion (Rectus femoris)

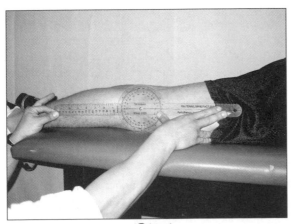

Start

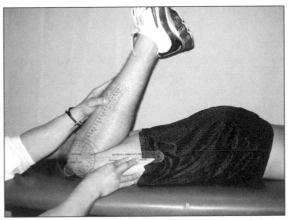

Finish

Knee Extension (Hamstring)

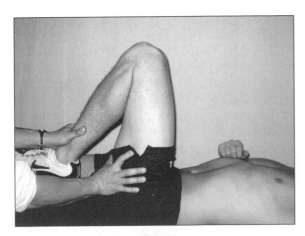

Start

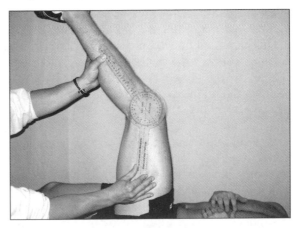

Finish

Ankle Dorisflexion (Gastrocnemius)

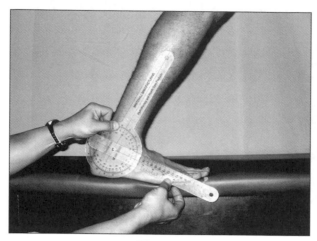

Finish

Programming

Programming for flexibility, like other fitness components, requires the organization of aggregate factors in a structured, premeditated format. The goal of flexibility training is to attain chronic adjustments in the tissue's ability to lengthen using progressively applied stretching applications. These applications should emphasize reducing the resistance within a muscle that is lengthening, while encouraging the greatest yield from the elastic properties of the tissue. The following text will review different techniques that have shown efficacy in promoting enhancements in flexibility.

The first step to implementing a flexibility program is to ensure that the tissue is in optimal condition to be stretched. This suggests participation in appropriate warm–up activities to encourage a reduced tissue viscosity and promote extensibility. Employing myofascial release techniques can also reduce fascial restriction that may limit the optimal elastic properties of the tissue. Applying acupressure or foam rolling a tender area following a general warm-up of the tissue can add to the flexibility performance. Warm-up modalities should be performed before all stretching activities.

Several techniques can be used to enhance range of motion. They are classified into one of two groups: active stretching or passive stretching. In active stretching, the client being stretched supplies the force to lengthen the tissue. In passive stretching, an external force supplies the means for moving the body segments. This force may be generated from a partner, gravity, or a stretching device.

Two categories of flexibility techniques exist within these classifications. The categories include static flexibility, meaning the tissue is lengthened and held for a designated period of time, and dynamic flexibility, which includes activities that require movement throughout the range of motion. Static flexibility is the largest category of techniques and includes static stretching, active-assisted stretching, proprioceptive neuromuscular facilitation, and active isolation. Dynamic flexibility includes dynamic performance stretching, slow speed dynamic stretching, and ballistic stretching. All hold merit to some degree for improving flexibility. The method selected will depend on one's level of knowledge and expertise with a given technique, client appropriateness, time for implementation, and where the activity falls within the exercise program.

Static Stretching

Static stretching is likely the most popular technique employed for flexibility. The basic protocol requires a person to lengthen the tissue in a slow, controlled manner to its terminal range of motion. It is important to perform the movement slowly to avoid eliciting the stretch reflex that will inhibit the attainment of full range of motion. Once the desired position has been reached, the client should concentrate on relaxing the tissue. Slow, controlled breathing techniques may help manage the discomfort experienced by some clients and aid in improving the relaxation state of the tissue. The stretch should be maintained for 30 seconds for optimal effect. Studies have analyzed different durations of static holds and 30 seconds works as effectively as longer durations.

Static stretching is ideally performed at the end of a workout routine rather than at the beginning, when strength and power activities are traditionally prescribed. Static stretching reduces power output when performed before resistance training or power-based activities. Even relatively short bouts of static stretching before strength and power events can be detrimental to performance. At the end of the workout, static stretching yields positive results following the cool down and may aid in recovery.

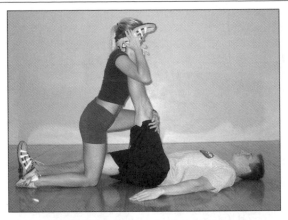

Example of Active-Assisted Stretching

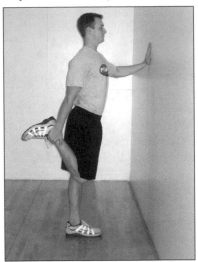

Example of Static Stretching

Active-Assisted Stretching

Active-assisted stretching utilizes the same basic premise as the static stretch, but it employs added force to increase the attainable range. The force may come from using the arms to pull the limb or body segment in a direction that increases the elongation of the tissue, a partner adding pressure to the body to increase the stretch, or the utilization of an external device to provide greater range attainment. The duration of the static hold is the same, 30 seconds. Caution must be taken so as not to overstretch the tissue. This is particularly true when a partner contributes to the additional force. Communication must be clear and concise so that only a healthy range is assumed. If a personal trainer is going to employ active-assisted stretching techniques with his or her clients, he or she should first explain the process and convey the importance of ongoing communication to avoid potential injury. Static stretching without assistance should be practiced before utilizing the active-assisted technique, so the client becomes comfortable with the protocol and identifies his or her respective limitations.

Proprioceptive Neuromuscular Facilitation (PNF)

Proprioceptive neuromuscular facilitation (PNF) is basically a hybrid between static and dynamic

flexibility because it utilizes different aspects from each protocol. The technique is widely used in clinical settings for rehabilitation of injuries but has gained popularity among fitness professionals due to its marked effects. PNF stretching is generally employed using a partner. Due to the risks associated with the technique, an appropriate level of expertise is required. PNF stretching should only be performed by individuals well versed in the technique.

PNF protocols have slight variations in the techniques used to attain a maximal range of motion. The basic technique utilizes a passive stretch to full tolerable range, which is then held for 10 seconds. At the end of the 10 second hold, the partner applies active–assisted pressure, which the client must resist by contracting the stretched muscle. This static tension segment is held for 6 seconds. The excessive tension stimulates the Golgi tendon organs, causing autogenic inhibition. At the end of the 6 second contraction, the limb is again passively stretched by the partner to the furthest attainable range and then held for the tolerable limit or 30 seconds.

In a slightly different contract–relax sequence, the client actively or passively reaches a full range of motion. Once the full tolerable range of motion is attained, the partner stabilizes the body segment in the stretched position. This position is held for 10 seconds. At the end of the 10 seconds, the client contracts the stretched muscle against the partner. The client should not change any body positions to gain leverage. Equally important, the partner assisting the stretch should have a sturdy position to prevent the body segment from moving or knocking them off balance. In many cases, the stronger movements of the body will slightly move the partner from the original position. The contract phase should last 6 seconds. Again, the partner should passively stretch the limb to the fullest attainable range and the position should be held for the tolerable limit or 30 seconds. In some techniques, the final passive stretch is assisted by an active contraction of the opposing muscle

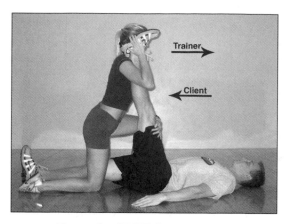

Example of PNF Stretching

group by the client to further move the body segment in the direction of the stretch. This method takes advantage of reflex inhibition and seems to present the greatest flexibility gains related to PNF techniques.

Although PNF provides notable results, the technique has its limitations. The procedure requires a competent partner and the procedures must be strictly adhered to in order to reduce the risk of injury. Even when the protocol is followed precisely, injury is more likely to occur with PNF than with a traditional static stretch. Clients must be thoroughly instructed to listen to their body and comply with an appropriate pain threshold. Some clients strive to perform so well, they ignore warning signs and may injure themselves in the process. Additionally, some clients do not like the technique due to the severity of discomfort. If this is the case, the procedure should be exchanged for a more acceptable one.

Active isolation is another hybrid model that uses a combination of active stretching and passive stretching. This technique requires the client to actively reach a full range of motion by contracting the antagonist muscle group (opposite of the muscle being stretched). Once full range of motion is reached, the partner holds the body segment. Now stabilized, the client again contracts the agonist muscle in an attempt to increase the stretch, which the partner lightly assists. The position is held for 6 seconds. The contraction is then released and a passive stretch is applied to the tolerable range and held for 15 seconds. This method also works on the premise of reciprocal innervation.

Dynamic Flexibility

The other group of stretches does not utilize the static hold position because they are dynamic in nature. **Dynamic flexibility** works in the same way that all physical activity encourages better movement ability. When tissues are routinely moved through a full range

of motion, they maintain their elastic properties. Dynamic flexibility is advantageous because it allows the body to gain flexibility from movements that can be employed before or during an exercise program. Dynamic flexibility gained popularity in track and field events and was adopted by many other sports as an effective model for preparation before an event or practice. It has also migrated into exercise programs as a way to improve flexibility during a limited duration exercise session. Dynamic flexibility is often used following a warm-up, and in some cases is used as a specific warm-up modality, mimicking the activities to follow.

Dynamic performance stretching uses a variety of movements that are similar to a particular sport or utilize the muscle emphasized in a specific activity. The movements often are exaggerated to facilitate motion in the greatest attainable range. Some common examples are high knee or straight leg marches, step-unders or step-overs using a hurdle, and long step lunges. These movements are performed in a controlled fashion so as not to elicit a response from the muscle spindles, which will limit the stretch.

Slow speed dynamic stretching is very similar to the dynamic performance stretching technique but uses slower movements that are more isolated. Some common examples are slow deep squats, single leg lunges, and floor to ceiling reaches. The technique often uses a designated time or count to complete each repetition to ensure a controlled eccentric and concentric contraction is performed without any reflex response. Slow speed dynamic stretching can utilize any movement through a full range of motion, so the options are limitless. If the movements are not being used as a specific warm-up modality, it makes sense to select movements that are not normally performed. Utilizing actions that are performed infrequently will help maintain flexibility in all the planes of movement.

Ballistic Stretching

Ballistic stretching is often considered a contraindicated method of stretching due to its potential risk for injury. The technique requires the body segment to move through a full range of motion while under momentum force. Bouncing toe touches and lunges, leg and arm swings, and high knee thrusts are all common examples. Karate and ballet have centered on ballistic stretching as a key component to flexibility enhancement. The technique does improve range of motion but with significant risk for injury. Proponents suggest the technique mimics the actions used in the events an individual trains for, whereas opponents to the technique cite the destructive nature of the movements

Key Terms

Proprioceptive neuromuscular facilitation (PNF) – A stretching technique that uses a combination of passive stretching and isometrics in which a muscle is passively stretched and then contracted to obtain an increased ROM in the joint.

Dynamic flexibility – A form of flexibility training, utilizing controlled movement performed through a full range of motion.

on the tissue and joints. The main argument against ballistic stretching, beside the stress it causes to the muscle, connective tissue, and joints, is that the velocities used never allow the tissue to relax. The fast, jerky movements employed cause the stretch reflex to create tension in the muscle, which is the direct opposite of the desired effect. With all the viable techniques available for safe flexibility training, including ballistic stretching in a personal training program is not necessarily the most sensible decision.

Flexibility Programming

Numerous factors determine the flexibility routine for a client. Each must be considered to optimize the effectiveness of the routine. Each factor requires careful consideration when designing the flexibility program. As with all programming, addressing the deficiencies first in the flexibility routine is important. Muscle imbalances in either strength or flexibility often lead to injury; therefore concentrating on the major issue will help to prevent further decline and consequences associated with the condition. Time is also an issue that may set limitations on the program. Optimal duration for most stretches is 30 seconds. Therefore, selecting a sequence of stretches that address all the major movements is a good idea. If the time available for flexibility is relatively short, the routine may focus on a particular area of interest. One key point is not to disregard any particular area for any length of time.

Movements that have demonstrated a healthy range of motion may become more difficult over time if not addressed on a frequent enough basis. It is much easier to maintain flexibility than to improve it.

If the client presents orthopedic problems, injuries, or disease related joint issues, only select flexibility activities that do not pose a threat to the injury or that will not exacerbate the problem. If a client prefers a particular flexibility technique over another, it is sensible to utilize that method in the program. Working within the client's comfort range increases the likelihood of compliance and adherence to the program.

If none of the aforementioned factors is relevant, then the flexibility routine can be fairly diverse in its offerings. General guidelines should be followed for safe and effective flexibility programming.

General Prescription Guidelines

Mode: Static or Dynamic

Volume: 10-12 movements, 2-4 sets, 15-30 sec static holds, 5-10 sec contraction durations for PNF and 6-12 sec holds

Dynamic: accumulate 1-2 minutes of stretch time per muscle group

Intensity: Tolerable discomfort, No pain

Duration: 15-30 minutes

Frequency: Minimum 2-3 days/week, most days if possible

Flexibility Training Protocols

Explain the techniques and protocols to the client and establish open communication.

Perform an appropriate warm-up.

Select at least one activity per major muscle group or joint action.

Order deficient areas first and perform others in order of need.

Perform 2-4 sets of 30 second holds or accumulate the duration with multiple sets.

Start slow and progress to greater ranges.

Use multiple planes of movement with each muscle group.

Exercise duration of 15-30 minutes.

Require strict protocol adherence.

Use dynamic flexibility before static flexibility.

Establish static stretching proficiency before including PNF.

Stretch to tolerable discomfort, not pain.

Use controlled breathing in a rhythmic pattern.

Record any pains experienced during the movements and look for compensatory actions

These recommendations can help guide the exercise decisions regarding the inclusion of flexibility in an exercise program. In some cases, the flexibility routine will be performed independently of other activities; in other cases, it will join aerobic and/or anaerobic exercises in a more comprehensive program matrix. If the flexibility routine is built into a single day program for a personal training client, all the same guidelines apply, even if the volume changes. Attempt to stretch each muscle group twice per week and alternate the stretches to vary the planes of movement. If limited time to stretch is a constant barrier, build the dynamic activities into the workout. A weighted squat immediately followed by slow speed, dynamic squats using only body weight is one example of how this can be done. Additionally, if maximal force output is not a concern, clients can stretch during the rest intervals of strength training exercises. Stretching the antagonist muscle group following a lift can take advantage of transitory reciprocal innervation and maximize the time in the training session.

Flexibility Training Techniques

Common Hip and Knee Stretches

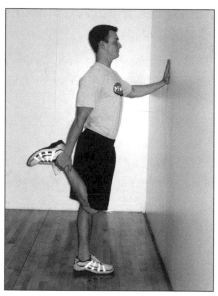

Standing Quadriceps Stretch

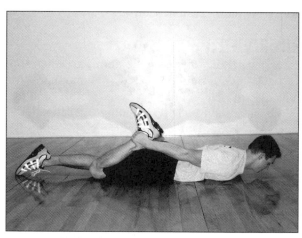

Prone Quadriceps Stretch

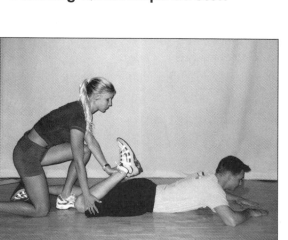

Partner-assisted Quadriceps Stretch

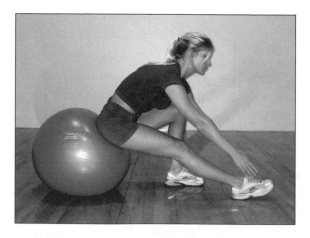

Seated Hamstring Stretch

Common Hip and Knee Stretches Continued

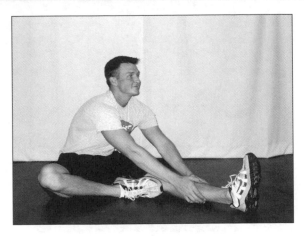

Modified Hurdler's Stretch

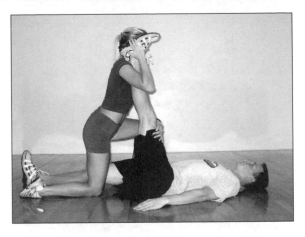

Partner-assisted Hamstring Stretch

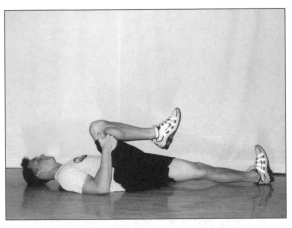

Prone Hip Extensor Stretch

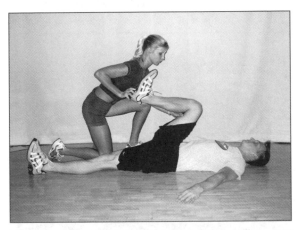

Partner-assisted Hip Extensor Stretch

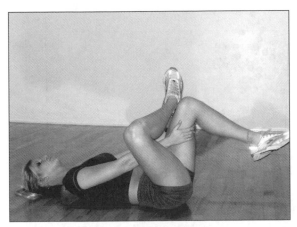

Piriformis Stretch

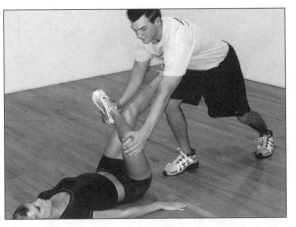

Partner-assisted Piriformis Stretch

Common Hip and Knee Stretches Continued

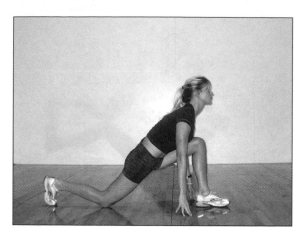

Hip Flexor Stretch

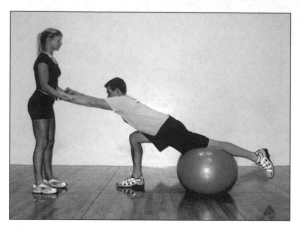

Partner-assisted Hip Flexor Stretch

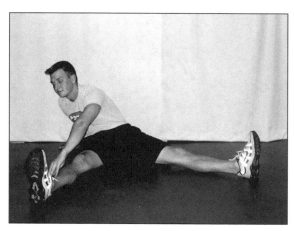

Seated V Stretch (Hip Adductor)

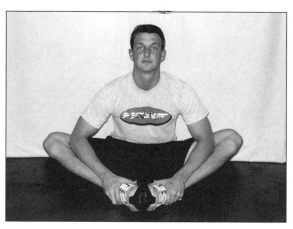

Butterfly Stretch (Hip Adductor)

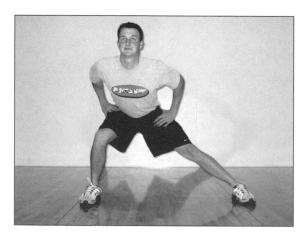

Standing Hip Adductor Stretch

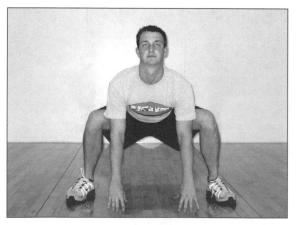

Hip Adductor/Extensor Squat Stretch

Common Ankle Stretches

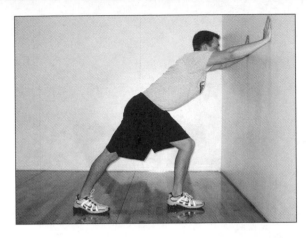

Standing Gastrocnemius Stretch

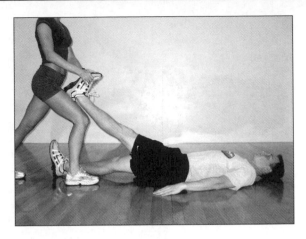

Partner-assisted Gastrocnemius Stretch

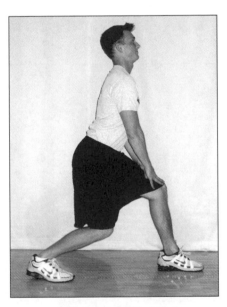

Standing Soleus

Common Trunk Stretches

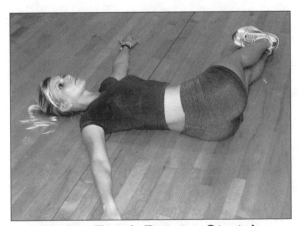

Supine Trunk Rotator Stretch

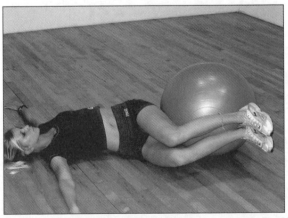

Supine Trunk Rotator Stretch with Ball

Common Trunk Stretches Continued

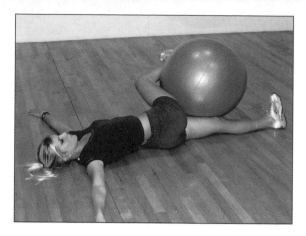

Split Leg Supine Trunk Rotator Stretch

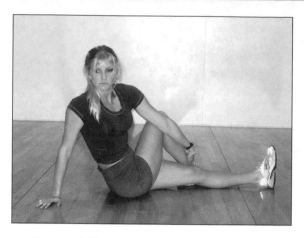

Seated Trunk Rotator Stretch

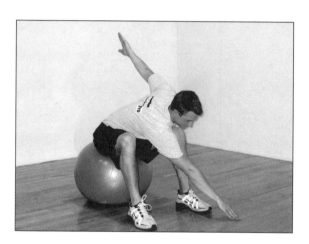

Seated Reach Trunk Rotator Stretch

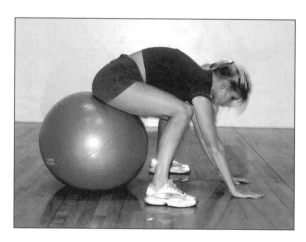

Seated Trunk Extensor Stretch

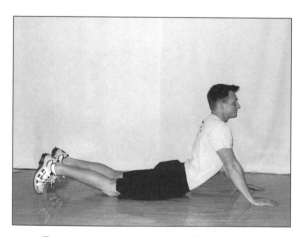

Prone Trunk Flexor Stretch

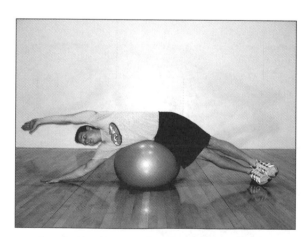

Lateral Trunk Flexor Stretch

Common Trunk Stretches Continued

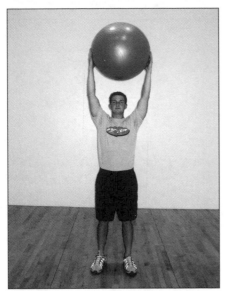 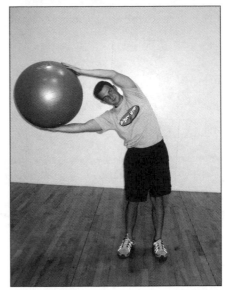

Start   **End**

Standing Lateral Trunk Flexor Stretch

Common Upper Body Stretches

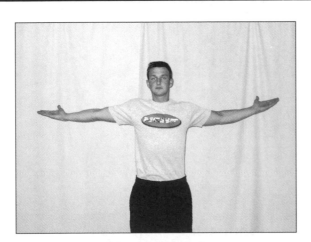 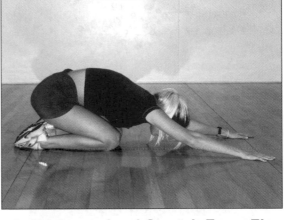

T-Chest Stretch   **Latissimus dorsi Stretch From Floor**

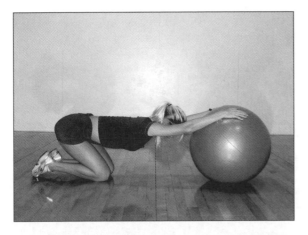 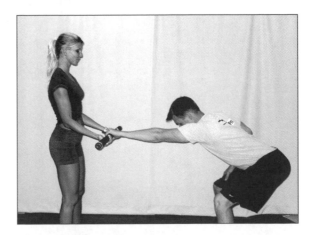

Latissimus dorsi Stretch with Ball   **Standing Latissimus dorsi Stretch**

Common Upper Body Stretches Continued

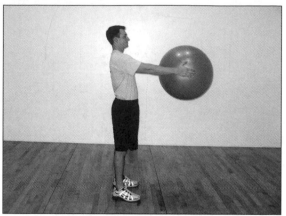

Rotator Cuff Stretch Starting Position

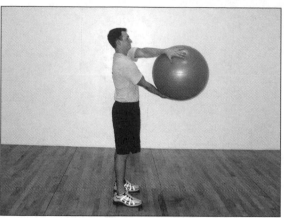

Rotator Cuff Stretch Ending Position

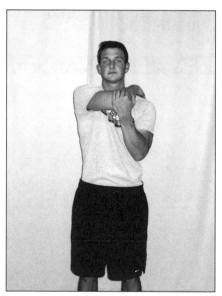

Upper Back Stretch

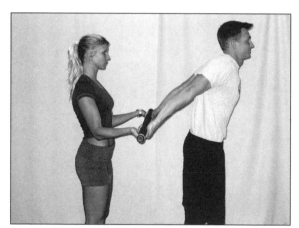

Shoulder Flexor Stretch

Chapter Sixteen References

1. **Almekinders LC and Temple JD**. Etiology, diagnosis, and treatment of tendonitis: an analysis of the literature. *Med Sci Sports Exerc* 30: 1183-1190, 1998.

2. **Anderson RU, Wise D, Sawyer T and Chan C**. Integration of myofascial trigger point release and paradoxical relaxation training treatment of chronic pelvic pain in men. *J Urol* 174: 155-160, 2005.

3. **Baker JH and Matsumoto DE**. Adaptation of skeletal muscle to immobilization in a shortened position. *Muscle Nerve* 11: 231-244, 1988.

4. **Baker JH and Matsumoto DE**. Adaptation of skeletal muscle to immobilization in a shortened position. *Muscle Nerve* 11: 231-244, 1988.

5. **Blalock SJ, DeVellis BM, Holt K and Hahn PM**. Coping with rheumatoid arthritis: is one problem the same as another? *Health Educ Q* 20: 119-132, 1993.

6. **Blecher AM and Richmond JC**. Transient laxity of an anterior cruciate ligament-reconstructed knee related to pregnancy. *Arthroscopy* 14: 77-79, 1998.

7. **Bradley PS, Olsen PD and Portas MD**. The effect of static, ballistic, and proprioceptive neuromuscular facilitation stretching on vertical jump performance. *J Strength Cond Res* 21: 223-226, 2007.

8. **Carlson CR and Curran SL**. Stretch-based relaxation training. *Patient Educ Couns* 23: 5-12, 1994.

9. **Carlson CR and Curran SL**. Stretch-based relaxation training. *Patient Educ Couns* 23: 5-12, 1994.

10. **Cavagna GA, Heglund NC and Mantovani M**. Muscle work enhancement by stretch. Passive visco-elasticity or cross-bridges? *Adv Exp Med Biol* 453: 393-407, 1998.

11. **Cavagna GA, Heglund NC and Mantovani M**. Muscle work enhancement

by stretch. Passive visco-elasticity or cross-bridges? *Adv Exp Med Biol* 453: 393-407, 1998.

12. **Charlton WP, Coslett-Charlton LM and Ciccotti MG**. Correlation of estradiol in pregnancy and anterior cruciate ligament laxity. *Clin Orthop Relat Res* 165-170, 2001.

13. **Clyman B**. Exercise in the treatment of osteoarthritis. *Curr Rheumatol Rep* 3: 520-523, 2001.

14. **Dyck DD, Jr. and Boyajian-O'Neill LA**. Plantar fasciitis. *Clin J Sport Med* 14: 305-309, 2004.

15. **Feldman D, Shrier I, Rossignol M and Abenhaim L**. Adolescent growth is not associated with changes in flexibility. *Clin J Sport Med* 9: 24-29, 1999.

16. **Frankel JE, Bean JF and Frontera WR**. Exercise in the elderly: research and clinical practice. *Clin Geriatr Med* 22: 239-256, 2006.

17. **Frost HM**. Skeletal structural adaptations to mechanical usage (SATMU): 4. Mechanical influences on intact fibrous tissues. *Anat Rec* 226: 433-439, 1990.

18. **Gajdosik RL**. Passive extensibility of skeletal muscle: review of the literature with clinical implications. *Clin Biomech (Bristol, Avon)* 16: 87-101, 2001.

19. **Girouard CK and Hurley BF**. Does strength training inhibit gains in range of motion from flexibility training in older adults? *Med Sci Sports Exerc* 27: 1444-1449, 1995.

20. **Goffaux J, Friesinger GC, Lambert W, Shroyer LW, Moritz TE, McCarthy M, Jr., Henderson WG and Hammermeister KE**. Biological age--a concept whose time has come: a preliminary study. *South Med J* 98: 985-993, 2005.

21. **Granata KP and England SA**. Stability of dynamic trunk movement. *Spine* 31: E271-E276, 2006.

22. **Hawkins RJ and Kennedy JC**. Impingement syndrome in athletes. *Am J Sports Med* 8: 151-158, 1980.

23. **Hawkins RJ and Kennedy JC**. Impingement syndrome in athletes. *Am J Sports Med* 8: 151-158, 1980.

24. **Heslinga JW, te KG and Huijing PA**. Growth and immobilization effects on sarcomeres: a comparison between gastrocnemius and soleus muscles of the adult rat. *Eur J Appl Physiol Occup Physiol* 70: 49-57, 1995.

25. **Hessert MJ, Gugliucci MR and Pierce HR**. Functional fitness: maintaining or improving function for elders with chronic diseases. *Fam Med* 37: 472-476, 2005.

26. **Hessert MJ, Gugliucci MR and Pierce HR**. Functional fitness: maintaining or improving function for elders with chronic diseases. *Fam Med* 37: 472-476, 2005.

27. **Hong CZ and Simons DG**. Pathophysiologic and electrophysiologic mechanisms of myofascial trigger points. *Arch Phys Med Rehabil* 79: 863-872, 1998.

28. **Hurschler C, Loitz-Ramage B and Vanderby R, Jr.** A structurally based stress-stretch relationship for tendon and ligament. *J Biomech Eng* 119: 392-399, 1997.

29. **Hurschler C, Loitz-Ramage B and Vanderby R, Jr.** A structurally based stress-stretch relationship for tendon and ligament. *J Biomech Eng* 119: 392-399, 1997.

30. **Ingraham SJ**. The role of flexibility in injury prevention and athletic performance: have we stretched the truth? *Minn Med* 86: 58-61, 2003.

31. **Ishiwata S, Shimamoto Y, Suzuki M and Sasaki D**. Regulation of muscle contraction by Ca2+ and ADP:

focusing on the auto-oscillation (SPOC). *Adv Exp Med Biol* 592: 341-358, 2007.

32. **Iwasawa T, Iwasaki K, Sawada T, Okada A, Ueyama K, Motomura S, Harata S, Inoue I, Toh S and Furukawa KI**. Pathophysiological role of endothelin in ectopic ossification of human spinal ligaments induced by mechanical stress. *Calcif Tissue Int* 79: 422-430, 2006.

33. **Kanbur NO, Duzgun I, Derman O and Baltaci G**. Do sexual maturation stages affect flexibility in adolescent boys aged 14 years? *J Sports Med Phys Fitness* 45: 53-57, 2005.

34. **Kell RT, Bell G and Quinney A**. Musculoskeletal fitness, health outcomes and quality of life. *Sports Med* 31: 863-873, 2001.

35. **Kiefhaber TR and Stern PJ**. Upper extremity tendinitis and overuse syndromes in the athlete. *Clin Sports Med* 11: 39-55, 1992.

36. **Klassbo M, Harms-Ringdahl K and Larsson G**. Examination of passive ROM and capsular patterns in the hip. *Physiother Res Int* 8: 1-12, 2003.

37. **Koopman FS, Edelaar M, Slikker R, Reynders K, van der Woude LH and Hoozemans MJ**. Effectiveness of a multidisciplinary occupational training program for chronic low back pain: a prospective cohort study. *Am J Phys Med Rehabil* 83: 94-103, 2004.

38. **Krivickas LS**. Anatomical factors associated with overuse sports injuries. *Sports Med* 24: 132-146, 1997.

39. **Krombholz H**. Physical performance in relation to age, sex, birth order, social class, and sports activities of preschool children. *Percept Mot Skills* 102: 477-484, 2006.

40. **Kuan TS, Hong CZ, Chen JT, Chen SM and Chien CH**. The spinal cord connections of the myofascial trigger spots. *Eur J Pain* 2006.

41. **Lieber RL and Friden J**. Functional and clinical significance of skeletal muscle architecture. *Muscle Nerve* 23: 1647-1666, 2000.

42. **Linari M, Bottinelli R, Pellegrino MA, Reconditi M, Reggiani C and Lombardi V**. The mechanism of the force response to stretch in human skinned muscle fibres with different myosin isoforms. *J Physiol* 554: 335-352, 2004.

43. **Marx RG, Sperling JW and Cordasco FA**. Overuse injuries of the upper extremity in tennis players. *Clin Sports Med* 20: 439-451, 2001.

44. **McMahon PJ and Lee TQ**. Muscles may contribute to shoulder dislocation and stability. *Clin Orthop Relat Res* S18-S25, 2002.

45. **McQuade KJ, Turner JA and Buchner DM**. Physical fitness and chronic low back pain. An analysis of the relationships among fitness, functional limitations, and depression. *Clin Orthop Relat Res* 198-204, 1988.

46. **Mikkelsson LO, Nupponen H, Kaprio J, Kautiainen H, Mikkelsson M and Kujala UM**. Adolescent flexibility, endurance strength, and physical activity as predictors of adult tension neck, low back pain, and knee injury: a 25 year follow up study. *Br J Sports Med* 40: 107-113, 2006.

47. **Moore JC**. The Golgi tendon organ: a review and update. *Am J Occup Ther* 38: 227-236, 1984.

48. **Mutungi G and Ranatunga KW**. Tension relaxation after stretch in resting mammalian muscle fibers: stretch activation at physiological temperatures. *Biophys J* 70: 1432-1438, 1996.

49. **Mutungi G and Ranatunga KW**. The visco-elasticity of resting intact mammalian (rat) fast muscle fibres. *J Muscle Res Cell Motil* 17: 357-364, 1996.

50. **Mutungi G and Ranatunga KW**. Sarcomere length changes during end-held (isometric) contractions in intact mammalian (rat) fast and slow muscle fibres. *J Muscle Res Cell Motil* 21: 565-575, 2000.

51. **Myers JB, Laudner KG, Pasquale MR, Bradley JP and Lephart SM**. Glenohumeral range of motion deficits and posterior shoulder tightness in throwers with pathologic internal impingement. *Am J Sports Med* 34: 385-391, 2006.

52. **O'Grady M, Fletcher J and Ortiz S**. Therapeutic and physical fitness exercise prescription for older adults with joint disease: an evidence-based approach. *Rheum Dis Clin North Am* 26: 617-646, 2000.

53. **O'Grady M, Fletcher J and Ortiz S**. Therapeutic and physical fitness exercise prescription for older adults with joint disease: an evidence-based approach. *Rheum Dis Clin North Am* 26: 617-646, 2000.

54. **Pathare NC, Stevens JE, Walter GA, Shah P, Jayaraman A, Tillman SM, Scarborough MT, Parker GC and Vandenborne K**. Deficit in human muscle strength with cast immobilization: contribution of inorganic phosphate. *Eur J Appl Physiol* 98: 71-78, 2006.

55. **Peat G, Croft P and Hay E**. Clinical assessment of the osteoarthritis patient. *Best Pract Res Clin Rheumatol* 15: 527-544, 2001.

56. **Rassier DE, Herzog W and Pollack GH**. Dynamics of individual sarcomeres during and after stretch in activated single myofibrils. *Proc Biol Sci* 270: 1735-1740, 2003.

57. **Rayan GM, Brentlinger A, Purnell D and Garcia-Moral CA**. Functional assessment of bilateral wrist arthrodeses. *J Hand Surg [Am]* 12: 1020-1024, 1987.

58. **Renkawitz T, Boluki D and Grifka J**. The association of low back pain, neuromuscular imbalance, and trunk extension strength in athletes. *Spine J* 6: 673-683, 2006.

59. **Renstrom P and Johnson RJ**. Overuse injuries in sports. A review. *Sports Med* 2: 316-333, 1985.

60. **Renstrom P and Johnson RJ**. Overuse injuries in sports. A review. *Sports Med* 2: 316-333, 1985.

61. **Sady SP, Wortman M and Blanke D**. Flexibility training: ballistic, static or proprioceptive neuromuscular facilitation? *Arch Phys Med Rehabil* 63: 261-263, 1982.

62. **Schwartz MH, Leo PH and Lewis JL**. A microstructural model for the elastic response of articular cartilage. *J Biomech* 27: 865-873, 1994.

63. **Schwartz MH, Leo PH and Lewis JL**. A microstructural model for the elastic response of articular cartilage. *J Biomech* 27: 865-873, 1994.

64. **Semble EL, Loeser RF and Wise CM**. Therapeutic exercise for rheumatoid arthritis and osteoarthritis. *Semin Arthritis Rheum* 20: 32-40, 1990.

65. **Sharman MJ, Cresswell AG and Riek S**. Proprioceptive neuromuscular facilitation stretching : mechanisms and clinical implications. *Sports Med* 36: 929-939, 2006.

66. **Simons DG and Mense S**. [Diagnosis and therapy of myofascial trigger points]. *Schmerz* 17: 419-424, 2003.

67. **Singh AS, Chin APM, Bosscher RJ and van Mechelen W**. Cross-sectional relationship between physical fitness components and functional performance in older persons living in long-term care facilities. *BMC Geriatr* 6: 4, 2006.

68. **Smith LK, Lelas JL and Kerrigan DC**. Gender differences in pelvic motions and center of mass displacement during walking: stereotypes quantified. *J Womens Health Gend Based Med* 11: 453-458, 2002.

69. **Smith LL, Brunetz MH, Chenier TC, McCammon MR, Houmard JA, Franklin ME and Israel RG**. The effects of static and ballistic stretching on delayed onset muscle soreness and creatine kinase. *Res Q Exerc Sport* 64: 103-107, 1993.

70. **Stewart M, Adams R, Alonso A, Van Koesveld B and Campbell S**. Warm-up or stretch as preparation for sprint performance? *J Sci Med Sport* 2006.

71. **Stone MH, Fleck SJ, Triplett NT and Kraemer WJ**. Health- and performance-related potential of resistance training. *Sports Med* 11: 210-231, 1991.

72. **Sun JS, Hou SM, Hang YS, Liu TK and Lu KS**. Ultrastructural studies on myofibrillogenesis and neogenesis of skeletal muscles after prolonged traction in rabbits. *Histol Histopathol* 11: 285-292, 1996.

73. **Tamai K, Kurokawa T and Matsubara I**. In situ observation of adjustment of sarcomere length in skeletal muscle under sustained stretch. *Nippon Seikeigeka Gakkai Zasshi* 63: 1558-1563, 1989.

74. **Thacker SB, Gilchrist J, Stroup DF and Kimsey CD, Jr.** The impact of stretching on sports injury risk: a systematic review of the literature. *Med Sci Sports Exerc* 36: 371-378, 2004.

75. **Toft E, Espersen GT, Kalund S, Sinkjaer T and Hornemann BC**. Passive tension of the ankle before and after stretching. *Am J Sports Med* 17: 489-494, 1989.

76. **Trombitas K and Pollack GH**. Elastic properties of the titin filament in the Z-line region of vertebrate striated muscle. *J Muscle Res Cell Motil* 14: 416-422, 1993.

77. **Trost SG, Pate RR, Dowda M, Saunders R, Ward DS and Felton G**. Gender differences in physical activity and determinants of physical activity in rural fifth grade children. *J Sch Health* 66: 145-150, 1996.

78. **Tseng CN, Chen CC, Wu SC and Lin LC**. Effects of a range-of-motion exercise programme. *J Adv Nurs* 57: 181-191, 2007.

79. **Urso ML, Clarkson PM and Price TB**. Immobilization effects in young and older adults. *Eur J Appl Physiol* 96: 564-571, 2006.

80. **Wang SC, Brede C, Lange D, Poster CS, Lange AW, Kohoyda-Inglis C, Sochor MR, Ipaktchi K, Rowe SA, Patel S and Garton HJ**. Gender differences in hip anatomy: possible implications for injury tolerance in frontal collisions. *Annu Proc Assoc Adv Automot Med* 48: 287-301, 2004.

81. **Whitehurst MA, Johnson BL, Parker CM, Brown LE and Ford AM**. The benefits of a functional exercise circuit for older adults. *J Strength Cond Res* 19: 647-651, 2005.

82. **Whitehurst MA, Johnson BL, Parker CM, Brown LE and Ford AM**. The benefits of a functional exercise circuit for older adults. *J Strength Cond Res* 19: 647-651, 2005.

83. **Williford HN, East JB, Smith FH and Burry LA**. Evaluation of warm-up for improvement in flexibility. *Am J Sports Med* 14: 316-319, 1986.

84. **Wilson GJ, Wood GA and Elliott BC**. The relationship between stiffness of the musculature and static flexibility: an alternative explanation for the occurrence of muscular injury. *Int J Sports Med* 12: 403-407, 1991.

85. **Yap EC**. Myofascial pain - an overview. *Ann Acad Med Singapore* 36: 43-46, 2007.

86. **Zakas A, Doganis G, Zakas N and Vergou A**. Acute effects of active warm-up and stretching on the flexibility of elderly women. *J Sports Med Phys Fitness* 46: 617-622, 2006.

Chapter 17

Programming for Cardiovascular Fitness

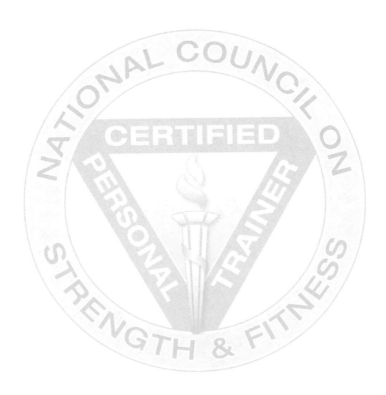

Introduction

It has been well documented that cardiorespiratory fitness (CRF) is one of the single most important factors that influences lifespan and quality of life (42). These reasons alone support routine participation in aerobic activities to encourage adequate fitness throughout the duration of person's life. In Chapter 6, "Cardiovascular Physiology" the structures and organs responsible for maintaining adequate flow of blood and oxygen to the tissues were identified. The ability of the body to efficiently deliver oxygen-rich blood to all its tissues, and the tissues' ability to use the oxygen to make energy is the foundation of aerobic fitness and will be the basis for the following text.

Based on statistical norms, previously sedentary and even physically active clients new to exercise are not likely to start off with a high level of CRF due to the lack of aerobic activity common amongst most Americans (22; 23). But as with any health component, there exists considerable variation among clients and numerous factors to determine a person's fitness level. Evaluation of a client's aerobic capacity is required to ascertain their relative ability to use oxygen and to establish exercise tolerance, interests, and starting points for the exercise program.

Assessing Cardiovascular Fitness

Following the screening process for exercise participation, a client should be tested in some capacity to identify his or her relative CRF. The test selection decisions will be based on the previously reviewed factors, including the client's specific characteristics, a trainer's knowledge and experience in testing, and other logistical concerns. Submaximal tests are far more common in personal training settings, compared to maximal tests and provide useful data for the exercise prescription when administered properly. For clients who are new to the exercise environment and have little experience with aerobic training, the test criteria should cater to these points. For instance, it would be unintelligent to ask a new exerciser to perform a 1-mile maximal run test. They would likely perform poorly, experience significant distress and might even become injured. It is very easy to turn a person off from exercise participation by being overly aggressive with the selected assessment activities. In addition, given their relative psychological states, new exercisers are likely to be somewhat anxious and may possess some level of intimidation related to the new experience, particularly if they have not performed well in similar activities in the past.

Selecting the appropriate test for a client does not need to be complicated. Each test has criteria distinctions that designate it as a viable option for the client or not. Submaximal test modalities offer different advantages and disadvantages, depending on the characteristics of the client. Matching the test with the client's capabilities will provide quality data through improved validity.

If the test selection is appropriate for the client and the protocol is strictly adhered to, the tests should provide quality data. In some cases, the data will provide a prediction of oxygen consumption capabilities (VO$_2$max). In others, the performance is charted and a category of fitness is determined. In either case, the exercise prescription will likely be based on heart rates for intensity determination rather than VO$_2$ or **MET** intensities, as the latter two require specific knowledge of oxygen usage by premeditated calculations or the use of equipment that calculates intensity via those means. Although it serves as an accurate method to determine aerobic training intensities, using percentage of VO$_2$max for the purposes of prescribing exercise is usually limited to cardiac rehabilitation programs.

Cardiorespiratory Test Comparisons

Step tests - Easy to implement and perform; limited equipment needs; valid for general population but often overpredict fit individuals; metronome paced tests are superior to non-paced protocols; should not be used with moderate to high-level obese, or very deconditioned clients. Leg strength is a factor, as is rhythm during cadence tests.

Walk/jog tests- Easy to implement and perform; limited equipment; viable for deconditioned or new exercisers with no experience; validity affected by motivation and exercise tolerance, as well as measured distance accuracy; overpredicts fit populations.

Run tests - Easy to implement and perform; limited equipment; viable for fit or conditioned individuals; validity affected by test experience due to pace, client motivation, running economy, and measured distance accuracy; recommended for the fit populations only.

Bike tests - More difficult to implement; equipment dependent; technicial expertise required; viable for multiple populations but some level of fitness required; validity is high with strict protocol adherence; leg strength a factor.

Measuring Intensity Through Heart Rate

Heart rate is the ideal measure to determine intensity because it has a linear relationship with aerobic work. During aerobic training, the harder a person exerts him or herself, the more oxygen is required to satisfy the demand. Consequently, the heart must pump more frequently to correspond with the increased need for oxygenated blood. This relationship allows intensity to be measured indirectly by tracking heart rate response to exercise. The term **heart rate training zone (HRTZ)** is used to define the heart rate range that a person should work in to maximize their adaptation response to aerobic exercise.

The first step in determining the heart rate training zone is to measure or predict the maximum heart rate of an individual. A direct measurement is always the best for true validity, but it is not practical for most training situations. Direct measurement requires a person to perform a maximal aerobic test, which is most commonly a **graded exercise test (GXT)** performed on a treadmill. The problem with maximal GXTs is the equipment, expertise, and client effort required often create logistical issues for the average personal trainer. For this reason, predictive formulas are far more commonly employed to determine a heart rate maximum. The classic formula to predict maximum heart rate is to subtract a person's age from 220 (220-age). The value is considered the highest attainable heart rate for an individual at a given age. The problem with this formula is that it suggests that everyone at a certain age has the exact same maximum heart rate,

which is not correct (38). The standard deviation for the equation is 10-12 beats · min^{-1}. Using bell curve theory, this would make the formula accurate for 68% of the population at a given age. Using the same theory, the remaining 32% of the population's maximum heart rate would either be under or over the predicted value by at least 10-24 beats · min^{-1}, depending on where they fall along the curve. This is hardly a precise prediction, and therefore, may throw off the accuracy of the training zone, consequently leading to reduced effectiveness of the training (19).

Rate of Perceived Exertion (RPE)

One way to improve the Max HR formula is to compare the heart rate measures with the values of the Rate of Perceived Exertion Scale. **Rate of perceived exertion (RPE)** is based on Borg's research to monitor exercise by perception of effort, rather than cardiovascular measures. Borg found that when local factors, such as perceived strain and discomfort, and the central factors, including respiration rate and heart rate were combined, they could be used to identify relative work level. In his original scale, the numbers 6-20 reflected heart rates of 60-200 beats · min^{-1}. A correlation exists between the scale defined for perceived effort and the intensity of the exercise (15; 36). A value of 12-14 on the RPE scale correlates with 60-80% of the heart rate reserve with 13-14 being closely related to lactate threshold (35). Using the combined method of age predicted max heart rate based training zones and RPE,

Key Terms

Metronome – An instrument used to indicate the exact tempo at which work should be performed during certain tests (i.e. Step test).

MET – A unit of measure used to describe the amount of oxygen one consumes at a given intensity.

Heart Rate Training Zone (HRTZ) – The heart rate range that a person should work between in order to maximize their adaptation response to aerobic exercise.

Graded Exercise Test (GXT) – A maximal aerobic test used to determine an individual's heart rate training zone.

Rate of Perceived Exertion (RPE) – A scale, usually numbered 6-20, that is used to monitor a client's own perception of their exertion during exercise.

Borg RPE Scale

6	No exertion at all
7	Extremely light
8	
9	Very light
10	
11	Light
12	
13	Somewhat hard
14	
15	Hard (heavy)
16	
17	Very hard
18	
19	Extremely hard
20	Maximal exertion

a person expected to be within a specific target zone should match the zone defined by perceived exertion when training above an intensity of 50% HRmax (13). When the zones align, the measured heart rates can be documented for improved accuracy to generate the exercise prescription.

Researchers have come up with other formulas that may increase the accuracy for heart rate prediction for specific populations. Research findings have indicated that age, obesity, fitness, and smoking status all contribute to prediction error when using the traditional heart rate max formula (54). Therefore, modified formulas to predict max heart rates have surfaced, each of which holds statistical merit for the respective population it is designed for. The following formulas can be used in place of the heart rate max formula for the select populations.

Even with the improved accuracy associated with the below formulas, standard deviations still exist that can reduce the accuracy of the predicted training zone. Personal trainers should utilize the rate of perceived exertion scale and other indicators to contend with the inherent variability associated with the prediction of heart rate max.

Talk Test

Another informal, subjective method of qualifying predicted heart rate max values is to employ the talk test. The method requires subjects to exercise at an intensity at which conversation is comfortable. The intensity is gradually increased until the exerciser has difficulty maintaining regular conversation. At this point, the individual is at, or near, ventilatory threshold. Ventilatory threshold describes a non-linear increase in respiration that corresponds with higher levels of

Multifactor General Population Formula for Max Heart Rate

Men

Max HR = 203.9 - (0.812 x age) + (0.276 x RHR) - (0.084 x kg) - (4.5 x smoking code)

Women

Max HR = 204.8 - (0.718 x age) + (0.162 x RHR) - (0.105 x kg) - (6.2 x smoking code)

Age = years
RHR = resting heart rate
Kg = body weight in kilograms
Smoking code = (1) for smoker, (0) nonsmoker

Obese Individuals

Max Hr = 200 - (0.5 x age)

Older Adults

Max HR = 208 - (0.7 x age)

Example

68 Year old male
161 lbs
RHR 75 bpm
Current Smoker

Max HR = 203.9 - (.812 x 68) + (.276 x 75) - (.084 x 73) - (4.5 x 1)
Max HR = 203.9 - 55.2 + 20.7 - 6.1 - 4.5
Max HR = 159 bpm

exercise intensity due to increased blood temperature and reduction of pH. Respiration increases fairly linearly with intensity until the ventilatory threshold is reached, at which time the increase in respiration breaks the linear progression. Research has demonstrated a close correlation between the Talk Test, VO_2, ventilatory threshold, and heart rate (30; 56). The Talk Test can be used with the RPE scale to increase accuracy of training heart rates. An RPE value of 14 generally equates to the value found in the Talk Test performance when conversation becomes difficult (55).

Heart Rate Training Zones

The predicted maximum heart rate can be used to prescribe exercise intensity by creating heart rate training zones. Different formulas can be used to calculate the training zones. The two most widely used formulas are the Heart Rate Max Formula and the **Heart Rate Reserve** method. The heart rate max formula is very easy to implement, and it is the method used to create most exercise intensity charts found on popular brands of cardiovascular equipment. This formula, though, has major drawbacks. Because it is simply a percentage of the max heart rate, any error in the determination of the max heart rate value will skew the range. Other problems include an underestimation of the required training heart rate, unless an upward adjustment is made, and it estimates the same value for all individuals in the same age range (51). It is inappropriate to assume all people of the same age will have similar heart rates at the same respective training intensities.

Heart Rate Max Method

Training HR = Max HR x Training Intensity Percentage

Heart Rate Reserve Method

The Heart Rate Reserve method is considered a superior technique to the Heart Rate Max method for defining heart rate training zones because it factors in an additional cardiovascular variable; resting heart rate. In Chapter 6, the relationship between resting heart rate and cardiorespiratory efficiency was established, and it was further identified that lower resting heart rates indicate higher stroke volume. The formula uses this relationship to make individual adjustments in the training heart rate estimates. Heart rate reserve (HRR) is calculated by subtracting a person's resting heart rate from their predicted maximum heart rate, using the above mentioned maximum heart rate formula. The value is then entered into the formula to estimate training heart rates, based on a selected intensity.

Heart Rate Max Method

Max Heart Rate Formula
20 Year Old Male
$$220 - 20 \text{ Years} = 200 \text{ beats} \cdot \text{min}^{-1}$$
$$\text{Predicted Max HR} = 200 \text{ beats} \cdot \text{min}^{-1}$$
HR Max Method
$$200 \text{ beats} \cdot \text{min}^{-1} \times 0.75 = 150 \text{ beats} \cdot \text{min}^{-1}$$
$$200 \text{ beats} \cdot \text{min}^{-1} \times 0.90 = 180 \text{ beats} \cdot \text{min}^{-1}$$
$$\text{Training Zone} = 150\text{-}180 \text{ beats} \cdot \text{min}^{-1}$$

The Heart Rate Reserve method requires that the HRR be multiplied by the desired training intensity. The resting heart rate is then added back into the equation to estimate the training intensity heart rate value. Heart rate reserve works on the logical premise that training heart rates must lie somewhere between the resting heart rate value and the maximal heart rate value. Due to individual variations, that range will be different for most people; therefore, it needs to be determined to accurately estimate the training intensities for exercise.

Adequate stimulus for cardiovascular improvements varies by the individual. General guidelines suggest that the intensity must be at least 40% of VO_2max for any cardiovascular adaptations to occur (61). This value though, is insufficient for performance improvements for most of the population. The following ranges will be appropriate for improvements in health and fitness in the majority of the population.

The specific intensity used will be based on a variety of factors, including current fitness level, exercise tolerance, and risk factors for disease. VO_2 and HRR do not correlate as well at lower intensity as they do at the

---

Recommended Training Intensities

Training Intensity Ranges for Deconditioned Individuals
40-60% VO2max
50-60% Heart Rate Reserve
60-70% Heart Rate Max

Training Intensity Ranges for Healthy Individuals
60-80% Heart Rate Reserve or VO2max
75-90% Heart Rate Max

Heart Rate Reserve Method

Heart Rate Reserve = Max HR - Resting HR

Training HR = (HRR x Training Intensity expressed as a percentage) + RHR

Example: 20 year old male, Max HR 200 beats min^{-1}, RHR 60 beats min^{-1}

$$200 \text{ beats} \cdot \text{min}^{-1} - 60 \text{ beats} \cdot \text{min}^{-1} = 140 \text{ beats} \cdot \text{min}^{-1}$$

$$(140 \text{ beats} \cdot \text{min}^{-1} \text{ x } 0.60) + 60 \text{ beats} \cdot \text{min}^{-1} = 144 \text{ beats min}^{-1}$$

$$(140 \text{ beats} \cdot \text{min}^{-1} \text{ x } 0.80) + 60 \text{ beats} \cdot \text{min}^{-1} = 172 \text{ beats} \cdot \text{min}^{-1}$$

$$\text{Training Zone} = 144\text{-}172 \text{ beats} \cdot \text{min}^{-1}$$

---

an effective method for attaining higher exercise intensities. It is based on the premise that the body will adapt to the highest perceived stress, even though the time spent in the higher intensity range is fairly limited compared to the total duration of the activity. It is much easier to push the body at high intensities for short periods of time, compared to attempting to maintain higher steady-state levels for the duration of the exercise session. Using intervals, a client can reach exercise intensities they otherwise would not be able to experience or maintain. It is suggested that interval training yields a greater adaptation response compared to steady-state training performed for the same period of time when applied properly (53).

higher intensities, so mild adjustments for deconditioned individuals are made in the intensity selection for this population (59). Deciding on the exact intensity to employ for a client is similar to other health related components. A period of acclimation is recommended to familiarize clients with exercise and to help in the adoption of routine engagement in the activity. When creating the exercise prescription, the exercise principles should be properly applied so that the progressive overload is appropriate for the client. Starting or progressing too aggressively can lead to attrition and possible injury.

Types of Aerobic Training

Different types of aerobic training can be used to elicit the desired adaptation response. In general, aerobic training is performed using steady-state heart rates or varying interval heart rates. Steady-state is probably the most common method for aerobic training. It requires exercisers to perform at a set pace without varying the resistance or movement factors. The term steady-state refers to the consistency of the heart rate during the performance of work. Adjustments less than 5 beats per minute suggest the aerobic pathways are maintained at a constant level due to the fact that oxygenated blood supply is meeting the demand.

Interval Training

Interval training, on the other hand, uses variation in heart rate and resistance or speed. The heart rates fluctuate based on the intensity of the work at a given time. Interval training is

High Intensity vs. Low Intensity Training

Intensity selection is also based on desired outcome. Higher intensity training optimizes the cardiovascular system for performance and contributes significantly to caloric expenditure (39). Moderate intensities are useful for health attainment, caloric expenditure, disease

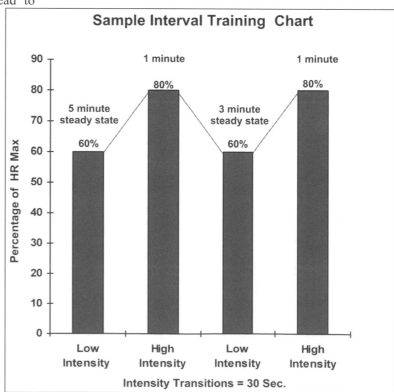

~Quick Insight~

Fat Burning Zone

When aerobic activity is used for weight loss, all attempts should focus on the caloric expenditure, even though training in the "fat-burning zone" is often recommended by some professionals to encourage weight loss. Low and low-moderate intensity training do yield a higher percentage of calories metabolized from fat compared to moderate and high intensity training, but again these training intensities do not measure up when total caloric expenditure is compared (26; 43).

Example based on a 150 lb person

3 mph walking	30 minutes	117 kcal expended	64 fat kcal expended
6 mph running	30 minutes	357 kcal expended	117 fat kcal expended

As you can see, the elevated intensity not only burned more than two times the total calories, but also utilized more fat during the exercise bout, even though the percentage of calories burned from fat was higher with the lower intensity exercise (70). In fact, the amount of calories expended from fat while running equated to the total calories burned while walking. In addition, higher intensities increase post-exercise metabolism (10-13% of total calories expended), further contributing to weight loss potential (44; 71).

prevention, and reduced risk for injury, compared to high intensity training (40). Additionally, many exercisers prefer moderate intensity activity because it is more tolerable for sustained periods of time compared to training at higher intensities (29). Low intensity aerobic training helps acclimate clients to exercise, and is indicated for those with health issues that prevent the use of more elevated intensity levels.

In some circles, low intensity exercise has been recommended for weight loss due to the emphasis on lipid metabolism. Although it is true that sleep, rest, and low intensity activity utilize fat preferentially for aerobic metabolism, the total calories expended during activities of low metabolic demand are considerably less than the expenditures associated with higher intensity activities (41). Therefore, although the percentage of calories burned from fat is higher with low intensity exercise, the total number of fat calories burned is actually lower (68). Individuals who attempt to lose weight by training in the "fat-burning zone" are actually limiting their ability to burn calories, which is the primary factor affecting weight loss (45). If the "fat-burning zone" was the optimal weight loss zone simply based on the percentage of fat used for fuel, then sleeping would be the best choice for weight loss activity, as it uses the highest percentage of fat for energy. Clearly this logic is skewed because a low number of calories are expended per minute while sleeping. In other words, a large percentage of a small number equates to an even smaller number in the end. Compared to moderate and high intensities, low intensity exercise reduces caloric expenditure, reduces cardiovascular adaptations, and in some cases (duration being the variable) reduces the total amount of fat utilized during the exercise bout (69).

Consistent with exercise intensity, the desired outcomes of the program will dictate the training frequency and duration. Unlike other types of exercise, aerobic training requires frequent and consistent participation to optimize results (16). It is recommended that for optimal health improvements, aerobic activities should be performed most days of the week and equal 14-20 calories per kilogram of body weight per week (9; 32). The same can be said when training for performance. The minimal frequency that aerobic activity should be performed is three or four days per week (8). For improvements in CRF, it is recommended that deconditioned individuals accumulate 30 minutes of aerobic activity most days of the week, while healthy individuals should engage in aerobic exercise for 30 or more minutes, 3-5 days per week (11; 66). In addition, vigorous intensity activities should be performed for 10-15 minutes at least twice per week by healthy individuals. Interestingly, deconditioned participants show almost equal benefit when the 30 minute time period is divided up into multiple sessions throughout the day (3 x 10 minutes), as long as the heart rates remain above the minimum threshold for CRF improvements (10). Additionally, deconditioned individuals have shown improvements with a participation of 2-3 sessions per week (65).

From an overall health standpoint, training at higher intensities most days of the week may initiate a cost-benefit imbalance due to the elevation in risk for musculoskeletal injury seen with more frequent and longer bouts of aerobic exercise. Likewise, training beyond 80% VO_2max has been correlated with greater risk for injury (37; 64). Longer duration bouts and high intensities are, in fact, necessary for higher end performance and competition level training. But, if the goal is optimal health, then training at roughly 80% of VO_2max, 4-5 days per week, for approximately thirty minutes is well justified.

General Aerobic Training Guidelines

Goal	Frequency	Duration
General Health	Most days	Accumulate 30 min/day
Fitness	3-5 days	30-60 min
Performance	5-7 days	45-90 min

Energy Expenditure

An energy expenditure of 200-400 kcal per a day is a marker for CRF improvement consistent with the other aerobic prescription guidelines for health (46; 62). It has been observed that when aerobic exercise is performed for a duration and intensity that meets or exceeds 14 kcal per kilogram of body weight per week, the body experiences improved health. Calories per training bout or those expended when performing aerobic activity seem to be part of the multifactorial threshold for health (31). The relationship between calories and aerobic training stems from the oxidation value of energy. Approximately 5 kcal of energy is released per liter of oxygen used. Therefore, measuring calories expended in an exercise bout or the oxygen used by the body during the exercise period will each identify the work performed. In fact, energy expenditure can be represented in numerous ways that all reflect the amount of oxygen or calories used while performing activity.

Understanding METs

The different ways to express energy expenditure allow for multiple variables to predict how much work is being done and how much oxygen and calories are needed to perform the activity. One of the more common ways to convey the demands of an activity is through a unit referred to as a MET, or metabolic equivalent. The MET intensity of an activity reflects the magnitude of work performed by the body relative to rest. Therefore, one MET is the value of oxygen used when the body is resting and equals the derived unit 3.5 ml of oxygen per kg of body weight per minute (3.5 ml $\cdot$ kg^{-1} $\cdot$ min^{-1}). This value is the same for every person. The way it becomes relative to a particular person is by factoring in the individual's weight and the time they spend at that relative oxygen demand. If an activity is performed above a resting level, then the MET value changes to reflect the oxygen demand. For instance, casual walking is generally performed at 2.8 METs, working at a desk is 1.5 METs, while washing and waxing a car is 4.5 METs. Each of these values can be multiplied by the 3.5 ml $\cdot$ kg^{-1} $\cdot$ min^{-1} unit to convert it to the specific oxygen demand. Once the total amount of oxygen utilized has been determined, the amount of calories expended can be calculated given that each liter (L) of oxygen used equates to 5 kcal burned.

MET Example One

Example: 220 lb. (100 kg) man sitting in a chair for 60 minutes (1 MET)

$$3.5 \text{ ml} \cdot kg^{-1} \cdot min^{-1} \times 100 \text{ kg} = 350 \text{ ml} \cdot min^{-1}$$

$$350 \text{ ml} \cdot min^{-1} \times 60 \text{ min} = 21{,}000 \text{ ml}$$

$$21000 \text{ ml} \times \frac{.001 \text{ L}}{\text{ml}} = 21 \text{ L}$$

$$21 \text{ L} \times 5 \text{ kcal} \cdot L^{-1} = 105 \text{ kcal}$$

The example above shows that when the relative variables of an individual are factored in, the MET value can be expressed as a measure of oxygen use and calories expended. In the case of the 220 lb. man sitting in the chair for an hour, he would require 21 liters of oxygen, or 105 calories for his tissues to function. This ability to express the values based on known variables allows for the identification of how much oxygen or energy is needed to perform a particular task. The equation used above can also be used to identify oxygen demand and calories for any level of work when the necessary variables are known. In fact, this is the same formula that aerobic exercise equipment uses to provide exercisers with the calories they expend during a workout.

One of the first values requested of an exerciser when they start on an aerobic machine is his or her weight. The machine quickly converts the pounds entered into kilograms and adds this value into the equation. The next value the machine often requests is the amount of time the exercise will be performed. This number is also entered into the equation. The last bit of

Common Expressions of Energy Expenditure

Liters of oxygen per minute	$L \cdot min^{-1}$
Calories per minute	$Kcal \cdot min^{-1}$
Milliliters of oxygen per kilogram of bodyweight per minute	$ml \cdot kg^{-1} \cdot min^{-1}$
Metabolic equivalent of oxygen	METs
Calories per kilogram of bodyweight per minute	$Kcal \cdot kg^{-1} \cdot hr^{-1}$

information used is the speed setting or intensity level selected. The machine has MET intensities built into its default program data, based on the level or speed selected. The following example demonstrates the machine's conversion of information to provide the user with a caloric value.

MET Example Two

Example: 220 lb (100 kg) male exercising at level 8 on a Stairclimber for 30 minutes.

Weight : $220 \text{ lbs} \div \dfrac{1 \text{ kg}}{2.2 \text{ lbs}} = 100 \text{ kg}$

Intensity: Level 8 = 10 METs (Default value based on resistance and speed)

Time: 30 minutes

1 MET = $3.5 \text{ ml} \cdot \text{kg}^{-1} \cdot \text{min}^{-1}$

$10 \text{ MET} \times \dfrac{3.5 \text{ ml} \cdot \text{kg}^{-1} \cdot \text{min}^{-1}}{1 \text{ MET}} = 35 \text{ ml} \cdot \text{kg}^{-1} \cdot \text{min}^{-1}$

$35 \text{ ml} \cdot \text{kg}^{-1} \cdot \text{min}^{-1} \times 100 \text{ kg} = 3500 \text{ ml} \cdot \text{min}^{-1}$

$3500 \text{ ml} \cdot \text{min}^{-1} \times 30 \text{ min} = 105{,}000 \text{ ml}$

$105{,}000 \text{ ml} \times \dfrac{.001 \text{ L}}{\text{ml}} = 105 \text{ L}$

$105 \text{ L} \times 5 \text{ kcal} \cdot \text{L}^{-1} = 525 \text{ kcal}$

This equation works for any activity that has been scientifically measured for work. Clinicians have analyzed hundreds of activities to provide MET intensities for use in determining oxygen demand and energy expenditure. In some cases, the activities are weight-bearing, like the Stairclimbing example, where the exerciser must lift his or her body weight as part of the work. In others, such as biking, the weight of an individual is not a relevant factor to determining the oxygen demand. Activities where bodyweight is a factor when determining work express the value as $\text{ml} \cdot \text{kg}^{-1} \cdot \text{min}^{-1}$, whereas in non-weight-bearing activities the oxygen is expressed as $\text{L} \cdot \text{min}^{-1}$.

The exercise bike uses revolutions per minute and the selected resistance to determine the MET intensity. The subsequent energy expenditure is based on how long that MET intensity is performed. This explains why a person who weighs 150 lbs. exercising at level 5 on the stationary bike will burn the same calories as a person weighing 200 lbs. exercising at the same intensity for the same period of time. Based on size, the smaller exerciser is performing more relative work when the liters of oxygen are converted to milliliters per kilogram of body weight per minute.

During weight-bearing exercise the amount of bodyweight determines the work being performed. The person's weight most often represents the vertical and horizontal resistive force that must be overcome to perform the movement. This variable becomes a factor when exercisers working out on this type of equipment lean on the guide rails or support bars to make the exercise easier. Any weight alleviated from the resistance to the movement and applied to the machine guide rails is not actually contributing to the vertical or horizontal component of work necessitated by running or climbing. If 30% of the body weight is removed from the leg's resistance force, the resultant calories displayed by the machine are 30% higher than the actual number burned. Commonly, exercisers set the machine on high training levels and compensate by resting on the machine to manage the work rate. This causes people to perceive a caloric expenditure during the exercise that may be as much as 50% above what they actually burned.

Similar pitfalls exist for non-weight-bearing machines. The MET value determined by the selected training level is based on a default RPM speed (rotations per minute), normally about 70 RPM's (numbers may vary). When exercisers select training levels that are too difficult they compensate by peddling slower, which negates the workload. Most machines are not technologically advanced enough to identify the change and recalculate the value, even though a light often flashes to signify a low RPM rate. Logically, most people should realize that if the exercise becomes easier by cheating, then it must not burn the same calories. However, most exercisers will acknowledge their work rate as consistent with the machine's data display, which is often an over-prediction of actual calories burned.

When METs are applied to a person's predicted or measured VO_2max, the amount of work they can tolerate becomes increasingly evident. The math required to convert VO_2max into METs is simple. One MET equals $3.5 \text{ ml} \cdot \text{kg}^{-1} \cdot \text{min}^{-1}$, and relative VO_2max is expressed using the same units. Therefore, to identify a person's maximum MET intensity capabilities, all one has to do is divide the VO_2max by $3.5 \text{ ml} \cdot \text{kg}^{-1} \cdot \text{min}^{-1}$. Once this maximal MET value is identified, it can be used to determine the individual's realistic energy expenditure capacity.

For example, if a 37 year old male weighing 200 lbs. was identified through aerobic testing to have a VO_2max of $43 \text{ ml} \cdot \text{kg}^{-1} \cdot \text{min}^{-1}$ his maximal MET intensity would be 12.25 METs.

$$43 \text{ ml} \cdot \text{kg}^{-1} \cdot \text{min}^{-1} \div \frac{3.5 \text{ ml} \cdot \text{kg}^{-1} \cdot \text{min}^{-1}}{1 \text{ MET}} = 12.25 \text{ METs}$$

If the individual wanted to lose weight, the length of time it would take can easily be figured out based on their respective capacity. A healthy person is expected to train at an intensity between 60% and 80% HRR or VO$_2$max. The individual's VO$_2$max was 43 ml · kg^{-1} · min^{-1}, or 12.25 METs.

$$60\% \text{ x } 12.25 \text{ METs} = 7.35 \text{ METs}$$
$$80\% \text{ x } 12.25 \text{ METs} = 9.8 \text{ METs}$$

The training intensity value suggests this individual should perform aerobic exercise at a work rate between 7.35 and 9.8 METs. Assuming this person could sustain the lower level for 30 minutes, the predicted aerobic training contribution to weight loss can be calculated.

$$7.35 \text{ MET x } \frac{3.5 \text{ ml} \cdot \text{kg}^{-1} \cdot \text{min}^{-1}}{1 \text{ MET}} = 25.7 \text{ ml} \cdot \text{kg}^{-1} \cdot \text{min}^{-1}$$

$$25.7 \text{ ml} \cdot \text{kg}^{-1} \cdot \text{min}^{-1} \text{ x } 91 \text{ kg} = 2,338 \text{ ml} \cdot \text{min}^{-1}$$

$$2,338 \text{ ml} \cdot \text{min}^{-1} \text{ x } 30 \text{ min} = 70,140 \text{ ml}$$

$$70,140 \text{ ml x } \frac{.001 \text{ L}}{\text{ml}} = 70.1 \text{ L}$$

$$70.1 \text{ L x } 5 \text{ kcal} \cdot \text{L}^{-1} = 350 \text{ kcal}$$

Based on these findings, it would be realistic to expect this healthy male individual to be able to burn 350 kcal in an aerobic exercise bout in the early stages of the training program. This prediction is very helpful because the expected caloric expenditure helps to identify the rate at which weight loss can occur via exercise capacity and the amount of dietary adjustments that must be made to compensate for the value. When clients have a 12 MET capacity or higher, it is easier to elicit the desired training response and reach weight loss goals because they have a high capacity to expend energy. When clients are deconditioned and present MET

capacities lower than 10 METs, it becomes increasingly difficult to reach the same weight loss goals (12).

METs & Daily Caloric Expenditure

METs can also be used in the energy balance equation to identify daily caloric expenditure. As stated above, the average daily caloric expenditure is more relevant than any single segment of high energy expenditure with regard to weight management. Therefore, identifying the mean energy expenditure value helps to identify the need for additional physical activity if weight loss and health are to be attained. In the same way one can use food logs to identify the caloric intake for a day, activity logs can be used to calculate the caloric expenditure. Recording the activity and the participation duration provides the data necessary to calculate the daily energy expenditure. The chart below is an example of a 24-hour activity recall for a 39 year old female weighing 152 lbs.

The example represents a total daily oxygen use of 475 liters of oxygen or 1.65 kcal · min^{-1}. Adding additional activity to this individual's lifestyle would increase the calories expended per day. Simply increasing daily oxygen use by an average of only one liter per hour would increase the caloric expenditure by 120 kcal. Encouraging more movement throughout the day can dramatically enhance the likelihood for a successful weight loss program (27). Additionally, those individuals who attain a minimum expenditure of 1,000-2,000 kcal per week from physical activity notably increase their health and reduce their risk for disease (47; 60).

Using METs to Determine Daily Caloric Expenditure

Time	Activity	MET	Kcal
8:00 – 8:30 am	Showered and dressed	2.5	91
8:30 – 8:50 am	Ate breakfast	1.5	36
8:50 - 9:30 am	Drove to work w/traffic	2.0	97
9:30 – 9:40 am	Walk to office	3.0	36
9:30 – 10:45 am	Sat at desk	1.5	136
10:45 – 12:00 am	Meeting	1.5	136
12:00 - 1:00pm	At lunch	1.5	109
1:00 – 2:30 pm	Sat at desk	1.5	163
2:30 – 2:50 pm	Walk to other office	3.0	72
2:50 – 5:00 pm	Presentation (standing)	2.3	361
5:00 – 5:15 pm	Walk to car	3.0	54
5:15 – 5:35 pm	Drove home	2.0	48
5:35 – 6:00 pm	Washed-up and changed	2.5	76
6:00 – 6:45 pm	Ate dinner	1.5	82
6:45 – 11:00 pm	Watch TV	1.0	308
11:00 – 11:10 pm	Self-care	1.0	12
11:10 pm – 8:00 am	Sleep	0.9	576

Total Energy Expenditure   2,393

Mode

Physical activity can come from a variety of different modalities. Aerobic exercise activities aimed at improving CRF include numerous modes that are equally effective. The key factors are the duration, intensity, frequency, and the energy expended per session. This suggests that any continuous, rhythmic activity that utilizes large muscle groups can be included in the CRF program. The exercise or mode selected should be based on the client's capabilities, interests, and experience. Each mode has advantages and disadvantages which should be evaluated and matched to the client. Identifying the activities that the client finds to be fun or most tolerable will help ensure compliance and adherence to the training prescription. If several modes are of interest to the client, the exercise prescription should include a mixture of activities. Commonly referred to as cross-training, varying aerobic activities reduces boredom, risk of overuse injury, and emphasizes different muscle groups. These modes can even be combined in a single training session. Running, rowing, and biking, for instance, can each be utilized in 10 minute segments for a 30 minute workout. The variation in mode and musculature used allows for higher training intensity due to improved mental focus. Boredom becomes a factor in any long duration activity performed on a frequent basis. Therefore, varying the modes reduces the consequences of mental staleness commonly experienced with single-mode, steady-state training.

Systems of Training

Within any of the selected modes of aerobic training, different systems exist to elicit improved adaptation responses. Each system varies by specific factors that modify the intensity, such as speed, terrain, or resistance. These systems can be used independently or in a coordinated fashion depending on the goals of the program and the interests of the client. Some common systems include lactate threshold, or tempo training, cross-training, cardio-circuits, and Fartlek training.

Lactate Threshold Training

Lactate threshold training employs tactics that vary the amount of anaerobic contribution during the aerobic exercise bout. This technique is used by conditioned individuals to push training levels for improvements in stamina and lactate tolerance. Anaerobic, or lactate threshold, is the point where lactic acid production is equal to the rate of lactate clearance. This state uses contributions from both energy systems (aerobic and anaerobic), but the effects of the anaerobic system are accommodated for via buffering mechanisms, which allow steady-state heart rate to be maintained and the

work to be performed without consequence. When the pace is increased beyond the lactate threshold, the contribution from anaerobic metabolism can no longer be compensated for via the buffering mechanisms used for lactate turnover. This causes lactic acid to accumulate, which increases discomfort, ventilation rate, and perceived exertion, eventually forcing the exerciser to slow down to a recovery pace, or to stop. It is suggested that exercisers should attempt to train using a pace at, or just below, lactate threshold for optimal cardiorespiratory adaptations (20; 24). This type of training is called "tempo training." Many endurance athletes will use steady-state tempo pace on certain training days and then cross the lactate threshold, using intervals to push the energy system to tolerate greater demands and to improve VO_2max on other days. Lactate intervals generally last between 2-5 minutes, depending on the intensity reached and the condition of the exerciser. This method of training should only be used by individuals acclimated to the training intensity (25).

Cross Training

Cross training, as mentioned earlier, utilizes different modes of exercise for aerobic improvements. In some cases, the mode of exercise varies by exercise session. In other cases, different modes of exercise are used within the same workout. The benefits include reduced risk of overuse of a particular muscle or group, reduced risk of boredom, utilization of different muscle groups for improved condition, and better mental focus during the exercise session. Cross training can also be employed in cycles to help maximize the efficiency of a particular mode of exercise. Over a 12-week training cycle, three different modes may be used for each four-week period. Biking can be used for the first segment, attempting to improve aerobic conditioning in the legs without impact, before switching to stair climbing in the second four-week period, and then jogging for the last segment of the cycle. This method allows adaptations specific to the mode to take place and encourages improvement in neural efficiency.

Cardio Circuit Training

Cardio circuit training is a type of aerobic conditioning that utilizes different exercise modalities and often total body contributions during the exercise session. Cardio-circuits require exercisers to perform steady-state aerobic activity with intermittent resistance training activities. A common example would be a parcourse, which employs jogging at a set pace and stopping at designated locations along the route to perform calisthenics, pull-ups, push-ups, or other anaerobic activities, before continuing on the jog at the steady-state pace to the next activity stop. Parcourses often

Example of Cardio Circuit Training

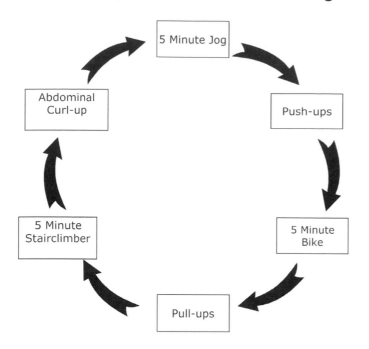

exist at local community parks. These courses can be mimicked in the fitness facilities by switching from aerobic activity to resistance training movements with only transitional rest. In most cases, an exercise will be selected for each body part and performed every three minutes during the exercise routine. Cardio-circuits work very well in the personal training environment because they can be used to address several facets of the exercise program in an on-going, aerobic-based exercise session.

Fartlek Training

Fartlek is Swedish for "speed play." **Fartlek training** is essentially a type of interval training that uses steady-state pace with periodic variations in speed and grade. The biggest difference compared to standard interval training is the variation in speeds and distances used within the interval segment, along with the changes in the surface angle. Fartlek training uses flat surfaces, uphill running and sprints, and downhill over-speed segments at different intervals in between steady-state pace. The distances used and segment speeds will be determined by the goals of the training and the capabilities of the client.

Aerobic Training Considerations

Genetics

Participants in routine aerobic exercise are generally able to increase their VO_2max by 10-30% with an average improvement of approximately 15% (5; 6). The amount of improvement is dependent upon pre-training

status, exercise tolerance, level of participation, and genetics. Of these factors, the largest variation is attributed to genetics, which accounts for as much as 35% of the differences (2; 28). This is largely attributed to adaptational responses in maximal cardiac output and oxygen extraction capabilities. Individuals with larger stroke volumes, greater concentrations of type I fibers, mitochondria, and capillaries, higher myoglobin concentrations, and more efficient neural and metabolic pathways show the greatest improvements (52; 73). Certain individuals are physiologically more efficient in aerobic pathways and therefore, present the most dramatic improvements in training (52; 74).

Age

Healthy, sedentary adults experience a decline of approximately 1% per year in maximal aerobic capacity. The combination of inactivity, weight gain, and age-related decline in muscle mass and maximal heart rate are all implicated in the loss of aerobic efficiency (4). In trained individuals, the rate of loss decreases in males to approximately 0.5% per year, but female aerobic decline remains consistent with their sedentary counterparts (1; 7; 63). Individuals who attain higher levels of aerobic fitness early in life and consistently work to maintain those levels will obviously experience higher values throughout their lifespan, thereby preventing the early onset of functional decline. When previously sedentary, older adults engage in aerobic activity, they experience similar improvements compared to younger individuals (10-20%) (72). However, due to their lower starting

Key Terms

Heart rate reserve (HRR) – The difference between heart rate maximum and resting heart rate (Max HR-Resting HR).

Fartlek training – A type of interval training that uses steady-state pace with periodic variations in speed and grade.

Radiation – One of the body's cooling methods in which heat from the body passes through the air into colder solids within close proximity.

Convection – The body's process of cooling, in which heat from the body is transferred into the air.

Conduction – The process in which heat is transferred from the body to a colder object upon contact.

Evaporation – The process by which water is passed through the skin and is converted to water vapor, causing a cooling effect.

values, older adults have difficulty reaching high levels of aerobic fitness. The adaptations in older men and women are different, as older men show improvement in both maximal cardiac output and oxygen extraction from increased capillary and mitochondria density. Improvements in aerobic efficiency in older women are solely limited to improvements in oxygen extraction (33).

Environmental Factors

The body is subjected to stress from external factors, including the environmental conditions it is exposed to. Heat, humidity, and altitude all exert potential adverse effects on the body during physical activity. Heat provides considerable stress to the body's internal environment because it increases the body's thermoregulatory response. When the tissues contract, they produce heat, which must be released from the body to prevent dangerous elevation of core temperatures. The human body cools itself via four methods: **radiation**, **convection**, **conduction**, and **evaporation**. Radiation causes heat from the body to pass through air into colder solids within close proximity. It works in the same fashion that light from the sun warms the earth. Convection works in a similar way, but the heat is transferred into the air. When it is windy, heat is mobilized from the skin into the air that passes over the body. Conduction represents heat loss to a colder object that comes in contact with the body or heat transferred from deep tissues to the skin. Jumping into cold water illustrates this concept very well. In fact, heat loss to water is 25 times that of heat loss to air at the same temperature. The last method of heat loss is the primary defense used by the body to prevent overheating. Evaporation is the process by which water is passed through the skin and evaporated into the air, causing a cooling effect. Heat is also lost through respiratory water vapor. All four mechanisms cooperate to keep body temperature regulated.

If environmental conditions are hot, heat loss via radiation, convection, and conduction becomes less effective, or even halts. This leaves evaporation as the only functioning mechanism to remove heat from the body. The body begins to mobilize extracellular fluid to the skin for evaporation. This leads to dehydration, causing the water content of the blood to decrease. Exercise in the heat becomes more difficult as blood volume is reduced. The reduction in blood plasma makes the heart work harder, thereby making exercise more difficult, even though the pace remains the same.

This problem is exacerbated when heat combines with high humidity. When the humidity is high, the process of evaporation decreases significantly because the ambient air/water vapor pressure is consistent with that of the skin. Sweat is produced, but it cannot evaporate into the air. This forces the body to increase sweat rate and further contributes to water loss. Exercise in high heat and humidity can be dangerous, as it increases risk of heat illness and thermoregulatory shut-down.

Altitude

Altitudes will also affect aerobic performance. At higher altitudes, the oxygen concentration of air is lower, leading to a reduction in available oxygen that can be extracted during respiration. When physical activity is performed at higher altitude, the stress becomes apparent as an individual's respiratory and heart rate must increase to deliver the same amount of oxygen to peripheral tissues. Due to the progressive decline in the partial pressure of oxygen as elevations rise, the higher a person climbs, the more difficult it becomes to perform all activities, including breathing.

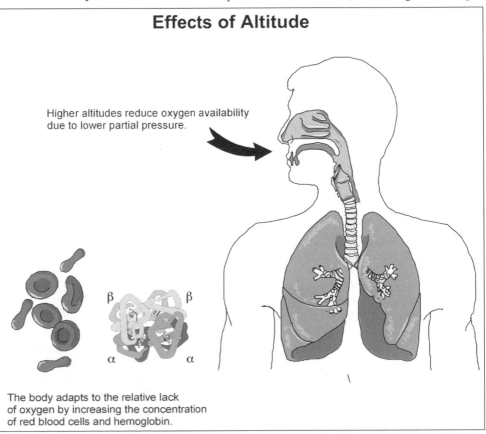

Effects of Altitude

Higher altitudes reduce oxygen availability due to lower partial pressure.

β   β

α   α

The body adapts to the relative lack of oxygen by increasing the concentration of red blood cells and hemoglobin.

At extreme heights, such as Mt. Everest in Nepal, climbers have died from hypoxia as their blood oxygen concentrations drop into lethal ranges.

The disadvantage of altitude becomes an advantage when the body is acclimated to the environment. Slow progressions in activity at higher altitudes over several weeks cause physiological adjustments in hemoglobin and red blood cell concentrations that become advantageous upon return to sea level (14; 58). Many athletes train in Colorado to acclimate to the high altitudes. When they return to lower terrestrial levels, these athletes are better able to remove carbon dioxide, experience higher red blood cell concentrations, allowing for higher arterial oxygen levels and also increase muscle capillary and mitochondrial density (48). All of these factors improve aerobic performance.

Acclimation to Heat

Acclimation also occurs when the body is exposed to heat over an extended period of time. With on-going exposure, the body makes physiological adjustments that provide greater heat tolerance. Sweat rate threshold decreases, while sweat production increases and expands the sweat distribution across a broader surface, allowing for greater evaporation (3). Correspondingly, plasma volumes increase to account for the improvements in sweat efficiency and the sodium concentration in sweat is reduced. The cardiovascular system also improves circulation and cutaneous blood flow to distribute more heat to the skin. These adaptations allow the body to more efficiently remove heat and enhance performance in hot environments.

Gender

Gender differences account for about a 15% disparity between VO_2max measures in adult men and women. The physiological differences found between genders accounts for the discrepancy between maximal attainable values (34). Females have smaller hearts, lower stroke volume, lower hemoglobin concentrations, and less muscle mass relative to size. In addition, females maintain higher body fat values compared to men (49). During submaximal work at the same absolute VO_2, females experience higher heart rates and higher cardiac output to compensate for the gender-related differences (67). Notably however, females do experience the same relative improvements to aerobic training as do men (21).

Recovery

Recovery needs to be a consideration any time the body performs work at elevated intensities due to damage of the tissue and changes in the cellular environment associated with increased metabolic activity. When exercise is performed at steady-state between 50-60% HRR, the metabolic conditions are not significantly disrupted. Hydrogen ion accumulation is attenuated via a slower rate of ATP hydrolysis, and a greater reliance is placed on lipid metabolism. Therefore, the resynthesis of high-energy phosphate (ATP), oxygen replenishment, and other mechanisms of recovery occur rather quickly with rest. When greater concentrations of lactate accumulate due to high volumes of glycogen and high energy phosphate utilization during high intensity work, the recovery process benefits from a longer, active cool down. Active recovery increases blood flow to the working myocytes to increase the rate of lactate transfer to neighboring aerobic muscle cells and increases mobilization of blood lactate to the liver, thereby increasing the rate of glycogen re-synthesis.

Muscle fatigue is another factor in recovery. Repeated bouts of exercise utilizing the same muscle groups can cause repetitive microtrauma in tissue not acclimated to the training, which increases requirements of rest for recovery. New exercisers can benefit from the one day on, one day off method, as progressions are steadily applied over an early training cycle. Individuals who train for aerobic performance often use six or seven consecutive days of training, which creates significant stress on the tissue. To compensate for the stress, variations in distance and speed are used to aid in recovery from one bout to the next. A full day of rest every 7-9 days is a generally accepted practice for individuals focusing on endurance performance enhancement. Using cross training techniques can also aid in recovery if multiple days are used without rest. Non-weight-bearing activities, such as swimming and biking, can be used to replace running, as the eccentric component of these activities, a major contributor to recovery requirements, is less intense than that experienced with running.

Detraining

The absolute cessation of aerobic activity has deleterious effects on aerobic endurance in a relatively short period of time. Trained individuals show a decline in aerobic performance within the first few weeks of detraining, due primarily to a reduction in blood plasma and consequent stroke volume diminution (17; 50; 57). If training is stopped for three or more weeks, oxygen extraction is reduced due to mitochondria loss in the muscle cell (18). When training volumes decrease, similar reductions are experienced but at a slower rate. To prevent periods of reduced volume from affecting VO_2max, intensities must be elevated to provide an overload stimulus on the system. Reductions in volume from 6 days to 3 days can be relatively negated by increasing the intensity to maximal tolerable levels. For example, if a training volume of 4 days per week at 70% HRR for 30 minutes is reduced to two days per week, the intensity should increase to 80-85% HRR. This can be accomplished using interval training and lactate threshold steady-states. Even if the intensities cannot be maintained for long periods of time, the body must experience this level of stress to maintain its current condition.

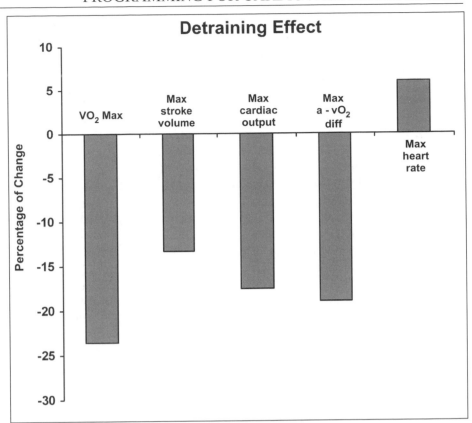

Preventing Common Overuse Injuries

Inherent to any increase in physical activity is the risk of injury. Due to the repetitive nature of aerobic training, overuse injuries are not uncommon. These injuries often stem from a variety of factors. Some of the more common variables that contribute to problems include starting off too aggressively, abruptly increasing progressions, muscle imbalances and lack of range of motion, incorrect footwear, and uneven running surfaces. Common injuries associated with aerobic training include **chondromalacia**, plantar fasciitis, **IT Band syndrome**, acute low back pain, and shin splints.

Chondromalacia

Chondromalacia is a common injury associated with impact aerobic activities. The condition occurs from damage to the articular cartilage of the knee. It can be caused by trauma, overuse, poor joint alignment, or muscle imbalances. It often occurs from the knee cap rubbing against the lower end of the thigh, damaging the cartilage underneath the knee cap. The level of damage varies from slight surface abnormalities in the cartilage surface to complete wear of the tissue, exposing the bone. Chondromalacia can also occur from blunt trauma, which tears off either a small piece of articular cartilage or a large fragment containing a piece of bone. This often requires invasive surgery to fix.

Chondromalacia can be treated using closed-chain exercises that strengthen the medial quadricep, and other connecting structures at, and around, the joint. Non-impact aerobic exercises can be used for aerobic conditioning if the knee is not bent more than 90 degrees. Therapuetic modalities include rest, anti-inflammatory medication, and ice therapy. If these treatments fail to improve the condition, arthroscopic surgery may be used to smooth the surface of the articular cartilage and remove cartilage fragments that cause irritation.

Plantar Fasciitis

Plantar fasciitis is the most common cause of heel pain from aerobic activity. A flat ligament band connects the calcaneous to the toes, called the plantar fascia, which supports the arch of the foot. When the tissue becomes strained, it becomes swollen and irritated, causing pain in the heel or bottom of the foot when weight is placed upon it. The exact cause of the tissue damage is not known, but it is likely attributed to repeated small tears in the plantar fascia during normal stride when the plantar fascia stretches upon foot strike. Plantar fasciitis can be caused by a tight achilles tendon, abrupt increase in repetitions from exercise, or improper arch support. Remedies for plantar fasciitis include stretching the fascia, myofascial release using a tennis ball or similar object, anti-inflammatory medication, massage, foot splints, arch supports, and rest.

Iliotibial Band Syndrome

Iliotibial band syndrome (ITBS) is common among runners and is responsible for more than 10% of all running-related overuse injuries. The injury occurs in the ligament that runs along the lateral aspect of the thigh, connecting the top of the hip to the lateral side of the knee. The tissue can become inflamed by uneven gait caused by running on a banked surface, tightness in the quadratus lumborum in the back, or may be attributed to inadequate warm-up or by increasing training distances too quickly.

The condition can usually be improved in a matter of weeks by stretching the IT band, myofascial release therapy, and ice and heat therapies. Additionally, it is importatnt to avoid the situations that caused the problem in the first place. It is recommended that therapies be employed for up to six weeks, even if the pain subsides.

Low Back Pain

Aerobic exercise may cause low back pain (LBP) in some particpants. Causes range from muscle imbalances, lack of flexibility, poor movement biomechanics, and poor movement postures, to general deconditioning or any combination of the aforementioned. Individuals new to exercise are often predisposed to acute pain response when they attempt prolonged activities that have not previously been experienced. The muscles in the back are often ill-prepared for the stress from the postural positions maintained during continuous exercise. Gait discrepacies during walking and running may also contribute to the problem.

In most cases, acute low back pain is treated using traditional therapies for LBP from other causes. Stretching the back and tight hip muscles, strengthening the abdominals and related structures, and heat therapies can all improve the condition. If exercise using erect posture is the probable cause, switching to biking or swimming may alleviate the symptoms.

Shin Splints

Shin splints, or medial tibial stress syndrome, is a common condition that includes pain and tenderness over the middle or lower part of the shin bone. The condition is usually caused by overuse, leading to inflammation of the anterior tibialis muscle and the lateral-anterior muscle compartment. Shin splints can be caused by a variety of different factors, including sudden increases in training volume, running on uneven surfaces, improper foot wear, and general overtraining. The exact location of the pain may also vary between the medial or lateral aspect of the shin. Medial shin splints are usually caused by excessive pronation or flat feet, and are common with activities that cause repetitive pounding.

Shin splints are often treated using rest, massage, ice therapy, and stretching and strengthening techniques. Stretching and strengthening the muscles of the lower leg help reduce incidence from muscle imbalance and tightness. Ice therapy and longer warm-ups have shown to be effective as well. Footwear and running surfaces should also be evaluated as possible causes. If the injury persists, it is cause for medical refereral to assess if a stress fracture has occurred.

Key Terms

Chondromalacia – Abnormal degeneration of the cartilage of the joints, especially in the knee, commonly associated with impact aerobic activities.

IT Band syndrome – An overuse injury, commonly associated with running, in which the iliotibial band running along the lateral aspect of the thigh becomes irritated due to the inflammation in the area.

Shin splints – Also known as medial tibial stress syndrome, which is a condition that is commonly associated with overuse and is characterized by pain and tenderness over the middle or lower part of the shin bone.

Chapter Seventeen References

1. American College of Sports Medicine Position Stand. Exercise and physical activity for older adults. *Med Sci Sports Exerc* 30: 992-1008, 1998.

2. **An P, Perusse L, Rankinen T, Borecki IB, Gagnon J, Leon AS, Skinner JS, Wilmore JH, Bouchard C and Rao DC.** Familial aggregation of exercise heart rate and blood pressure in response to 20 weeks of endurance training: the HERITAGE family study. *Int J Sports Med* 24: 57-62, 2003.

3. **Armstrong LE and Maresh CM.** Effects of training, environment, and host factors on the sweating response to exercise. *Int J Sports Med* 19 Suppl 2: S103-S105, 1998.

4. **Atomi Y and Miyashita M.** Effect of training intensity in adult females. *Eur J Appl Physiol Occup Physiol* 44: 109-116, 1980.

5. **Blumenthal JA, Emery CF, Madden DJ, George LK, Coleman RE, Riddle MW, McKee DC, Reasoner J and Williams RS.** Cardiovascular and behavioral effects of aerobic exercise training in healthy older men and women. *J Gerontol* 44: M147-M157, 1989.

6. **Blumenthal JA, Matthews K, Fredrikson M, Rifai N, Schniebolk S, German D, Steege J and Rodin J.** Effects of exercise training on cardiovascular function and plasma lipid, lipoprotein, and apolipoprotein concentrations in premenopausal and postmenopausal women. *Arterioscler Thromb* 11: 912-917, 1991.

7. **Bortz WM and Bortz WM.** How fast do we age? Exercise performance over time as a biomarker. *J Gerontol A Biol Sci Med Sci* 51: M223-M225, 1996.

8. **Braun LT.** Exercise physiology and cardiovascular fitness. *Nurs Clin North Am* 26: 135-147, 1991.

9. **Braun LT.** Exercise physiology and cardiovascular fitness. *Nurs Clin North Am* 26: 135-147, 1991.

10. **Braun LT.** Exercise physiology and cardiovascular fitness. *Nurs Clin North Am* 26: 135-147, 1991.

11. **Braun LT.** Exercise physiology and cardiovascular fitness. *Nurs Clin North Am* 26: 135-147, 1991.

12. **Brooks AG, Withers RT, Gore CJ, Vogler AJ, Plummer J and Cormack J.** Measurement and prediction of METs during household activities in 35- to 45-year-old females. *Eur J Appl Physiol* 91: 638-648, 2004.

13. **Buckley JP, Sim J, Eston RG, Hession R and Fox R.** Reliability and validity of measures taken during the Chester step test to predict aerobic power and to prescribe aerobic exercise. *Br J Sports Med* 38: 197-205, 2004.

14. **Burtscher M, Nachbauer W, Baumgartl P and Philadelphy M.** Benefits of training at moderate altitude versus sea level training in amateur runners. *Eur J Appl Physiol Occup Physiol* 74: 558-563, 1996.

15. **Chen MJ, Fan X and Moe ST.** Criterion-related validity of the Borg ratings of perceived exertion scale in healthy individuals: a meta-analysis. *J Sports Sci* 20: 873-899, 2002.

16. **Cox MH.** Exercise training programs and cardiorespiratory adaptation. *Clin Sports Med* 10: 19-32, 1991.

17. **Coyle EF, Hemmert MK and Coggan AR.** Effects of detraining on cardiovascular responses to exercise: role of blood volume. *J Appl Physiol* 60: 95-99, 1986.

18. **Coyle EF, Martin WH, III, Bloomfield SA, Lowry OH and Holloszy JO.** Effects of detraining on responses to submaximal exercise. *J Appl Physiol* 59: 853-859, 1985.

19. **Davis JA and Convertino VA.** A comparison of heart rate methods for predicting endurance training intensity. *Med Sci Sports* 7: 295-298, 1975.

20. **Denis C, Dormois D, Castells J, Bonnefoy R, Padilla S, Geyssant A and Lacour JR.** Comparison of incremental and steady state tests of endurance training. *Eur J Appl Physiol Occup Physiol* 57: 474-481, 1988.

21. **Deschenes MR, Hillard MN, Wilson JA, Dubina MI and Eason MK.** Effects of gender on physiological responses during submaximal exercise and recovery. *Med Sci Sports Exerc* 38: 1304-1310, 2006.

22. **Duncan GE, Sydeman SJ, Perri MG, Limacher MC and Martin AD.** Can sedentary adults accurately recall the intensity of their physical activity? *Prev Med* 33: 18-26, 2001.

23. **Escolar Castellon JL, Perez Romero de la Cruz and Corrales MR.** [Physical activity and disease]. *An Med Interna* 20: 427-433, 2003.

24. **Faria EW, Parker DL and Faria IE.** The science of cycling: physiology and training - part 1. *Sports Med* 35: 285-312, 2005.

25. **Faria EW, Parker DL and Faria IE.** The science of cycling: physiology and training - part 1. *Sports Med* 35: 285-312, 2005.

26. **Friedlander AL, Jacobs KA, Fattor JA, Horning MA, Hagobian TA, Bauer TA, Wolfel EE and Brooks GA.** Contributions of working muscle to whole body lipid metabolism are altered by exercise intensity and training. *Am J Physiol Endocrinol Metab* 292: E107-E116, 2007.

27. **Gal DL, Santos AC and Barros H**. Leisure-time versus full-day energy expenditure: a cross-sectional study of sedentarism in a Portuguese urban population. *BMC Public Health* 5: 16, 2005.

28. **Gaskill SE, Rice T, Bouchard C, Gagnon J, Rao DC, Skinner JS, Wilmore JH and Leon AS**. Familial resemblance in ventilatory threshold: the HERITAGE Family Study. *Med Sci Sports Exerc* 33: 1832-1840, 2001.

29. **Glass SC and Stanton DR**. Self-selected resistance training intensity in novice weightlifters. *J Strength Cond Res* 18: 324-327, 2004.

30. **Goldberg L, Elliot DL and Kuehl KS**. Assessment of exercise intensity formulas by use of ventilatory threshold. *Chest* 94: 95-98, 1988.

31. **Gordon NF, Scott CB, Wilkinson WJ, Duncan JJ and Blair SN**. Exercise and mild essential hypertension. Recommendations for adults. *Sports Med* 10: 390-404, 1990.

32. **Gordon NF, Scott CB, Wilkinson WJ, Duncan JJ and Blair SN**. Exercise and mild essential hypertension. Recommendations for adults. *Sports Med* 10: 390-404, 1990.

33. **Hagberg JM, Goldberg AP, Lakatta L, O'Connor FC, Becker LC, Lakatta EG and Fleg JL**. Expanded blood volumes contribute to the increased cardiovascular performance of endurance-trained older men. *J Appl Physiol* 85: 484-489, 1998.

34. **Harms CA**. Does gender affect pulmonary function and exercise capacity? *Respir Physiol Neurobiol* 151: 124-131, 2006.

35. **Irving BA, Rutkowski J, Brock DW, Davis CK, Barrett EJ, Gaesser GA and Weltman A**. Comparison of Borg- and OMNI-RPE as markers of the blood lactate response to exercise. *Med Sci Sports Exerc* 38: 1348-1352, 2006.

36. **Irving BA, Rutkowski J, Brock DW, Davis CK, Barrett EJ, Gaesser GA and Weltman A**. Comparison of Borg- and OMNI-RPE as markers of the blood lactate response to exercise. *Med Sci Sports Exerc* 38: 1348-1352, 2006.

37. **Jones BH, Cowan DN and Knapik JJ**. Exercise, training and injuries. *Sports Med* 18: 202-214, 1994.

38. **Katch V, Weltman A, Sady S and Freedson P**. Validity of the relative percent concept for equating training intensity. *Eur J Appl Physiol Occup Physiol* 39: 219-227, 1978.

39. **Kemi OJ, Haram PM, Loennechen JP, Osnes JB, Skomedal T, Wisloff U and Ellingsen O**. Moderate vs. high exercise intensity: differential effects on aerobic fitness, cardiomyocyte contractility, and endothelial function. *Cardiovasc Res* 67: 161-172, 2005.

40. **Kemi OJ, Haram PM, Loennechen JP, Osnes JB, Skomedal T, Wisloff U and Ellingsen O**. Moderate vs. high exercise intensity: differential effects on aerobic fitness, cardiomyocyte contractility, and endothelial function. *Cardiovasc Res* 67: 161-172, 2005.

41. **Knechtle B, Muller G and Knecht H**. Optimal exercise intensities for fat metabolism in handbike cycling and cycling. *Spinal Cord* 42: 564-572, 2004.

42. **Kohut ML, McCann DA, Russell DW, Konopka DN, Cunnick JE, Franke WD, Castillo MC, Reighard AE and Vanderah E**. Aerobic exercise, but not flexibility/resistance exercise, reduces serum IL-18, CRP, and IL-6 independent of beta-blockers, BMI, and psychosocial factors in older adults. *Brain Behav Immun* 20: 201-209, 2006.

43. **Kuo CC, Fattor JA, Henderson GC and Brooks GA**. Lipid oxidation in fit young adults during postexercise recovery. *J Appl Physiol* 99: 349-356, 2005.

44. **Lacour JR**. [Lipid metabolism and exercise]. *Rev Prat* 51: S36-S41, 2001.

45. **Laforgia J, Withers RT, Shipp NJ and Gore CJ**. Comparison of energy expenditure elevations after submaximal and supramaximal running. *J Appl Physiol* 82: 661-666, 1997.

46. **Leaf DA and Reuben DB**. "Lifestyle" interventions for promoting physical activity: a kilocalorie expenditure-based home feasibility study. *Am J Med Sci* 312: 68-75, 1996.

47. **Lee IM, Sesso HD, Oguma Y and Paffenbarger RS, Jr**. Relative intensity of physical activity and risk of coronary heart disease. *Circulation* 107: 1110-1116, 2003.

48. **Levine BD and Stray-Gundersen J**. A practical approach to altitude training: where to live and train for optimal performance enhancement. *Int J Sports Med* 13 Suppl 1: S209-S212, 1992.

49. **Lewis DA, Kamon E and Hodgson JL**. Physiological differences between genders. Implications for sports conditioning. *Sports Med* 3: 357-369, 1986.

50. **Madsen K, Pedersen PK, Djurhuus MS and Klitgaard NA**. Effects of detraining on endurance capacity and metabolic changes during prolonged exhaustive exercise. *J Appl Physiol* 75: 1444-1451, 1993.

51. **Malek MH, Housh TJ, Berger DE, Coburn JW and Beck TW**. A new non-exercise-based Vo2max prediction equation for aerobically trained men. *J Strength Cond Res* 19: 559-565, 2005.

52. **Maughan RJ**. The limits of human athletic performance. *Ann Transplant* 10: 52-54, 2005.

53. **McManus AM, Cheng CH, Leung MP, Yung TC and Macfarlane DJ**. Improving aerobic power in primary school boys: a comparison of continuous and interval training. *Int J Sports Med* 26: 781-786, 2005.

54. **Narita K, Sakamoto S, Mizushige K, Senda S and Matsuo H**. [Development and evaluation of a new target heart rate formula for the adequate exercise training level in healthy subjects]. *J Cardiol* 33: 265-272, 1999.

55. **Persinger R, Foster C, Gibson M, Fater DC and Porcari JP**. Consistency of the talk test for exercise prescription. *Med Sci Sports Exerc* 36: 1632-1636, 2004.

56. **Persinger R, Foster C, Gibson M, Fater DC and Porcari JP**. Consistency of the talk test for exercise prescription. *Med Sci Sports Exerc* 36: 1632-1636, 2004.

57. **Petibois C and Deleris G**. Effects of short- and long-term detraining on the metabolic response to endurance exercise. *Int J Sports Med* 24: 320-325, 2003.

58. **Rusko HK, Tikkanen HO and Peltonen JE**. Altitude and endurance training. *J Sports Sci* 22: 928-944, 2004.

59. **Scharff-Olson M, Williford HN and Smith FH**. The heart rate VO2 relationship of aerobic dance: a comparison of target heart rate methods. *J Sports Med Phys Fitness* 32: 372-377, 1992.

60. **Smekal G, Pokan R, Baron R, Tschan H and Bachl N**. [Amount and intensity of physical exercise in primary prevention]. *Wien Med Wochenschr* 151: 7-12, 2001.

61. **Swain DP and Franklin BA**. VO(2) reserve and the minimal intensity for improving cardiorespiratory fitness. *Med Sci Sports Exerc* 34: 152-157, 2002.

62. **Sykes K, Choo LL and Cotterrell M**. Accumulating aerobic exercise for effective weight control. *J R Soc Health* 124: 24-28, 2004.

63. **Tanaka H, Desouza CA, Jones PP, Stevenson ET, Davy KP and Seals DR**. Greater rate of decline in maximal aerobic capacity with age in physically active vs. sedentary healthy women. *J Appl Physiol* 83: 1947-1953, 1997.

64. **Walther M, Reuter I, Leonhard T and Engelhardt M**. [Injuries and response to overload stress in running as a sport]. *Orthopade* 34: 399-404, 2005.

65. **Wenger HA and Bell GJ**. The interactions of intensity, frequency and duration of exercise training in altering cardiorespiratory fitness. *Sports Med* 3: 346-356, 1986.

66. **Wenger HA and Bell GJ**. The interactions of intensity, frequency and duration of exercise training in altering cardiorespiratory fitness. *Sports Med* 3: 346-356, 1986.

67. **Wiebe CG, Gledhill N, Warburton DE, Jamnik VK and Ferguson S**. Exercise cardiac function in endurance-trained males versus females. *Clin J Sport Med* 8: 272-279, 1998.

68. **Yoshioka M, Doucet E, St Pierre S, Almeras N, Richard D, Labrie A, Despres JP, Bouchard C and Tremblay A**. Impact of high-intensity exercise on energy expenditure, lipid oxidation and body fatness. *Int J Obes Relat Metab Disord* 25: 332-339, 2001.

69. **Yoshioka M, Doucet E, St Pierre S, Almeras N, Richard D, Labrie A, Despres JP, Bouchard C and Tremblay A**. Impact of high-intensity exercise on energy expenditure, lipid oxidation and body fatness. *Int J Obes Relat Metab Disord* 25: 332-339, 2001.

70. **Yoshioka M, Doucet E, St Pierre S, Almeras N, Richard D, Labrie A, Despres JP, Bouchard C and Tremblay A**. Impact of high-intensity exercise on energy expenditure, lipid oxidation and body fatness. *Int J Obes Relat Metab Disord* 25: 332-339, 2001.

71. **Yoshioka M, Doucet E, St Pierre S, Almeras N, Richard D, Labrie A, Despres JP, Bouchard C and Tremblay A**. Impact of high-intensity exercise on energy expenditure, lipid oxidation and body fatness. *Int J Obes Relat Metab Disord* 25: 332-339, 2001.

72. **Young A**. Exercise physiology in geriatric practice. *Acta Med Scand Suppl* 711: 227-232, 1986.

73. **Zhang CF, Wang L, Zhang T and Jin F**. [Human genetics of physical performance]. *Yi Chuan Xue Bao* 31: 317-324, 2004.

74. **Zhang T, Zhang CF, Jin F and Wang L**. [Association between genetic factor and physical performance.]. *Yi Chuan* 26: 219-226, 2004.

Chapter 18

Anaerobic Training

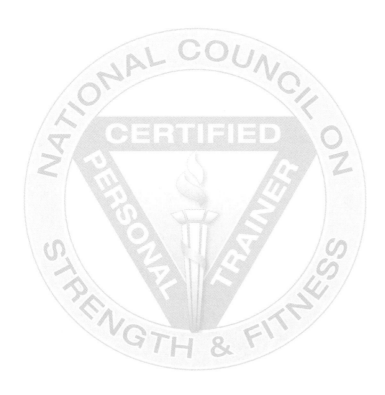

Introduction

Anaerobic exercise encompasses activities in which oxygen cannot satisfy the energy demands of the working muscle. As a result, muscle fibers have to derive their contractile energy from stored substrates like glycogen, ATP, and creatine phosphate (CP). This differs from aerobic exercise, where the muscles continuously generate ATP to drive the muscular contractions via the citric acid cycle. The difference between the two energy systems lies in the intensity. Anaerobic exercise employs higher amounts of force production (greater intensity) than aerobic exercise. For this reason, greater resistance and contractile velocity is required to facilitate adaptations in muscular power and fitness. Although aerobic training offers numerous health benefits, anaerobic training is necessary for improvements and adaptations that cannot be attained from participation in aerobic training alone.

Training that utilizes the anaerobic energy system challenges the body via resistive forces. The resistance may be any force the body must overcome to perform a task that exceeds the energy production capabilities of the aerobic system. Gravity, dumbbells, resistive machines, and medicine balls are all common examples of resistance that increases the force demands of movement. When the body must overcome resistance to move or to perform normal movements in an accelerated manner, the systems utilized to produce the force are challenged or stressed. When the stress is routinely and appropriately applied, the body adapts in a fashion specific to the demand. These adaptations lead to enhancement in the body's ability to perform efficiently under the stress of varied conditions. The benefits of resistance training are universal and clients of all age groups should be encouraged to participate on a routine basis.

Benefits of Resistance Training

- Increased muscular strength, power, and endurance
- The maintenance of, or increase in, lean mass
- Increased metabolism
- Increased bone density
- Improved athletic performance
- Improved movement economy
- Improved body composition
- Improved insulin sensitivity
- Improved range of motion
- Improved function and quality of life

Muscle strength, power, and endurance are all related to the force production capacity of the neuromuscular system. Therefore, activities that place resistive stress upon muscle tissue stimulate adaptations, which improve the neuromuscular system's efficiency in a manner consistent with the stress. Exercise programs should include activities that address each of these components, as appropriate levels of strength, power, and endurance are necessary to carry out routine tasks and to support performance in physical activities. Inadequate measures of these fitness components can lead to physical deficiencies and age-related decline.

Role of Resistance Training

The loss of lean mass, or muscle atrophy, is associated with a reduction in strength and anaerobic power. As stated earlier, these physical attributes are necessary for proper human function. The loss of skeletal muscle mass in older Americans is a common occurrence that is significantly and independently associated with functional impairment and disability, particularly in older women. In fact, lean mass decline can begin as early as 25 years of age in sedentary populations (102). Sarcopenia was previously discussed as the age-related disorder characterized by a loss of muscle mass, leading to functional decline and culminating in an early loss of independence (6). These observations provide strong support for the prevailing views that sarcopenia may be an important and potentially reversible cause of morbidity and mortality in older persons.

Resistance training can play a significant role in preventing the onset of sarcopenia (4). If applied appropriately, resistance training activities can be used to maintain or increase muscle mass. Studies have shown that strength, balance, agility, and jump training (especially in combination) prevent functional decline in the elderly (5; 25). In addition, studies have demonstrated a positive effect in the structure of the weight-loaded tibia bone, indicating that exercise may also play a role in preventing bone fragility (3; 60). These studies emphasize that an adequate maintenance of muscle strength, particularly in the lower limbs, is crucial for proper body balance, and suggest that dynamic balance is an independent predictor of a standardized quality of life estimate.

In addition to decline in functional capabilities, fear of falling is pervasive among older people and is an independent risk factor for decreased mobility and loss of quality of life (118). Lack of physical confidence can have severe implications for physical and health-related deficits in very functional older adults due to a reduction in movement from fear of falling. The marked deficits in the strength and health status found among independent and healthy seniors who report being fearful of falling underscores the seriousness of this psychological barrier as a potential risk factor in healthy, older adults (11). Individuals who engage in strength training self-report greater confidence in physical capabilities, which may negate the psychological impact age can have on activity participation (66).

Resistance Training & EPOC

Resistance training has been shown to improve strength and increase muscle mass. The addition of lean mass causes a proportionate increase in metabolism. Each pound of muscle mass provides an additional 11-15 kcal increase in resting metabolism per day (49). This value becomes more significant when the tissue is actively stressed, contributing to enhancement in total-body oxygen utilization. The added mass forces the body to perform more work every time it moves, further increasing daily energy expenditure. Resistance training offers an added advantage, as it is also associated with an increased post-exercise metabolism (EPOC) (94). When exercise VO_2 and exercise duration were matched, circuit resistance training was associated with a greater metabolic expenditure during the early phases of EPOC (9). The overall 2-hour EPOC corresponded to an 18.6% elevation over resting state (8). Further significance of the finding was that respiration exchange ratio or **respiratory quotient (RQ)** decreased from 0.85 to 0.75, demonstrating greater reliance on fat utilization following circuit resistance exercise compared to the RQ at a normal resting rate. The effect resistance training has on the body has been demonstrated in numerous studies. Although exercise duration is a factor, high intensity anaerobic training demonstrates the most significant impact on post-exercise oxygen consumption (7). From this information, it can be surmised that routine participation in high intensity resistance exercise can have a notable and positive effect on mean resting metabolic rate (RMR) values.

Resistance Training & Bone Density

Earlier text stressed the importance of weight-bearing and resistance exercises in preventing reductions in bone mass with

age. Strong evidence correlates bone mass with the strength of the attached musculature (104; 109). Bone loss can occur at any age, but the onset of bone mass decline is fairly consistent among adults after the age of 30, with the most significant loss occurring in older age (59; 116). Resistance training aimed at improving total body strength can provide considerable benefit in reducing the risk of premature bone loss and the development of osteopenia and osteoporosis. These improvements are not limited by age. Pre-pubescent children, adolescents, and adults have all demonstrated improvements in bone mass with weight-bearing exercise. Physical activities continue to stimulate increases in bone diameter throughout the lifespan when adequate stress is routinely applied. These exercise-stimulated increases in bone diameter diminish the risk of fractures by mechanically counteracting the thinning of bones and may halt bone porosity (108). Recommendations for resistance exercise aimed at

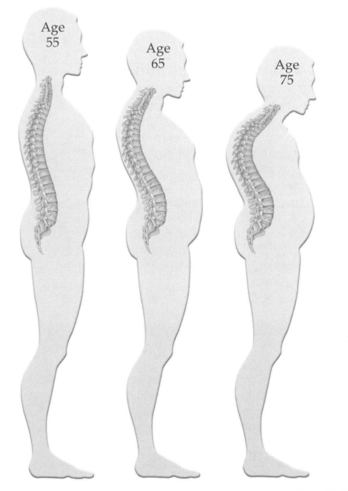

Progressive Spinal Deformity in Osteoporosis

Bone loss can occur at any age, but the onset of bone mass decline is fairly consistent among adults after the age of 30, with the most significant loss occurring in older age.

improving bone mass or preventing increased bone porosity include selecting dynamic, ground-based activities that exceed threshold intensity and occur with a regular frequency (19). Additionally, using an unusual loading pattern on the bones can contribute to improved adaptation by stimulating different muscle group recruitment. The activities should be supported by adequate energy intake, calcium, and vitamin D (40).

Conditioning for Sports Performance

Resistance training has gained popularity as an integral part of conditioning for sports performance. Enhancements in strength and power associated with resistance exercise have demonstrated improvements in sports performance of varying energy systems. Anaerobic and aerobic athletes alike have experienced performance augmentation with a variety of anaerobic training modalities. When appropriately applied, the subsequent neuromuscular adaptations are associated with faster speeds of movement, improved movement economy, greater power output, reduced rate of fatigue at submaximal levels, and improved muscle balance (46; 51; 79; 89).

Improved Movement Economy

Improvements in movement economy are attributed to both athletic and functional performance increases associated with resistance training. Trained distance runners for instance, have shown improvements of up to 8% in running economy following participation in resistance training programs (52; 73). The limited economy adjustments caused significant improvements in marathon performance (50). These improvements were likely related to neuromuscular characteristics, including motor unit recruitment, and faster firing rates, which reduced ground contact time. Improvements in running economy have also been observed in sprinters who employ resistance training activities as part of their performance preparation. Similarly, improvements were demonstrated in movement gait economy in the elderly. Resistance training led to an average 17% increase in lower body strength, which enhanced several walking gait variables, particularly peak mediolateral velocity and base of support related stability (mediolateral stability) (12). These findings indicate that locomotion economy can be improved with resistance training, regardless of movement speed.

Improved Body Composition

Resistance training has demonstrated importance in several ways related to body composition and weight management. Obesity presents significant health consequences, particularly related to central adiposity.

Therefore, weight control is an essential factor in decreasing the risk for metabolic syndrome. However, weight loss often comes with an associated decline in lean tissue when caloric restriction is used as a sole means for creating a negative caloric balance (106). Consequential decreases of lean tissue can hinder the progress of weight loss or perpetuate difficulty in long-term maintenance. Resistance training has been shown to enhance lean mass, which represents a key determinant of the magnitude of resting metabolic rate. With respect to long-term effectiveness of weight-loss programs, lean mass is a vital component in aiding the initial efforts and in continuing the maintenance phase once the fat has been appropriately reduced (23).

Studies analyzing the effects of resistance training on body composition have found resistance training to be associated with an increase in energy expenditure and lean mass, thus promoting changes in body composition and body weight when energy intake is maintained at a constant (21; 71). Other studies have identified that resistance training yields positive effects on body composition, but does not cause significant changes in fat mass (42; 86). The greatest effects have been demonstrated when aerobic exercise, resistance training, and caloric control were combined (41). These results may be due to higher caloric expenditure, although body composition was positively affected, indicating that lean mass was maintained or increased with a simultaneous reduction of fat mass.

Improved Insulin Sensitivity

Strength training enhances insulin sensitivity and improves lean and adipose tissue insulin responsiveness (93). This is particularly relevant for obese individuals, who experience a low-grade inflammatory state, which is suggested to lead to an increased insulin resistance. Several research trials have indicated that obese subjects who engage in routine, dynamic strength training experience improvement in whole-body insulin sensitivity (10; 20; 55). This has also been shown to be true for children (100). Insulin resistance is considered the primary defect in the pathophysiology of obesity-related disorders in children, such as type II diabetes (99). Performing resistance training twice a week for a 16-week period significantly increased insulin sensitivity and strength in overweight Latino adolescent males, independent of changes in body composition (101).

The augmentation of insulin sensitivity is valuable for non-obese elderly as well. As mentioned earlier, aging is associated with a loss of muscle mass, and consequently, the metabolic quality of skeletal muscle tissue, often leading to the development of sarcopenia and reduced daily function. In addition, age-related muscle changes lead to an increased risk for development of insulin resistance and type II diabetes (32). A primary threat is physiological decline, associated with an age-related decrease in the physical activity level. Strength training has been shown to improve insulin-stimulated glucose uptake in both healthy elderly individuals and patients with diabetes (33). In addition, resistance training improved muscle strength in healthy individuals, healthy elderly individuals, and in elderly individuals with chronic disease (20; 121). Older hypertensive men demonstrated significant improvement of insulin-mediated glucose uptake and lean body mass using a 4-month resistance training program (92).

Improved Range of Motion

Resistance training has been shown to enhance flexibility in older adults (27; 31). Several clinical trials indicate that resistance training programs using 60-80% of 1RM are effective at improving range when performed for 6 to10 week periods (26). Positive, but less dramatic effects were demonstrated when less resistance was used. In a similarly structured study examining healthy young adults, the improvements in flexibility were found to be insignificant. Interestingly, Olympic weight lifters in the same age range demonstrate impressive flexibility in hip, shoulder, and trunk range of motion (37).

The improvements in flexibility associated with resistance training seem to be related to the range of motion employed during the exercise bout (107). In older adults, improvement in range may be associated with a general increase in physical activity, which explains why young, healthy individuals do not show the same improvements. Some evidence suggests that resistance training may be able to increase range of motion in a number of joints of inactive older

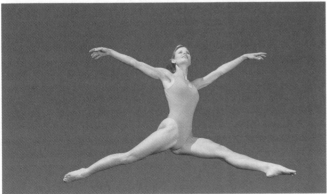

The improvements in flexibility associated with resistance training seem to be related to the range of motion employed during the exercise bout.

individuals due to an improvement in muscle strength (30). This conclusion is plausible, as total strength and strength balance both can affect joint range of motion.

Improved Quality of Life & Function

Adequate strength and power strongly correlate to functional independence in older adults. Research findings demonstrate that resistance exercise can lead to improvements in multiple domains of functional fitness, even among previously sedentary elderly individuals (13; 43). When disabled older women with CHD participated in an intense resistance training program, they experienced improved physical capacity over a wide range of household physical activities. Researchers found that benefits extend beyond strength-related activities; as endurance, balance, coordination, and flexibility were also improved. In another study, a strong dose-response relationship was found between resistance training intensity and strength gains in older adults, and subsequently, between strength gains and functional improvements (44; 47). These findings were consistent with others which support supervised moderate and high intensity (60-80% 1RM) training for healthy older adults. Low and low-moderate intensity resistance training may not be sufficient to achieve optimal improvements in functional performance. Supervised, high intensity, free weight-based resistance training for healthy older adults appears to be as safe as lower intensity training, but is much more effective for physiological and functional improvements (53).

Resistance Training & Energy Pathways

Anaerobic training encompasses a vast number of modalities, training systems, and exercise techniques due to the higher force capabilities of the anaerobic energy system. As stated earlier, any activity requiring force production above what the aerobic metabolic system can manage requires anaerobic energy. Recall from Chapter 5, anaerobic metabolism has two primary pathways: the phosphagen system, including stored adenosine triphosphate (ATP) and phosphocreatine (CP), and the glycolytic system that relies on glucose and glycogen. The unique differences between the energy systems ultimately determine when they are emphasized for a particular task or training technique. Based on this fact, the energy system pathways will be one of the aspects considered when making program decisions for specific results.

The anaerobic phosphagen system provides for the greatest magnitude of force due to the high energy phosphate bonds. When large quantities of force are required, the phosphagen system is utilized to accomplish the task. The inherent problem with the immediate energy system is its rapid depletion. Therefore, it is ideal for short bout, high force output activities lasting less than 10 seconds, such as sprinting, heavy weight lifting, and power training.

If the activity requires longer durations, the body must utilize the glycolytic pathways. The use of sugar for fuel allows moderately high force output and longer durations of training due to greater storage within the muscle. The key factor that controls this energy system is not the rate of depletion but rather the rate of lactate production and cellular **ischemia**. The higher the force output, the more energy required. Therefore, utilizing heavy resistance causes the rapid build up of lactate due to a production-removal rate imbalance, ultimately causing contractile inhibition. This fact indicates that the amount of force needed to perform a task will ultimately determine the duration the activity can be performed. When the glycolytic pathway becomes the primary energy system, activities may last up to approximately 90 seconds at maximal output.

Training for a Desired Outcome

A second aspect to consider when deciding on the appropriate type of anaerobic training is the desired outcome of the activity, or goal of the training. The neuromuscular system adaptations related to anaerobic training are specific to the force production requirements of the body. If the goal of the training is power, then by definition, the work being performed must be completed at the fastest possible rate. This suggests that the activities will be performed rapidly and for a relatively short period of time. Power employs a neural-dominant emphasis of the neuromuscular system due to the velocity of the contraction. This is supported by the fact that one of the predominant adaptations to power training is an increase in neural firing rate.

If strength is the desired outcome, it too will require heavy emphasis on the neural component of the muscle contraction. However, strength training also utilizes specific characteristics of the muscle fiber to contribute to the slower production of maximal force. Both maximal power and strength rely on the phosphagen energy system, thereby making the performance bout short in duration.

Key Terms

Respiratory Quotient (RQ) – The ratio of carbon dioxide produced by tissue metabolism to oxygen consumed in the same metabolism.

Ischemia – An insufficient supply of oxygen to a certain area of the body.

On the contrary, training for an increase in muscle size (hypertrophy) requires increased time under tension and moderately-high force output. The demands necessary for proper stimulus require the muscle to be stressed for longer periods of time, which places the energy demands primarily upon the glycolytic pathways. The slower application of force requires recruitment of more muscle fibers to sustain the force over the entire duration of the exercise. Therefore, the emphasis is on recruitment patterns, with the preponderance of stress on the muscle tissue. Hypertrophy training incorporates techniques that attempt to recruit and overload as many muscle fibers as possible to stimulate anabolic activity.

Muscle endurance training is similar, as the adaptations are more muscle tissue based and glycolytic dependent, but utilizes lower force outputs. When endurance is a desired outcome, the muscle tissue must become more efficient in the tolerance and removal of lactic acid, and the recruitment emphasis is on sustaining a necessary contractile force, rather than producing an abundance of force. The lower force requirements allow the muscle to perform for longer periods of time before fatiguing.

Another consideration in the anaerobic exercise decision making process concerns the performance capabilities and identified needs of the client based on their fitness test scores. Power, strength, and endurance each have independent and interdependent characteristics. A person can perform well in measures of power but may not have the same level of performance in measures of endurance. Likewise, a person can demonstrate impressive measures of strength but not have very good power output capabilities. For these reasons and others, exercise testing should be performed to aid in the program decision making process.

Fitness Testing

Utilizing tests that measure each of the aforementioned components of fitness aid in the development of a neuromuscular profile of the client. Chapter 14 provides several testing modalities for each of the respective components. Consistent with earlier reading, all tests must be age and population appropriate and match the client's capabilities and related characteristics. Tests of power, for instance, may range from a vertical jump test for a high school volleyball player to the 30 second chair stand test for an older adult client. The same is true for measures of muscular strength and anaerobic endurance. Client appropriate test selections are very important with regard to safety, validity, and subsequent reliability.

In addition to client-specific factors, testing for these parameters is also subject to similar considerations that were reviewed for flexibility testing. The power, strength, and endurance of a muscle group are fairly independent on other muscles from other regions of the body. For this reason, power should be measured in the upper and lower body independently, strength testing should be performed on all major muscle groups, and endurance tests should include a lower body, trunk, and upper body assessment. Additionally, agonist/antagonist relationships are relevant in anaerobic training, particularly in the prevention of injury. Muscle imbalances or identified deficiencies should be prioritized in the exercise program. Applying

individual-specific considerations related to the findings will help define the appropriateness of the exercise modalities and techniques used in the program.

Needs Analysis

As previously discussed, several assessments must be made before an exercise program can be developed. Test scores that identify deficiencies are always prioritized first on the list of needs to be addressed. Pursuing goal-oriented adaptation response without addressing deficiencies commonly leads to injury or presents barriers to improvements later in the exercise program. If tests for power, strength, and endurance all indicate low scores, then the exercise prescription

Needs Analysis Example

Category	Need	Remedy	Solution
Strength			
Hip extension	x	Strengthen glutes	Mod. Deadlift
Hip flexion			
Knee extension			
Knee flexion	x	Strengthen hamstrings	Leg curls
Plantar flexion			
Trunk flexion	x	Strengthen abdominals	Ab curl-ups
Trunk extension	x	Strengthen back extensors	Good morning
Shoulder flexion	x	Strengthen anterior deltoids	Front raise
Shoulder extension			
Shoulder adduction			
Shoulder abduction	x	Strengthen medial deltoids	DB press
Shoulder hor. flexion			
Shoulder hor. extension	x	Strengthen posterior deltoids	Rear delt pull
Shoulder internal rotation			
Shoulder external rotation	x	Strengthen external rotators	Band rotation
Power			
Lower body			
Upper body	x	Increase upper body power	MB chest pass
Endurance			
Upper body			
Lower body	x	Increase endurance hip ext.	Body squats
Trunk	x	Increase endurance ab flexion	Trunk drill
Program Goal			
Increased muscle tone	x	Resistance exercise	60-70% 1 RM
Weight loss	x	Caloric expenditure	Circuit training

should include methods to improve upon each component. Anaerobic exercise programs can utilize all three fitness components in the same training bout as long as they are sequenced logically.

Issues of muscle imbalance should also fall under the category of deficiency, as the respective relationship between muscles acting at a joint is very relevant for joint health. These muscle groups should receive appropriate attention in the exercise selection process. In most cases, the deficiencies and imbalances can be blended with goal-oriented activities in an efficient manner, with only limited disruption to the overall program's integrity.

The final additions to the list of needs are the client-specific goals of the training. Strength, hypertrophy, sports performance, weight loss, and any other goal that can be affected by anaerobic training should be listed. These particular needs, in addition to the others identified through testing must then be analyzed for the program decision making process. Proper understanding of the energy systems and the stress required to address the items on the needs list is pertinent to making the correct decisions.

The identification of the primary needs of the resistance program allows for suitable actions to address each problem. The remedies are often broad in scope so that client-specific characteristics can be applied to find the best solution to the problem. If a client presents weak knee flexors, for instance, then any exercise that they can perform safely that resists the hamstring muscle can be considered. The number of exercises at the personal trainer's disposal allows for answers to any number of problems or situations. At this point, it becomes a matter of what is best for the client. Recalling early considerations, the exercise decisions will be based on presence of disease or injury, physical condition, range of motion capabilities, training status, training experience, and age. Additional considerations may be presented and should be addressed accordingly.

The needs analysis will direct the program decision making process to create suitable remedies and plausible solutions for the identified goals, or problems, a client may present. The exercise program components are identified based on the specific requirements of the desired adaptations. Exercise selection, training volume, intensity, rest interval, duration, frequency, and the specific system of training must be consistent with the intended goals. If any of these parameters is not correctly applied, the intended results may not occur.

Training Systems

It has been clearly demonstrated that different demands placed on the muscular system present different adaptation responses within the tissue. Identifying the specific demand-result relationship is valuable in improving the magnitude of the adaptations and enhancing the efficiency by which those adaptations occur. Within resistance training, several training systems have demonstrated effectiveness in producing desired results in one or more of the anaerobic-based fitness components.

Popular Training Systems

- Priority system
- Pyramid system
- Superset system
- Contrast system
- Complex system
- Drop set system
- Circuit system
- Lactate tolerance system
- Negative set system

Each system offers unique characteristics that elicit specific responses from the neuromuscular system. The rationale for including a particular system depends on the particular emphasis of the demand. In some cases, the systems may be concomitantly employed in an exercise bout, whereas other systems may not be used at all. The decision to implement any of the systems will depend upon the same considerations as the other program components.

Priority System

The priority system is a very logical approach to exercise. It suggests performing exercises for deficient muscle groups first in an exercise bout to ensure they receive appropriate attention and are performed with maximal energy availability. Muscles that are subject to imbalance and weakness are placed high in the exercise order, even if they normally would be trained later in an exercise bout due to their respective characteristics. The priority system makes particular sense for new clients, or those who have experienced negative consequences due to their musculoskeletal deficiencies.

Pyramid System

The pyramid system utilizes the principle of neural preparation similar to a specific warm-up. The original

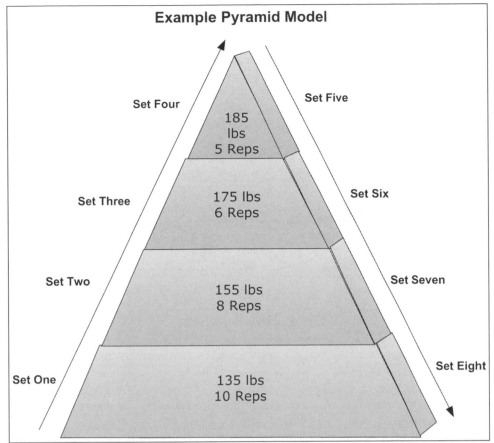

Example Pyramid Model

Set Four

Set Five

185 lbs 5 Reps

Set Three

175 lbs 6 Reps

Set Six

Set Two

155 lbs 8 Reps

Set Seven

Set One

135 lbs 10 Reps

Set Eight

allows for a wider range of repetitions and resistive stress compared to traditional work sets, which commonly use the same number of repetitions for each set, 3 sets of 10 repetitions for instance.

Superset System

The superset system is simplistic in design but can be very effective for accomplishing multiple goals. The general concept is to perform one set of exercise, immediately followed by a different exercise, with only transitional rest between the sets. Due to the fact that any two exercises can be placed together, a plethora of combinations can be created. The intended adaptations will determine the exercises selected for the superset. If hypertrophy is the goal, the superset can combine two exercises that target the same muscle group as the prolonged stress on the tissue will stimulate

pyramid system utilized a very high volume, requiring exercisers to increase weight while decreasing repetitions in subsequent sets. Once the defined lowest end of the repetition range was met, the sets ascended back in an opposite manner, decreasing the weight while increasing the repetitions. This process is not very practical for most training goals and would be inappropriate for personal training due to time and frequency limitations.

The more common system is actually a half pyramid and works by increasing the resistance while lowering the repetitions performed. The repetitions and amount of resistance used depend upon the defined strength goal. In some cases, the early sets are not performed to volitional failure in preparation for the heavier workloads. Other techniques utilize resistance selected for maximal performance of each set within the defined repetition scheme. Pyramid training is very effective for strength gains and may be used for hypertrophy training when set schemes descend from 12 to 8 repetitions. The actual number of repetitions selected for the pyramid system will vary based on the client's capabilities and intended goals. For new clients, a schematic similar to the example may be used with a repetition range starting with 20 repetitions and ending with 12 or 15 repetitions. One advantage to this method is that it

greater muscle fiber recruitment. If the goal is strength improvement, then the superset will combine opposite muscle groups, or lower and upper body exercises, so the prime mover does not become fatigued from the previous set. If general fitness or caloric expenditure is the desired outcome, then any combination consistent with the program goals can be used.

Sample Super Set System

Hypertrophy	Bench press	Superset with push-ups
Strength	Back squat	Superset with seated row
Fitness	Tricep dips	Superset with bicep curls

Supersets may become more complex by adding a third exercise, sometimes referred to as the Tri-set system. When additional stress is added, considerations should be made for fatigue and any respective stability requirements. Utilizing three exercises that stress the same postural muscle groups or articular stabilizers may lead to fatigue and performance breakdown. Therefore, the requirements of the three exercises should be reviewed before they are joined in a program. This is particularly true when heavy resistance or high movement complexity is used. Exercise combinations for less trained clients should split the body into its respective thirds. This suggests using an exercise for each of the upper, lower, and trunk musculatures. If a client is well-conditioned, other combinations can be utilized based on his or her performance capabilities.

Sample Tri-Set System

	First Exercise	Second Exercise	Third Exercise
Beginner	Seated floor reach	Body squats	Side raise
Intermediate	Step ups	Push-ups	Ab-curl up
Advanced	Pull-ups	Lunge	Body dips

The repetition ranges can vary between exercises to cater to increasing demands or remain constant. The supersets may be performed by time segments rather than repetition ranges to allow exercisers to pace their efforts. Individuals who train at higher intensities will likely pass ventilatory threshold, making the perceived effort rather high on the Borg scale. Individual variables will ultimately serve as the defining factor for the program activity selection.

Contrast System

The contrast system is based on the superset concept, but as the name suggests, contrasts exist in the exercise parameters. The system is commonly used for performance enhancement, emphasizing the combination of neuromuscular crossover between strength and power. The first set of an exercise is performed using a non-select number of repetitions to volitional failure. Upon completion, the exerciser performs a duplicate movement using less resistance, applied at a faster speed.

The slow, heavy component recruits fibers based on the

Sample Contrast System

1. Weighted Back Squat superset with Jump Squats
2. Bench Press superset with Medicine Ball Chest Pass
3. Dumbbell Pullovers superset with Medicine Ball Chop Rebounds

application of strength, while the fast, light component utilizes more powerful movements. These techniques are physiologically demanding and often require rest periods similar to heavy resistance training. It should be noted that some texts refer to contrast training as crossing energy systems rather than working in a consistent system.

Complex System

Complex training also has been defined differently, depending on the source, but for the purpose of this text, it will be viewed as a grouping of movement patterns. Complex training is a combination of agonist, or agonist/antagonist, exercises used in a grouping with varying rest periods. The grouping may include a single

muscle group aimed at fatiguing a particular area to stimulate increased muscle fiber recruitment for hypertrophy, or cover an array of movements at a particular joint for endurance and fitness improvements. The rest periods may be as short as transitional rest or up to a minute to employ heavier resistance. Training complexes cause more work to be done in shorter periods of time. The rest interval is often defined "as tolerable" for the client to maintain proper form throughout the complex. Set and repetition schematics should match the desired effect.

Sample Complex System

Exercise One	Exercise Two	Exercise Three	Exercise Four
Front Squat	Step-up	Lunge	Leg extension
Triceps dip	Straight bar curl	Tricep pushdown	Dumbbell curl
Shoulder press	Push-up	Front raise	Flyes

Drop Set System

Drop sets, sometimes called strip sets, are another hypertrophy technique that increases the demands on a particular muscle. The system uses the same exercise performed for a set of repetitions to volitional failure. The weight is then immediately lowered and the next set begins without a rest interval. This may go on for three or four sets as the muscle fatigues.

Performing thirty repetitions with the same exercise may seem like endurance training, but the intensity is near maximal at the time of the performance, which triggers an endocrine response based on the high concentration of lactate in the tissue. This is a completely different response than

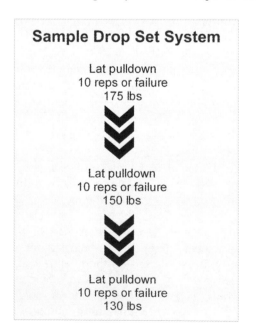

Sample Drop Set System

Lat pulldown
10 reps or failure
175 lbs

Lat pulldown
10 reps or failure
150 lbs

Lat pulldown
10 reps or failure
130 lbs

performing the thirty repetitions using the same weight for the entire set, as the system is based on the maximal tolerable intensity.

Circuit System

The circuit training system has gained popularity in many fitness facilities due to the high caloric expenditure, tolerable resistance, and relatively short workout duration. In most resistance training circuits, 12-15 exercises are performed for a predefined time period or repetition range before moving to the next exercise. Essentially, it is a total body complex system or long string of supersets. When used for fitness training, the exercise selection commonly employs one exercise for each major muscle group. Rest periods are normally 15-30 seconds or the transitional time between exercises. The circuits may be performed continuously for a designated time period or done for a certain number of cycles. The client's exercise tolerance is often the best gauge. Some circuits mix cardiovascular activities in between the resistance training exercises to encourage elevated heart rates and muscle recovery. When using the circuit system any exercises can be introduced into the exercise sequence as long as they are appropriate for the client.

Lactate Tolerance System

An interesting twist to the circuit training concept is the lactate tolerance system. With this unique system, a group of exercises is selected with a designated number of repetitions. The goal of the training is to complete all the repetitions of all the exercises in the shortest period of time. The difficulty lies in tolerating the lactic acid produced during the performance of high repetitions. In some cases, a client will be able to complete the exercise in two or three sets; in other cases, it may take 4 or 5 sets due to the onset of fatigue. In either case, the training system allows for a complete bout of exercise in a very short period of time. The duration of any rest period between sets depends upon the exerciser's ability to recover and/or tolerate discomfort. This allows the same training bout to be individualized, based on relative condition.

The number of exercises and repetitions selected will be determined by the client's capabilities. One of the hardest components of the training is pacing the body so that fatigue does not hinder exercise technique or force the participant to stop. The client determines how many repetitions to perform, based on rate of perceived exertion before moving to a different exercise. A good introduction of the system is to designate a maximum number of repetitions per set so the client does not over-fatigue themselves attempting to perform all the repetitions in a single exertion and then require

Sample Lactate Tolerance System

Exercise	Reps
Body Squat	100 reps
Push-ups	80 reps
Modified Pull-ups	60 reps
Lunge	80 reps
Tricep Dips	60 reps
Step-up	60 reps
Calf Raise	100 reps

prolonged rest before continuing. This training system is designed for well-conditioned clients and athletes. The same exercise bout can be used repeatedly throughout a multi-week training cycle with a goal to reduce the time to completion.

Negative Set System

The negative set system was popularized by strength athletes in an attempt to maximize force production for specific lifts. The concept behind the training technique is the body's ability to produce more force during the eccentric contraction than it can during the concentric phase of the movement. The technique requires exercisers to lift a resistance that is greater than their 1RM, usually 105%-125% of maximum, by performing a controlled eccentric movement, followed by a spot-assisted, concentric movement (22).

The negative system is generally not appropriate for personal training clients as described above, but it can be used in some more appropriate situations. For instance, a spot-assisted concentric phase of the pull-up followed by an unsupported eccentric contraction is safe and can yield positive results. Likewise, assistance of an older adult in the concentric phase of the bench-squat followed by a controlled eccentric phase is another viable example of this technique in personal training.

Goals of Resistance Training

Each desirable adaptation response to resistance exercise has particular defining characteristics required of the stress used for its attainment. Resistance training outcomes are similar to the outcomes that occur when cooking. If all the ingredients called for by the recipe are included in correct portion, the food will come out as desired. However, if any ingredients are changed, reduced, or forgotten, the outcome is not always

Key Terms

Priority System – A training approach, particularly for new clients, that suggests performing exercises for deficient muscle groups first in an exercise bout.

Pyramid System – A training approach that utilizes the principle of neural preparation similar to a specific warm-up which requires exercisers to increase weight while decreasing repetitions in subsequent sets.

Superset System – A training approach in which the general concept is to perform one set of exercise immediately followed by a different exercise, with only transitional rest between sets.

Contrast System – A training approach based on the superset concept, used primarily for performance enhancement, emphasizing the combination of neuromuscular crossover between strength and power by performing a select number of repetitions to volitional failure followed by a similar exercise with less resistance at a faster speed.

Complex System – A training approach using a combination of agonist, or agonist/antagonist exercises used in a grouping with varying rest periods.

Drop Set System – A training approach, also referred to as strip sets, that is a hypertrophy technique that increases the demands on a particular muscle by using a set of repetitions to volitional failure then reduces the weight and begins the subsequent set without a rest interval.

Circuit System – A training approach usually comprised of a total body complex training system consisting of 12-15 exercises. Each is performed for a predefined time period or repetition range before moving to the next exercise.

Lactate Tolerance System – A training approach in which a group of exercises are selected with a designated number of repetitions with a goal to complete all the repetitions of the exercises in the shortest period of time. The rest period is dependent upon the exerciser's ability to recover.

Negative Set System – A training approach which requires exercisers to lift a resistance that is greater than their 1 RM, usually 105%-125% of maximum, by performing a controlled eccentric movement followed by a spot-assisted, concentric movement.

Human Growth Hormone (HGH) – A hormone secreted by the pituitary gland which is responsible for promoting bone and muscle growth in the body.

desirable or predictable. Resistance training adaptations work the same way. To cause the appropriate adaptation using resistance training, the correct recipe of exercise is required. If any part of the recipe is changed, the adaptation response is affected. The following section provides the evidence-based training stress necessary for the intended adaptation.

Hypertrophy Training

Hypertrophy training is used to increase the mass of a muscle. Although there are numerous systems and techniques that can be used to cause the muscle to grow, they all must follow a consistent theme. For a muscle to increase in size, it must be stimulated by anabolic hormones. Recalling from Chapter 4, anabolic hormones are released by specific types of stress. The more muscle tissue that is targeted by the hormones, the greater the hypertrophic response, assuming there is adequate energy and nutrition to support the tissue's growth. This identifies the need to stimulate the recruitment of many fibers when training for increases in muscle size. This is necessary to increase the process of muscle remodeling in large quantities of tissue, as described in earlier chapters.

The specific requirements for hypertrophy training mandate that exercises be performed to volitional failure with 8-12 repetitions, using 70-85% 1RM intensity. The rest periods must be short to avoid full recovery. This combination of stress has shown to augment **human growth hormone** and subsequent gains in mass above any other training stress arrangement. The main reason that exercisers fail to see the results they desire from hypertrophy training is that the rest intervals are often much too long. The low blood pH attained with shorter rest periods is one variable that stimulates the hormone response (58). To ensure that the appropriate rest interval is followed, a stop watch should be used between sets. More intense sets of exercise can utilize the 60 second recovery (up to 90 seconds if near maximal resistance is used), but moderate intensity sets should use only 30 seconds (117). The short rest periods make body building physiologically very uncomfortable, explaining why most exercisers take too much time between sets, and consequently don't experience the anabolic effects.

Additionally, gains in muscle mass are consistent with higher intensity total body movements. Exercises involving larger muscle groups (i.e. legs and back) elicit a greater hormonal response. Since muscle hypertrophy depends on hormone response and the hormone response is systemic, exercises involving larger muscle groups will also benefit the small muscle groups. For example, a person who performs lifts for their arms only

Hypertrophy Training Guidelines

Exercises	8-12
Volume	30-40 sets, 3-5 sets per exercise, 8-12 repetitions
Intensity	70-85% 1RM
Rest interval	30-60 seconds
Frequency	4-6x/week
Recovery	1-3 rest days per week
Emphasis	Muscle fiber recruitment, muscle isolation
Training system	Supersets, drop sets, pyramid sets

will not see improvements in hypertrophy to the same extent as if they perform compound lifts for their legs and back as well. This suggests that back squats, deadlifts, bench press, military press, bent-over rows, and other compound movements should be employed as often as possible. The heaviest lifts are often benefited by pyramid sets for neural preparation. If increased muscle mass is intended for personal training clients, then these variables should be found in the exercise prescription. The limiting factor with most personal training situations is the low weekly work volume. Body building two or three times per week is insufficient for large gains in mass. Interestingly, training experience also has implications for rate of growth. Experienced body builders show greater mass gains following 18 months of training compared to the initial 18 months. Gaining muscle mass is a slow, arduous task that requires high volume, fairly heavy resistance, and elevated discomfort tolerance.

Hypertrophy for the personal training client is definitely attainable, but it comes with limitations. Utilizing the aforementioned guidelines for hypertrophic response will increase mass on a previously untrained client with only two or three days of training per week. This hypertrophic response is usually evident within approximately 4-6 weeks (98). In significantly detrained individuals, this response may occur more rapidly. With regard to hypertrophic improvements, the difficulty lies in continuing to make progress in mass gains following the initial adaptation, based on the previously mentioned time restrictions. Clients who are deconditioned will reap greater improvements in mass in a relative time period, compared to a client who has been trained for several months or years. Additionally, although personal training is about reaching client goals, many other important needs warrant priority in the exercise session. Solely emphasizing hypertrophy training may limit the attainment of more important health pursuits within the program.

One common concern related to hypertrophy or resistance training is the fear of getting too massive. The trepidation is more common in women, which often leads to the avoidance of resistance training altogether. Due to the low levels of testosterone in females, adding muscle mass is very challenging for females compared to males. In fact, an addition of 1-2 lbs. of muscle with an equal weight loss from fat will actually make a person smaller even though bodyweight remains unchanged. Additionally, increased mass is most associated with the 8-12 repetition scheme and moderately heavy weight. Higher repetition ranges do not yield the same hypertrophic results and therefore, can be used as a viable option to encourage resistance training in women.

Hypertrophy workouts attempt to train the muscle as frequently as tolerable, based on recovery demand. In most cases, the training utilizes each muscle group at least twice per week; however, many body builders do not set their programs up over the seven day week. Variations in training are common, and the seven day cycle often does not fit with the volume and recovery periods needed to maximize the anabolic effect. The level of intensity used often dictates the number of work days performed without rest. Heavy resistance training increases the recovery demands, particularly when higher volumes are used.

Strength Training

Strength is the ability to produce a maximal contractile force. Therefore, resistance to movement that challenges the maximal capabilities of the tissue will yield the greatest adaptation response. Training for maximal strength requires heavy resistance and full recovery between exercise sets. The maximal force requirements place a rapid drain on the phosphagen energy system, limiting the duration of the performance. This suggests that repetition ranges are relatively low, often less than 6-7 repetitions. Longer rest periods are necessary to fully rephosphorylate the energy system, requiring 2-5 minutes of rest between maximal bouts. Based on these facts, increasing muscle strength is more a factor of the nervous system compared to hypertrophy training, due to the short duration of time that resistance is applied to the tissue. Although the stimulation of tissue growth is more limited with heavy resistance training, increases in mass do take place. Strength increases proportionately with increased muscle cross-sectional area. Therefore, increases in mass equate to improvements in force production. Interestingly, body

~Quick Insight~

From an adaptation standpoint, recovery between training sessions can be considered just as important as the stress of the exercise. Physiological adaptations mainly occur when the tissue is in a vegetative state. During rest and sleep, the tissue has a reduced responsibility to work, which allows it to focus on the healing process. The cells of the body address the injury caused by the tissues' work distress during exercise. Resistance training places significant strain upon the muscle tissue, which causes microtrauma in the myofibrils along the sarcomere. The healing of this trauma leads to increases in mass and strength. If the tissue is given inadequate time to recover and heal, it will remain damaged. Consistent stress without adequate recovery causes dysfunction, which acutely presents as overstraining before progressing to overtraining syndrome.

Hypertrophy training and strength training cause particularly high amounts of tissue damage and, therefore, require additional recovery time: anywhere from 48-72 hours before training that muscle group again. New exercisers should take a full day of rest between workout sessions that contain resistance training activities. The more resistance lifted and the greater the total volume, the more important recovery requirements become. Increasing training volume and frequency while lifting significant resistance requires planned recovery strategies. Utilizing specific muscle group training and offsetting upper and lower body workouts can aid in recovery efforts. For hypertrophy training and strength training, muscle splits can be used to emphasize particular areas while the other areas rest. Although it is still necessary to take complete rest periods, balancing muscle group activity can increase the number of exercise bouts performed per week.

Hypertrophy		Strength	
Day 1	Chest, Shoulder, Triceps	Day 1	Upper body
Day 2	Quads, Hamstrings, Glutes	Day 2	Lower body
Day 3	Back, Biceps, Calves	Day 3	Off
Day 4	Off		

Sample Hypertrophy Workout

Day 1	**Day 2**	**Day 3**	**Day 4**
Bench press	Back squat	Bent-over row	Off
Incline press	Leg press	Pull-ups	
Chest flye	RDL	Seated row	
s/s push-ups	Lateral lunge	Lat pulldown	
DB press	Step-up	Pull-over	
Upright row	Leg extension	s/s Rev. grip pull	
Front raise	s/s Leg curl	Straight bar curl	
s/s Rear delt pulls	Hip Adduction	Preacher curl	
Close grip press	Calf raise	Hammer curl strip set	
Tricep dips	Seated calf raise	Forearm curl	
Tricep extension			

Other examples

Day 1	Chest, back	Day 1	Quads, biceps
Day 2	Legs	Day 2	Chest, triceps
Day 3	Shoulders, arms	Day 3	Back, shoulders
		Day 4	Hamstrings, calf, forearms

S/S = Superset

builders do not exhibit the highest strength levels, even though they attain the largest mass. This illustrates the role of the nervous system in strength gains. Muscle tissue often has untapped potential due to the dynamics of muscle fiber recruitment, firing rate, and synchronicity. Individuals who emphasize absolute strength training actually create more efficient force production using less tissue than individuals who perform hypertrophy training. Again, the stress stimulus is specific to the adaptation of the tissue.

The effect the nervous system has on force production enhancements becomes even more evident when previously sedentary individuals begin a strength training program. Initial strength gains are significant and occur fairly rapidly. Neural motor patterning occurs through the performance of repeated resisted movements, which causes the nervous system to become efficient at producing force through the movement range. In the first 3-5 weeks of training, the nervous system is primarily responsible for resultant improvements in strength (74; 97). This is valuable for personal training because it demonstrates noticeable improvements that the clients can observe, adding to motivation.

Sample Strength Training Program

Day 1	Day 2	Day 3
Bench press	Deadlift	Off
Military press	Front squat	
Incline press	Weighted lunge	
Upright row	Seated row	
Body dips	Leg curl	
Front raise	One arm row	
Tricep extension	Calf raise	
Shrugs	Hammer curls	

The movements used for strength training are often compound in nature, thereby stimulating large amounts of mass to move the resistance. The use of large muscles for high intensity training stimulates the release of testosterone in larger quantities, compared to small muscle group use. This factor aids in the development of greater strength. Additionally, closed-chain, cross-joint exercises strengthen the muscles used for stabilization to a much greater degree, compared to exercise performed on resistance exercise machines. Both ground based and non-ground based exercises that require additional body control for proper performance increase stability and lead to improved strength performance. Some examples include the squat, deadlift, military press, pull-up, and body weight dips. These movements require the prevention of body sway,

Training Intensities vs. Desired Outcome

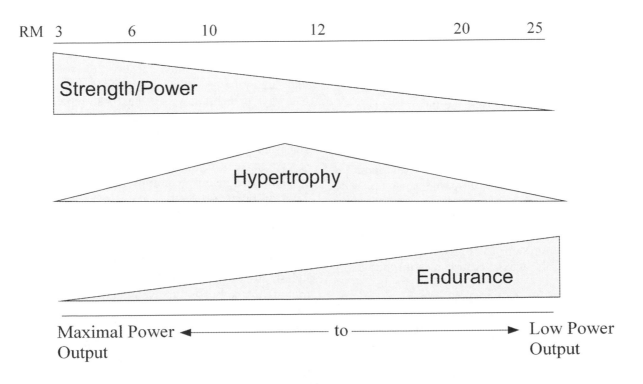

Strength Training Guidelines

Exercises	6-8
Volume	18-30 sets, 3-5 sets per exercise, 3-10 repetitions
Intensity	75-95% 1RM
Rest interval	2-5 minutes
Frequency	3-5x/week
Recovery	2-4 rest days per week
Emphasis	Neural efficiency, compound lifts
Training systems	Pyramid sets, negative sets

so forces can be more efficiently directed to the vertical component of the lift. Muscles of the trunk are key stabilizers for these movements.

Strength training used for new clients should be modified from the absolute strength prescription. As with any new stress, clients should be appropriately acclimated and properly instructed before progressing. Inexperienced exercisers should focus on mastery of skill and movement proficiency. Increasing repetition ranges and emphasizing technique will still lead to strength improvements, even if the number of sets is limited to accommodate individual exercise tolerance. Employing too much resistance early in the training program is a common error and leads to adjustments in movement mechanics to manage the weight. All exercises should be performed proficiently before a new overload is considered.

Power Training

Training for power is very different than training for hypertrophy or strength. The difference lies in the rate of acceleration. Power training uses momentum forces and reflex action to generate large amounts of force. The movements are performed rapidly, thereby placing large amounts of stress upon the tissue. Even light resistance can cause considerable force demands upon the muscle and connective tissues due to the high velocities attained during power training. Recalling from Chapter 2, if a light object is accelerated, the force required to decelerate or stop it is much more than the accelerating force of the mass because it is magnified by the rate of movement or velocity. A 5 lb. medicine ball is easy to press off the body, but to project it across the room would require much more force. Likewise, the person catching the mass must provide a deceleration force much greater than the 5 lbs. of its mass. The same is true when the body is accelerated. Squatting with bodyweight requires much less acceleration and deceleration force compared to jump squats, which must

significantly overcome gravity to propel the body in the air and to decelerate it when the feet again make contact with the ground.

Training for improved power uses two different, distinct categories: heavy-low-rate power and light-high-rate power. Do not let the terms low and light suggest their dictionary meaning when being viewed as an application of power training. Heavy-low-rate power is actually performed at near-maximal or maximal velocity. The weight slows down the movement due to its mass, but the rate of action is still far more rapid than the rate used for traditional resistance training. For instance, weighted jump shrugs with 40 lb. dumbbells are performed much more slowly than the same movement with 8 lb. dumbbells. The rate may be maximal in both cases, but the forces the muscles must overcome are different, and therefore, the velocity of the movement is different. Heavy-low-rate movements require excessive force and cause rapid fatigue in the tissue. In many cases, these movements can only be performed for a low number of repetitions. The light-high-rate movements utilize very high velocities, but the onset of fatigue is much slower due to the lower force or power (measured in watts) required for the movement, even when performed at maximal rates.

The energy systems used during each respective type of power training are specific to the load or intensity. As stated earlier, heavy lifts deplete the phosphagen system rapidly and in many cases, the energy demands cannot be met via the glycolytic pathways. For this reason, low repetitions are used, often between 2-6 repetitions. The light-high-rate power is supported by the glycolytic pathways, which allows for the 10-20 repetitions often used with the training. From an adaptation standpoint, the heavy-low-rate power training is mainly neural, consistent with high intensity strength training. This should make sense since the repetition schemes are similar. The neural recruitment patterns though, are very different between heavy strength training and heavy power training due to the differences in velocity used to execute the movement. A 1RM squat is considerably slower than a 1RM power clean, for example. Similarities and differences also exist between light-high-rate power and hypertrophy training. Both training methods use the glycolytic pathways and fairly similar repetition schemes, therefore stressing the muscle tissue similarly, but the velocities used in power training cause a greater neural adaptation response compared to what is observed with hypertrophy training.

Hybrid Power Model

Heavy-Low-Rate Power		Light-High-Rate Power
Day 1	**Day 2**	**Day 3**
Power clean from floor	Off	Depth jumps
Split jerk		Tuck jumps
Hang pull		Triple bounds
Single arm snatch		Lateral cone hops
		Medicine ball chest pass
		Medicine ball chops
		Clap push-ups

The modes of training for power include the Olympic lifts, plyometric training, weighted throws, and resistance swing exercises. With power training, a common movement pattern is hip extension and hip flexion due to the magnitude of accelerating force potential within the muscles that cause these movements. The exercise modalities are not commonly used in many personal training settings, but are widespread in programs directed at athletic performance. When traditional power training is used, the sets and repetitions are consistent with the resistance and the speed of the movement. Olympic lifts and high intensity plyometrics often use low repetition schemes, whereas the light weight, high speed movements use much higher repetition schemes. The volumes of the training also vary by the same factors. In many cases, power-based exercises are mixed in with strength exercises to cover different training stress in the same workout.

Power can be adapted into personal training programs directed at multiple populations by simply changing the velocity of the movement. An older adult client may be asked to rapidly rise from a seated position on a chair or bench for example, or single-leg box step-ups can be performed at an accelerated rate. Both cases increase the power component due to the increased rate of movement. A hybrid model can be applied, which uses rapid concentric contractions with controlled eccentric movements for increased safety. In the example of the older adult performing the rapid chair stands, the hybrid model would require the client to rise from the chair as quickly as possible and then return to the seated position using a traditional, controlled rate of descent during the eccentric phase. Another example of the hybrid model can be seen with a medicine ball chest pass. The client can accelerate the ball from the chest to pass it to his or her trainer who then quickly hands it back to him or her to repeat the action. Thus, the power phase is done through concentric acceleration without the demands or safety issues associated with the eccentric deceleration component. More advanced clients can certainly perform fitness/skill level-appropriate plyometrics, medicine ball throws, and Olympic lift variations. Again client specific considerations will apply.

Heavy-Low-Rate Power

Exercises	4-5
Volume	12-20 sets, 3-4 sets per exercise, 3-6 repetitions
Intensity	85-95% 1RM
Rest interval	2-4 minutes
Frequency	3-4x/week
Recovery	3-4 rest days per week
Emphasis	Speed of movement, hip extension and flexion
Training systems	Plyometrics, Olympic lifts

Light-High-Rate Power

Exercises	7-10
Volume	20-30 sets, 2-3 sets per exercise, 10-20 repetitions
Intensity	50-75% 1RM
Rest interval	30-60 seconds
Frequency	2-4x/week
Recovery	3-5 rest days per week
Emphasis	Speed of movement
Training systems	Contrast, plyometrics

Endurance Training

The definition of muscular endurance implies that the rate of force decline ultimately determines a muscle's ability to perform prolonged work. Anaerobic endurance is affected by several factors, including exposure to long durations of resistive stress, the muscle's strength, neural efficiency, aerobic capacity, and anaerobic energy system efficiency. Endurance athletes, like those who compete in the Olympic marathon or the Tour de France, experience high levels of prolonged resistive stress from the force demands associated with running or biking. So which athlete would have better anaerobic endurance in their legs? Both

~Quick Insight~

Plyometric Exercise

Plyometrics are a very effective type of training for increased power output. The training employs the stretch-shortening cycle, which exploits the spring-loaded potential of the muscle. Proprioceptors create tension during the eccentric component that is magnified when combined with a rapid concentric contraction. Essentially, the muscle is stretched and then shortened. This combination increases tension potential and when performed quickly enough, will generate greater kinetic force. This force may also be attributed to a reflex reaction that increases the firing rate of the motor neurons in the active tissue.

The benefit of the stretch-shortening cycle on force production enhancement can be easily illustrated using a vertical jump. A person who positions the body in a pre-jump stance and accelerates upward without additional flexion of the knees or hips immediately prior to the jump will not attain the same height compared to a start in a standing ready position, immediately and rapidly flexing the knees and hips before jumping upward. The second technique uses a rapid eccentric or lowering phase (counter movement) and equally rapid concentric phase that combine to create more upward acceleration force than the static start trial (non-counter movement). The stored elastic energy from the eccentric movement and the reflex innervations of the tissue increase the force output by 20-30% (112).

Jump studies have demonstrated that plyometric training can lead to significant improvements in power in just 5-8 weeks of training (69). These adaptations were possibly associated with the force and velocity characteristics of the training exercises but do not seem to be specific to the movement patterns. This suggests that as long as the rate of the movement is performed with appropriate velocity, numerous exercises can be equally effective. If the rate is slow, the transition time from the eccentric to the concentric contraction is insufficient to elicit the stretch-shortening response. For this reason, appropriate heights and resistance are necessary for the improvement of power using this technique. As a rule of thumb, resisted jumps should use loads that are <12% of body weight and jump heights less than 110 cm (43.3 inches). When depth jumps from heights of 0.12, 0.24, 0.36, 0.46, 0.58, and 0.68 m were performed, the results showed that the best performance in all measured parameters was for the drop height of 0.12 m, or 30.5 inches, suggesting the lower height allowed for more rapid concentric contractions (61). In most cases, the jump height used will be considerably lower than 30-40 inches but still offer significant gains in power. This is also true for resisted jumps. It is important to note that the transition rate of the stretch shortening cycle is of primary concern (shortest ground contact period), not the height or load used.

Common Plyometric Exercise Categories
Depth jumps
Box jumps
Bounds
In place jumps
Rebounds

have incredible measures of aerobic capacity, and both have undoubtedly efficient neural pathways, but upon reviewing all the factors that affect endurance, the likely answer is the Tour de France competitor. Due to the amount of force necessary to bike over varying terrain and the significant anaerobic contribution during hill climbs, the biker's legs will likely be stronger and have better anaerobic efficiency in the glycolytic pathways.

Each factor plays a role in the body's ability to sustain force. Many people are surprised to find out that muscular strength plays a large role in muscle endurance, but when analyzed for relevant variables, the reason becomes very clear. The stronger a muscle becomes, the less intense submaximal work is perceived. For instance, if 50 lbs. is used for a test of upper body endurance on the bench press, who would perform more repetitions, a person who bench presses 150 lbs. or a person who bench presses 300 lbs.? The likely answer lies in their respective strength. The 50 lb. resistance would be 33% of the 150 lb. bench press maximum, whereas it would only represent 16% of the 300 lb. bench press maximum. It is obviously easier to lift 16% of a maximum for a high number of repetitions compared to lifting 33% of the maximum. Notably, this would not be the only factor in local muscle endurance, as alluded to above. The efficiency of the glycolytic pathway and the individual's respective aerobic capacity would also come into play. The ability to remove lactate from the blood and tissue is necessary to continue producing force. If lactate production

Sample Endurance Training Program

Day 1	Day 2	Day 3
Squat to press	Off	Deadlift
Modified pull-up		Incline bench press
Cable press		Seated row
Walking lunge		DB press
Lat pulldown		Lateral squat
Push-up		Cable torso rotation
Leg curl		T-bar row
One arm row		Close grip push-up
Front raise		Leg curl on ball
s/s back extension		s/s calf raise
Step-ups		Leg extension
Tricep pushdowns		Ab-curl up
s/s Bicep curl		s/s hammer curl

S/S = Superset

dominates lactate removal, fatigue will cause force output to decline quickly.

If anaerobic endurance is a goal of the resistance training program, the factors that affect endurance performance must be considered. This suggests performing activities that challenge the glycolytic pathways, improve strength, and enhance nervous efficiency in the trained muscle groups. Endurance training uses low-moderate resistance with high repetition ranges. The exercises are performed with minimal rest, therefore placing reliance on increased aerobic assistance to manage the training stress. The volumes used in endurance training are high, to ensure the tissue experiences prolonged stress. Characteristics of endurance training include the following.

Endurance Training Guidelines

Exercises	10-15
Volume	30-45 sets, 2-4 sets per exercise, 12-25 repetitions
Intensity	50-70% 1RM
Rest interval	20-30 seconds
Frequency	3-5x/week
Recovery	2-4 rest days per week
Emphasis	Lactate tolerance
Training systems	Strip sets, Complex

Utilizing components of endurance training is very useful for many personal training clients. Endurance training is a very viable option for new exercisers, so they can become proficient at resisted movements while developing a base for future progressions. Many women

clients prefer the lower resistance because it does not increase mass the way strength and hypertrophy training potentially may, however, endurance athletes often use anaerobic endurance training to complement their aerobic activities. Although this mode is an appropriate supplement, research has demonstrated strength and power training yield better performance results in endurance events (45; 68).

Endurance training may emphasize the whole body in a single workout, or it may select muscle groups for a particular day. The goal is to utilize a muscle group at least twice within the same week. Areas that are weaker should use heavier resistance to help attain adequate strength. Muscle balance is of particular importance and should be emphasized in the training. If a particular sport or activity requires endurance performance from a select group of muscles, they may be emphasized within the training bout. Likewise, endurance activities can be mixed with strength and power activities depending on need. When endurance training utilizes the lower intensity range, trained individuals can use the same muscle group two days in a row, due to the low relative training volume of each particular muscle group.

Fitness Training

Resistance training for fitness does not necessarily have the same defining characteristics as the previously mentioned training categories, as its adaptation focus is on all the components of fitness. This suggests that muscular strength, endurance, and power are all employed to some degree within the training program, with the addition of some effort toward improving balance, coordination, and speed. Fitness components have a spectrum of values that, beyond those needed for normal function, are individual specific. The primary goal of fitness training is to have appropriate levels of fitness within each of the respective components. Beyond those values, individual needs related to desire and the activities engaged in determine the training requirements. This being said, there is no single fitness program that is perfect for everyone, but there can be some generalized markers to ensure each component of fitness is addressed.

Using the parameters associated with each of the previous training categories, a blend of activities can be placed within the program in logical order. For the average person looking to use fitness training for overall

Fitness Training Guidelines

Exercises	10-15
Volume	30-45 sets, 2-4 sets per exercise, 8-15 repetitions
Intensity	65-80% 1RM
Rest interval	30-90 seconds
Frequency	3-5x/week
Recovery	2-4 rest days per week
Emphasis	Multiple Demands
Training systems	Any

health purposes, some easy to follow guidelines can aid in the development of the program. The first guideline is consistent with normal exercise order: power should be placed before strength, and strength training should precede endurance exercise. The individual capabilities and needs of the client will determine the number of exercises used from each training category, as well as the intensity and total volume prescribed. As a minimum, fitness training should be performed at least three days per week. Commonly, a total body work out is used on Monday, Wednesday, Friday, or on a Tuesday, Thursday, Saturday split. This allows for one day of recovery between exercise sessions. Workouts can be performed on consecutive days as well but require muscle group management to allow for adequate recovery. The options within the fitness program are rather prolific, so any number of variables can be adjusted to match the client's schedule.

The ambiguity of the emphasis and training systems defined for the exercise program allows for creative application of stress. It is appropriate to utilize any of the aforementioned training systems, so long as they logically fit into the exercise program and are within the client's capabilities. Due to the fact that body composition is part of the health related components of fitness, the total caloric output should be considered. Many clients use the training for weight loss purposes, and therefore employing supersets, strip sets, and circuits can aid in this effort. A goal of the fitness training program is to maximize the work performed per session. Varying intensity, sets, and utilizing activities that combine two exercises into one can be very effective in improving rate of progress toward goal attainment.

Although numerous options are available for ever-changing workouts, the stress should still allow for enough frequency so adaptations can occur. Making too many changes within a workout may limit success because the body never has a chance to become proficient at the movements. The neuromuscular system adapts based on a dose–response, so a particular exercise or movement should be performed for at least 3 weeks before altering it or changing it to a different exercise completely. Clients want to see improvements, and the nervous system yields the most rapid adaptation response.

Exercise Considerations

Concurrent Training

Although it is true that many different types of modalities and techniques can be included in a comprehensive fitness or performance regimen, some conflicts exist that warrant consideration. Recalling the principles of training specificity from Chapter 15, resistance and aerobic endurance training induce distinct neuromuscular adaptations. The adaptation response is energy system specific, which is where the problem lies when using combined training for simultaneous adaptation response. Endurance training, for example, decreases the activity of the glycolytic enzymes but increases intramuscular oxidative enzyme concentrations, capillaries, and mitochondria. In contrast, resistance or strength training reduces mitochondrial density and may cause marginal impact upon capillary density and oxidative enzyme activities but yields much greater increases in activity and concentration of the glycolytic enzymes. Both training modalities will induce the transformation of type IIb muscle fibers into type IIa fibers (91). Although both stimulate the transformation, they have opposing effects on the fibers' size. Resistance training increases type II fiber size, whereas endurance training has the opposite effect (90). This is the result of different hormonal responses to the two training modalities,

Sample Fitness Training Program

Monday	Wednesday	Friday
Warm-up	Warm-up	Warm-up
Bench stands to MB press	Incline MB pass	Jump rope
Physioball chest press	Lunges w/ torso twist	Assisted pull-ups
Step-ups to high knee	Military press	Squat to plate raise
Modified pull-up	Physioball leg curls	Alternating press
Cable overhead reach	Single-arm cable row	Romanian deadlift
Leg curl	Side raise	Bench push-ups
Rear delt raise	DB squat to bicep curl	Machine row
s/s calf raise	Pullover	Weighted curl-up
Cable triceps kick back	s/s Front raise	s/s back extension
s/s Bicep DB curl	Calf raise strip set	Bicep strip set

where anaerobic training elicits a greater response in growth hormone and **testosterone** release, aerobic training stimulates adrenal hormone release. Aerobic training is complemented by resistance training for strength and power as seen by improvements in both short- and long-term endurance capacity in sedentary and trained individuals alike (14; 80). Resistance training may also improve lactate threshold in some individuals (110).

On the contrary, aerobic training is detrimental to maximal measures of power and strength and will negatively affect muscle mass. The performance decreases associated with continuous aerobic training occur as a result of the impact it has on neuromuscular adaptations, neural recruitment pathways, an increased catabolic hormonal profile, and reduced recovery capacity from the training. Individuals looking to increase mass, strength, and power should avoid long bouts of aerobic training. Essentially, the magnitude of the training should be consistent with the desired outcome. If improvements in 5k or 10k running time are the goal, then anaerobic power and strength training should be used to complement the endurance training, but if hypertrophy and strength are the basis of the training, less aerobic training volume should be considered. This is not to suggest that a person should avoid aerobic training altogether, as it is fundamental to health, but rather cater the volumes to acceptable levels to allow for the desired adaptations to become dominant.

Age

Earlier text has covered issues of lean mass loss with age (sarcopenia) and the consequential effect is has on power and strength production. The effects of age on anaerobic measures have been analyzed in both healthy young and older persons using both open- and closed-chain exercises. Age differences in specific strength were observed even when adjustments were made for total lean mass. Older adults demonstrated 24-41% lower power output across varying loads (85). Additionally, older adults experienced a faster rate of fatigue, with a 24% decline in peak velocity over a 10 repetition performance (84; 88). Other studies have reported similar results, suggesting older adults have less capacity to sustain maximum concentric velocity during repetitive contractions, compared to younger adults (15; 48). Velocity impairments are a possible contributor to mobility loss, difficulty in rising from seated and supine positions, and fall risk among older adults.

When compared by gender, women demonstrate similar decline in strength and power at both slow and fast velocities (96). Age-related reductions in concentric and eccentric maximal contractile force occur in men and women alike, with no differences between the gender groups at any particular velocities (87; 95). It is suggested that gender specific age-related decline in strength (peak torque) is 30% for concentric contractions and 19% for eccentric contractions in men, and 28% for concentric contractions and 11% for eccentric contractions in women (65; 83). Interestingly, women demonstrate a reduced rate of decline in eccentric peak torque with age, while experiencing an enhanced capacity to store and utilize elastic energy, compared with similarly aged matched men.

Age related decline in muscle strength and power are mainly attributed to muscle atrophy and changes in the muscle architecture, leading to lower muscle quality (81). The loss of type II fibers, reduction in myosin ATPase, and loss of myosin heavy chain proteins within the contractile unit are the primary causes of age-related decline in muscle strength, power, and size (82; 122). Resistance training performed by older adults produces similar improvements in muscle strength, compared to young adults. Muscle fiber cross-sectional improvements are generally between 10-30%. Strength may improve to a more significant magnitude, with previously untrained individuals experiencing >100% increase in 1RM (67). Likewise, men and women demonstrate a similar ability to increase strength with age. It is suggested that the earlier resistance training begins in life, the better the muscle quality related to the contractile element in later years.

Gender

Gender differences exist in both the ability to produce force and the magnitude of the adaptation response experienced with resistance training. This being said, exercise programs for males and females do not differ, related to the activities and prescriptions used for a desired anaerobic adaptation. An adult female's average maximal total body strength is approximately 40% less than the average male's (115). When compared by upper and lower body, interesting differences are identified. An average female's upper body force capabilities are slightly greater than half (55%) of the average man, whereas lower body measures of strength show less disparity between genders (36; 38). The average female's lower body strength is close to 75% of the average male's strength (35). Even more interesting, that value increases 30% more when men and women are compared by lean mass values. This suggests that female lower body strength is at least comparable if not equal when expressed relative to lean mass.

The measured strength differences between average men and women remain consistent with those values found in elite male and female weightlifters when compared by body weight (114). This suggests that compared differences between trained women and men remain fairly constant with those measures between untrained men and women. Additionally, the rate at which women and men add strength is similar between genders, relative to lean mass.

The observed distinction between men and women is likely based on the mass distribution associated with hormone differences. Men show larger upper body muscle mass than women, but when lower body lean mass is compared, the differences are again reduced (72). Women maintain higher fat mass values compared to men, which contributes to the discrepancy found in relative measures at similar body weights. The additional lean mass contributes to greater force output capabilities in men.

When gains in mass are compared, proportionate, but insignificant, lean mass changes over the initial eight weeks of resistance training show no gender difference. This observation is consistent with the duration of time before hypertrophic adaptations take place, as well as the role the nervous system plays in early strength improvements. When longer studies were used, women showed much less ability to add mass, compared to men, particularly in the upper body. Female circumference measures following prolonged resistance training showed only small changes in mass gain (.16 - .2 inch) (18; 57; 70). Researchers conclude that added muscle mass is met by a fairly proportionate mass reduction in body fat at measured regions. These findings suggest that most women can perform routine resistance training with little worry of increasing body segment circumference measures. Women who do show larger than average increases in mass may experience genetic and non-genetic related factors, including higher than normal resting or exercise anabolic hormone levels, high testosterone to estrogen ratio, genetic predispositions, and/or greater resistance exercise tolerance (103).

Anabolic hormones increase notably via training in both genders, but the concentration difference between men and women is significant. Men show a 15-25x greater testosterone concentration compared to women in response to the same resistance workout but are fairly similar with regard to growth hormone release (17). The difference in testosterone levels and muscle hormone receptor concentration at target tissues likely accounts for the major differences in muscle hypertrophy between men and women. The role testosterone plays in muscle hypertrophy may be illustrated by the mass attained by female body builders who use anabolic hormones, thereby negating the normal hormonal gender differences.

Detraining

Detraining effects in response to cessation in resistance training cause a de-conditioning process that reverses the adaptations gained from previous exercise participation. In some cases, the adaptation reversal process begins due to reductions in volume and intensity, even though resistance training is still performed. Once the application of stress is taken away, the muscle begins to return to its pre-trained state. Detraining due to the cessation of resistance stress causes reduction in muscle mass and fiber size, increased capillary and mitochondrial density, increased body fat percentage, increased aerobic enzyme with concurrent reductions in anaerobic enzyme concentration, loss of muscle strength, power, and endurance, and a reduction in neuromuscular efficiency (2; 24; 119). The degree to which any of these myophysiological characteristics changes depends upon the starting level, quantity and intensity of other activities performed, and the duration of time for whom the resistance activity is ceased. Unlike aerobic training, resistance training adaptations exhibit a slower reversal process rate, which depends upon the magnitude of the adaptations and the intensity used during the training. Individuals trained at high intensities return to pre-training values at a slower rate (28). In fact, whereas aerobic detraining effects can occur in one week, a week off from resistance training has shown improvements in strength and power in certain individuals following a long training cycle. These improvements are likely due to the adaptations associated with resistance training that occur during recovery. Overtraining is very common with resistance training, due to the heavy stress placed on the tissue. Therefore, extended rest intervals can be placed at the end of 8-12 week training cycles with positive effects.

When training stops, the initial effects are not dramatic, however following 3 weeks of detraining, peak power output and mean power output decrease by approximately 9% and 10%, respectively (56; 64). Force production declines at a slower rate but is notably effected. Strength experiences an initial decline, but usually remains above control values for very long periods (75). This suggests that strength outputs are relatively sustained even with the concurrent loss in power. Training-induced changes in fiber cross-sectional area are reversed, but strength performance decline related to the muscle atrophy is limited, suggesting that, at least initially, little change in neural pathway efficiency occurs. Fiber distribution remains during the initial weeks of inactivity, but oxidative fibers may increase within 8 weeks of detraining (77; 78). Hormonal changes include a reduction in insulin sensitivity, possible changes in testosterone and growth hormone levels, and a reversal of short-term, training-induced adaptations in fluid-electrolyte-regulating hormones.

Following 12 weeks of detraining, significant decline in muscle fiber cross-sectional area occurs, with a noted shift of type II fibers from fast glycolytic to fast oxidative-glycolytic fibers (125). This shift is likely one of the contributing factors to the observed muscle atrophy. Peak torque remains above initial values, but upper body measures have demonstrated significant reductions in strength by as much as 6-10% in young adults and 11-15% in older adults. Interestingly, long duration studies of detraining (>30 weeks) suggest a considerable decline in strength occurs following 3 months of detraining, compared to the rate of decline in the initial 12 weeks of detraining in men (1; 63). This suggests that a detraining threshold may exist before the magnitude of the decline becomes accelerated. Older women show particular sensitivity to detraining from resistance exercise programs.

In both previously untrained and trained adults who participate in a structured resistance program, the adaptation related muscular characteristic changes that occurred in response to the training remain above initial values following short periods of detraining. Strength performance, in general, is readily maintained for up to 4 weeks post exercise termination in highly trained individuals, but sport-specific power may be significantly reduced, particularly if recently acquired (62). Even after 3 months of detraining, maximal muscle strength and EMG remain preserved during eccentric contraction, but concentric contraction peak torque significantly reduces (16). The magnitude of decline is individual-specific and depends upon the training experience of the individual and the total volume and intensity used for the training. The effects of detraining seem to be more pronounced with age, which may be due to the reduced quality and quantity of muscle, hormonal differences, and/or reduced physical activity participation, particularly with resistive stress (111).

The negative effects associated with detraining can be avoided, or at least limited, by employing a reduced-training strategy. The volume of training can be reduced as long as training intensity is maintained at the highest attainable level (29). Marked reduction in volume requires the use of heavy, total body, cross-joint exercises to maintain mass, power, and strength. This is also true for hypertrophy training. Muscle isolation should also be avoided during periods of low frequency, and exchanged for compound, higher intensity lifts.

The worst situation for detraining is immobility (123). Muscle tissue declines at the most rapid rate when immobilized (113; 120). For instance, a casted limb will lose as much as 7% or more of its total strength in the first week, due to the magnitude of the atrophy and reduction in neural stimulation associated with immobility (34; 105). When a limb is unilaterally immobilized, the contralateral limb should be trained to help reduce the detraining effect in the tissues of the immobilized area (39). The existence of a cross-transfer effect between ipsilateral and contralateral limbs has been demonstrated (54; 76). One study analyzed the blood flow in the left (untrained or contralateral) forearm during exhaustive training of the right arm using an arm ergometer. Researchers found blood flow increased gradually with increasing training periods, and that after 6 weeks of training, grip strength, muscle endurance, and peak blood flow of the forearm increased significantly not only in the trained forearm but also in the untrained forearm (124).

Common Injuries

Muscle Strains

Muscle strains account for many of the common injuries associated with physical activity participation. Muscle strains occur when the muscle tissue is stretched into significant deformation or the fibers tear due to excessive tension. Muscle strains, commonly referred to as pulled muscles, may occur in response to anything that places sudden or unaccustomed stress on the muscle tissue. Common causes include lifting heavy objects, unstable joint segments during exertion, poor lifting mechanics, muscle imbalance, exertion in an unfamiliar position, and the placement of deconditioned muscle groups under high stress. Additional factors that increase susceptibility to muscle strain include being overweight, inflexible, physically inactive, or in poor overall physical condition. Although evidence is equivocal, the lack of a warm-up before exertion may increase risk for injury.

Strains are often recognized by an immediate sharp pain at the site of an injury. In the hours that follow, the tissue becomes swollen, stiff, and tender to contact due to inflamation. If the muscle is torn, bruising and discoloration occur in and around the injury site. Strains are usually evaluated by degree of severity. A first degree strain causes localized pain and discomfort that usually subsides in about a week or two. General healing time for a first degree strain is approximately 6 weeks. Second degree strains occur when the tissue is damaged and are associated with increased pain and tenderness. These injuries often sideline or limit activity for several weeks. In many cases, the tissue heals in about 2-3 months depending on severity. Third degree strains are also called tears. They present significant trauma to the tissue, with pain persisting for several weeks to months following the injury. The susceptibility of re-strain is very high during the recovery process. Once the pain subsides, many people feel they are healed, which is not true, and can often lead to exertion beyond the tissues' capacity, resulting in reinjury.

Early management of a muscle strain includes the application of ice packs and maintenance of the strained muscle in a stretched position. Ice applications should be done for 15-20 minutes several times per day following the injury but should not be applied directly to the skin. Heat is not an acute therapy but can be used later in the treatment when moving back to activity. Over-the-counter, anti-inflamatory medications, including aspirin, can be used to manage pain and improve mobility but should not be used to manage pain for a premature return to exercise. Other strategies to manage the injury include PRICE therapy. Protection, rest, ice, compression, and elevation (known as the PRICE formula) can help the affected muscle. Protecting the strained muscle from further injury and resting the tissue allows the healing process to occur. Ice can be directly applied early on and followed by ice massage later in the treatment. Ace bandages, or compression wraps, can help support the tissue and reduce swelling. Avoid tightly wrapping the bandage to allow for adequate blood flow. Elevation helps reduce the swelling simply due to the effect of gravity. When returning to activity, use longer warm-ups and acclimate the tissue before jumping back into intense training.

Ligament Sprain

Ligament sprains are another common soft tissue injury that often occur during participation in physical activity. Whereas strains affect the muscle tissue, connective tissue sprains affect joints. Damage to ligaments usually occurs when the joint becomes unstable during exertion, or after a fall or sudden movement that violently pulls or twists a body segment. The ankle joint is a common site for sprains, particularly when decelerating force is applied to uneven surfaces during running or jumping.

When the connective tissue becomes significantly deformed under excessive tension, or tears due to violent force, immediate localized pain and rapid swelling of the joint occur. Significant ligament trauma causes small blood vessel tears, which lead to bruising. The natural defense mechanism of the body to protect the injury leads to excessive joint stiffness, tenderness, and difficulty moving the injured joint. When a joint injury occurs, it should be immediately treated with the PRICE therapies. The sooner ice can be applied, the better swelling and stiffness can be managed. Similar to strains, sprains are also categorized by severity. Due to the semi-avascular nature of ligaments compared to

PRICE Formula

Protection: Immediately following an injury, it is important to protect the injured body part from further damage.

Rest: Avoid painful activities involving the injury site.

Ice: The application of ice or cold to the injured body part reduces inflammation.

Compression: A means of reducing swelling and excessive bleeding in the injured area.

Elevation: Elevation of the area above the level of the heart immediately following an injury helps to minimize the amount of swelling and pain.

muscle tissue, healing takes more time. First degree and mild second degree sprains often heal themselves given adequate time and rest. Severe tearing or complete rupture of the ligaments often require surgical repair, as damage caused by a sprain can lead to significant instability, improper alignment, and tissue damage, making the joint particularly vulnerable to future injury. Ligament tears require medical attention. Therefore, if significant pain and instability is experienced, particularly with bruising, clients should be referred to their physician for diagnosis and treatment.

Low Back Pain

Low back pain can be triggered by a variety of situations in resistance training. In most cases, the tissue is predisposed for injury due to a combination of overuse, particularly from biomechanically compromised movements, muscle imbalances, lack of flexibility, and general deconditioning. The resultant repetive microtrauma leads to spinal muscle strain, or injury to the ligaments that support the spine. Over time, muscle strain and stretched ligaments may lead to structural alterations and spinal positions that increase potential for further injury and chronic pain.

Acute and chronic back pain can lead to greater suseptibility to further damage. Back pain causes people to change normal movements to relieve the distress. Variations in lifting posture can lead to undesirable lifting mechanics. In many cases, compensatory actions cause non-injured tissues of the back to absorb additional stress, adding to increased risk for injury. Genetic vertebra defects, such as **spondylolysis** and **spondylolisthesis**, may cause vertebral sliding and discomfort when aggravated, and **scoliosis** may contribute to pain with certain activities.

The therapy for low back pain will depend on the cause, and in many cases, acute lower back pain will go away with rest in 7-10 days. Pain persisting beyond a week warrants medical evaluation, as a serious injury may be present. Additonally, lower back injuries that cause numbness or weakness in a limb should be evaluated immediately by a physician. Low back pain is the most debilitating injury in persons under the age of 45. Therefore, appropriate attention and management upon early onset is important to prevent a chronic syndrome.

Shoulder Impingement Syndrome

Shoulder impingement syndrome is a common condition affecting the glenohumeral joint, often seen in sports and activities which employ repetitive overhead movements. The prevelance of the condition increases with age. Repeated movement of the arm overhead can cause the rotator cuff to contact the outer end of the shoulder blade where the collarbone is attached, called the acromion. When this happens, the rotator cuff becomes inflamed and swollen, a condition called tendonitis. The swollen rotator cuff can get trapped and pinched under the acromion. All these conditions can inflame the bursa in the shoulder area. As mentioned previously, a bursa is a fluid-filled sac that provides a cushion between the bone and tissues, such as skin, ligaments, tendons, and muscles. An inflammation of the bursa is known as bursitis. Acromium impingement can occur as a result of improper lifting technique or from increased joint pressure, causing tissue compression and friction. Impingement often leads to pain with overhead movement. Chronic impingement syndrome can lead to significant muscle damage and dysfunction. In some cases, bone spurs or changes in the normal contour of the bone may be present.

If pain occurs during shoulder movements, the activity should be discontinued and replaced with actions that do not present discomfort. If shoulder discomfort continues, ice, rest, and anti-inflammatory medicines can be used. If the pain continues past 10 days, a medical professional should evaluate the injury. Therapeutic exercises for shoulder strengthening and stretching may improve the condition and can be prescribed by a therapist. Persistent symptoms may warrant a cortisone (a type of steroid) injection. Most people who experience impingement syndrome find relief with medication, stretching exercises, and temporary avoidance of repetitive overhead activity. Those suffering from chronic impingement syndrome should be evaluated for a rotator cuff injury.

Rotator Cuff Injury

The four muscles that make up the rotator cuff (supraspinatus, infraspinatus, subscapularis and teres minor) are subject to injury in both active and sedentary populations. Active indidvuals usually experience inflammation, calcium build-up in the tendon, and tears due to multiple contributing factors such as muscle imbalance. This is particularly true in sport movements when high force acceleration is associated with inadequate decelerator control. Age-related rotator cuff disorders are often caused by impingement syndrome where the tendon rubs on the bone.

In most cases, rotator cuff injuries are not caused by an independent factor but rather a combination of contributing factors. Repetitive stress from overuse often leads to impingement, causing tissue abrasion and inflammation. The damaged tissue causes compression syndrome and further erosion, which weakens the tissue and can lead to tears. Repetitive activities, including volleyball, baseball, tennis, and swimming are all associated with rotator cuff problems. Improper weight lifting technique and inadequate rotator strengthening activities can also lead to problems with resistance trained individuals.

Rotator cuff injuries can be managed using ice, rest, and therepuetic exercise and stretching. Avoiding the activities that cause the problem is necessary in preventing further damage. If the tissue is torn, surgery may be necessary to correct the damage. Ongoing pain and movement limitation warrant medical referral for proper diagnosis and treatment. The majority of rotator cuff injuries can be prevented with adequate strengthening exercises for the rotator cuff muscles.

Tendonitis

Tendonitis is an inflammation of the tendon, which often occurs due to repetitive overuse or excessive strain, or may stem from sudden trauma caused by unmanageable force vectors. Tendonitis is most often an overuse injury from repetitive actions or sport movements, including those performed while weight training, playing tennis, golf, and throwing sports.

With resistance training, tendonitis may occur due to muscle imbalance, repetitive biomechanical error, or other soft tissue disorders. Likewise, joint disorders, including arthritis and gout, can increase one's propensity for developing tendonitis. Tendonitis is more common in adults over 40 years of age. The reduction in the functional quality of aging tendons caused by reduced force tolerance and elasticity make these individuals more susceptible to tears.

Treatment of tendonitis is consistent with other soft tissue injuries. Initial treatment includes avoiding activities that aggravate the problem, anti-inflammatory medications, utilizing ice therapy, and resting the injured area. Avoiding any activity that led to the problem or causes discomfort is very important to prevent a chronic syndrome. If conditions do not improve, a physician may recommend cortisone injections or physical therapy. Surgery is rarely needed.

Key Terms

Testosterone – A hormone secreted by the testes responsible for the development and maintenance of male secondary sex characteristics.

Muscle strains – A stretching of the muscle into significant deformation or torn fiber due to excessive tension.

Ligament sprains – A stretching of the ligaments usually occurring when the joint becomes unstable during exertion, or after a fall or sudden movement that violently pulls or twists the body.

Spondylolysis – A condition in which there is a defect in the vertebrae, usually the lower lumbar, typically caused by a stress fracture to the bone.

Spondylolisthesis – A condition marked by an instability between two involved vertebrae caused by genetic inheritance or a trauma to the upper of the two vertebrae.

Scoliosis – An abnormal lateral curvature of the spine.

Chapter Eighteen References

1. **Andersen LL, Andersen JL, Magnusson SP, Suetta C, Madsen JL, Christensen LR and Aagaard P**. Changes in the human muscle force-velocity relationship in response to resistance training and subsequent detraining. *J Appl Physiol* 99: 87-94, 2005.

2. **Andersen LL, Andersen JL, Magnusson SP, Suetta C, Madsen JL, Christensen LR and Aagaard P**. Changes in the human muscle force-velocity relationship in response to resistance training and subsequent detraining. *J Appl Physiol* 99: 87-94, 2005.

3. **Barlet JP, Coxam V and Davicco MJ**. [Physical exercise and the skeleton]. *Arch Physiol Biochem* 103: 681-698, 1995.

4. **Biolo G, Ciocchi B, Stulle M, Piccoli A, Lorenzon S, Dal M, V, Barazzoni R, Zanetti M and Guarnieri G**. Metabolic consequences of physical inactivity. *J Ren Nutr* 15: 49-53, 2005.

5. **Bonnefoy M, Constans T and Ferry M**. [Influence of nutrition and physical activity on muscle in the very elderly]. *Presse Med* 29: 2177-2182, 2000.

6. **Bonnefoy M, Constans T and Ferry M**. [Influence of nutrition and physical activity on muscle in the very elderly]. *Presse Med* 29: 2177-2182, 2000.

7. **Borsheim E and Bahr R**. Effect of exercise intensity, duration and mode on post-exercise oxygen consumption. *Sports Med* 33: 1037-1060, 2003.

8. **Braun WA, Hawthorne WE and Markofski MM**. Acute EPOC response in women to circuit training and treadmill exercise of matched oxygen consumption. *Eur J Appl Physiol* 94: 500-504, 2005.

9. **Braun WA, Hawthorne WE and Markofski MM**. Acute EPOC response in women to circuit training and treadmill exercise of matched oxygen consumption. *Eur J Appl Physiol* 94: 500-504, 2005.

10. **Brooks N, Layne JE, Gordon PL, Roubenoff R, Nelson ME and Castaneda-Sceppa C**. Strength training improves muscle quality and insulin sensitivity in Hispanic older adults with type 2 diabetes. *Int J Med Sci* 4: 19-27, 2006.

11. **Brouwer B, Musselman K and Culham E**. Physical function and health status among seniors with and without a fear of falling. *Gerontology* 50: 135-141, 2004.

12. **Buchner DM, Cress ME, de Lateur BJ, Esselman PC, Margherita AJ, Price R and Wagner EH**. The effect of strength and endurance training on gait, balance, fall risk, and health services use in community-living older adults. *J Gerontol A Biol Sci Med Sci* 52: M218-M224, 1997.

13. **Chiba A**. [Positive effects of resistance strength training on QOL in the frail elderly]. *Nippon Koshu Eisei Zasshi* 53: 851-858, 2006.

14. **Chtara M, Chamari K, Chaouachi M, Chaouachi A, Koubaa D, Feki Y, Millet GP and Amri M**. Effects of intra-session concurrent endurance and strength training sequence on aerobic performance and capacity. *Br J Sports Med* 39: 555-560, 2005.

15. **Coggan AR, Abduljalil AM, Swanson SC, Earle MS, Farris JW, Mendenhall LA and Robitaille PM**. Muscle metabolism during exercise in young and older untrained and endurance-trained men. *J Appl Physiol* 75: 2125-2133, 1993.

16. **Colliander EB and Tesch PA**. Effects of detraining following short term resistance training on eccentric and concentric muscle strength. *Acta Physiol Scand* 144: 23-29, 1992.

17. **Consitt LA, Copeland JL and Tremblay MS**. Endogenous anabolic hormone responses to endurance versus resistance exercise and training in women. *Sports Med* 32: 1-22, 2002.

18. **Cureton KJ, Collins MA, Hill DW and McElhannon FM, Jr**. Muscle hypertrophy in men and women. *Med Sci Sports Exerc* 20: 338-344, 1988.

19. **Daly RM and Bass SL**. Lifetime sport and leisure activity participation is associated with greater bone size, quality and strength in older men. *Osteoporos Int* 17: 1258-1267, 2006.

20. **Dela F and Kjaer M**. Resistance training, insulin sensitivity and muscle function in the elderly. *Essays Biochem* 42: 75-88, 2006.

21. **Demling RH and DeSanti L**. Effect of a hypocaloric diet, increased protein intake and resistance training on lean mass gains and fat mass loss in overweight police officers. *Ann Nutr Metab* 44: 21-29, 2000.

22. **Doan BK, Newton RU, Marsit JL, Triplett-McBride NT, Koziris LP, Fry AC and Kraemer WJ**. Effects of increased eccentric loading on bench press 1RM. *J Strength Cond Res* 16: 9-13, 2002.

23. **Donnelly JE, Smith B, Jacobsen DJ, Kirk E, Dubose K, Hyder M, Bailey B and Washburn R**. The role of exercise for weight loss and maintenance. *Best Pract Res Clin Gastroenterol* 18: 1009-1029, 2004.

24. **Elliott KJ, Sale C and Cable NT**. Effects of resistance training and detraining on muscle strength and blood lipid profiles in postmenopausal women. *Br J Sports Med* 36: 340-344, 2002.

25. **Evans W**. Functional and metabolic consequences of sarcopenia. *J Nutr* 127: 998S-1003S, 1997.

26. **Fatouros IG, Kambas A, Katrabasas I, Leontsini D, Chatzinikolaou A, Jamurtas AZ, Douroudos I, Aggelousis N and Taxildaris K**. Resistance training and detraining effects on flexibility performance in the elderly

are intensity-dependent. *J Strength Cond Res* 20: 634-642, 2006.

27. **Fatouros IG, Kambas A, Katrabasas I, Leontsini D, Chatzinikolaou A, Jamurtas AZ, Douroudos I, Aggelousis N and Taxildaris K**. Resistance training and detraining effects on flexibility performance in the elderly are intensity-dependent. *J Strength Cond Res* 20: 634-642, 2006.

28. **Fatouros IG, Kambas A, Katrabasas I, Nikolaidis K, Chatzinikolaou A, Leontsini D and Taxildaris K**. Strength training and detraining effects on muscular strength, anaerobic power, and mobility of inactive older men are intensity dependent. *Br J Sports Med* 39: 776-780, 2005.

29. **Fatouros IG, Kambas A, Katrabasas I, Nikolaidis K, Chatzinikolaou A, Leontsini D and Taxildaris K**. Strength training and detraining effects on muscular strength, anaerobic power, and mobility of inactive older men are intensity dependent. *Br J Sports Med* 39: 776-780, 2005.

30. **Fatouros IG, Taxildaris K, Tokmakidis SP, Kalapotharakos V, Aggelousis N, Athanasopoulos S, Zeeris I and Katrabasas I**. The effects of strength training, cardiovascular training and their combination on flexibility of inactive older adults. *Int J Sports Med* 23: 112-119, 2002.

31. **Fatouros IG, Taxildaris K, Tokmakidis SP, Kalapotharakos V, Aggelousis N, Athanasopoulos S, Zeeris I and Katrabasas I**. The effects of strength training, cardiovascular training and their combination on flexibility of inactive older adults. *Int J Sports Med* 23: 112-119, 2002.

32. **Ferrara CM, Goldberg AP, Ortmeyer HK and Ryan AS**. Effects of aerobic and resistive exercise training on glucose disposal and skeletal muscle metabolism in older men. *J Gerontol A Biol Sci Med Sci* 61: 480-487, 2006.

33. **Ferrara CM, Goldberg AP, Ortmeyer HK and Ryan AS**. Effects of aerobic and resistive exercise training on glucose disposal and skeletal muscle metabolism in older men. *J Gerontol A Biol Sci Med Sci* 61: 480-487, 2006.

34. **Frimel TN, Kapadia F, Gaidosh GS, Li Y, Walter GA and Vandenborne K**. A model of muscle atrophy using cast immobilization in mice. *Muscle Nerve* 32: 672-674, 2005.

35. **Frontera WR, Hughes VA, Lutz KJ and Evans WJ**. A cross-sectional study of muscle strength and mass in 45- to 78-yr-old men and women. *J Appl Physiol* 71: 644-650, 1991.

36. **Frontera WR, Hughes VA, Lutz KJ and Evans WJ**. A cross-sectional study of muscle strength and mass in 45- to 78-yr-old men and women. *J Appl Physiol* 71: 644-650, 1991.

37. **Fry AC, Ciroslan D, Fry MD, LeRoux CD, Schilling BK and Chiu LZ**. Anthropometric and performance variables discriminating elite American junior men weightlifters. *J Strength Cond Res* 20: 861-866, 2006.

38. **Fuster V, Jerez A and Ortega A**. Anthropometry and strength relationship: male-female differences. *Anthropol Anz* 56: 49-56, 1998.

39. **Gabriel DA, Kamen G and Frost G**. Neural adaptations to resistive exercise: mechanisms and recommendations for training practices. *Sports Med* 36: 133-149, 2006.

40. **Gibson JH, Mitchell A, Harries MG and Reeve J**. Nutritional and exercise-related determinants of bone density in elite female runners. *Osteoporos Int* 15: 611-618, 2004.

41. **Hansen D, Dendale P, Berger J, van Loon LJ and Meeusen R**. The effects of exercise training on fat-mass loss in obese patients during energy intake restriction. *Sports Med* 37: 31-46, 2007.

42. **Hansen D, Dendale P, Berger J, van Loon LJ and Meeusen R**. The effects of exercise training on fat-mass loss in obese patients during energy intake restriction. *Sports Med* 37: 31-46, 2007.

43. **Hartman MJ, Fields DA, Byrne NM and Hunter GR**. Resistance training improves metabolic economy during functional tasks in older adults. *J Strength Cond Res* 21: 91-95, 2007.

44. **Hartman MJ, Fields DA, Byrne NM and Hunter GR**. Resistance training improves metabolic economy during functional tasks in older adults. *J Strength Cond Res* 21: 91-95, 2007.

45. **Hoff J, Gran A and Helgerud J**. Maximal strength training improves aerobic endurance performance. *Scand J Med Sci Sports* 12: 288-295, 2002.

46. **Holviala JH, Sallinen JM, Kraemer WJ, Alen MJ and Hakkinen KK**. Effects of strength training on muscle strength characteristics, functional capabilities, and balance in middle-aged and older women. *J Strength Cond Res* 20: 336-344, 2006.

47. **Hruda KV, Hicks AL and McCartney N**. Training for muscle power in older adults: effects on functional abilities. *Can J Appl Physiol* 28: 178-189, 2003.

48. **Izquierdo M, Hakkinen K, Ibanez J, Garrues M, Anton A, Zuniga A, Larrion JL and Gorostiaga EM**. Effects of strength training on muscle power and serum hormones in middle-aged and older men. *J Appl Physiol* 90: 1497-1507, 2001.

49. **Jequier E**. Energy metabolism in human obesity. *Soz Praventivmed* 34: 58-62, 1989.

50. **Joyner MJ**. Modeling: optimal marathon performance on the basis of physiological factors. *J Appl Physiol* 70: 683-687, 1991.

51. **Judge LW, Moreau C and Burke JR**. Neural adaptations with sport-specific resistance training in highly skilled athletes. *J Sports Sci* 21: 419-427, 2003.

52. **Jung AP**. The impact of resistance training on distance running performance. *Sports Med* 33: 539-552, 2003.

53. **Kalapotharakos VI, Michalopoulos M, Tokmakidis SP, Godolias G and Gourgoulis V**. Effects of a heavy and a

moderate resistance training on functional performance in older adults. *J Strength Cond Res* 19: 652-657, 2005.

54. **Kamen G**. Neural issues in the control of muscular strength. *Res Q Exerc Sport* 75: 3-8, 2004.

55. **Klimcakova E, Polak J, Moro C, Hejnova J, Majercik M, Viguerie N, Berlan M, Langin D and Stich V**. Dynamic strength training improves insulin sensitivity without altering plasma levels and gene expression of adipokines in subcutaneous adipose tissue in obese men. *J Clin Endocrinol Metab* 91: 5107-5112, 2006.

56. **Kraemer WJ, Koziris LP, Ratamess NA, Hakkinen K, TRIPLETT-McBRIDE NT, Fry AC, Gordon SE, Volek JS, French DN, Rubin MR, Gomez AL, Sharman MJ, Michael LJ, Izquierdo M, Newton RU and Fleck SJ**. Detraining produces minimal changes in physical performance and hormonal variables in recreationally strength-trained men. *J Strength Cond Res* 16: 373-382, 2002.

57. **Kraemer WJ, Nindl BC, Ratamess NA, Gotshalk LA, Volek JS, Fleck SJ, Newton RU and Hakkinen K**. Changes in muscle hypertrophy in women with periodized resistance training. *Med Sci Sports Exerc* 36: 697-708, 2004.

58. **Kraemer WJ and Ratamess NA**. Hormonal responses and adaptations to resistance exercise and training. *Sports Med* 35: 339-361, 2005.

59. **Lamichhane AP**. Osteoporosis-an update. *JNMA J Nepal Med Assoc* 44: 60-66, 2005.

60. **Layne JE and Nelson ME**. The effects of progressive resistance training on bone density: a review. *Med Sci Sports Exerc* 31: 25-30, 1999.

61. **Lees A and Fahmi E**. Optimal drop heights for plyometric training. *Ergonomics* 37: 141-148, 1994.

62. **Lemmer JT, Hurlbut DE, Martel GF, Tracy BL, Ivey FM, Metter EJ, Fozard JL, Fleg JL and Hurley BF**. Age and gender responses to strength training and detraining. *Med Sci Sports Exerc* 32: 1505-1512, 2000.

63. **Lemmer JT, Hurlbut DE, Martel GF, Tracy BL, Ivey FM, Metter EJ, Fozard JL, Fleg JL and Hurley BF**. Age and gender responses to strength training and detraining. *Med Sci Sports Exerc* 32: 1505-1512, 2000.

64. **Lemmer JT, Hurlbut DE, Martel GF, Tracy BL, Ivey FM, Metter EJ, Fozard JL, Fleg JL and Hurley BF**. Age and gender responses to strength training and detraining. *Med Sci Sports Exerc* 32: 1505-1512, 2000.

65. **Lindle RS, Metter EJ, Lynch NA, Fleg JL, Fozard JL, Tobin J, Roy TA and Hurley BF**. Age and gender comparisons of muscle strength in 654 women and men aged 20-93 yr. *J Appl Physiol* 83: 1581-1587, 1997.

66. **Liu-Ambrose T, Khan KM, Eng JJ, Lord SR and McKay HA**. Balance confidence improves with resistance or agility training. Increase is not correlated with objective changes in fall risk and physical abilities. *Gerontology* 50: 373-382, 2004.

67. **Macaluso A and De Vito G**. Muscle strength, power and adaptations to resistance training in older people. *Eur J Appl Physiol* 91: 450-472, 2004.

68. **Marcinik EJ, Potts J, Schlabach G, Will S, Dawson P and Hurley BF**. Effects of strength training on lactate threshold and endurance performance. *Med Sci Sports Exerc* 23: 739-743, 1991.

69. **Markovic G**. Does plyometric training improve vertical jump height? A meta-analytic review. *Br J Sports Med* 2007.

70. **Martel GF, Roth SM, Ivey FM, Lemmer JT, Tracy BL, Hurlbut DE, Metter EJ, Hurley BF and Rogers MA**. Age and sex affect human muscle fibre adaptations to heavy-resistance strength training. *Exp Physiol* 91: 457-464, 2006.

71. **McCarty MF**. Optimizing exercise for fat loss. *Med Hypotheses* 44: 325-330, 1995.

72. **Miller AE, MacDougall JD, Tarnopolsky MA and Sale DG**. Gender differences in strength and muscle fiber characteristics. *Eur J Appl Physiol Occup Physiol* 66: 254-262, 1993.

73. **Morgan DW, Martin PE and Krahenbuhl GS**. Factors affecting running economy. *Sports Med* 7: 310-330, 1989.

74. **Moritani T**. Neuromuscular adaptations during the acquisition of muscle strength, power and motor tasks. *J Biomech* 26 Suppl 1: 95-107, 1993.

75. **Mujika I and Padilla S**. Detraining: loss of training-induced physiological and performance adaptations. Part I: short term insufficient training stimulus. *Sports Med* 30: 79-87, 2000.

76. **Mujika I and Padilla S**. Detraining: loss of training-induced physiological and performance adaptations. Part II: Long term insufficient training stimulus. *Sports Med* 30: 145-154, 2000.

77. **Mujika I and Padilla S**. Detraining: loss of training-induced physiological and performance adaptations. Part II: Long term insufficient training stimulus. *Sports Med* 30: 145-154, 2000.

78. **Mujika I and Padilla S**. Muscular characteristics of detraining in humans. *Med Sci Sports Exerc* 33: 1297-1303, 2001.

79. **Myer GD, Ford KR, Palumbo JP and Hewett TE**. Neuromuscular training improves performance and lower-extremity biomechanics in female athletes. *J Strength Cond Res* 19: 51-60, 2005.

80. **Nader GA**. Concurrent strength and endurance training: from molecules to man. *Med Sci Sports Exerc* 38: 1965-1970, 2006.

81. **Nair KS**. Age-related changes in muscle. *Mayo Clin Proc* 75 Suppl: S14-S18, 2000.

82. **Nair KS**. Age-related changes in muscle. *Mayo Clin Proc* 75 Suppl: S14-S18, 2000.

83. **Neder JA, Nery LE, Silva AC, Andreoni S and Whipp BJ**. Maximal aerobic power and leg muscle mass and strength related to age in non-alethic males and

females. *Eur J Appl Physiol Occup Physiol* 79: 522-530, 1999.

84. **Newton RU, Hakkinen K, Hakkinen A, McCormick M, Volek J and Kraemer WJ**. Mixed-methods resistance training increases power and strength of young and older men. *Med Sci Sports Exerc* 34: 1367-1375, 2002.

85. **Newton RU, Hakkinen K, Hakkinen A, McCormick M, Volek J and Kraemer WJ**. Mixed-methods resistance training increases power and strength of young and older men. *Med Sci Sports Exerc* 34: 1367-1375, 2002.

86. **Nindl BC, Harman EA, Marx JO, Gotshalk LA, Frykman PN, Lammi E, Palmer C and Kraemer WJ**. Regional body composition changes in women after 6 months of periodized physical training. *J Appl Physiol* 88: 2251-2259, 2000.

87. **Petrella JK, Kim JS, Tuggle SC, Hall SR and Bamman MM**. Age differences in knee extension power, contractile velocity, and fatigability. *J Appl Physiol* 98: 211-220, 2005.

88. **Petrella JK, Kim JS, Tuggle SC, Hall SR and Bamman MM**. Age differences in knee extension power, contractile velocity, and fatigability. *J Appl Physiol* 98: 211-220, 2005.

89. **Porter MM**. Power training for older adults. *Appl Physiol Nutr Metab* 31: 87-94, 2006.

90. **Putman CT, Xu X, Gillies E, MacLean IM and Bell GJ**. Effects of strength, endurance and combined training on myosin heavy chain content and fibre-type distribution in humans. *Eur J Appl Physiol* 92: 376-384, 2004.

91. **Putman CT, Xu X, Gillies E, MacLean IM and Bell GJ**. Effects of strength, endurance and combined training on myosin heavy chain content and fibre-type distribution in humans. *Eur J Appl Physiol* 92: 376-384, 2004.

92. **Reynolds TH, Supiano MA and Dengel DR**. Resistance training enhances insulin-mediated glucose disposal with minimal effect on the tumor necrosis factor-alpha system in older hypertensives. *Metabolism* 53: 397-402, 2004.

93. **Ryan AS, Hurlbut DE, Lott ME, Ivey FM, Fleg J, Hurley BF and Goldberg AP**. Insulin action after resistive training in insulin resistant older men and women. *J Am Geriatr Soc* 49: 247-253, 2001.

94. **Schuenke MD, Mikat RP and McBride JM**. Effect of an acute period of resistance exercise on excess post-exercise oxygen consumption: implications for body mass management. *Eur J Appl Physiol* 86: 411-417, 2002.

95. **Seiler KS, Spirduso WW and Martin JC**. Gender differences in rowing performance and power with aging. *Med Sci Sports Exerc* 30: 121-127, 1998.

96. **Seiler KS, Spirduso WW and Martin JC**. Gender differences in rowing performance and power with aging. *Med Sci Sports Exerc* 30: 121-127, 1998.

97. **Seynnes OR, de Boer M and Narici MV**. Early skeletal muscle hypertrophy and architectural changes in response to high-intensity resistance training. *J Appl Physiol* 102: 368-373, 2007.

98. **Seynnes OR, de Boer M and Narici MV**. Early skeletal muscle hypertrophy and architectural changes in response to high-intensity resistance training. *J Appl Physiol* 102: 368-373, 2007.

99. **Shaibi GQ, Cruz ML, Ball GD, Weigensberg MJ, Salem GJ, Crespo NC and Goran MI**. Effects of resistance training on insulin sensitivity in overweight Latino adolescent males. *Med Sci Sports Exerc* 38: 1208-1215, 2006.

100. **Shaibi GQ, Cruz ML, Ball GD, Weigensberg MJ, Salem GJ, Crespo NC and Goran MI**. Effects of resistance training on insulin sensitivity in overweight Latino adolescent males. *Med Sci Sports Exerc* 38: 1208-1215, 2006.

101. **Shaibi GQ, Cruz ML, Ball GD, Weigensberg MJ, Salem GJ, Crespo NC and Goran MI**. Effects of resistance training on insulin sensitivity in overweight Latino adolescent males. *Med Sci Sports Exerc* 38: 1208-1215, 2006.

102. **Short KR, Vittone JL, Bigelow ML, Proctor DN, Coenen-Schimke JM, Rys P and Nair KS**. Changes in myosin heavy chain mRNA and protein expression in human skeletal muscle with age and endurance exercise training. *J Appl Physiol* 99: 95-102, 2005.

103. **Solomon AM and Bouloux PM**. Modifying muscle mass - the endocrine perspective. *J Endocrinol* 191: 349-360, 2006.

104. **Soot T, Jurimae T, Jurimae J, Gapeyeva H and Paasuke M**. Relationship between leg bone mineral values and muscle strength in women with different physical activity. *J Bone Miner Metab* 23: 401-406, 2005.

105. **Stevens JE, Walter GA, Okereke E, Scarborough MT, Esterhai JL, George SZ, Kelley MJ, Tillman SM, Gibbs JD, Elliott MA, Frimel TN, Gibbs CP and Vandenborne K**. Muscle adaptations with immobilization and rehabilitation after ankle fracture. *Med Sci Sports Exerc* 36: 1695-1701, 2004.

106. **Stiegler P and Cunliffe A**. The role of diet and exercise for the maintenance of fat-free mass and resting metabolic rate during weight loss. *Sports Med* 36: 239-262, 2006.

107. **Stone MH, Fleck SJ, Triplett NT and Kraemer WJ**. Health- and performance-related potential of resistance training. *Sports Med* 11: 210-231, 1991.

108. **Suominen H**. Muscle training for bone strength. *Aging Clin Exp Res* 18: 85-93, 2006.

109. **Taaffe DR and Marcus R**. The muscle strength and bone density relationship in young women: dependence on exercise status. *J Sports Med Phys Fitness* 44: 98-103, 2004.

110. **Takeshima N, Rogers ME, Islam MM, Yamauchi T, Watanabe E and Okada A**. Effect of concurrent aerobic and resistance circuit exercise training on fitness in older adults. *Eur J Appl Physiol* 93: 173-182, 2004.

111. **Toraman NF**. Short term and long term detraining: is there any difference between young-old and old people? *Br J Sports Med* 39: 561-564, 2005.

112. **Toumi H, Best TM, Martin A, F'Guyer S and Poumarat G**. Effects of eccentric phase velocity of plyometric training on the vertical jump. *Int J Sports Med* 25: 391-398, 2004.

113. **Urso ML, Clarkson PM and Price TB**. Immobilization effects in young and older adults. *Eur J Appl Physiol* 96: 564-571, 2006.

114. **Vanderburgh PM and Dooman C**. Considering body mass differences, who are the world's strongest women? *Med Sci Sports Exerc* 32: 197-201, 2000.

115. **Vanderburgh PM, Kusano M, Sharp M and Nindl B**. Gender differences in muscular strength: an allometric model approach. *Biomed Sci Instrum* 33: 100-105, 1997.

116. **Vlasova IS, Ternovoi SK, Sorokin AD, Gorbatov MM and Vozhagov VV**. [Age-related changes of vertebral bone mineral density in Russian population]. *Vestn Rentgenol Radiol* 28-33, 1998.

117. **Willardson JM**. A brief review: factors affecting the length of the rest interval between resistance exercise sets. *J Strength Cond Res* 20: 978-984, 2006.

118. **Wilson MM, Miller DK, Andresen EM, Malmstrom TK, Miller JP and Wolinsky FD**. Fear of falling and related activity restriction among middle-aged African Americans. *J Gerontol A Biol Sci Med Sci* 60: 355-360, 2005.

119. **Winters KM and Snow CM**. Detraining reverses positive effects of exercise on the musculoskeletal system in premenopausal women. *J Bone Miner Res* 15: 2495-2503, 2000.

120. **Witzmann FA, Kim DH and Fitts RH**. Hindlimb immobilization: length-tension and contractile properties of skeletal muscle. *J Appl Physiol* 53: 335-345, 1982.

121. **Wojtaszewski JF and Richter EA**. Effects of acute exercise and training on insulin action and sensitivity: focus on molecular mechanisms in muscle. *Essays Biochem* 42: 31-46, 2006.

122. **Yarasheski KE**. Exercise, aging, and muscle protein metabolism. *J Gerontol A Biol Sci Med Sci* 58: M918-M922, 2003.

123. **Yasuda N, Glover EI, Phillips SM, Isfort RJ and Tarnopolsky MA**. Sex-based differences in skeletal muscle function and morphology with short-term limb immobilization. *J Appl Physiol* 99: 1085-1092, 2005.

124. **Yuza N, Ishida K and Miyamura M**. Cross transfer effects of muscular endurance during training and detraining. *J Sports Med Phys Fitness* 40: 110-117, 2000.

125. **Yuza N, Ishida K and Miyamura M**. Cross transfer effects of muscular endurance during training and detraining. *J Sports Med Phys Fitness* 40: 110-117, 2000.

Chapter 19

Resistance Training Techniques

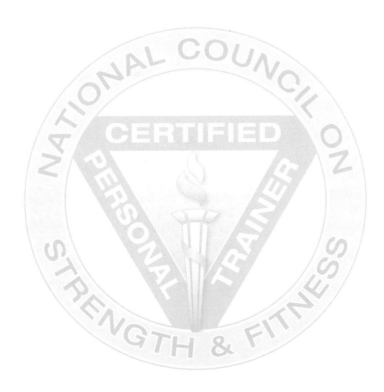

Types of Strength Training

The diversity in resistance training prescription options is matched by the number of different modalities which can be used to create the resistance. Each resistive modality has characteristics that determine its applicability within the program matrix. The goal of the training and the desired adaptations define the particular resistance training technique and equipment used to provide the resistive stress. Resistance training equipment may vary by the stability requirements necessary to use it, range of attainable motion, applicable rate of the movement, and physical properties, such as shape, size, and material (7). Some of the more common categories of resistance training include:

> Bodyweight
> Free weight
> Machine training
> Free motion bands and cables
> Stability equipment

The selection of a particular modality should match the need and capabilities of the client. Movement proficiency is a key consideration for proper movement mechanics and the effectiveness of the training. Some resistance equipment is more difficult to use compared to other types due to variations in the neuromuscular requirement it places upon the body's systems for proper movement execution. Each modality will necessitate proper instruction and practice before being used within the exercise program. In many cases, an assortment of equipment will be used in the same workout to address different issues and goal-oriented adaptation responses. Strength equipment can be viewed as tools of the personal training trade. Similar to any other job, there is a specific tool designed to perform a particular job. A plumber could not successfully address all plumbing issues with just a wrench, nor can a personal trainer remedy every situation with a dumbbell. Identifying the right piece of equipment to create the appropriate stress enhances the efficiency of the adaptation response.

Bodyweight Training

Bodyweight training utilizes the natural force of gravity to create resistance to movement. It can be a very effective source of resistance for numerous movements when the exercise techniques are performed correctly. One advantage of body weight exercise is the fact that it enhances the efficiency by which the body can move its own mass, an adaptation that transfers into improved movement capability for everyday tasks (2; 5). It is of particular interest for programs used to improve functional performance, especially for obese and older

adult clients (1). Some of the more common body weight exercises include pull-ups, push-ups, ab curl-ups, squats, lunges, dips, and an assortment of plyometric and callisthenic activities. The amount of body weight applied to the exercise can be manipulated by changing the direction at which the force is accelerated. Due to the fact that gravity pulls straight down, vertical force application directly opposite the line of gravitational pull provides the greatest magnitude of resistance. To reduce the effects of gravity, the exercises can be modified to increase the horizontal component, thereby making the exercise easier for the client. Performing a push-up from the floor is much more difficult than performing the same exercise off of an elevated bench. A client may have difficulty performing a desired repetition range of push-ups from the floor, but when elevated to the bench, they are able to complete the designated number successfully. The change in position reduces the trunk stabilization requirements and reduces the vertical resistance component, as the weight migrates away from the upper body position into the lower body/ground contact location. The greater the horizontal component of the push or pull of the body weight exercise, the easier it becomes.

Another advantage to body weight exercise is the reduced requirement to manage external resistance, which can aid in the rate of neuromuscular movement patterning or motor learning. Bodyweight squats, lunges, and similar exercises should be learned and perfected before applying weight, so that the technique is always performed properly. The addition of external force increases neural activity for stability and force production, which may cause inappropriate biomechanical adjustments to compensate for the added resistance, particularly if used prematurely in an exercise prescription. This can lead to poor body

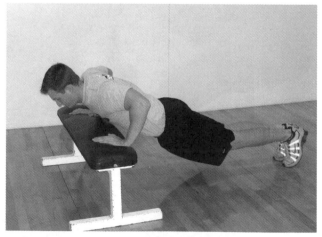

Bodyweight training utilizes the natural force of gravity to create resistance to movement.

mechanics and often results in injury. Body weight exercises can be used to focus on the proficiency of stabilizers and prime movers to improve functional movement performance. Once the movements have been adequately mastered, application of external resistance can be considered.

Manual Resisted Training

Manual resistance can serve as an extension of body weight training. This resistance exercise technique requires the trainer to provide the resistance to the movement. Manual resistance can serve as a progression from movement technique practice to controlled, accommodating resistance in an attempt to maximize the efficiency of the neuromuscular movement patterns before additional external loads are used. Accommodating resistance suggests that the application of resistive force changes with the body's natural strength curve and rate of fatigue. A common example would be the seated side raise exercise, targeting the deltoids. The client initiates an upward movement from the starting position while the trainer stands behind the client and applies stress to the forearms. The amount of stress applied is adjusted so the movement maintains the same controlled rate of speed. At the top of the movement, the client continues to exert a level of resistance, as the trainer pushes down upon the arms, returning them to the starting position under the eccentric load. Manual resistance can be applied for leg curls, triceps, and bicep exercises using a towel, for abdominal activities, or any other appropriate exercise. When implemented correctly, the technique can be very demanding on the tissue. In fact, manual resistance training is very common in the sports training environment due to its effectiveness in eliciting an adaptation response.

Free Weight Training

Free weight training adds external resistance to the body's natural movements. In many cases, once a bodyweight movement has been perfected, the addition of free weight is used for progressive overload. **Free weight** is a fairly encompassing term that generally describes resistance that is a free-body; essentially, it has no attachment to a machine or the earth and the resistive force is provided by the gravitational pull on the object (25). Common examples of free weight equipment include dumbbells, barbells, weight plates, kettlebells, weighted bars, sand bags, and medicine balls.

Each type of free weight equipment provides a level of uniqueness which defines its respective aptitude for different training objectives. For instance, medicine balls work more effectively for weighted throwing

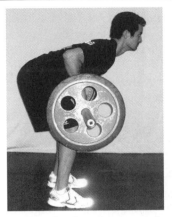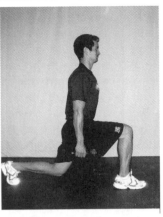

Due to the fact that most free weight movements require the application of vertical acceleration, the exercises above demonstrate that body position must change in order to adjust for different muscle group training.

exercises compared to barbells or dumbbells, which would compromise safety. Similarly, dumbbells increase the stabilization requirements of many lifts by allowing for unilateral resisted movements, compared to performing the same exercise bilaterally with a barbell. For the same reason, dumbbells are an excellent choice when addressing bilateral strength differences between two extremities (i.e. right and left biceps). Barbells though, offer the ability to lift greater loads by employing synchronized movements via bilateral force application.

During most traditional free weight exercises, barbells and dumbbells dominate their equipment selected to resist the movement. Medicine balls, sand bags, and weight vests can be used in a similar application as dumbbells and barbells but provide for increased diversity in the exercise program. Due to the fact that dumbbells, weight plates, and barbells are metal, they are limited in how they can be held and can be cumbersome for some movements. On the contrary, softer, varied shaped resistance devices do not have the same grip limitations and reduce risk for injury when they contact the body. Sand bags and weight vests are often used with plyometric exercises, or in activities which are performed at a faster pace because they act as a weighted extension of the body due to the close proximity to the trunk. Weight vests have an added advantage because they free up arm movement. Medicine balls provide an additional dimension by allowing for planned throws, catches, and bounce or swing actions. These devices can be used to address strength or power, depending on the rate of movement.

Free weights use a vertical force vector because gravity is the basis of resistance which is either an advantage or disadvantage, depending on how it is viewed. Due to the fact that most free weight movements require the application of vertical acceleration, the body's position must change to adjust for different muscle group training. This fact provides an added advantage, as it allows for a variety of ground based, closed-chain exercises. This provides for an integration of muscle groups to stabilize the body segments along the kinetic chain, while the prime movers apply acceleration force. Many of the traditional free weight lifts fall under this description, including weighted squats, deadlifts, bent-over rows, and military press. The use of the whole body during resistance training enhances endocrine response, muscle stabilization, and coordination of body segment movement, all of which are valuable adaptations.

Resistance Machine Training

Machine resistance training can also be used to complement other activities in a resistance program (26). The advantage that machines hold over free weight and body weight movements is that they can be performed safely and effectively with minimal instruction, as they often require limited stabilization, balance, and coordination. Most machines are designed to isolate the prime mover in the linear application of force. Due to the properties of muscle isolation, machine resistance training works very well for hypertrophy training (28). The stable environment allows for increased force in a single direction, which can be used to overload the targeted tissue and increase muscle fiber recruitment within the trained muscle group. This advantage can also be a disadvantage when viewed from other perspectives. Machine resistance training does not allow for functional enhancements related to improvements in body segment coordination and stability (27). The stable isolation reduces reliance on other muscle groups and conditions the muscle to

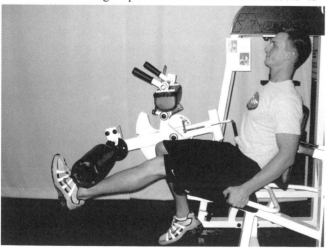

Machine resistance training requires some knowledge in ergonomics to properly set the seat height and movement arms for proper use by clients of varying sizes.

resisted movement patterns in a single plane at a consistent angle. Therefore, the muscle becomes very efficient at producing force in a single, narrow environment. Adding free weight training to machine resisted exercise can aid in negating the limitations created by the linear application of force experienced with machine training alone.

Machine resistance training requires some knowledge in ergonomics to properly set the seat height and movement arms for proper use by clients of varying sizes. The first step to adjusting a resistance machine to the client's dimensions is to align the axis of rotation of the working joint with the axis of rotation of the machine. Aligning the rotational points allows for smooth movement without undesirable stress on the joint. The adjustable components of the machine, such as seat height, swing arm, or back support, should all cater to the particular physical properties presented by the client's frame. Very tall or short clients may have difficulty using some machines due to limb length discrepancies. If the axis of rotation does not properly align, or the full range causes an undesirable body position, select a different exercise. In addition to proper set up and instruction, trainers should also evaluate the cables and other moving parts for wear and tear for added safety. If a cable breaks while a person is exerting force, he or she may be severely injured.

One decision that a personal trainer must make regarding resistance training is with which clients to use machine training. New exercisers and older adults are often steered to machine training, due to the ease of use and limited skill acquisition necessary for successful performance. Although the machines allow for a smooth transition into strength training, they do not provide appropriate stress to help people become more efficient at the movements they perform everyday. An argument exists in some circles between starting off on machines or using body weight and assistive training to teach improved movement economy before using machines. It generally makes the most sense to use both. The complement of machine strength training with select body weight and assistive exercises for neuromuscular efficiency and preparation for advanced training techniques can serve both strength and functional needs simultaneously.

Free Motion Training

Free motion resistance equipment is the polar opposite of traditional selectorized machines. Free motion suggests that the training device does not limit the direction or range of the movement beyond the resistance used (14). Common examples include cable machines and resistance bands that allow for an unlimited number of resisted movements. In most cases, the adjustable height of the band or cable determines the movement direction. Unlike gravitational pull, which is vertical, the adjustability of the machines and related equipment allows for variations in horizontal and vertical force vectors, and a broad range of movements in varying directions, based on changes to the settings (13).

Free motion equipment requires increased stabilization compared to traditional machines, which have select pivot points or a set axis of rotation. Although workout benches, physioballs, and other utility devices can be used to create different exercises, ground-based training with cables can be particularly effective due to the increased activity of the trunk and assistive stabilizers. A large number of movement combinations which utilize pressing, pulling, and rotation can be performed, as well as more isolated actions for specific muscle group attention. This suggests that exercises for strength, stability, and applications of general function can all be performed with this type of equipment. A number of attachments can be added to provide additional variations to the training. Different shaped bars, ropes, and handles can add further diversity to the exercise and contribute to the large number of exercise options.

Stability Equipment

Stability equipment is not technically classified as resistance equipment like the aforementioned training tools but enhances the application of resistance. When used in conjunction with free weights and free motion equipment, stability devices increase the stress placed upon the body by increasing stabilization and neuromuscular coordination (3). Physioballs, stability discs, balance boards, and related apparatuses replace the traditional stable surfaces on which resisted lifts are performed. Chest press on a physioball, for instance, requires stabilization of the body while exerting prime mover acceleration. Performing squats on stability discs likewise increases the balance and stabilizing demands of the body for successful completion (4). The addition of these devices to a training program can expand the adaptation potential of the training (29).

Teaching Weight Training Exercise

Resistance training instruction is very similar to teaching any other motor skill. Start off simple and create a very strong platform to support additional learning or added complexity. Whenever the body experiences something new, a learning process occurs in which the nervous system tries to figure out the best way to manage the situation. The nerves are an extension of the brain, and therefore, are the vehicle of

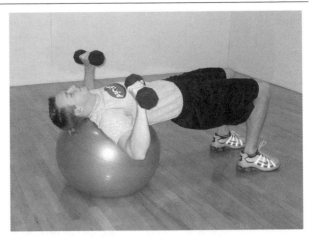

When used in conjunction with free weights and free motion equipment, stability devices increase the stress placed upon the body by increasing stabilization and neuromuscular coordination (3).

physical intelligence. They learn by experiencing a problem and working on a solution. The more often the problem is presented, the more efficient the nerves become at coming up with the appropriate response. When humans learn math, they do not start off with algebra, but rather basic addition and subtraction. As the brain becomes proficient at the basics, newer and harder math problems can be presented and solved. The nerves function similarly, and this is called motor learning. An example of this process is swinging a golf club. When starting off for the first time, the movement is awkward and cumbersome. However, after repeated drilling, the motor neural pathways are reinforced, and execution of the movement becomes second nature.

Skill Acquisition

The term skill acquisition applies to the process of learning how to perform a movement task. The easier the task is, the faster the body will be able to successfully manage it. This suggests that when instructing clients on how to perform resistance training activities, the learning process should be made easy. Initiating skill acquisition usually means teaching the movement without any resistance. In some cases, a light resistance can be assistive in the learning process, but more often than not, it is much easier to master the movement when no additional stress is added to the motor pattern. For upper body movements, passively moving the client's body in the manner in which the exercise is performed teaches the nerves exactly how the limb should move through the full range of motion. Performing five or six passive movements before asking the client to continue duplicating the action often leads to rapid comprehension.

When lower body movements are instructed, it is usually difficult to apply passive assistance, so physical and verbal cues should be used to account for each of the body's segments during the movement. Physical cueing suggests the use of physical contact or manipulation of the body segment that needs adjustment. Sometimes simple contact provides the client additional information via neural pathways to correct the error. A good illustration of this phenomenon can be seen when teaching scapular retraction. The trainer places two fingers between the right and left scapula against the spine, and asks the client to squeeze the two scapulae together to form a muscular clamp upon the fingers, by engaging the **rhomboids**. The physical contact allows the tissue to identify which muscles to activate to control the movement. Verbal cues are descriptions of actions or instructions that aid in the movement performance. Describing body adjustments such as "raise the chest," "do not look down," or "bend the knee" can help the client attain the correct position. In many cases, a combination of verbal and physical cues can be used to develop quality movement techniques by the client.

Practicing the movement in a repeated fashion allows for the nervous system to refine its action. This is commonly seen in sports preparation. Repetitive performance of a movement during practice encourages efficiency, so that in a game situation, the action is executed with precision. Resistance training instruction should employ the same tactics. Teach the movement in its respective parts before joining the parts into a smooth movement. Once the desired movement is attained, repeat it for the purposes of motor patterning. A person should be able to perform the exercise with complete proficiency before adding a resistive progression.

Proper Breathing

Breathing is another consideration during the initial stages of movement development. Many people have a tendency to hold their breath during movements, as it naturally adds to stability. Holding one's breath while exerting force is referred to as the valsalva maneuver (17). It increases intra-abdominal pressure and acute blood pressure response (21). Breathing is a fundamental part of proper movement execution, as respiration is part of the pressure control mechanisms and buffering system within the body (18). Clients should be instructed to inhale during the eccentric contraction and exhale during the concentric contraction. A very short duration breath hold can take place on the transition from eccentric to concentric contraction for initial stabilization but should be released upon the concentric phase. Holding one's

breath can lead to dizziness or light headedness upon exertion. Hypertensive clients and the elderly should closely regulate their breathing technique to adequately manage internal pressures (16; 19).

~Quick Insight~

Speed of Movement

An often overlooked component of resistance training exercise is the speed or velocity of the movement. Most exercises have a specific speed associated with their performance. This speed should be continuous and controlled during resistance activities, unless the goal or exercise requires accelerated movement for proper performance or is specific to improvements in power (22). For instance, medicine ball passes require a certain velocity to be performed correctly, while leg presses should be controlled and deliberate. Quite often, increased speed of movement is used when an exerciser cannot manage the load assignment due to inadequate muscle strength. This occurs when momentum forces are generated to assist in lifting the resistance. When this occurs, the quality of the movement is sacrificed and risk for injury increases. Common biomechanical compensatory movements include hip extension during side raises and bicep curls, hip flexion during leg curls and tricep pushdowns, and back and/or hip extension during pulls and closed-chain overhead presses. The use of slower, controlled speeds increases the duration of time stress is placed on the muscle tissue and increases muscle fiber recruitment. With most traditional resistance training, a 2 to 3 second eccentric contraction phase is followed by a 2 to 3 second concentric phase (10).

Movement Compensation

If, during the performance of an exercise, improper movement is observed, it should be quickly addressed. Personal trainers should not allow incorrect technique at any time while they are providing supervision of an exercise. If improper movements are allowed to occur, those movements are reinforced with repetitive application making it more difficult to correct. It is common for clients to adjust their actions when a new stress is applied due to neuromuscular inefficiency. Trainers should cue proper correction strategies to compensate for the adjustment errors. If a person is unable to comply with the instructions or physical cues, the resistive progression should be removed, lessened, or exchanged for a different strategy.

Movement compensation most commonly occurs when a person's level of conditioning is not adequate to manage the new stress. Simply reducing the weight often helps correct the problem. In some cases, the performance error occurs after several repetitions have been performed. If this is the case, the activity should migrate back to an easier action by fusing the stresses together within the same set. If, for instance, a person is expected to perform ten repetitions per leg in the weighted step-up exercise but is only able to perform six step-ups with a resistance before compromising technique, he or she should drop the resistance upon volitional failure and continue the exercise to the designated number of repetitions using their body weight. Likewise, if a person can only perform 10 out of a designated 15 abdominal curl-ups with resistance before errors begin, the client should perform ten with the resistance, unload, and then immediately continue without the added workload. This technique allows for adequate overload at an individual-specific progression rate without the sacrifice of correct movement mechanics.

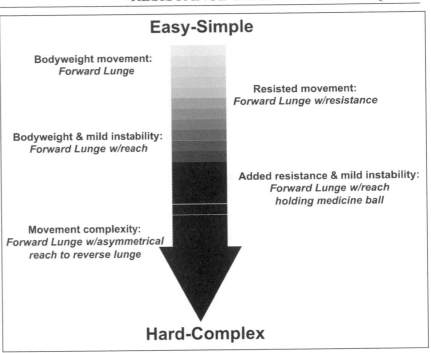

Progressions

The use of proper progressions in resistance training is vital to successfully programming the **central nervous system (CNS)** for desired movement patterns and advancing adaptations. Due to the complex relationship between the CNS and the different segments of the musculoskeletal system, the body must learn through a developmental building-block approach in order to enhance movement economy (20). This is particularly true if the body is to react appropriately to the simultaneous application of gravity, contact reaction, and momentum forces (6). Progressions within an exercise program may be as diverse as the exercises themselves but should remain criteria-based to reflect the individuality of the client and the program. The decision to select a progressive variation should be based on considerations regarding physiological indicators, task performance proficiency, and goal-oriented planning.

The specific criteria for ascertaining a progression sequence employ characteristics of both the client and program goal. As previously stated, the development of movement proficiency initiates the progression sequence. Once the basic movement can be accomplished efficiently, additional physiological demands can be added to challenge the neuromuscular system (12). The goal is to increase the overload in some manner, without compromising the quality of the movement.

Employing proper progressions requires an on-going, building-block approach. As the body develops kinesthetic awareness through **proprioception**, advancements in the training system can be made (9). Movement starting points should be simple and performed in a physiological environment that requires low neuromuscular demands, so proper motor learning can take place (11). The resistance should be limited, so the client can perform repeated, controlled movements. The base of support should be stable to account for center of gravity changes with little difficulty. As the movement patterns become more efficient, the exercises can become more complex. As the movements become more complex, the environment begins to change from low to moderate to high neuromuscular demand, based on increasing force and proprioceptive requirements (8). Static movements become more dynamic, resistance increases, and stability requirements become more proprioceptively challenging. The progression may take advantage of one or more of these external demands to make the exercise more difficult.

Although adding weight is sometimes the easiest way to apply progressive overload, it may not be the correct solution for the intended outcome. Progression models can vary rather significantly as long as they add a new perceived stress to the body. Changing load locations or lifting the resistance asymmetrically challenges the neuromuscular system without the addition of more resistance. Likewise, adding complexity, varying the speed of movement, or changing the movement surface height, angle, or stability all present new progressive challenges.

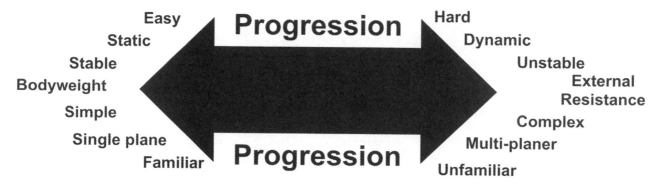

No matter where the new stress is created, the progressions must remain consistent with the goals of the training. If the goal is strength, the addition of resistive loads is necessary and complemented by mild increases of stability. Too much stability training though, may take away from the emphasis on strength. Therefore, an appropriate balance of progressive techniques should be programmed. If the emphasis is on increasing muscle mass, the progressions must reflect increased training volume. Hypertrophy training warrants placing greater stress upon an isolated area with appropriate increases in resistance. Adding stability training, in this case, would limit success. If sports performance is the goal, the progressions should mirror the sport specific behavior, speed, and complexity of the activities performed during the competition. Keep in mind that most sport activities require multi-planar movements; therefore, isolated muscular contractions may not be the most beneficial. Each desired outcome should have a linear progression from the physiological baseline, or starting point, to the new level of physiological improvement, or designated goal. The building-block approach provides for continuous improvements at a physiologically tolerable progression rate.

Spotting Techniques

Resistance training, as with any physical activity, brings with it a level of risk. Because some exercises place the body in compromised positions or use non-forgiving resistance placed above the head and neck, personal trainers must always keep a watchful eye on the client during the performance of any exercise. Spotting is the term used to describe the supervision and hands-on management of an exercise performance. Spotting each exercise does not necessarily mean physical action initiated by movement failure. Rather, it conveys the trainer's responsibility to control the client's lift, so it is performed correctly during each and every repetition without risk for injury. The trainer is responsible for the safety of his or her client by job description, so the promotion of safe training can never be overstated.

~Quick Insight~

Hand Positions

Hand positions used when performing resistance exercises are important for proper technique. Improper hand position changes the joint angles and can add undue stress to the wrist, elbow, and shoulder joints. Three types of hand positions are generally used during resistance training exercise: a supinated grip, a pronated grip, and a neutral grip. Each holds merit for specific exercises or may be varied to provide a different emphasis of tissue activation within the prime mover. For instance, a pull-up utilizes a pronated grip to emphasize activation of the **latissimus dorsi**. When the grip is changed to supinated, the exercise is referred to as a chin-up, modifying the back musculature employed and increasing contribution from the **biceps brachii**. Rowing exercises experience a similar stress alteration when different hand positions are used. Changes in grip and arm position will move the predominance of the resistive stress to different locations in the back musculature. Varying hand position when performing push-down exercises also modifies the activation of the **triceps brachii**, placing different levels of stress on the respective heads of the muscle.

An alternate hand grip may also be used in some cases. The deadlift exercise uses an alternate grip to increase activation of the leg musculature. If a pronated grip is utilized during the deadlift movement, the hip extensors assume more responsibility. Changing hand positions, where appropriate, can be used to provide muscle tissue activation diversity, so more of the muscle is trained without changing the volume. If three sets of a particular movement are performed, it may make sense to use a different grip or hand position for each set. In other cases, the overload may be directed into a designated location to enhance the training stress on a particular area of the tissue, specific for hypertrophy or strength purposes. Variations in hand position should be used to reflect the purpose of the exercise.

Each type of lift has a specific spotting technique used to help ensure that the movement is successfully completed and that the lifter is not injured during the performance of the exercise. It is important to realize that spotting is not intended for the purposes of lifting the weight for the client, except when a lift-failure situation arises. Constantly lifting resistance for the client suggests that the weight is too heavy for the movement. In some cases, it is necessary to lift the resistance from a client due to fatigue. Personal trainers should always assume a ready position in the event a movement fails during its performance. Injuries to the client and/or trainer can occur when the trainer is not in the right position at the time aid is needed. Spotting positions should be broad-based and stable, and allow for maximal control over the situation. Variations in spotting techniques exist based on lift specific characteristics. The actual technique employed should reflect the dynamics of the movement and type of resistance used for the exercise.

Properly spotting overhead lifts varies by the type of resistance used and the position of the body during the movement. The standing military press can be spotted by the trainer standing behind the lifter. When assistance is needed, the trainer can supply support by lifting or decelerating the distal end of the humerus near the elbow. When dumbbells are used in a seated position, the trainer can spot the lift by grasping the distal end of the forearms at the wrists. This allows the lifter to continue through their functional ROM and prevents undesired movements and asymmetrical arm acceleration. When a bar is used in the seated position, the trainer can spot by supporting the bar rather than the lifter's wrists. In all cases, it is the trainer's responsibility to watch for deviations in body alignment, improper movement, and signs of fatigue. At the first sign of execution deviation, such as a rapid decrease in speed or loss of stability, a personal trainer should be prepared to assist.

Learning how to spot exercises performed over the face is very important for the safety of the client. Instability, fatigue, and improper technique can put a person in a precarious situation if not attended to in time. For this reason, exercises performed over the face require constant, uninterrupted attention. As with overhead spotting, the technique is resistance modality specific. Exercises using a straight bar, as seen in the different types of bench press techniques, require both a lift off and lift back on to the rack, so the exerciser does not lift the bar while the arm is externally rotated and also necessitate bar management to avoid uneven pressing and undesirable bar movements. This is usually initiated by the spotter assisting the lift off with an alternating grip in between the lifter's hand location on the bar. The

spotting technique then requires close monitoring with the hands supinated or alternated in a position that travels with the bar but does not make contact until fatigue slows or stops the ascent or the point of termination of the lift. At this time, the bar is assisted back onto the rack, making sure it rests properly in position.

When presses are performed with a dumbbell, the spotter should spot from the distal end of the forearm as described for the seated overhead dumbbell lifts. Using this method, the spotter can control the stabilization component and assist when fatigue affects the movement execution. For exercises such as the supine tricep extension, sometimes referred to as skull crushers (for obvious reasons), the spotter can maintain a static position with hands pronated at the terminal ROM, usually just above the lifter's forehead. For added control, the spotter can hold the elbows and use their upper arm as the terminal ROM limiter. This position requires the spotter to make light contact with the distal upper arm of the lifter, with the spotter's arms extended under the bar. As the bar descends, the trainer's forearms or biceps can stop the bar from being lowered too far toward the forehead. This technique is best for lighter lifts. Heavier resistance may require better mechanical advantage, so the spotting technique may shift to mirror the bench press technique.

Spotting pulling movements is sometimes more difficult than presses, as often nothing exists for the trainer to grasp. Generally, a trainer can assist the lifter by physically cueing body alignment for exercises such as seated cable rows and bent-over rows and can aid in the pulling movement by helping to initiate scapular retraction through physical cueing. Rows pulled downward from a cable machine, including variations of bar rows and lat pull-downs, can be spotted by assisting the bar movement at the beginning of the exercise to get the exerciser in proper position and during periods of momentary failure and fatigue. The trainer should stand behind the lifter for proper assistance and safety. Likewise, pull-ups and chin-ups can be spotted effectively with the trainer standing behind the exerciser. Using this spotting technique, the trainer provides assistance by lifting from the waist or upper trunk. In this manner, the trainer can feel the necessary assistance requirements and can control body swing. This position also offers better control and mechanical advantage than spotting from the ankles. Spotting from the ankles does not provide assistance where it is needed most, and can lead to injury by forcing a position of **lordosis** upon the exerciser when the trainer lifts up on the ankles. Spotting the trunk also helps in assisting the start position and final descent to the floor, as commonly seen with gymnastic spotting.

Spotting deadlifts and squats also uses an upper trunk hand placement technique. These lifts require concentration and constant attention because the back can easily be injured if the exercise is performed incorrectly. The spotter's hands should be placed on the outside of the lifter's rib cage, just under the chest, with the spotter standing behind the lifter. When spotting the squat, assume the position beginning with the lift off of the rack and walk the person to the starting position. As the descent of the lift occurs, the spotter should also squat, mirroring the lifter's form and speed. When assistance is needed, the trainer should lift upward with the legs to elevate the chest. This allows the hips to extend and move the lifter safely into an upright position. When spotting a female, the trainer can modify the technique by transferring the hands slightly backward on the rib cage to avoid breast contact. Again, the trainer will maintain a stable position and squat with the lifter. When the lift is complete, walk the client back to the rack and watch to make sure the weight is racked correctly.

Some trainers have been incorrectly taught to place one hand on the low back of the client with the other supporting the chest. This technique is contraindicated because it can cause spinal rotation under axial loaded conditions, will not effectively support the body, and does little good if the exerciser completely fails on a lift. As with any spotting technique, the spotter is there in case something happens - not to perform the lift for the client. If the client fails early in the lift or the trainer has to constantly apply stabilizing assistance to the client, the resistance is too heavy.

It takes a little practice for most trainers to determine how much and when to provide assistance. In most cases, clients will need just enough assistance to complete a repetition, but sometimes, the trainer assumes responsibility for the entire load. Trainers should know the correct amount of resistance to prescribe through routine evaluations and must be able to lift the full amount of the resistance if complete muscle failure occurs. Additionally, communication for assistance should be discussed with every client prior to engaging in resistance activities. It must be communicated that the client continues to stay with the lift until the bar is racked. Some clients will release tension or let go of the resistance as soon as the trainer grabs the bar, which could be a serious error. When spotting, always attempt to move smoothly and avoid jerking the bar. As stated earlier, a trainer must always

be ready to assume the full weight of the lift, so make sure the spotting position is stable and mechanically advantageous. Trainers are susceptible to injury when spotting; therefore, focus and preparation, along with proper technique, should be employed at all times.

Identifying Training Intensities

Identifying the appropriate amount of weight to be used with an exercise is necessary for the proper application of overload and to ensure the designated number of repetitions can be performed correctly. A relationship exists between percentage of 1RM and the resistance associated with a respective number of repetitions (24). For instance, 70% of 1RM correlates to 100% of the 10RM. Each repetition accounts for an approximately 2%-3% difference of the 1RM load. Based on this information, inferences can be made that increase the accuracy of resistant load prediction for a designated number of repetitions (15). Using the following formula or predefined charts will help ensure that the client is experiencing the appropriate stress from the resistance training exercise.

Appropriate resistance = 1 RM ÷ {1 + (0.03 x desired number of repetitions)}

Appropriate resistance = 130 lbs. ÷ {1 + (0.03 x 10 repetitions)}

Appropriate resistance = 130 lbs. ÷ {1 + (0.3)}

Appropriate resistance =130 lbs. ÷ 1.3

Appropriate resistance = 100 lbs.

100 lbs. ÷ 130 lbs. = .76 or 76% of 1 RM

If the 1RM for a bench press equals 130 lbs. and the designated number of repetitions to be used in the program equals 10, the resistance load to be used for the exercise set would equal 100 lbs. Likewise, the predicted 1 RM can be calculated any time a number of repetitions are performed to volitional failure. Simply reversing the predictive equation, as demonstrated in Chapter 14, will identify the 1RM equivalent of the exercise performance.

1RM = Resistance used x {1 + (0.03 x Repetitions performed)

1RM = 100 lbs. x {1 + (0.03 x 10 repetitions)}

1RM = 100 lbs. x {1 + (0.3)}

1RM = 100 lbs. x 1.3

1RM = 130 lbs.

In this case, the 1RM is not known, but can be calculated using the predictive equation. This technique can dramatically enhance program effectiveness and serves as a constant measuring device for improvements in strength performance. The formula is accurate but not an exact science. It has best predictability when lower numbers of repetitions are performed to failure. High numbers of repetitions can still be used, but the formula does not account for the decreased stability requirements when less resistance (% of 1RM) is used in the prediction (23).

Repetition to Percentage of 1RM Predictions

2 repetitions = 95%

3 repetitions = 92.5%

4 repetitions = 90%

5 repetitions = 87.5%

6 repetitions = 85%

7 repetitions = 82.5%

8 repetitions = 80%

9 repetitions = 77.5%

10 repetitions = 75%

12 repetitions = 70%

Timed-Intensity Technique

Due to the psychology of repetition lifting and daily variations in performance capabilities, resistance training exercises may use time to failure rather than a defined repetition scheme. This technique requires some trial and error but can be used effectively to maximize training effort. If the optimal resistance for the 10 RM is not known, a prediction can be made to designate a weight. Using the timed lift technique, the client should attempt to perform as many controlled lift repetitions in the desired energy pathway, measured by time. For ten repetitions, this would be about 30 seconds. This technique forces the client to perform to volitional failure rather than stopping at a defined number, even though proper overload did not occur. For instance, if a client is told to lift ten pounds for ten repetitions, they will do so, even if they could have performed 14 repetitions with the same weight. In this case, the repetition number limits the performance. Instead, if the client were asked to perform as many controlled repetitions as possible in a 30 second period, he or she would likely reach volitional failure and attain the desired overload effect.

Key Terms

Manual resistance – A resistance technique in which the trainer applies resistance to the movement in a lifting exercise.

Free weight – Resistance that has no attachment to a machine and its resistive force is provided by the gravitational pull on the object.

Ergonomics – The science of equipment set-up intended for maximal work efficiency and safety.

Rhomboids – Rhombus-shaped muscles of the back that are chiefly responsible for scapular retraction.

Central Nervous System (CNS) – Consists of the brain, spinal cord, and connecting nerves.

Latissimus dorsi – Broad, triangular shaped muscles connecting from the vertebral column to the humerus, responsible for shoulder extension and humeral adduction.

Biceps brachii – A muscle of the upper arm (anterior) mainly responsible for flexing the elbow and supinating the forearm.

Triceps brachii – A muscle of the upper arm (posterior) mainly responsible for extending the arm and forearm.

Lordosis – An abnormal increase in the natural curvature of the spine in the lumbar region.

Timed-Intensity Technique – A lifting technique using a time-to-failure strategy to designate a proper weight.

Estimated Training Intensities

% of 1 RM	100	93.5	91	88.5	86	83.5	81	78.5	76	73.5	71	68.5	66	63.5	61
Repetitions Completed	1	2	3	4	5	6	7	8	9	10	11	12	13	14	15
Weight Lifted (lb)															
	5	4.7	4.5	4.4	4.3	4.2	4.1	3.9	3.8	3.7	3.6	3.5	3.3	3.2	3.1
	10	9.4	9.1	8.9	8.6	8.4	8.2	7.9	7.6	7.4	7.1	6.85	6.6	6.35	6.1
	15	14	13.7	13.3	12.9	12.5	12.2	11.8	11.4	11	10.7	10.3	9.9	9.5	9.2
	20	18.7	18.2	17.7	17.2	16.7	16.2	15.7	15.2	14.7	14.2	13.7	13.2	12.7	20.6
	25	23.4	22.8	22.1	21.5	20.9	20.2	19.6	19	18.4	17.8	17.2	16.5	15.9	15.3
	30	28.1	27.3	26.6	25.8	25.1	24.3	23.6	22.8	22.1	21.3	20.6	19.8	19.1	18.3
	35	32.7	31.9	31	30.1	29.2	28.4	27.5	26.6	25.7	24.9	24	23.1	22.2	21.4
	40	37.4	36.4	35.4	34.4	33.4	32.4	31.4	30.4	29.4	28.4	27.4	26.4	25.4	24.4
	45	42.1	41	39.8	38.7	37.6	36.5	35.3	34.2	33.1	32	30.9	29.7	28.6	27.5
	50	46.8	45.5	44.3	43	41.8	40.5	39.3	38	36.8	35.5	34.3	33	31.8	30.5
	55	51.4	50.1	48.7	47.3	45.9	44.6	43.2	41.8	40.4	39	37.7	36.3	34.9	33.6
	60	56.1	54.6	53.1	51.6	50.1	48.6	47.1	45.6	44.1	42.6	41.1	39.6	38.1	36.6
	65	60.8	59.2	57.5	55.9	54.3	52.7	51	49.4	47.8	46.2	44.5	42.9	41.3	39.7
	70	65.5	63.7	62	60.2	58.5	56.7	55	53.2	51.5	49.7	48	46.2	44.5	42.7
	75	70.1	68.3	66.4	64.5	62.6	60.8	58.9	57	55.1	53.3	51.4	49.5	47.6	45.8
	80	74.8	72.8	70.8	68.8	66.8	64.8	62.8	60.8	58.8	56.8	54.8	52.8	50.8	48.8
	85	79.5	77.4	75.2	73.1	71	68.9	66.7	64.6	62.5	60.4	58.2	56.1	54	51.9
	90	84.2	81.9	79.7	77.4	75.2	72.9	70.7	68.4	66.2	63.9	61.7	59.4	57.2	54.9
	95	88.8	86.5	84.1	81.7	79.3	77	74.6	72.2	69.8	67.5	65.1	62.7	60.3	54.9
	100	93.5	91	88.5	86	83.5	81	78.5	76	73.5	71	68.5	66	63.5	61
	105	98.2	95.6	92.9	90.3	87.7	85.1	82.4	79.8	77.2	74.6	71.9	69.3	66.7	64.1
	110	102.9	100.1	97.4	94.6	91.9	89.1	86.4	83.6	80.9	78.1	75.4	72.6	69.9	67.1
	115	107.5	104.7	101.8	98.9	96	93.2	90.3	87.4	84.5	81.7	78.8	75.9	73	70.2
	120	112.2	109.2	106.2	103.2	100.2	97.2	94.2	91.2	88.2	85.2	82.2	79.2	76.2	73.2
	125	116.9	113.8	110.6	107.5	104.4	101.3	98.1	95	91.9	88.8	85.6	82.5	79.4	76.3
	130	121.6	118.3	115.1	111.8	108.6	105.3	102.1	98.8	95.6	92.3	89.1	85.8	82.6	79.3
	135	126.2	122.9	119.5	116.1	112.7	109.4	106	102.6	99.2	95.9	92.5	89.1	85.7	82.4
	140	130.9	127.4	123.9	120.4	116.9	113.4	109.9	106.4	102.9	99.4	95.9	92.4	88.9	85.4
	145	135.6	132	128.3	124.7	121.1	117.5	113.8	110.2	106.6	103	99.3	95.7	92.1	88.5
	150	140.3	136.5	132.8	129	125.3	121.5	117.8	114	110.3	106.5	102.8	99	95.3	91.5
	155	144.9	141.1	137.2	133.3	129.4	125.6	121.7	117.8	113.9	110.1	106.2	102.3	98.4	94.6
	160	149.6	145.6	141.6	137.6	133.6	129.6	125.6	121.6	117.6	113.6	109.6	105.6	101.6	97.6
	165	154.3	150.2	146	141.9	137.8	133.7	129.5	125.4	121.3	117.2	113	108.9	104.8	100.7
	170	159	154.7	150.5	146.2	142	137.7	133.5	129.2	125	120.7	116.5	112.2	108	103.7
	175	163.6	159.3	154.9	150.5	146.1	141.8	137.4	133	128.6	124.3	119.9	115.5	111.1	106.8
	180	168.3	168.3	163.8	154.8	150.3	145.8	141.3	136.8	132.3	127.8	123.3	118.8	114.3	109.8
	185	173	168.4	163.7	159.1	154.5	149.9	145.2	140.6	136	131.4	126.7	122.1	117.5	112.9
	190	177.7	172.9	168.2	163.4	158.7	153.9	149.2	144.4	139.7	134.9	130.2	125.4	120.7	115.9
	195	182.3	177.5	172.6	167.7	162.8	158	153.1	148.2	143.3	138.5	133.6	128.7	123.8	119
	200	187	182	177	172	167	162	157	152	147	142	137	132	127	122
	205	191.7	186.6	181.4	176.3	171.2	166.1	160.9	155.8	150.7	145.6	140.4	135.3	130.2	125.1
	210	196.4	191.1	185.9	180.6	175.4	170.1	164.9	159.6	154.4	149.1	173.9	138.6	133.4	128.1
	215	201	195.7	190.3	184.9	179.5	174.2	168.8	163.4	158	152.7	147.3	141.9	136.5	131.2
	220	205.7	200.2	194.7	189.2	183.7	178.2	182.7	167.2	161.7	156.2	150.7	145.2	139.7	134.2
	225	210.4	204.8	199.1	193.5	187.9	182.3	176.6	171	165.4	159.8	159.8	148.5	142.9	137.3

Estimated Training Intensities

% of 1 RM	100	93.5	91	88.5	86	83.5	81	78.5	76	73.5	71	68.5	66	63.5	61
Repetitions Completed	1	2	3	4	5	6	7	8	9	10	11	12	13	14	15
Weight Lifted (lb)															
	230	215.1	209.3	203.6	197.8	192.1	186.3	180.6	174.8	169.1	163.3	157.6	151.8	146.1	140.3
	235	219.7	213.9	208	202.1	196.2	190.4	184.5	178.6	172.7	166.9	235.7	155.1	149.2	143.4
	240	224.4	218.4	212.4	206.4	200.4	194.4	188.4	182.4	176.4	170.4	164.4	158.4	152.4	146.4
	245	229.1	223	216.8	210.7	204	198.5	192.3	186.2	180.1	174	167.8	161.7	155.6	149.5
	250	233.8	227.5	221.3	215	208.8	202.5	196.3	190	183.8	177.5	171.3	165	158.8	152.5
	255	238.4	232.1	225.7	219.3	212.9	206.6	200.2	193.8	187.4	181.1	174.7	168.3	161.9	155.6
	260	243.1	236.6	230.1	223.6	217.1	210.6	204.1	197.6	191.2	184.6	178.1	171.6	165.1	158.6
	265	247.8	241.2	234.5	227.9	221.3	214.7	208.1	201.4	194.8	188.2	181.5	174.9	168.3	161.7
	270	252.5	245.7	239	232.2	225.5	218.7	212	205.2	198.5	191.7	185	178.2	171.5	164.7
	275	257.1	250.3	243.4	236.5	229.6	22.8	215.9	209	202.1	195.3	188.4	181.5	174.6	167.8
	280	261.8	254.8	247.8	240.8	233.8	226.8	219.8	212.8	205.8	198.8	191.8	184.8	177.8	170.8
	285	266.5	259.4	252.2	245.1	238	230.9	223.7	216.6	209.5	202.4	195.2	188.1	181	173.9
	290	271.2	269.9	256.7	249.4	242.5	234.9	227.7	220.4	213.2	205.9	198.7	191.4	184.2	176.9
	295	275.9	268.5	261.1	253.7	246.3	239	231.6	224.2	216.8	209.5	202.1	194.7	187.3	180
	300	280.5	273	265.5	258	250.5	243	235.5	228	220.5	213	205.5	198	190.5	183
	305	285.2	277.6	269.9	262.3	254.7	247.1	239.4	231.8	224.2	216.6	208.9	201.3	193.7	186.1
	310	289.9	282.1	274.4	266.6	258.9	251.1	243.4	235.6	227.9	220.1	212.4	204.6	196.9	189.1
	315	294.5	286.7	278.8	270.9	263	255.2	247.3	239.4	231.5	223.7	215.8	207.9	200	192.2
	320	299.2	291.2	283.2	275.2	267.2	259.2	251.2	243.2	235.2	227.2	219.2	211.2	203.2	195.2
	325	303.9	295.8	287.6	279.5	271.4	263.3	255.1	247	238.9	230.8	222.6	214.5	206.4	198.3
	330	308.6	300.3	292.1	283.8	275.9	267.3	259.1	250.8	242.6	234.3	226.1	217.8	210	201.3
	335	313.2	304.9	296.5	288.1	279.7	271.4	263	254.6	246.2	237.9	229.5	221.1	212.7	204.4
	340	317.9	309.4	300.9	292.4	283.9	275.4	266.9	258.4	249.9	241.4	159.5	224.4	215.9	207.4
	345	322.6	314	305.3	296.7	288.1	279.5	270.8	262.2	253.6	245	236.3	227.7	219.1	210.5
	350	327.3	318.5	309.8	301	292.3	283.6	274.8	266	257.3	248.5	239.8	231	222.3	213.5
	355	331.9	323.1	314.2	305.3	296.4	287.6	278.7	269.8	260.9	252.1	243.2	234.3	225.4	216.6
	360	336.6	327.6	318.6	309.6	300.6	291.6	282.6	273.6	264.6	255.6	246.6	237.6	228.6	219.6
	365	341.3	332.2	323	313.9	304.8	295.7	286.5	277.4	268.3	259.2	250	240.9	231.8	222.7
	370	346	336.7	237.5	318.2	309	299.7	290.5	281.2	272	262.7	253.4	244.2	235	225.7
	375	350.6	341.3	331.9	322.5	313.1	303.8	294.4	285	275.6	266.3	256.9	247.5	238.1	228.8
	380	355.3	345.8	336.3	326.8	317.3	307.8	298.3	288.8	279.3	269.8	260.3	250.8	241.3	231.8
	385	360	3350	340.7	331.1	321.5	311.9	302.2	292.6	283	273.4	263.7	254.1	244.5	234.9
	390	364.7	354.9	345	335.4	325.7	315.9	306.2	264.4	286.7	276.9	267.2	257.4	247.7	237.9
	395	369.3	359.5	349.6	339.7	329.8	320	310.1	300.2	290.3	280.5	270.6	260.7	250.8	241
	400	374	364	354	344	334	324	314	304	294	284	274	264	254	244
	405	378.7	368.6	358.4	348.3	338.2	328.1	317.9	307.8	297.7	287.6	277.4	267.3	257.2	247.1
	410	383.4	373.1	362.9	352.6	342.4	332.1	321.9	311.6	301.4	291.1	280.9	270.6	260.4	250.1
	415	388	377.7	367.3	356.9	346.5	336.2	325.8	315.4	305	294.7	284.3	273.9	263.5	253.2
	420	392.7	382.2	371.7	361.2	350.7	340.2	329.7	319.2	308.7	298.2	287.7	277.2	266.7	256.2
	425	397.4	386.8	376.1	365.5	354.9	344.3	333.6	323	312.4	301.8	291.1	280.5	269.9	259.2
	430	402.1	391.3	380.6	369.8	359.1	348.3	337.6	326.8	316.1	305.3	294.6	283.8	273.1	262.3
	435	406.7	395.9	385	374.1	363.2	352.4	341.5	330.6	319.7	308.9	298	287.1	276.2	265.4
	440	411.4	400.4	389	378.4	367.4	356.4	345.4	334.4	323.4	312.4	301.4	290.4	279.4	268.4
	445	416.1	405	393.8	382.7	371.6	360.5	349.3	338.2	327.1	316	304.8	293.7	282.6	271.5
	450	420.8	409.5	398.3	387	375.8	364.5	353.3	342	330.8	319.5	308.3	297	285.8	274.5

Upper Body Resistance Training

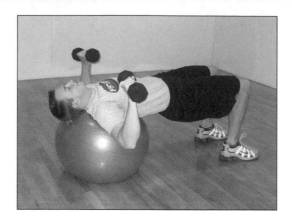 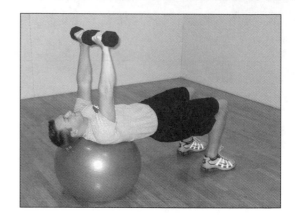

Exercise:	Dumbbell Chest Press
Joint Action:	Shoulder horizontal adduction, elbow extension
Muscles Involved:	Pectoralis major, anterior deltoid, triceps brachii
Modifications:	Dumbbell, cable, bands performed on a physioball, bench, or Bosu

Starting Position
Start in a supine position with a neutral spine. The elbows should be extended with the shoulders horizontally adducted. The palms should face the lifters feet (pronated grip).

Movement Phase
Start by lowering the resistance in a controlled manner downward toward the chest by flexing the arms and horizontally abducting the humerus so the wrists maintain alignment with the elbows. As the descent is made, the body should remain in a fixed stable position with no extraneous body movement. The weight should descend until the dumbbells are in a position lateral to either side of the chest. Any internal and/or external rotation of the shoulder or excessive elbow flexion should be avoided. Once the dumbbells reach full function ROM on the descent, the client should concentrically press the weight upward in the same plane of motion used during the descent phase. The resistance is pressed upward until the arms are fully extended but not locked.

Spotting
There are several methods of spotting this exercise. The first technique involves the spotter applying inward and upward force to the distal portion of the humerus. This technique can be hazardous as the triceps may fatigue first and loss of arm extension control may result in the dumbbell colliding with the client. The preferred technique involves the spotting of the wrist or distal end of the forearms. By grasping the lifters forearm, the spotter has more control over the movement and safety is not compromised.

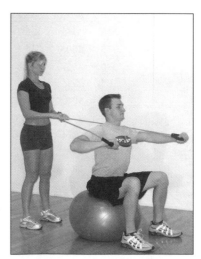

Training Considerations
Proper wrist and elbow positioning is important to the proper execution of this lift. Using dumbbells, as opposed to a bar or machine resistance, requires the lifter to possess a higher amount of motor control because each arm operates independent of one another and the resistance is not in a fixed path of motion. Performing the exercise on a physioball is more benign to the shoulder as the scapula can more easily retract.

Modification to Movement:
Seated Alternating Band Press

Upper Body Resistance Training

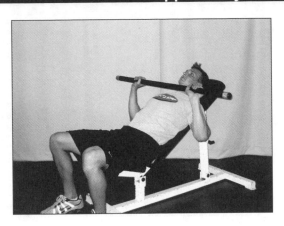 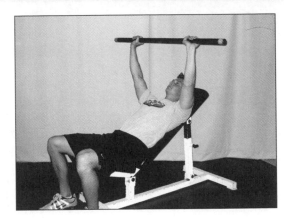

Exercise:	Incline Bench Press
Joint Action:	Shoulder horizontal flexion and adduction, elbow extension
Muscles Involved:	Pectoralis major (clavicular head), anterior deltoid, triceps brachii
Modifications:	Barbell, dumbbell, cable, bands, medicine ball performed on a bench or physioball

Starting Position
Starting in a supine position on an incline bench position both feet flat on the ground. Each joint segment should closely align and the spine should be in a neutral position. Position the hands just outside shoulder width using a closed (thumbs wrapped around bar) grip. Lift the bar off the rack with assistance from a spotter and position it over the chest with arms fully extended.

Movement Phase
Lower the bar in a slow and controlled manner downward toward the chest. The body should remain fixed during the descent with no extraneous body movement. The bar should descend in a controlled manner until it makes contact with the top portion of the chest, or within the defined functional range of the client. Once the bar has reached the lowest point of descent the client exerts concentric force on the bar in the same plane of motion as used during the descent phase. The bar should be pressed upward until the arms are fully extended.

Spotting
The spotter should lift the bar off the rack to the start position. This will reduce stress on the glenohumeral joint during the lift off. As the bar is lowered during the eccentric phase the trainer should spot the bar, cueing controlled deceleration to the chest. Upon the concentric contraction, the spotter should monitor the upward movement with hands supinated under the bar inside the lifter's grip position. When re-racking the bar it should be placed securely in the rack. If the rack has low rack arms, be sure the bar does not exceed the height of the rack. This is of particular concern for individuals with long limbs and during close grip lifts.

Training Considerations
At no time should the lifter bounce the bar off the chest. Injury can occur from the high compression forces placed on the rib cage. A common error is raising the hips off the bench during the ascent to increase mechanical advantage. If the lifter is unable to achieve the designated number of reps without lifting the hips, the weight should be reduced. Another common error is uneven bar extension. Uneven bar extension is either a symptom of diminished motor control, asymmetrical stabilizer fatigue or a muscle strength imbalance issue. Neural issues are easier to rectify than imbalances, whereby using a lighter weight and further practice should correct the problem. If a muscle imbalance is the issue, you may need to look more in depth at the following structures and issues: rotator cuff imbalance and weakness, latissimus dorsi weakness, triceps imbalance, or previous injury.

Upper Body Resistance Training

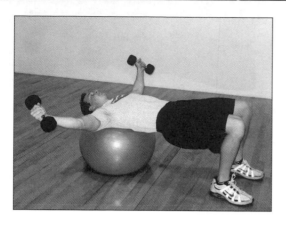
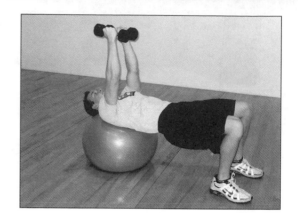

Exercise:	Chest Fly
Joint Action:	Shoulder horizontal adduction
Muscles Involved:	Pectoralis major, anterior deltoid
Modifications:	Dumbbell, cable, bands performed on a physioball, bench, or Bosu

Starting Position

Start in a supine position with a neutral spine. Horizontally adduct the shoulders and extend the arms, positioning the dumbbells lateral to the either side of the chest. The hands should be in the neutral position.

Movement Phase

Slowly lower the resistance by simultaneously flexing the elbows slightly and horizontally abducting the arms. In a slow arching motion lower the weight through full functional ROM with normal end range approximately at chest height. Once the descent reaches functional ROM, the client should be concentrically contracted, horizontally adducting the arms to the starting position. The movement is performed in the same plane of motion as the descent.

Spotting

Many potential injuries stem from performing this exercise incorrectly or with too much weight. The dumbbell flye exercise should be spotted either at the wrist or forearm. Spotting from the elbow during this exercise is not recommended as it reduces flexion control and may lead to hyperextension of the arm.

Training Considerations

The flye exercise should only be used if the client has healthy shoulder joint structures. It is a difficult lift to master because the lifter will often externally rotate the shoulder during the decent, which places excessive stress on the rotator cuff structures.

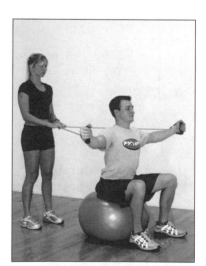

Modification to Movement:
Seated Band Fly

Upper Body Resistance Training

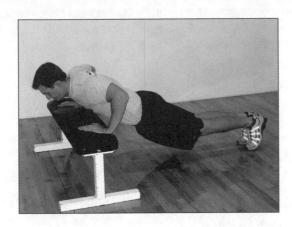 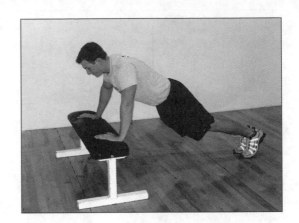

Exercise:	Bench Push-up
Joint Action:	Shoulder horizontal adduction, elbow extension
Muscles Involved:	Pectoralis major, anterior deltoid, triceps brachii
Modifications:	Performed on a physioball, bench, or Bosu

Starting Position
Start by placing both hands on the bench with arms extended and walk the feet back to an extended straight body position. The hands should be placed on the bench just outside shoulder width. The spine and hips should maintain a neutral position with legs together.

Movement Phase
Start by lowering the body in a controlled manner downward toward the bench by flexing the arms and horizontally abduct/extending the humerus so the wrists maintain alignment with the elbows. As the descent is made, the body should remain in a fixed stable position with no extraneous body movement. The body should descend until the chest reaches a position at or near the bench. Any changes in the spine or hip position should be avoided. Once the client reaches full function ROM on the descent, he or she should concentrically press the body upward in the same plane of motion used during the descent phase. The body is pressed upward until the arms are fully extended but not locked.

Spotting
The bench push-up can be spotted by the waist of the client, if necessary. The goal is to maintain a stable torso and hip position during the movement.

Training Considerations
Proper wrist and elbow positioning is important to the proper execution of this lift. Proper hand placement will ensure the wrist is not injured during the performance of the movement.

Upper Body Resistance Training

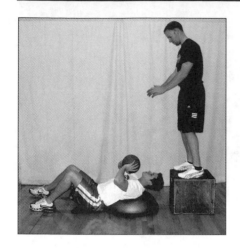 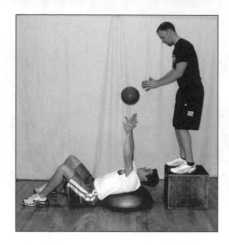 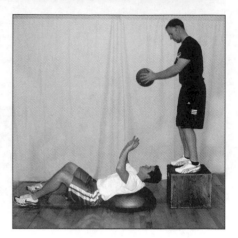

Exercise: Medicine Ball Drop Pass

Joint Action: Shoulder horizontal adduction, elbow extension

Muscles Involved: Pectoralis major, anterior deltoid, triceps brachii

Modifications: Performed on a physioball, bench, or Bosu

Starting Position

Lying in a supine position on a Bosu or similar object the client grasps a medicine ball and holds it at the chest using flexed arms and a neutral grip. The ball is held over the chest with the scapula retracted and the spine and hips in a neutral position with legs flexed and feet flat on the floor.

Movement Phase

The client initiates the movement by horizontally adducting and flexing the shoulder while extending the elbow. The ball is accelerated upwards and is released at full arm extension to the trainer standing overhead. Once received, the ball is released back to the client, who remains in the release position, ready to receive the returned ball. Upon receipt of the ball the client decelerates the ball back to the chest in the same plane of movement and rapidly repeats the movement.

Spotting

The medicine ball drop pass is spotted using verbal cues and the medicine ball is closely managed by the trainer.

Training Considerations

Due to the overhead position of the resistance the exercise has an increased risk of injury. The trainer must be in a position to control the ball at all times and the client must have experience in this type of training before using this exercise. The ball should be properly decelerated and never hit the client's chest, as an injury may occur.

Upper Body Resistance Training

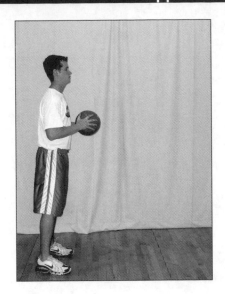 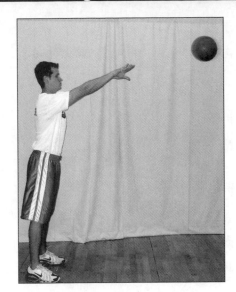

Exercise: Medicine Ball Chest Pass

Joint Action: Shoulder horizontal adduction, elbow extension

Muscles Involved: Pectoralis major, anterior deltoid, triceps brachii

Modifications: Performed standing, kneeling, or seated

Starting Position
Standing in an upright posture with feet shoulder width apart, the client grasps a medicine ball using a neutral grip. The arms are flexed next to the body so the ball is held at chest height. The spine should be neutral and the hips slightly flexed.

Movement Phase
The movement is initiated by the client concentrically pressing the ball forward by flexing and horizontally adducting the shoulder while extending the arms in the sagittal plane. The hips may flex slightly as the ball is accelerated from the body. The client should release the ball at shoulder height once the arms have been fully extended. The trainer should receive the ball and quickly return it to the client, who remains ready in the release position. The ball should be returned in a controlled manner and decelerated back to the start position upon receipt.

Spotting
The medicine ball chest pass is spotted using verbal cues and by speed control. The client should maintain body control throughout the release and receipt of the ball and the ball should be properly decelerated.

Training Considerations
The client should be acclimated to the ball weight and the deceleration requirements upon receipt. To reduce risk, the ball can be thrown to the trainer and handed back to the client to increase concentric power, while reducing the risk associated with the eccentric deceleration.

Upper Body Resistance Training

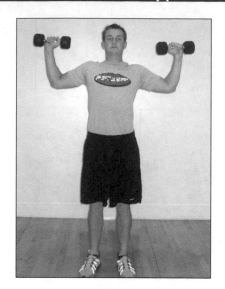
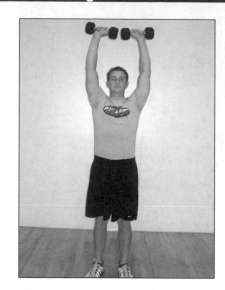

Exercise: Shoulder Press

Joint Action: Shoulder abduction, scapular rotation, elbow extension

Muscles Involved: Medial and anterior deltoid, supraspinatus, triceps brachii, trapezius, serratus anterior

Modifications: Barbell, dumbbell, cable, bands performed standing or seated on a physioball or bench

Starting position

Although the exercise can be performed from a seated or standing position, using different forms of resistance, the illustrated exercise is performed from a standing position using dumbbells. The client should stand in an upright posture with feet in a neutral position, separated to approximately hip width. The client's arms should be flexed with the wrists and elbows aligned. The dumbbells should be located at approximately ear level.

Movement Phase

Start the movement by concentrically contracting the deltoids while extending the elbow to press the resistance upward. As the resistance travels upward, a neutral spine position should be maintained. The client should press the resistance until the arms are fully extended. Once the arms are fully extended, but not locked, the resistance should be lowered to the starting position in the same plane of motion as the ascent phase. A neutral spine position should be maintained throughout the movement. Do not allow the weight to bounce at the bottom, as the natural tendency is to take advantage of the stretch reflex.

Spotting

The type of resistance used (dumbbell, bar, machine) will dictate which spotting technique to employ. Seated Position: If using dumbbells, the spotting technique is consistent with the dumbbell bench press; the wrists are often preferred. If using a straight bar or machine, spot the bar as opposed to the appendage performing the lift. Standing Position: spotting a standing press uses an assistance position at the distal end of the humerus. Providing assistance can be accomplished during both the concentric phase and eccentric phase by aiding in a steady movement of acceleration and deceleration.

Training Considerations

One of the more common mistakes personal trainers make is to have clients perform the shoulder press exercise even when the client does not possess acceptable shoulder ROM. This becomes ever more apparent as the resistance migrates into the sagittal plane. This causes a backward lean and stress on lumbar structures. The lift should never be performed behind the head. This causes excessive stress on the anterior capsule of the shoulder and increases risk for injury.

Upper Body Resistance Training

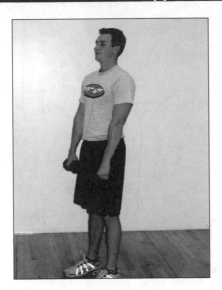 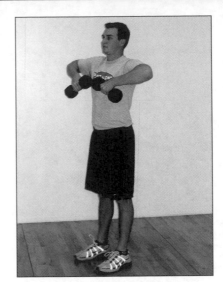

Exercise:	Upright Row
Joint Action:	Shoulder abduction, scapular elevation/rotation, arm flexion
Muscles Involved:	Medial and anterior deltoid, supraspinatus, levator scapulae, upper trapezius, brachialis, brachioradialis.
Modifications:	Barbell, dumbbell, cable, bands

Starting Position
The client should stand in an upright posture with feet in a neutral position separated to approximately hip width. The client's arms should be extended downward with the wrists and elbows in alignment. The palms should face the body in a pronated grip.

Movement Phase
Initiate the upward movement by contracting the deltoid and flexing the arms. As the resistance begins the ascent, the lifter should keep the elbows elevated. The elbows should remain superior to the wrists during all phases of the lift. The resistance will travel along the front of the body in a controlled fashion until the humerus is approximately parallel to the floor. Once the upward phase has reached functional ROM the resistance should be lowered to the starting position in the same plane of motion as the ascent phase. A neutral spine should be maintained throughout the entire movement. Do not allow the weight to bounce or jerk at end point ROM.

Spotting
The upright row exercise can be performed using different hand widths and forms of resistance (barbell, dumbbell, cable, bands, etc). This exercise is difficult to spot safely as the spotter does not want to change the ROM by over lifting the upper arm. When using a straight bar assistance can occur by standing in front of the lifter and spotting the bar. The trainer can be more useful by selecting an appropriate weight so the lifter can complete the sets with proper form.

Training Considerations
As the resistance is elevated it is not uncommon for the lifter to drop the elbows and/or shrug the shoulders. If proper shoulder abduction cannot be maintained or excessive shoulder elevation occurs, the trainer should decrease the resistance. Additionally, the client should not use momentum forces to complete repetitions as evidenced by bouncing and jerking the resistance and flexing and extending the knees and hips. Be cautious of the terminal end ROM. Some individuals are susceptible to impingement when the arms are abducted beyond 90 degrees.

Upper Body Resistance Training

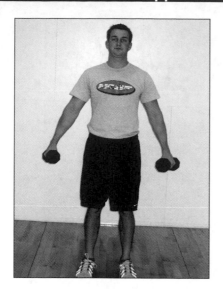 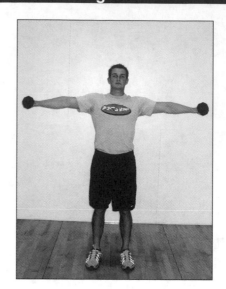

Exercise: Lateral Deltoid Raise

Joint Action: Shoulder abduction, scapular rotation

Muscles involved: Middle deltoid, supraspinatus, levator scapulae, upper trapezius, rhomboids, brachialis, brachioradialis

Modifications: Dumbbell, cable, bands in a seated or standing position

Starting Position
The client should stand in an upright posture with feet in a neutral position separated to approximately hip width. The client's arms should be extended downward at the sides of the body. The palms should face the body in a neutral grip. The arms are then extended and held approximately 4"- 6" from the sides of the body. The abducted starting position reduces supraspinatus activation and concentrates the resistance on the medial deltoid.

Movement Phase
Initiate the upward movement phase by abducting the arms in the frontal plane. During the ascent the arms should remain extended with slight elbow flexion while a neutral spine position is maintained. The client should abduct the arms to a point where the humerus is parallel with the floor. Once the upward end ROM has been reached the resistance should be lowered to the starting position in the same plane of motion as the ascent phase. Maintain the neutral spine position throughout the movement. The lowest point should be approximately 30 degrees from the hip. If the weight is lowered all the way down the neural activation and contraction of the deltoid is diminished, which reduces the effectiveness of the exercise.

Spotting
Spotting can be effectively performed by standing behind the lifter and applying assistance to the proximal forearm area when needed.

Training Considerations
It is not uncommon to see lifters performing this exercise using poor technique. Many lifters will compromise technique and safety to lift more weight. Common practices include bending the elbows, which reduces the length of the resistance arm and corresponding load on the target musculature, as well as using hip flexion and extension to capitalize on momentum forces generated by this action. This exercise can also be performed using manual resistance from the trainer.

Upper Body Resistance Training

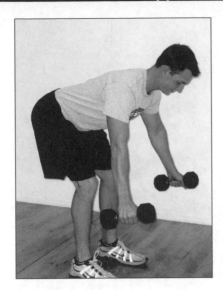 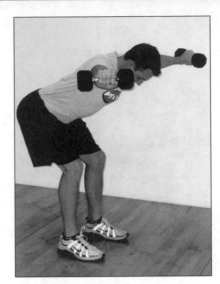

Exercise:	Rear Deltoid Raise
Joint Action:	Shoulder horizontal extension
Muscle Involved:	Posterior deltoid, teres major, infraspinatus, teres minor
Modifications:	Dumbbell, cable, bands in a seated or standing position

Starting Position
The client should assume a flexed hip position so the torso is parallel with the floor. The arms should be extended downward with the hands pronated.

Movement Phase
While maintaining a flat back position the arms should be horizontally abducted to a point where the arms are parallel with the floor. The path of motion for this movement is slightly anterior to the top of the shoulder. Once the full ROM has been attained the arms should be horizontally adducted back to the starting position following the same path of motion as the ascent phase. The client should maintain a flat back position and pronated grip throughout the entire motion. Do not allow the weight to bounce or jerk at end point ROM.

Spotting
Spotting can be performed from the front of the client by providing assistance to the forearm. It is imperative that the movement be performed with the torso in a position parallel with the floor to maintain true shoulder horizontal abduction.

Training Considerations
This exercise is important for the complete development of the deltoid, as the posterior head is often under trained which can lead to shoulder strength imbalances. Although the technique illustrated is demonstrating a closed chain standing form of the movement, the exercise can be taught from a seated position using bands or cables. Common mistakes during the execution of the exercise are incomplete shoulder abduction leading to an incorrect path of motion and failure of the client to maintain a flat back position.

Upper Body Resistance Training

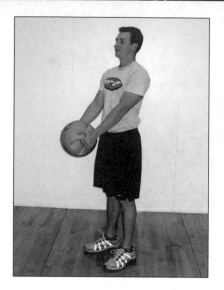 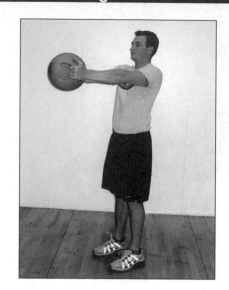

Exercise:	Front Raise
Joint Action:	Shoulder flexion
Muscles Involved:	Anterior deltoids
Modifications:	Dumbbell, medicine ball, cable, bands, Olympic plate

Starting Position

Standing in an upright posture with feet shoulder width apart the client grasps a medicine ball using a neutral grip. The elbows should be extended with the humerus flexed to approximately 10 degrees.

Movement Phase

With the palms facing inward, the client contracts the deltoids by flexing the shoulders while maintaining a straight back position. The client should maintain a neutral hip and spinal position avoiding any forward or backward movement to generate momentum forces during the lift. The shoulders should be flexed to 100 degrees. Upon attainment of full range of motion the resistance is lowered in a controlled fashion until it reaches the starting position. The client should maintain a flat back position as the weight is decelerated downward.

Spotting

Trainers should spot the resistance to assist in attainment of full range of motion. It is important that a stable body position is maintained throughout the movement.

Training Considerations

It is common for lifters to use too much weight during the front raise. Clients may "cheat" by swinging the weight. This can be detrimental as it often overstresses the shoulder and may lead to impingement. The neutral grip is favored over a pronated grip which increases risk for shoulder impingement at the top of the movement.

Upper Body Resistance Training

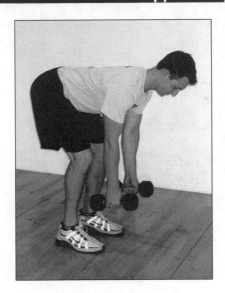 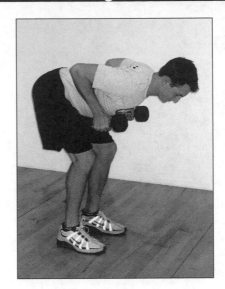

Exercise: Bent-Over Row

Joint Action: Shoulder horizontal extension, scapular retraction, arm flexion

Muscles Involved: Latissimus dorsi, teres major, trapezius, infraspinatus, teres minor, posterior deltoid, rhomboids, brachialis, biceps brachii, brachioradialis

Modifications: Barbell, dumbbell, cable, bands

Starting Position
The client should assume flexed hip position so the torso is parallel with the floor. The feet should be approximately hip width apart. The arms should be extended downwards with the hands in a neutral position.

Movement Phase
Start the movement by pulling the weight upward by simultaneously flexing the arms and retracting the scapula. It is important that the client maintains a flat back position with the torso parallel to the floor. Continue the upward movement phase until the scapula is fully retracted and the shoulder hyperextended so the dumbbells are at a point lateral to the lifters rib cage. Maintaining the flat back position, the weight is descended as the arms extend and the scapula is protracted. The resistance should descend in a controlled fashion to the start position.

Spotting
The spotting of the free weight movement is a little more difficult than that of a machine movement so it is best to assign appropriate weight and use verbal cueing throughout the lift. It is imperative that the lifter maintains the flat back position during the entire performance of the exercise. A common error is for the client to extend the hips to gain mechanical advantage.

Training Considerations
The row movement is an excellent exercise for the development of the back. The exercise is illustrated using dumbbells as the form of resistance however, the row movement can be performed using a bar, cables, machines or unilaterally and isolaterally. Consistent with other resistance training techniques, the lift is always performed in a slow and contolled manner. It is imperative that no "rounding" of any spinal segment occur and that the lifter does not flex and extend the hips and legs generating momentum forces to achieve the reps.

Upper Body Resistance Training

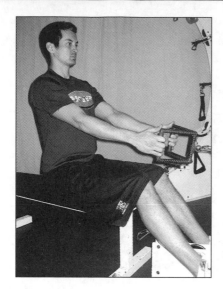 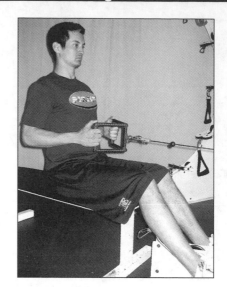

Exercise:	Seated Cable Row
Joint Action:	Shoulder horizontal abduction and extension, scapular retraction, elbow flexion
Muscles Involved:	Trapezius, rhomboids, latissimus dorsi, teres major, brachialis, biceps brachii, brachioradialis
Modifications:	One or two arms

Starting Position
The client should assume a seated position placing both feet on the footplate with knees slightly flexed. The client should grasp the handles using a neutral grip with arms extended, scapula slightly protracted, and spine in a neutral position.

Movement Phase
While maintaining a neutral spine position the client should simultaneously retract the scapula while extending and horizontally abducting the shoulder and flexing the elbows. The client should pull the handle to the mid point of the abdomen while keeping the back flat and chest elevated. The scapula should be fully retracted at end point ROM. Once the full ROM has been attained the client should extend the arms, flex the shoulder and protract the scapula back to the start of the movement. The motion should follow the same plane as in the pulling phase. The client should maintain the flat back position and not allow the weight to accelerate during the eccentric phase.

Spotting
Spotting is done verbally to assist in the maintenance of proper body alignment. As the movement begins, the trainer can place their hand between the lifters scapula as a cue for them to retract during the pulling phase and to prevent trunk extension.

Training Considerations
This exercise is often performed incorrectly as the lifter will lean forward, flexing the hip and then extending the hip and spine to generate momentum forces. The hip angle should be relatively unchanged while the spine remains in a neutral position throughout the lift. Another common mistake is the lifter utilizing primarily arm flexion and extension with minimal scapular action.

Upper Body Resistance Training

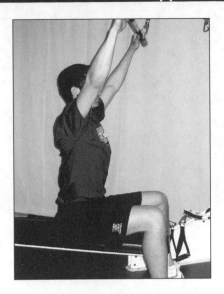 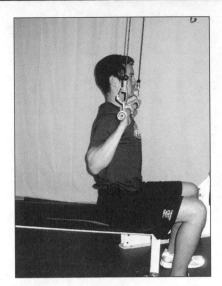

Exercise:	Wide Grip Lat Pull-Down
Joint Action:	Shoulder adduction, scapular medial rotation, elbow flexion
Muscles Involved:	Middle fibers of the trapezius, rhomboids, latissimus dorsi, teres major, brachialis, biceps brachii, brachioradialis
Modifications:	Cables, bands, using one arm or two

Starting Position
Similar to the pull-up exercise, the client grasps the bar with a closed pronated grip. (Grip width will vary, but for the normal execution of the lat pull down the grip should be a few inches wider than shoulder width.) The client should position his or her legs under the pad for stability. The selected machine will dictate the proper hip position so the bar can be pulled unabated to the chest.

Movement Phase
The client begins the movement by pulling the bar downward, simultaneously flexing the arms, adducting the humerus and inwardly rotating the scapula. The initial torso position should be maintained as the bar is pulled to the client's upper chest. Ensure the client does not perform back/hip extension to generate momentum forces. Once the bar has traveled through a full ROM the client should extend his or her arms, simultaneously outwardly rotating the scapula and extending the arms as the resistance is brought back to the start position. The motion should follow the same linear plane as the downward pulling phase.

Spotting
The spotter can apply the needed assistance to the bar while standing behind the lifter. Be sure to watch for undesirable movements particularly back extension for increased mechanical advantage. Again, the hip angle should be relatively unchanged throughout the lift.

Training Considerations
The movement should never be performed to the back of the head. This places excessive stress on the shoulder joint and increases risk of cervical spine injury.

Upper Body Resistance Training

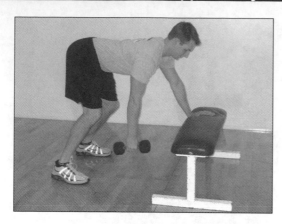 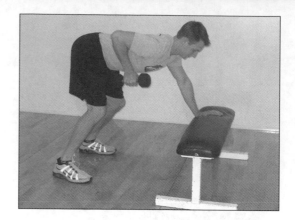

Exercise: One Arm Row

Joint Action: Shoulder horizontal extension, scapular retraction, arm flexion

Muscles Involved: Latissimus dorsi, teres major, trapezius, infraspinatus, teres minor, posterior deltoid, rhomboids, brachialis, biceps brachii, brachioradialis

Modifications: Hand on physioball, hands and knee on bench or with no support

Starting Position
The client should assume a flexed hip position so the torso is parallel with the floor. One arm should be extended downward with the hand in neutral position. The other hand should be placed on a bench in an extended position to support the upper body.

Movement Phase
The lifter initiates the upward movement by simultaneously flexing the arm, extending the shoulder, and retracting the scapula. The movement should be continued until the scapula is fully retracted, shoulder hyperextended, elbow flexed, and the dumbbell is at a point lateral to the client's rib cage. Do not extend the hip or rotate the spine, which is a common error with too much resistance. The client should lower the resistance by extending the arm and protracting the scapula. A flat back position must be maintained as the resistance is lowered toward the floor. Lower the weight in a controlled fashion to the start position.

Spotting
The one arm row is spotted using verbal cues. Spotters should watch the position of the spine to avoid rotation and rounding of the back. The weight should not be bounced at the bottom. The lift should be performed as a slow controlled movement.

Training Considerations
It is not uncommon for lifters to use too much weight and use momentum and ballistic style movement to complete the designated repetitions. This is commonly reflected when the lifter brings the torso downward to meet the rising dumbbell. The lifter will also utilize trunk rotation to enhance (undesirable) momentum forces.

Upper Body Resistance Training

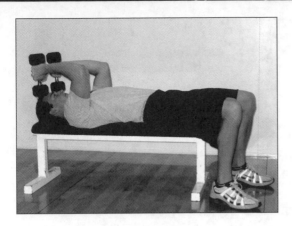 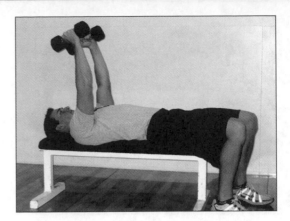

Exercise: Supine Triceps Extension

Joint Action: Elbow extension

Muscles Involved: Triceps brachii

Modifications: Dumbbell, barbell, cable, bands

Starting Position
Start in a supine position on a bench with the feet flat on the floor. Fully extend the arms so the elbow and wrist align with the shoulder joint. The hands will be in a neutral position with dumbbells, pronated if using a bar.

Movement Phase
The client should begin by flexing the elbow to lower the resistance as the upper arm remains perpendicular to the floor. The elbows should not move outward nor should the shoulders be additionally flexed. The client should continue to flex the arm until the forearms are approximately parallel to the floor. Once the descent has reached full ROM the client should extend the arms by concentrically contracting the triceps without extending the shoulder. The client should maintain a neutral spine and upper arm position as the resistance is lifted back to the start position.

Spotting
Spotting is performed from a position at the head of the lifter providing assistance as warranted by the movement. The spotter should establish an end ROM and guard against movements past this position. Be cautious of the resistance making contact with the lifter's head.

Training Considerations
This movement is very effective for isolating the triceps muscle group, however some people may experience discomfort in the wrist or elbow region, particularly if the shoulder is abducted during the execution phase. The trainer should look for technique errors, decrease the resistance, or change the form of resistance to accommodate the client.

Upper Body Resistance Training

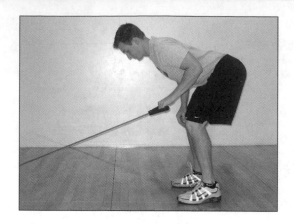 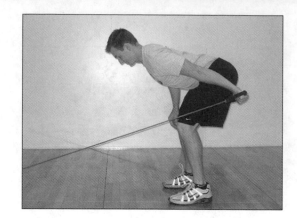

Exercise:	Tricep Kickback
Joint Action:	Elbow extension
Muscles Involved:	Triceps brachii
Modifications:	Cables, dumbbells, using one or two arms

Starting Position
The exercise begins with the client assuming a flexed hip position with feet approximately hip width apart. The spine should be neutral and approximately parallel to the floor. The client should grasp a cable or band in one or both hands using a pronated grip and extend the shoulder.

Movement Phase
While maintaining body position the client should extend the elbow moving the resistance backward and upward. Shoulder extension must be maintained as the resistance is being lifted solely through elbow extension. The humerus should remain close to the body throughout movement and the elbow positioning should remain unchanged as extension takes place. The elbow should be fully extended at end point ROM. Once full ROM has been reached the client should return to the start position. The arm should remain fixed as the elbow is flexed, returning the resistance to the start position.

Spotting
Spotting can effectively be performed from the side of the lifter by applying the necessary assistance to the forearm while providing mild support to the upper arm.

Training Considerations
Cables and bands are ideal resistance since the movement travels across gravitational pull. The exercise has been performed with dumbbells, but the resistance is compromised as gravity is the primary factor affecting the load. It is also important the lifter maintains a neutral spine position and does not swing the weight to take advantage of momentum forces.

Upper Body Resistance Training

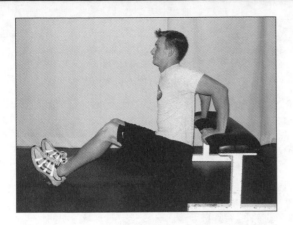 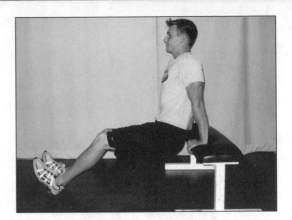

Exercise:	Tricep Bench Dips
Joint Action:	Elbow extension, shoulder flexion
Muscles Involved:	Triceps brachii, anterior deltoids, pectoralis major
Modifications:	Feet on bosu or physioball

Starting Position
The client begins in a seated position on the edge of a bench with the hands placed on either side of the hips. The legs should be extended in front of the body with the heels on the ground. The client should extend the elbows to the start position. Before descending, the lifter must shift the body forward to clear the bench on the decent.

Movement Phase
The client begins the descent by flexing the elbows and slightly extending the shoulders. As the elbows flex the client should maintain a neutral posture and should not allow the body to travel away from the bench. Forward travel will cause excessive extension of the shoulder and place stress on the anterior capsule. The body should descend straight down toward the floor in a slow and controlled movement. The lifter should descend to 90° of arm flexion. Using the same plane of motion as the descent, the client should contract the triceps to return to the start position. The client should maintain an upright torso position throughout ROM.

Spotting
There is no trainer spotting technique for this lift. If the lifter has their feet on the ground they can self-spot by extending flexed knees. The lift should be performed with minimal ground clearance at the lowest functional ROM so if the lifter slips or falls due to fatigue it is a very short distance to the ground.

Training Considerations
This lift is not recommended for individuals with shoulder pain, limited ROM or other related problems due to the shoulder extension component and the anterior capsule stress. If an individual is unable to perform the lift with the legs extended they can flex the knees placing the bottom of the feet on the ground. This decreases the resistance and allows them to self-spot by extending the legs during the execution. Wrist extension is another concern as some people may experience discomfort through the extended wrist position.

Upper Body Resistance Training

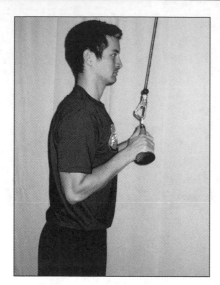 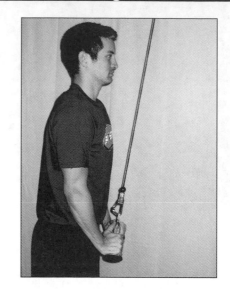

Exercise: Standing Triceps Pushdown

Joint Action: Elbow extension

Muscles Involved: Triceps brachii

Modifications: Single or double arm

Starting Position
Standing in a neutral spine position with feet shoulder width apart the client should grasp the bar with a closed pronated grip. The hands are placed shoulder width apart with the humerus against the lateral aspect of the body along the midaxillary line.

Movement Phase
Maintaining strict body and upper arm position the client should extend the elbows pushing the resistance downward toward the floor. The elbows should remain fixed against the sides of the body. The arms should be fully extended but not locked. While maintaining the flat back position, the client should flex the arms in a controlled manner to return to the start position. As the bar is raised the elbows should remain against the body.

Spotting
Spotting uses verbal cues to help the lifter maintain proper body position. The trainer can also apply assistance to the top of the bar accessory.

Training Considerations
A common tendency is to generate momentum by flexing the hips, laterally moving the elbows and/or flexing and extending the shoulder. To avoid any undesirable movements the lift should be performed in a slow controlled manner with appropriate resistance. The lift can also be performed using a wide variety of accessories. It is recommended to periodically change the accessory used to stimulate the muscle with new training angles.

Upper Body Resistance Training

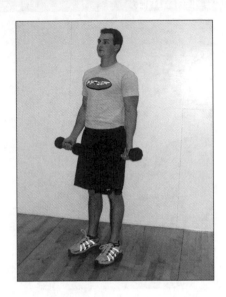 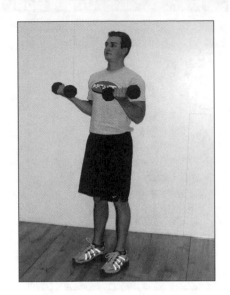

Exercise: Bicep Curls

Joint Action: Elbow flexion

Muscles Involved: Biceps brachii, brachialis, brachioradialis

Modifications: Dumbbell, barbell, cable, bands

Starting Position
Standing in an upright posture with feet shoulder width apart the client grasps a dumbbell in each hand with a supinated grip. The elbows should be extended with the humerus aligned along the mid-axillary line.

Movement Phase
The client initiates the upward movement by contracting the biceps to flex the arm. As the weight ascends the arm remains adducted and elbows remain positioned against the body. The weight ascends to full ROM without any shoulder flexion. Once full ROM is attained the resistance is slowly lowered to the starting position through extension of the elbows. The client should maintain a flat back position as the weight is lowered to the start position.

Spotting
Spotting can be effectively performed from the front of the lifter by providing assistance to the dumbbell or bar. Be sure the lifter maintains an erect posture with a neutral spine through verbal cues.

Training Considerations
It is common for lifters to use too much weight during bicep curl exercise and often "cheat" by swinging the weight. Often lifters will flex and extend the hips to generate momentum forces.

Upper Body Resistance Training

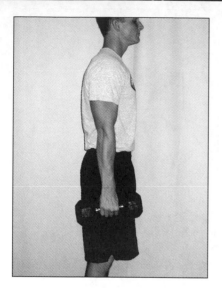 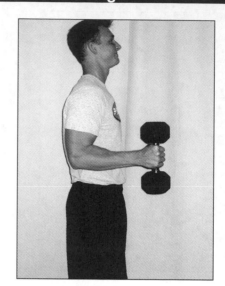

Exercise:	Hammer Bicep Curls
Joint Action:	Elbow flexion
Muscles Involved:	Biceps brachii, brachialis, brachioradialis
Modifications:	Dumbbell, cable, bands

Starting Position
Standing in an upright posture with feet shoulder width apart the client grasps a dumbbell in each hand with a neutral grip. The elbows should be extended with the humerus aligned along the mid-axillary line.

Movement Phase
With the palms facing inward, the client contracts the biceps flexing the elbows while maintaining the position of the humerus along the midaxillary line. The client should maintain a neutral hip and spinal position avoiding any forward or backward movement to generate momentum forces. The arms should be flexed to full ROM. The resistance is lowered in a controlled fashion until the elbows are extended. The client should maintain a flat back position as the weight is decelerated to the start position.

Spotting
There are numerous techniques for the bicep curl movement. The hammer curl will emphasize the forearm more than techniques that employ a supinated grip. Spotting can be effectively performed from the front of the lifter by providing assistance to the dumbbells.

Training Considerations
It is common for lifters to use too much weight during bicep curl exercises and often "cheat" by swinging the weight. Often lifters will flex and extend the hips to generate momentum forces.

Upper Body Resistance Training

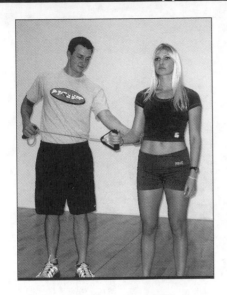
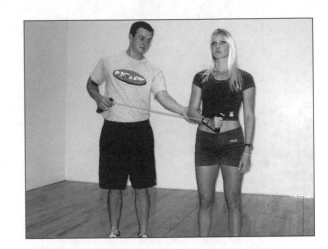

Exercise:	Internal Rotation
Joint Action:	Humeral internal rotation, elbow flexion
Muscles Involved:	Subscapularis, pectoralis major
Modifications:	Dumbbell, cable, bands performed on a physioball, bench, or standing

Starting Position

Start in an upright standing position. Adducted the shoulder and flex the arm positioning the humerus against the midaxillary line with the elbow approximately two inches lateral to the trunk. Grasp a cable or band handle using a neutral position.

Movement Phase

Maintaining the humeral position along the midaxillary line and elbow flexion, internally rotate the humerus bringing the hand to a point in front of the abdominals. Once full range of motion is attained, externally rotate the humerus back to the start position.

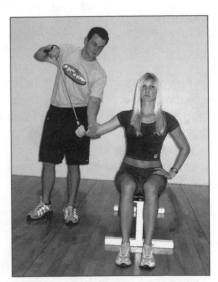

Spotting

The trainer can spot the exercise by using physical and verbal cues to ensure the humerus rotates along the midaxillary line.

Training Considerations

A common error is to employ shoulder flexion or arm extension rather than rotation. A towel can be placed in between the torso and humerus to ensure the position is maintained along the midaxillary line. If dumbbells are used the client must lie on his or her side to rotate against gravity.

**Alternative body position for
humeral internal rotation**

Upper Body Resistance Training

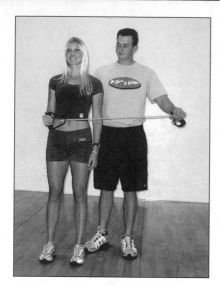 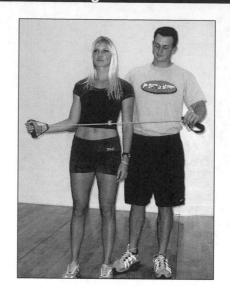

Exercise: External Rotation

Joint Action: Humeral external rotation, elbow flexion

Muscles Involved: Teres minor, infraspinatus

Modifications: Dumbbell, cable, bands performed on a physioball, bench, or standing

Starting Position
Start in an upright standing position. Adducted the shoulder and flex the arm positioning the humerus against the midaxillary line with the elbow approximately two inches lateral to the trunk. Grasp a cable or band handle using a neutral position.

Movement Phase
Maintaining the humeral position along the midaxillary line and elbow flexion, externally rotate the humerus bringing the hand to a point lateral to the trunk. Once full range of motion is attained, internally rotate the humerus back to the start position.

Spotting
The trainer can spot the exercise by using physical and verbal cues to ensure the humerus rotates along the midaxillary line.

Training Considerations
A common error is to employ shoulder extension or arm extension rather than rotation. A towel can be placed in between the torso and humerus to ensure the position is maintained along the midaxillary line. If dumbbells are used the client must lie on his or her side to rotate against gravity.

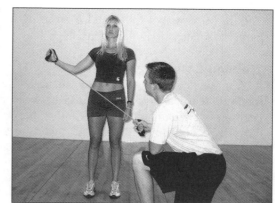

**Alternative body position for
humeral external rotation**

Lower Body Resistance Training

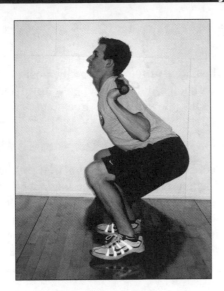 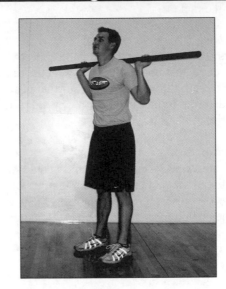

Exercise: Back Squat

Joint Action: Hip extension, knee extension

Muscles Involved: Gluteus maximus, rectus femoris, vastus lateralis, vastus intermedius, vastus medialis, biceps femoris, semimembranosus, semitendinosus

Modifications: Dumbbell, barbell, cable, bands, medicine ball performed on a stable or unstable surface

Starting Position
Prior to the performance of the exercise, the correct bar height must be established and set so that the client can safely position the bar on the traps and step clear of the bar holder (rack). To do this, the bar height should be set at approximately the height of the client's upper chest. The type of rack will determine the adjustment method.

Once the bar is set to the correct height, the client faces the bar and grasps it with a closed pronated grip. The hands should be placed slightly wider than shoulder width apart. The client then steps under the bar and positions it across the superior aspect of the scapula – on top of the trapezius. The bar should never be placed across the cervical spine. The scapula should be retracted to help provide rigidity to the upper spine.

To attain the correct starting position the client should extend the hips and knees to lift the bar off the rack. Once client has established control under load, they should position themselves away from the rack to avoid unintentional contact during the execution phase of the lift. A one to two foot clearance is all that is needed. The client's stance should be shoulders width apart with feet forward and slightly outward. The degree of outward rotation will be consistent with the stance width and natural standing gait of the individual; often dictated by hip complex anatomy.

Movement Phase
The client initiates the downward movement phase by flexing the hips, and flexing the knees. The torso should remain isometrically contracted, the head remains forward, and chest elevated as the lifter further flexes the hips and knees to continue in the descent phase. The ideal end-point ROM is the top of the thigh parallel with the floor, however this will be client specific. Flexibility limitations may cause an early posterior migration of the pelvis. Never descend beyond functional ROM or compromise ROM to increase weight. The knees should never cross the plane of the toe during any phase of the movement. Once end point ROM has been reached the client extends the knees and hips. As the weight ascends, the spinal position should be maintained, the femur should not adduct, and the hips and knees should extend at an equal rate. Upon returning to the starting position do not lock the knees – maintain a flat back position throughout the

movement. Once the designated number of repetitions has been completed, re-rack the bar checking to be sure the bar is resting safely on the rack.

Spotting

Spotting squats utilizes an upper trunk hand placement technique. The hands of the spotter should be placed on the outside of the rib cage, just under the chest with the trainer standing behind the lifter. Assume the position right at the lift off of the rack and walk the person to the starting position. The spotter should mirror the client's form and speed. When assistance is needed, the trainer should lift upward to raise the chest. This allows the hips to extend and move the client safely into an upright position.

Training Considerations

The term "squat" describes a movement and should not always reflect an externally loaded activity. The movement is one of the most functional actions a person can perform in a fitness setting regardless of the load. The movement calls upon a multitude of muscle groups requiring them to work synergistically with one another to produce the desired outcome. Whether helping an elderly person to more efficiently rise from the seated position or attempting to increase strength in a seasoned athlete, the squat exercise has application for a multitude of training populations. Note: Never place any objects under the heels of the client. It causes biomechanical shifts that place increased shear stress on the knees.

There are many common performance technique errors associated with the squat exercise. Listed below are just some of the improper techniques that fitness professionals should look for and correct.

- Knee travels out over the toes during the descent phase
- Movement is knee flexion dominant
- Weight centered over the front portion of feet
- Bar positioned too high on cervical spine
- Lumbar spine does not remain isometrically contracted
- Excess forward lean causing back extension
- Knees adduct during the onset of the concentric movement

A good way to initiate the correct squatting technique with a person who has either never performed the activity or is performing the activity incorrectly is to use a bench or box. This entails having the client stand with heels against the box. The client is instructed to push the glutes backward to initiate the movement while flexing the knees, the application of force should be focused through the heels of the client and the knees do not break the plane of the toes at any part during the movement. In many cases the client will lose stability and have to sit on the bench. Practice the movement until the client no longer loses stability. The trainer can physically cue this technique by holding on to the outstretched hand of the client during the initial skill acquisition.

Lower Body Resistance Training

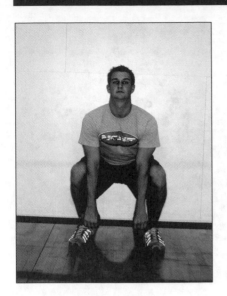 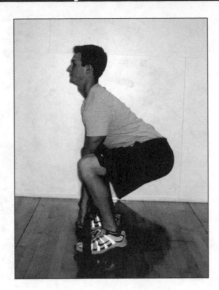 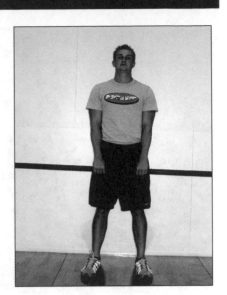

Exercise: Modified Deadlift

Joint Action: Hip extension, leg extension, back extension

Muscles Involved: Gluteus maximus, rectus femoris, vastus lateralis, vastus intermedius, vastus medialis, biceps femoris, semimembranosus, semitendinosus, erector spinae

Modifications: Barbell, dumbbell, medicine ball using one or two arms

Starting Position
The client assumes a slightly wider than shoulder width stance with the bar in front of the shins. Squatting down by flexing both the knees and hips the client should grip the bar with a closed pronated or alternating closed grip just inside the knees. The shoulders are positioned over the bar and back is set in a flat back position.

Movement Phase
The client begins the lift by elevating the chest, simultaneously extending the knees and hips. The majority of the force application should be transferred through the heels of the feet. The back must remain in a flat position as the bar is lifted from the floor. The client should extend the knees and hips until an erect standing posture is attained. The descent is made in the same plane of motion as the ascent. The client flexes the hip and knees to lower the bar in a slow controlled manner. As the bar is lowered, the back remains in a flat position. No rounding of any spinal segment should occur as injury may result. The descent is made in a slow controlled manner and the weight must not drop or bounce if floor contact is used.

Spotting
Spotting the deadlift can be performed similar to the squat technique. The spotter should stand behind the client supporting the upper torso as needed. The spotter should assume a squat position at the onset of the lift and watch for deviations in spinal alignment. To reduce the risk of back instability, mechanical advantage can be gained with a wider stance using an inside knee grip. Although modifying the lift increases leg adduction contribution, it is easier to keep a straight back position and to open the hips earlier during the movement.

Training Considerations
Like the squat, the deadlift is a very functional movement. However, it is not uncommon for individuals to perform the lift incorrectly. Common mistakes include rounding of the back, unsynchronized leg, hip, and back extension, and improper force transfer (the lifter does not push through the heels because either the resistance is too heavy or the knees are positioned in front of the toes during the initial starting position).

Lower Body Resistance Training

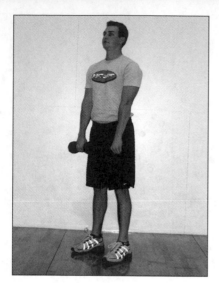
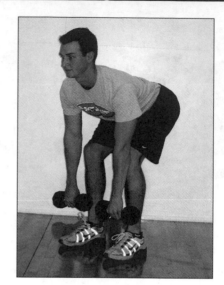

Exercise: Romanian Deadlift

Joint Action: Hip extension, back extension

Muscles Involved: Gluteus maximus, biceps femoris, semimembranosus, semitendinosus, erector spinae

Modifications: Barbell, dumbbell, cable, medicine ball using one or two arms, or one or two legs

Starting Position

The client stands in an upright posture, feet under the hips with the resistance grasped using a closed pronated or alternating grip at shoulder width and arms extended. The feet are placed hip width apart facing forward with knees slightly flexed.

Movement Phase

The client initiates the movement by flexing the hip while slightly flexing the knees. The bar descends downward with the bar held close to the body. The descent is made in a slow and controlled manner through flexion of the hips; the knees should remain in their initial flexed position. The back must remain flat as the bar is lowered until the greatest functional ROM is reached with a straight back. Hamstring flexibility will depict ROM. The hips should not drop during the descent once initially flexed. Once functional ROM has been attained, the lifter reverses the lift by elevating the chest and extending the hips. This is done through a concentric contraction of the hamstrings and glutes while the back musculature remains isometrically contracted. The knees should remain in slight flexion as the weight is returned to the start position.

Spotting

Spotting is done by verbal cueing, as this lift can cause strain in the low back if too much load is selected or the technique is performed incorrectly. The key points to make are the maintenance of a flat back, the knees slightly flexed – never locked, and the movement should be executed in a controlled manner by action of the glutes and hamstrings, not the back extensors. Do not allow the hips to descend toward the floor. The hips will travel in the sagittal plane only. Full ROM may be a few inches below the knees. Do not round the back or bend the knees further to achieve greater ROM.

Training Considerations

Many people often mistake this lift for a lower back exercise. It is true that the transversospinalis group will be innervated; however the lower back is isometrically contracted and is not the prime mover in the actual upward and downward movement. An excellent teaching cue is to tell the client to elevate the chest and "drive" the hips backward and slightly upward. Common errors are a round back, locked knees, and excessive knee flexion.

Lower Body Resistance Training

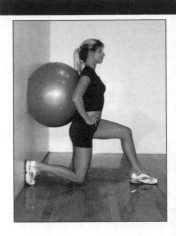 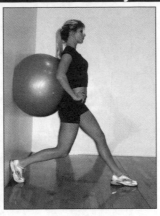 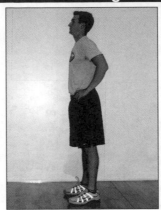 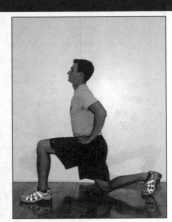

Exercise: Lunge

Joint Action: Hip extension, knee extension

Muscles Involved: Gluteus maximus, rectus femoris, vastus lateralis, vastus intermedius, vastus medialis, sartorius, biceps femoris, semimembranosus, semitendinosus

Modifications: Dumbbell, barbell, medicine ball held at different locations while static or walking

Starting Position

The client begins the movement in an erect standing posture with the hands on the hips and feet about hip width apart.

Movement Phase

The client takes a large step forward and attains balance in the split stance position. Approximately 60% of the bodyweight is transferred to the front leg with the force directed through the heel of the front foot. The knee of the front foot should be slightly flexed and the back foot should be in a dorsi flexed position with the weight on the ball of the foot. While keeping the toes pointed forward and the front foot flat on the floor, the lifter flexes the front and rear knees while simultaneously descending toward to the floor. At no time should the front knee cross the plane of the toes. The lifter descends to a point where the back knee is just above the floor. The knee should not make contact with the floor. The top of the forward leg should now be in a position parallel to the floor. Maintaining balance and an upright torso position, the lifter extends the knee of the front leg. The majority of the resistance is overcome by the extension of the front leg. The lifter must maintain balance and an upright posture as the ascent is made to the starting position.

Spotting

The spot for the lunge is managed from physical and verbal cues. The most common mechanical errors are too much movement of the front knee in the sagittal plane (excess dorsi flexion) caused by the subject not having a wide enough stance and not flexing the back knee early enough in the movement. The trainer can have the client perform the movement in a static split stance to practice the movement before making it more dynamic. To increase the intensity, the client can hold an external load or perform the movement in a different plane. To avoid excessive anterior movement the spotter should use verbal cues ensuring simultaneous knee flexion of the back leg as the lifter descends toward the floor. The movement should be controlled by early flexion of the back knee to lower the hips in the frontal plane as this will reduce excessive movement in the sagittal plane.

Training Considerations

The lunge is an excellent exercise to develop the muscles of the lower extremities. It is a compound movement that utilizes muscular action of the hip, knee, and ankle. The lunge can be performed a number of ways from stationary to walking to lateral movement with rotation. The basic mechanics of hip and knee positioning remain the same. The biggest determinant of lunge complexity is individual movement ability, particularly as it relates to balance and coordination. Do not progress to more advanced lunges until the basic stationary lunge mechanics can be performed without assistance.

Lower Body Resistance Training

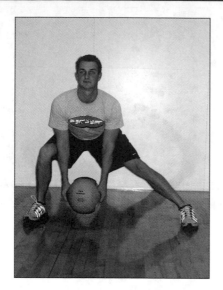 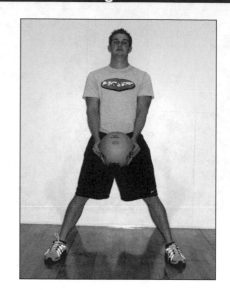

Exercise:	Lateral Lunge
Joint Action:	Hip extension, hip adduction, knee extension
Muscles Involved:	Gluteus maximus, hip adductors
Modifications:	Dumbbell, barbell, medicine ball

Starting Position
The client begins the movement in a standing upright posture with the feet positioned outside of hip width. The arm position will depend on the resistance used, but generally will fall within the base of support.

Movement Phase
The client simultaneously and unilaterally flexes the hip and knee while maintaining an upright torso position. The hip will move laterally and backward. The flexed knee will move in the frontal plane to a position above the heel of the foot. The other leg should remain extended as the body descends to a point of attainable range of motion. Once full ROM has been attained the client should ascend through the same line of motion by extending and adducting the hip. The back should remain flat throughout the movement.

Spotting
The spotting for the lateral lunge is similar to the squat or deadlift. The most common mechanical error is too much movement of the flexed knee in the frontal plane caused by the subject not having a wide enough stance and inadequate hip flexion. The trainer should always have the client perform the movement in a static wide stance to practice the movement before making it more dynamic. To increase the intensity the client can hold an external load or add upper body activity. Cueing adequate hip flexion will aid in preventing excessive frontal plane translation.

Training Considerations
The lateral lunge is very useful to encourage closed-chain movement in the frontal plane. It is a functional, compound movement that encourages muscle activation of the hip adductors above that seen in traditional sagittal plane movements. The movement, like other lunge activities, can be made more dynamic and diverse by changing the training variables.

Lower Body Resistance Training

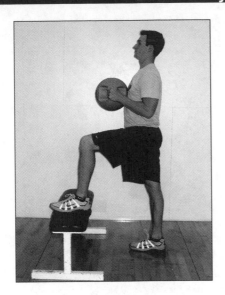 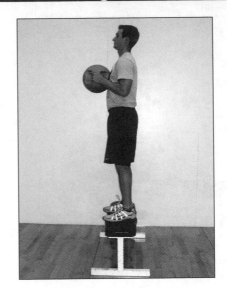

Exercise: Step-ups (with medicine ball)

Joint Action: Knee extension, hip extension

Muscles Involved: Gluteus maximus, rectus femoris, vastus lateralis, vastus intermedius, vastus medialis, sartorius, biceps femoris, semimembranosus, semitendinosus

Modifications: Barbell, dumbbell, sand bags

Starting Position
The client begins the movement by standing in front of the step, box, or bench placing one foot on the top of the step with the heel fully supported. The front knee should be flexed at approximately 90° and directly over the heel.

Movement Phase
To initiate the upward movement the client should shift the center of gravity forward bringing the chest over the top of the thigh of the flexed leg. The client extends the hip and leg on the step by applying force through the heel. The back should remain flat as the hip is extended and body elevates to a standing position on the box. Once balance is maintained, the lifter flexes the knee and slowly returns one foot to the floor. (The feet can be alternated if desired). The descent should be controlled and should follow the same path of motion as the ascent.

Training Considerations
Stepping is another very functional movement. Consistent with all the closed-chain leg movements outlined in this manual, the client's knees must not break the plane of the toes during the upward movement. This can be avoided by taking a broad step backwards and ensuring the front heel is fully on the step. Another common error is the lifter will generate force from the back leg which diminishes the role of the quadriceps and glutes of the front/top leg. This exercise can be done with barbells, dumbbells, medicine balls, or body weight and combined with any number of upper body movements. Fitness level will depict size of step, amount of resistance, as well as the total volume.

Lower Body Resistance Training

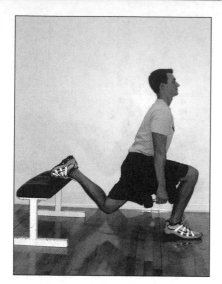 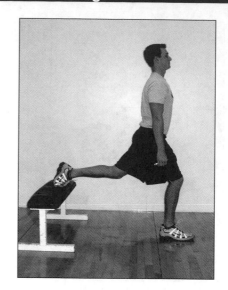

Exercise: Single-leg Squat

Joint Action: Hip extension, knee extension

Muscles Involved: Gluteus maximus, rectus femoris, vastus lateralis, vastus intermedius, vastus medialis, sartorius, biceps femoris, semimembranosus, semitendinosus

Modifications: Dumbbell, barbell, medicine ball

Starting Position

With spot assistance from the trainer the client begins the movement by placing one foot on a bench located behind the client. The front leg should be extended, with a foot position anterior to the hip. The arms should be extended at the sides of the body when dumbbells are used, but arm position may vary depending on the resistance used and balance requirements. The client's back should be flat with the head facing forward.

Movement Phase

The client initiates the movement by flexing the knee of the back leg, while flexing the hip and knee of the front leg to descend toward the floor. Approximately 70% of the bodyweight is transferred to the front leg with the force directed through the heel of the front foot. The knee of the front foot should flex directly above the heel. The back knee should be flexed until the thigh of the front leg is parallel to the floor. The body should not move anteriorly, so at no time should the front knee cross the plane of the toes. Maintaining balance and an upright torso position, the client should extend the hip and knee of the front leg.

Spotting

Spotting the single-leg squat is managed from the front or side of the client. In most cases, balance and lateral stability is the largest challenge to successful completion of the exercise. Spotting the lower rib cage will enable body control, but verbal cues and appropriate selection of resistance is equally valuable.

Training Considerations

The single-leg squat is a difficult exercise that challenges the body through increased stability requirements and mechanical disadvantage. The exercise encourages increased neuromuscular coordination, strength, and range of motion. The exercise requires adequate preparation, practice, and should only be used with suitable clients.

Lower Body Resistance Training

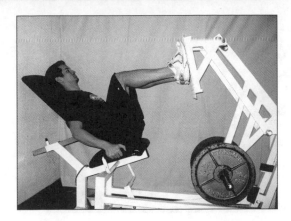 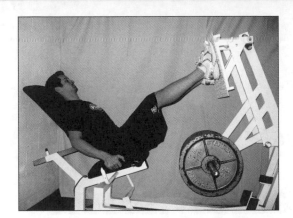

Exercise: Leg Press

Joint Action: Knee extension, hip extension

Muscles Involved: Rectus femoris, vastus lateralis, vastus intermedius, vastus medialis, sartorius, biceps femoris, gluteus maximus, semimembranosus, semitendinosus

Starting Position
The client starts with their back pressed flat against the support pad with their feet placed high on the footplate approximately shoulder width apart. The lumbar spine should be pressed firmly into the pad and the knees should be slightly flexed prior to disengaging the load from the machine.

Movement Phase
The client extends the legs slowly and disengages the weight (usually by a rotating handle). With the back pressed firmly against the back pad the weight is slowly lowered so the knees flex toward the client's chest. As the weight descends the lumbar spine and upper glutes must stay in contact with the back pad. The weight is lowered until full functional ROM has been reached. This will vary from person to person. Individual flexibility limitations within the glutes, low back, and hamstrings will depict specific endpoint ROM. At no point should the glutes rise off the back pad. Consistent with all compound leg movements, the knees should not be flexed more than 90° and at no point should the knees break the plane of the toes. Once full functional ROM has been attained or the knees have reached 90° of flexion, the client should apply additional force through the heels into the footplate and extend the legs. The ascent is continued to a point just before full knee extension. The knees are never placed into a "locked" position at any point during the execution.

Spotting
Spotting the leg press requires the trainer to stand on the side of the machine. Provide support to the movement plate at the lift off to be sure the client is ready and supporting the weight. Have them perform the repetitions while watching for controlled deceleration and smooth acceleration. If assistance is needed, supply force to the footplate and hold it at the end point while the client locks the weight into place with the handles.

Training Considerations
The leg press is a fairly simple movement, but it is easy to perform incorrectly. Common errors include incorrect foot placement (too low), pushing through the balls of the feet instead of the heels, not enough downward phase deceleration, and lifting the glutes off the pad and rounding the lower back – usually due to poor glute flexibility. Additionally, the leg press can be dangerous for individuals with high blood pressure. The combination of body compression with an elevated heart rate can more than double resting blood pressure, which increases the risk for further damage and possibly a cardiovascular incident in high risk clients.

Lower Body Resistance Training

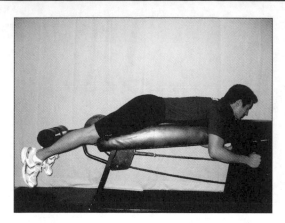 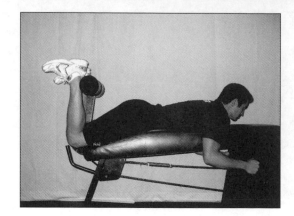

Exercise: Leg Curl

Joint Action: Knee flexion

Muscles Involved: Biceps femoris, semimembranosus, semitendinosus, gastrocnemius

Modification: Single leg or double leg

Starting Position

The client assumes a supine position on the machine. The ankles are placed behind the swing arm pad so that the pad rests against the distal aspect of the lower leg. The ankles are placed in neutral position and the legs are placed parallel to each other ensuring the axis of rotation of the knee joint lines up directly with the machine's axis of rotation.

Movement Phase

The client flexes the legs in a controlled manner by contracting the hamstring muscle group. The legs are flexed to full attainable range of motion. The ankles should remain in a neutral position during the ascent phase of the movement. Once full range of motion is attained the resistance is lowered back to the starting position in a controlled manner. The ankles should remain neutral throughout the ROM and hips should stay in contact with the machine pad. The lifter should not bounce or use momentum during any portion of ROM.

Spotting

Spotting the exercise can easily be performed by standing on the side of the machine and assisting the movement from the machine swing arm pad.

Training Considerations

The exercise can be performed with one or two legs to change the primary emphasis of the contractile force. The most common errors include excessive hip flexion, incorrect joint axis alignment, and use of limited range of motion. A quick clue that the resistance is too heavy is hip flexion upon initial exertion against the resistance.

Lower Body Resistance Training

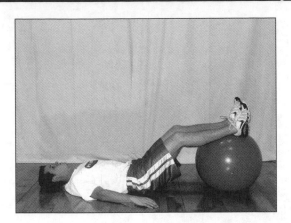 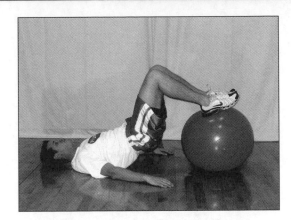

Exercise:	Physioball Leg Curl
Joint Action:	Knee flexion
Muscles Involved:	Biceps femoris, semimembranosus, semitendinosus, gastrocnemius
Modification:	Single leg or double leg

Starting Position
The client assumes a supine position on the ground with feet on the ball and arms extended at the sides of the body. A stable supine bridge position is established with the distal aspect of the lower leg on the ball. The ankles are held in a neutral position and the legs are positioned parallel to each other with a neutral pelvis and slight knee flexion.

Movement Phase
The client flexes the legs in a controlled manner by contracting the hamstring muscle group simultaneously extending the hip. The legs are flexed to full attainable range of motion while the hip is extended to maintain a neutral pelvic position. The ankles should remain in a neutral position during the ascent phase of the movement. Once full range is attained, the body is lowered back to the bridge position in a controlled manner. The ankles should remain neutral throughout the ROM and hips should remain extended.

Spotting
Spotting the exercise can easily be performed by standing in front of the ball and assisting the movement from the lateral aspect of the ball.

Training Considerations
The exercise can be performed with one or two legs to increase stability and force requirements. The most common error is not extending the hip while the knees are flexed.

Lower Body Resistance Training

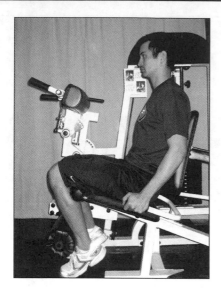 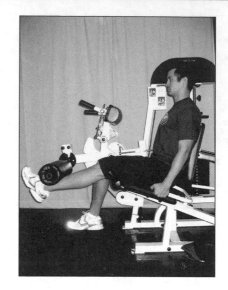

Exercise: Leg Extension

Joint Action: Knee extension

Muscles Involved: Rectus femoris, vastus lateralis, vastus intermedius, vastus medialis

Modification: Single leg or double leg

Starting position
The client assumes a seated position on the machine. The ankles are placed behind the swing arm pad so that the pad rests against the anterior portion of the lower leg. The ankles are then dorsi flexed and legs positioned parallel to each other ensuring the axis of rotation of the knee joint lines up directly with the machine's axis of rotation.

Movement phase
The client extends the legs in a controlled manner by contracting the quadriceps muscle group. The legs are extended to full range of motion. The ankles remain in a neutral position during the ascent phase of the movement. The resistance is lowered back to the starting position in a controlled manner. The ankles should remain neutral throughout the ROM. The lifter should not bounce or use momentum during any portion of ROM or allow the resistance to contact the weight stack.

Spotting

Spotting the exercise can easily be performed by standing on the side of the machine and assisting the movement from the machine swing arm pad.

Training considerations
Be sure the action is controlled and isolated, as this is the only reason to use this type of machine. The exercise can be performed with one or two legs to change the action of hip flexors and to reduce the shear forces created with the heavier weights associated with to leg lifting. Common errors include limited range of motion, incorrect joint axis alignment, use of momentum and elevation of the glutes off the pad to increase force production through leverage.

Lower Body Resistance Training

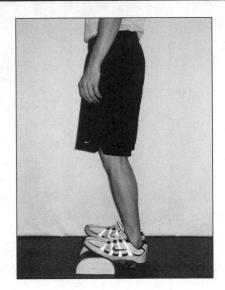 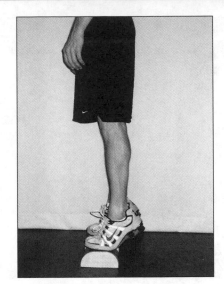

Exercise: Standing Heel Raise

Joint Action: Plantar flexion

Muscles Involved: Gastrocnemius, soleus, planaris

Modifications: Single or double leg, performed seated or standing

Starting Position
Begin movement by placing the ball of one or both feet on the elevated surface. The foot position should allow the ankles to be fully dorsi flexed. Toes should point straight ahead with knees slightly flexed.

Movement Phase
The client initiates the movement by plantar flexing the ankles. The resistance is transferred through the balls of the client's feet until the ankles are fully plantar flexed. The client should maintain slight knee flexion throughout ROM and perform the movement in a slow continuous manner. Upon reaching full plantar flexion the client should descend back to the start position by dorsi flexing the ankles using a controlled speed. Do not bounce at the bottom of the movement.

Spotting
Spotting is usually performed using verbal cues ensuring the client's knees do not lock and full ROM is achieved.

Training Considerations
The illustrated exercise is performed in a knee-extended position. In this position the gastrocnemius is emphasized over the soleus, as the soleus muscle does not cross the knee joint. If the soleus is the intended prime mover then the knee should be in a flexed position as is experienced in the seated calf raise exercise. Common mistakes to this lift include the use of ballistic movements and the lifter not moving through full functional ROM due to excessive resistance.

Lower Body Resistance Training

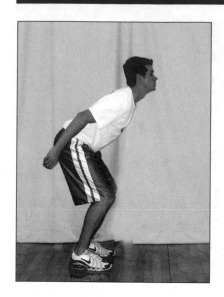 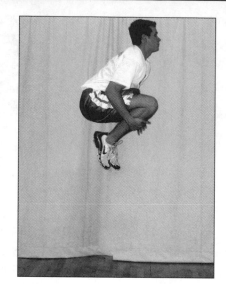 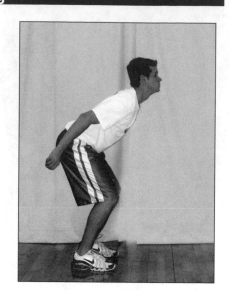

Exercise: Tuck Jumps

Joint Action: Hip extension, hip flexion, knee extension, knee flexion

Muscles Involved: Hip and knee extensors

Modifications: Single or double leg

Starting Position
The client starts in an athletic stance with hips and knees flexed. The shoulders are slightly extended with the arms partially flexed at the sides of the body. The feet should be under the hips and ankles slightly dorsi flexed.

Movement Phase
The client initiates the movement by extending the hips and knees while flexing the shoulders to jump upward. As the client fully extends to leave the ground the hips and knees should rapidly flex to attain a full tuck position at the apex of the jump. As the client begins to descend back toward the ground the hips and knees should be extended enough to create a shock absorbing position once the feet reach the ground. When the feet make contact with the ground the knees and hips should flex to absorb the impact but then immediately extend to take advantage of the stretch shortening cycle to assist in the acceleration back to the tuck position.

Spotting
The tuck jump can be spotted from behind where the trainer should stand ready to catch a client who becomes unbalanced upon the landing.

Training Considerations
The tuck jump requires adequate strength and power to be performed correctly. The landing requires significant deceleration force and should be practiced at half speed before fully attempting the exercise. Appropriate foot wear should be worn to prevent impact injuries.

Lower Body Resistance Training

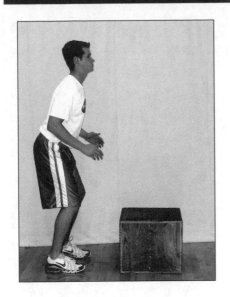 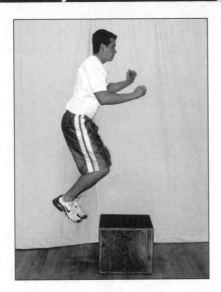 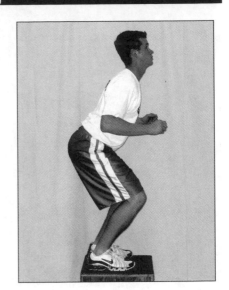

Exercise:	Box Jumps
Joint Action:	Hip extension, knee extension
Muscles Involved:	Hip and knee extensors
Modifications:	Single or Double leg

Starting Position
The client starts by standing in front of a box in an athletic stance with hips and knees flexed. The shoulders are slightly extended with the arms partially flexed at the sides of the body. The feet should be under the hips with the ankles slightly dorsi flexed.

Movement Phase
The client initiates the movement by extending the hips and knees while flexing the shoulders to jump upward. As the client fully extends and leaves the ground the hips and knees should begin to flex to increase foot height to land on the box. As the client reaches the apex of the jump the hips and knees should be flexed in a shock absorbing position. Once the feet make contact with the box the knees and hips should further flex to absorb the impact on the box. The client can then step down and re-establish the start position or jump down to rebound back upward depending on the exercise goal and relative aptitude of the client.

Spotting
Box jumps are spotted using verbal cues to help correct movement errors.

Training Considerations
Box jumps are particularly hazardous due to the object height. If the feet do not clear the box lip the client will fall and shin injury will likely occur. The landing requires significant deceleration force and should be practiced at low height before attempting higher elevations.

Lower Body Resistance Training

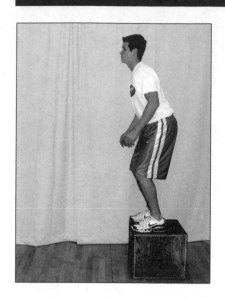 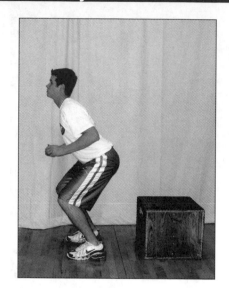 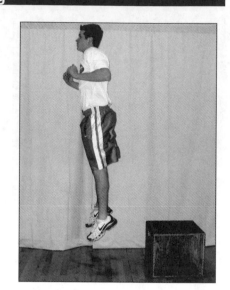

Exercise: Depth Jumps

Joint Action: Hip extension, knee extension

Muscles Involved: Hip and knee extensors

Modifications: Single or double leg with vertical, forward, or lateral jump

Starting Position
The client starts in an athletic stance atop a box or step with hips and knees flexed. The shoulders are slightly extended with the arms partially flexed at the sides of the body. The feet should be under the hips and ankles slightly dorsi flexed.

Movement Phase
The client initiates the movement by stepping off the box. Once the feet hit the ground the knees and hips should flex to absorb the impact, but then be rapidly extended while flexing the shoulders to jump upward. As the client begins to descend back toward the ground the hips and knees should be flexed enough to create a shock absorbing position once the feet reach the ground. When the feet make contact with the ground the knees and hips should flex to absorb the impact.

Spotting
The depth jump is spotted using verbal cues to control proper performance.

Training Considerations
Depth jump requires adequate strength and power to be performed correctly. The height of the box should be low to acclimate clients to the activity before higher heights are used.

Lower Body Resistance Training

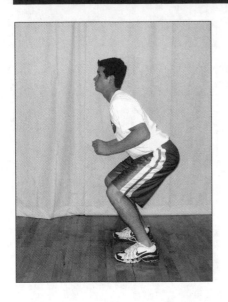 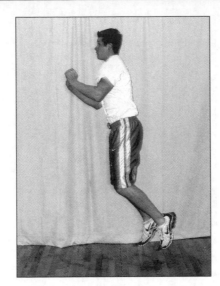 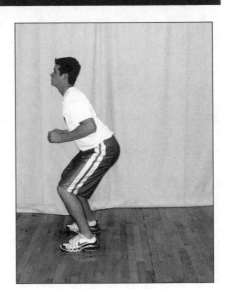

Exercise: Double Leg Bounds

Joint Action: Hip extension, knee extension

Muscles Involved: Hip and knee extensors

Modifications: Single or double leg

Starting Position
The client starts in an athletic stance with hips and knees flexed. The shoulders are slightly extended with the arms partially flexed at the sides of the body. The feet should be under the hips and ankles slightly dorsi flexed.

Movement Phase
The client initiates the movement by extending the hips and knees while flexing the shoulders to jump forward. As the client fully extends and leaves the ground the hips and knees should begin to flex at the apex of the jump. As the client begins to descend back toward the ground the hips and knees should be partially flexed in a shock absorbing position. When the feet make contact with the ground the knees and hips should flex to absorb the impact, but then immediately extend to take advantage of the stretch shortening cycle to assist in the acceleration to the next bound.

Spotting
Bounding is spotted using verbal cues to help correct movement errors.

Training Considerations
Bounding is simply repeated long jumps, but requires additional consideration due to the repeated changes in body movement at rapid speeds. The landing requires significant deceleration force and should be practiced at half speed before fully attempting the exercise. Appropriate foot wear should be worn to prevent impact injuries.

Lower Body Resistance Training

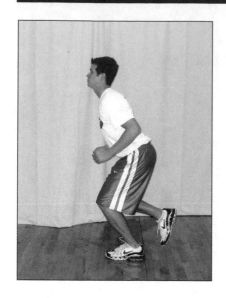 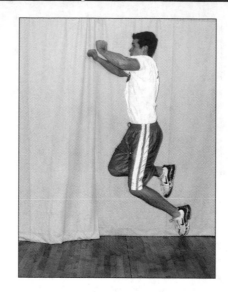 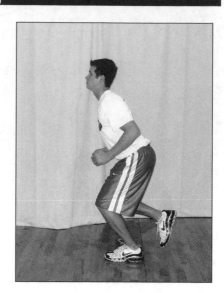

Exercise: Single Leg Bounds

Joint Action: Hip extension, knee extension

Muscles Involved: Hip and knee extensors

Modifications: Single or double leg

Starting Position
The client starts by standing on one foot in an athletic stance with hips and knees flexed. The raised leg will be slightly behind the body. The shoulders are slightly extended with the arms partially flexed at the sides of the body. The contact foot should be under the hip with the ankle slightly dorsi flexed.

Movement Phase
The client initiates the movement by extending the hips and knees while flexing the shoulders to jump forward. The suspended leg will swing through as the hips and contact leg extend to lift the client into the air. The hips and knees should begin to flex at the apex of the jump. As the client begins to descend back toward the ground, the hips and knees should be partially flexed in a shock absorbing position. Once the foot makes contact with the ground the knee and hips should flex to absorb the impact, but then immediately extend to take advantage of the stretch shortening cycle to assist in the acceleration to the next bound.

Spotting
Bounding is spotted using verbal cues to help correct movement errors.

Training Considerations
Single leg bounding is a difficult activity and requires significant preparation using single leg activities before jumping is initiated. The ankles are at particular risk for injury as the base of support is limited to one foot. Short shallow jumps should be practiced before single leg bounds are attempted.

Core Training

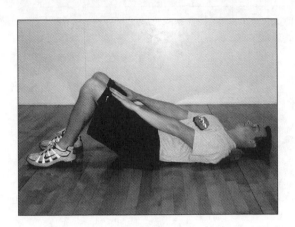 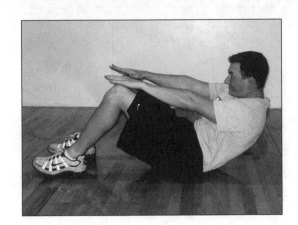

Exercise:	Abdominal Curl-up
Joint Action:	Trunk flexion
Muscles Involved:	Rectus abdominis
Modifications:	Change resistance arm length, add resistance to movement

Starting Position
The client begins the movement by lying in a supine position with knees flexed and feet flat on the floor. The arms should be extended forward with both hands placed on the thighs.

Movement Phase
The client initiates the movement by drawing in the umbilicus and posteriorly tilting the pelvis. The client flexes the abdominals as they slide their hands up the thighs to the top of the knee. Once the palms have reached the knees, or 30° of flexion has been attained, the client should descend in a controlled manner toward the starting position. The descent should last until the upper back makes contact with the ground, while the abdominals should remain contracted.

Spotting
Spotting is performed using verbal cues to ensure the client reaches full range of motion in a controlled manner.

Training Considerations
Clients commonly error by not initiating the movement using a posterior pelvic tilt, but rather emphasize hip flexor activation. Additionally, momentum forces are often used by increasing the rate of the movement and lifting the hips off the ground for mechanical advantage.

Core Training

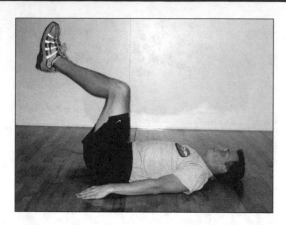 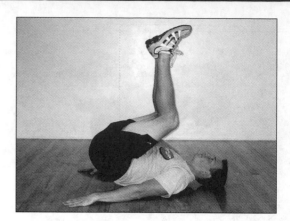

Exercise:	Reverse Abdominal Curl-up
Joint Action:	Trunk flexion
Muscles Involved:	Rectus abdominis
Modifications:	Perform on an incline or from hanging position

Starting Position
The client begins the movement by lying in a supine position with their knees and hips flexed. The arms should be extended at the sides of the body with palms facing down.

Movement Phase
The client initiates the movement by drawing in the umbilicus and posteriorly tilting the pelvis. The client flexes the abdominals pulling the glutes off the ground. The flexed knee position should remain unchanged throughout the movement. Once full range of motion has been attained the client should descend in a controlled manner. The descent phase should end once the upper glute makes contact with the ground.

Spotting
Spotting is performed using verbal cues to ensure the client reaches full range of motion in a controlled manner.

Training Considerations
The most common error during the reverse abdominal curl-up is the use of momentum from hip flexion and leg extension. Clients should be instructed to move in a controlled manner concentrating effort in the abdominal contraction and not the hip movement. The exercise can be made more difficult by performing the movement on an incline surface.

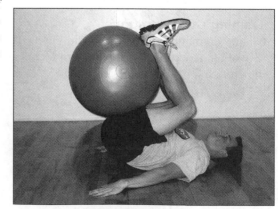

Modification to Movement:
Physioball to control lower limb joint alignment

Core Training

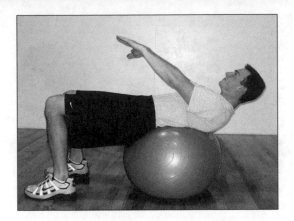
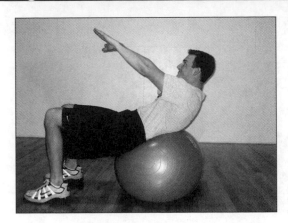

Exercise: Physioball Curl-up

Joint Action: Trunk flexion

Muscles Involved: Rectus abdominis

Modifications: Change resistance arm, add weight, use one leg

Starting Position
The client starts by lying in a supine position on a physioball with knees flexed and feet flat on the floor facing forward with the joints in alignment. The arms should be extended forward or crossed over the chest.

Movement Phase
The client initiates the movement by drawing in the umbilicus and posteriorly tilting the pelvis. The low back will push into the physioball as the client flexes the abdominals. Reaching forward further contributes to abdominal flexion when a posterior tilt is maintained. Once 30° of flexion has been attained the client should descend in a controlled manner toward the start position. The descent should last until the middle back makes contact with the ball; the abdominals should remain contracted throughout the movement.

Spotting
Spotting the abdominal curl-up on the physioball is done by managing any ball movement. Stabilizing the ball with contact makes the exercise easier and reduces the risk on falling off the ball.

Training Considerations
The physioball changes the dynamics of the movement by increasing the stability requirement and changes the starting angle due to the change in hip/shoulder relationship. The width of the feet also changes the difficulty by adding to, or reducing, the base of support.

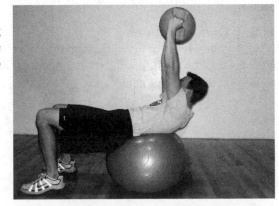

Modification to Movement:
Holding medicine ball for added resistance

Core Training

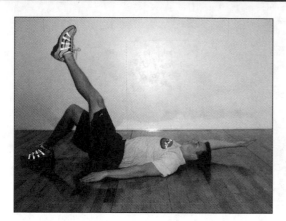 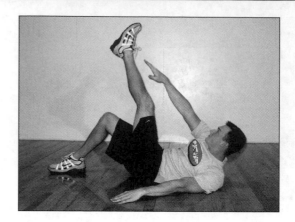

Exercise: Alternating Ankle Touches

Joint Action: Trunk flexion and rotation

Muscles Involved: Rectus abdominis, lateral obliques

Modifications: Add cable or band resistance, on Bosu

Starting Position
The client begins the movement by lying in a supine position with the hip flexed; one knee flexed with foot flat on the floor while the other leg is extended upward. The arm of the elevated leg should be extended forward next to the body while the contralateral arm is extended and abducted in a position lateral and superior to the top of the shoulder.

Movement Phase
The client initiates the movement by drawing in the umbilicus and posteriorly tilting the pelvis. The client then flexes the abdominals and rotates the spine by reaching the extended arm upward and across the body through the transverse plane toward the extended leg. Once full attainable range has been reached the client should descend in a controlled manner toward the starting position. The descent should last until the upper back makes contact with the ground, while the abdominals should remain contracted. To add further rotation to the movement the client can reach to a more lateral point outside the extended leg.

Spotting
Spotting is performed using verbal cues to ensure the client reaches full range of motion in a controlled manner.

Training Considerations
Clients commonly error by initiating the movement using an arm swing to generate momentum forces. Abdominal exercises should be controlled to prevent undesirable actions. Providing a hand target can further add to the technique by contributing to observation targeting.

Core Training

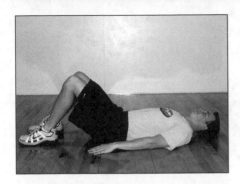 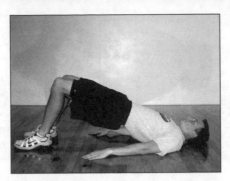 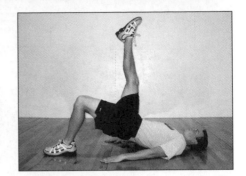

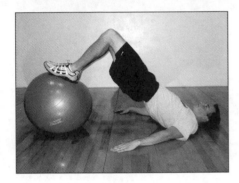 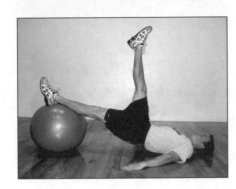 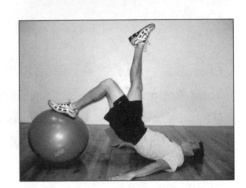

Exercise:	Floor Bridging
Joint Action:	Trunk extension, hip extension
Muscles Involved:	Back extensors, hip extensors
Modifications:	Ground, physioball, Bosu, dynadisc performed unilaterally or bi-laterally

Starting Position
The client starts by lying in a supine position with knees flexed and feet flat on the floor. The arms should be extended forward with both hands pronated on the ground.

Movement Phase
The client initiates the movement by drawing in the umbilicus and extending the hip. The client presses through the heels while contracting the glutes and low back. Once a straight hip and trunk position have been attained the client should descend in a controlled manner toward the start position without making ground contact with the glutes. The descent should last until the glutes are in close proximity to the ground; the torso should remain contracted.

Spotting
Spotting is performed using verbal cues to ensure the client reaches full range of motion in a controlled manner.

Training Considerations
Feet placement changes the emphasis of the movement. Closer feet cause more quadriceps activity, whereas wider feet increase glute mechanical advantage. The exercise can be made more difficult by performing the movement using one leg rather than two or performing the movement on a physioball or other stability device.

Core Training

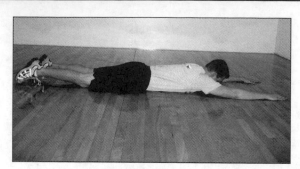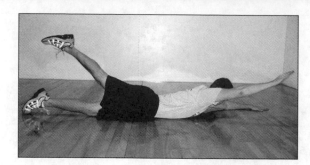

Exercise:	Opposite Raise
Joint Action:	Hip extension, trunk extension, shoulder flexion
Muscles Involved:	Gluteus maximus, back extensors, deltoids, mid-trapezius
Modification:	Floor, kneeling, physioball

Starting Position
The client begins the movement by lying in a prone position with arms extended forward in shoulder flexion while the legs lie parallel to each other in an extended position. The head should be neutral.

Movement Phase
The client initiates the movement by extending the hip of one side while flexing the shoulder of the contralateral arm and extending the trunk. The client should move their limbs through a full pain free range of motion. Once full range of motion is attained the client should return to the starting position and perform the same movement using the contralateral limbs.

Spotting
Spotting is performed using verbal cues to ensure the client reaches full range of motion in a controlled manner.

Training Considerations
The opposite raise should be performed in a slow controlled fashion with smooth transitions between contralateral movements. The exercise can be made more challenging by performing it from the kneeling position or on a physioball.

Core Training

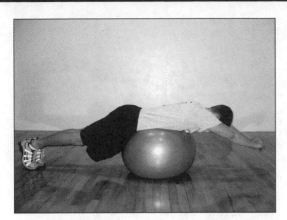 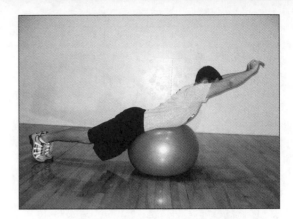

Exercise: Physioball Back Extension

Joint Action: Trunk extension, hip extension

Muscles Involved: Back extensors

Modifications: Perform on machine, use one leg or two

Starting Position
The client begins the movement by lying in a prone position on a physioball with legs extended and feet on the floor. The arms should be extended forward with shoulders flexed.

Movement Phase
The client initiates the movement by extending the trunk and hip to raise the stomach from the ball. The shoulder and arm position should be maintained or slightly exaggerated during the upward phase. Once full range of motion has been attained the client should descend in a controlled manner toward the starting position. The low back should remain contracted throughout the movement.

Spotting
Spotting can be performed by managing the ball or the client's legs.

Training Considerations
Errors with the back extension on the ball are similar to those made on the traditional machine. Commonly, momentum is used which increases risk of excessive extension which can lead to spinal disc compression. For added stability, and consequently greater range of motion, the client's feet can be pressed against a wall or manually held in place. The exercise can also be done using one unstable leg for added difficulty.

Core Training

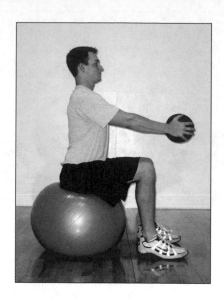 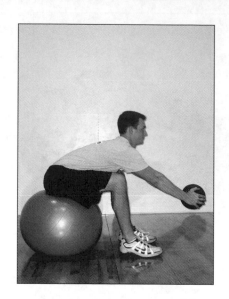

Exercise:	Medicine Ball Seated Reach
Joint Action:	Trunk extension
Muscles Involved:	Back extensors
Modifications:	Perform using one arm or two

Starting Position
The client begins by sitting on a bench or physioball with the hips slightly abducted, the knees flexed, and feet flat on the floor. The shoulders will be flexed with the arms extended forward.

Movement Phase
The client initiates the movement by flexing the hip and shoulder reaching forward and downward toward the floor. The client's back should remain flat while the hip is flexed and the arms are reached forward. Once full functional range is reached the client should extend the back and hip to return to the start position. The flat back position should be maintained throughout the movement range. The movement should be controlled and the client should not accelerate forward or bounce at the bottom of the movement.

Spotting
Spotting is performed using verbal cues to ensure the client reaches full range of motion in a controlled manner and the back remains flat.

Training Considerations
Clients commonly error by rounding the back and/or bouncing at the bottom to use momentum forces during the movement. This exercise should be performed in a controlled manner through the full range of motion.

Core Training

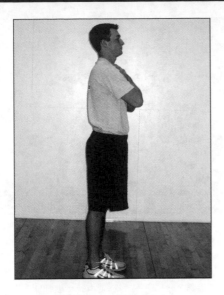
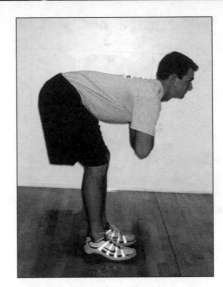

Exercise:	Goodmorning
Joint Action:	Trunk extension, hip extension
Muscles Involved:	Back extensors, hip extensors
Modifications:	Barbell, dumbbell, medicine ball, physioball

Starting Position
The client begins by standing in an upright posture with feet shoulder width apart. Arms will be crossed over the chest if no added resistance is being used. The spine and pelvis should be in neutral position.

Movement Phase
The client initiates the movement by flexing the hip and slightly flexing the knees, leaning forward and downward toward the floor. The client's back should remain flat while the hip is flexed and the shoulders slightly flexed. Once the back is parallel to the floor or full functional range is reached, the client should extend the back and hip to return to the start position. The flat back position should be maintained throughout the movement range. The movement should be controlled and the client should not accelerate downward or upward. The knees should remain fixed from the initially flexed position.

Spotting
Spotting is performed using verbal cues to ensure the client reaches full range of motion in a controlled manner and the back remains flat.

Training Considerations
Clients commonly error by flexing the knees due to hamstring tightness or rounding the back. This movement, like all low back exercises should be performed in a controlled manner through a full range of motion. To make the exercise more difficult the arms can be extended and shoulders flexed to lengthen the resistance arm.

Core Training

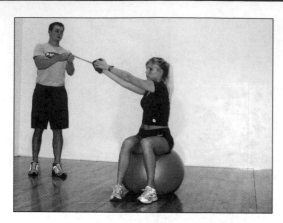 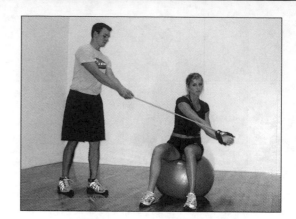

Exercise:	Seated Cable Chops
Joint Action:	Trunk rotation
Muscles Involved:	Obliques
Modifications:	Cables, medicine ball

Starting Position
The client begins by sitting on a bench or physioball with the hips slightly abducted, the knees flexed, and feet flat on the floor. The trunk will be rotated and shoulders will be flexed with the arms extended toward the line of the resistance with the resistance handle held using a neutral grip.

Movement Phase
The client initiates the movement by rotating and flexing the trunk while the shoulders slightly extend downward toward the floor. The client's back should remain flat while the trunk rotates and arms are reached forward. Once full functional range is reached the client should counter rotate back to the start position. The flat back position should be maintained throughout the movement range.

Spotting
Spotting is performed using verbal cues to ensure the client reaches full range of motion by rotating the trunk properly.

Training Considerations
Clients commonly error by moving the arms horizontally, rather than rotating the trunk to move the resistance. The shoulders should be isometrically contracted throughout the movement so the trunk serves as the prime mover.

Core Training

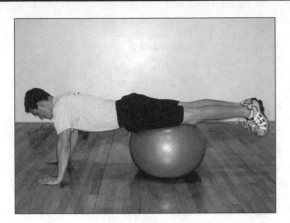 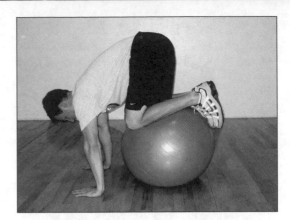

Exercise:	Physioball Roll-up
Joint Action:	Trunk flexion
Muscles Involved:	Rectus abdominis
Modifications:	Performed using one leg or two

Starting Position
Starting in a prone position on the ball the client walks the arms out into a push-up position to the point where the thighs are held in a parallel position on the ball. The torso and hips should be maintained in a neutral position with shoulders flexed and arms extended.

Movement Phase
The client initiates the movement by flexing the trunk, hips, and knees simultaneously. The client's back will round as the pelvis rolls into a posterior pelvic tilt and knees flex under the body. The physioball will roll forward toward the arms as the knees fully flex. The shoulders and arms should remain in the same position throughout the movement. Once full range of motion is attained the client should extend the trunk, hips, and knees to roll the ball back to the starting position. The back should be flat and pelvis neutral at the end position.

Spotting
Spotting is performed using verbal cues to ensure the client reaches full range of motion in a controlled manner and the back remains flat.

Training Considerations
Clients are required to maintain adequate upper body strength to hold the body in position during the exercise. Weakness or instability of the shoulders can lead to injury so clients should be screened and acclimated before attempting the exercise. Common errors occur from improper start position (knees too far forward) leading to incorrect body position and a lack of trunk flexion.

Core Training

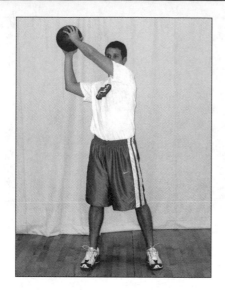 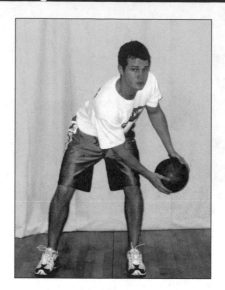

Exercise: Medicine Ball Chops

Joint Action: Trunk rotation and flexion

Muscles Involved: Obliques, rectus abdominis

Modifications: Change direction, use cables or bands

Starting Position
Standing in an upright posture with feet shoulder width apart grasp a medicine ball using a neutral grip with arms slightly flexed. Flex the shoulders, extend the hip and rotate the trunk to full range of motion. The ball should be held over the shoulder.

Movement Phase
The client initiates the movement by rotating the trunk and flexing the trunk and hips. The arms should remain in the slight flexed position as the ball moves through the transverse plane across the body toward the floor. The movement should be dominated by trunk rotation and flexion. Once the trunk is fully rotated the ball is either released to the ground or decelerated to a terminal range of motion. The client then returns to the start position in the same plane as the descent, decelerating the ball in a controlled manner at the start position.

Spotting
Spotting is performed using verbal cues to ensure the client reaches full range of motion with trunk rotation and properly decelerates the ball in a controlled manner.

Training Considerations
The medicine ball chop can be performed at different angles and even performed directly overhead into ground bounce pass activities for more sagittal work. When rotation is used the end points should be controlled so the client only moves through a safe range of motion.

Core Training

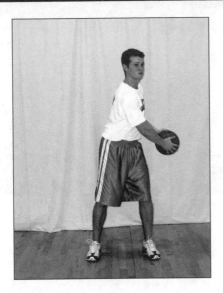
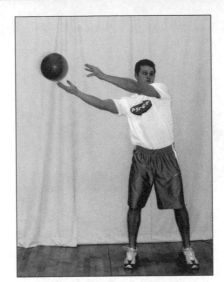

Exercise: Medicine Ball Side Pass

Joint Action: Trunk rotation

Muscles Involved: Obliques

Modifications: Change angles, stand on one or two legs

Starting Position
Standing in an upright posture with feet shoulder width apart grasp a medicine ball using a neutral grip with arms extended. Rotate the trunk to full range of motion with limited hip flexion and rotation.

Movement Phase
The client initiates the movement by rotating the trunk and extending the hips. The arms should remain extended as the ball moves through the transverse plane across the body. The movement should be dominated by trunk rotation. Once the trunk is fully rotated the ball is released to a partner who catches and rapidly returns the ball to the client readied at the release position. Upon receipt of the ball the client returns to the start position in the same plane as the throw, but decelerates the ball in a controlled manner.

Spotting
Spotting is performed using verbal cues to ensure the client reaches full range of motion with trunk rotation and properly decelerates the ball in a controlled manner.

Training Considerations
Clients often compensate lateral movement using excess horizontal shoulder action, foot movement, and hip rotation. The ball should be thrown and received in a controlled manner. If the ball is too heavy it may force a range of motion beyond the client's control and lead to injury.

Core Training

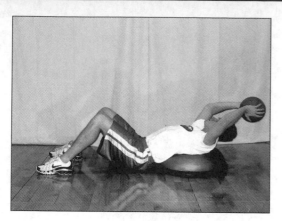
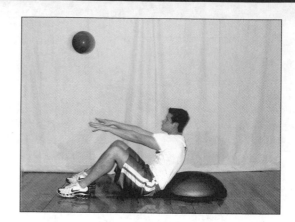

Exercise:	Medicine Ball Pullover Pass
Joint Action:	Trunk flexion, shoulder extension
Muscles Involved:	Rectus abdominis, latissimus dorsi
Modifications:	Use one or two legs on ground

Starting Position
The client lies in a supinated position on a Bosu or similar object with arms extended overhead in full shoulder flexion. The medicine ball should be held using a neutral grip. The hips and knees are flexed with feet flat on the floor.

Movement Phase
The client initiates the movement by flexing the trunk while extending the shoulders. The arms should remain extended as the ball moves through the sagittal plane over the body. The movement should be dominated by shoulder extension and trunk flexion although hip flexion will contribute to the movement. Once the trunk is fully flexed the ball is released to a partner who catches and rapidly returns the ball to the client readied at the release position. Upon receipt of the ball the client returns to the start position in the same plane as the throw, but decelerates the ball in a controlled manner maintaining abdominal contraction to avoid hyperextension.

Spotting
Spotting is performed using verbal cues to ensure the client reaches full range of motion with trunk flexion and properly decelerates the ball in a controlled manner to the start position.

Training Considerations
Ballistic activities increase the force requirement of deceleration so the ball should be returned at a controlled speed. If the ball is too heavy or thrown too hard, it may force a range of motion beyond the client's control and lead to injury. It is important to focus on the abdominal contraction so the hips do not assume the primary role.

Chapter Nineteen References

1. **Alexander NB, Galecki AT, Grenier ML, Nyquist LV, 5. Hofmeyer MR, Grunawalt JC, Medell JL and Fry-Welch D**. Task-specific resistance training to improve the ability of activities of daily living-impaired older adults to rise from a bed and from a chair. *J Am Geriatr Soc* 49: 1418-1427, 2001.

2. **Alexander NB, Galecki AT, Grenier ML, Nyquist LV, Hofmeyer MR, Grunawalt JC, Medell JL and Fry-Welch D**. Task-specific resistance training to improve the ability of activities of daily living-impaired older adults to rise from a bed and from a chair. *J Am Geriatr Soc* 49: 1418-1427, 2001.

3. **Anderson K and Behm DG**. Trunk muscle activity increases with unstable squat movements. *Can J Appl Physiol* 30: 33-45, 2005.

4. **Anderson K and Behm DG**. Trunk muscle activity increases with unstable squat movements. *Can J Appl Physiol* 30: 33-45, 2005.

5. **Baker DG and Newton RU**. An analysis of the ratio and relationship between upper body pressing and pulling strength. *J Strength Cond Res* 18: 594-598, 2004.

6. **Carson RG**. Changes in muscle coordination with training. *J Appl Physiol* 101: 1506-1513, 2006.

7. **Cotterman ML, Darby LA and Skelly WA**. Comparison of muscle force production using the Smith machine and free weights for bench press and squat exercises. *J Strength Cond Res* 19: 169-176, 2005.

8. **Davidson KL and Hubley-Kozey CL**. Trunk muscle responses to demands of an exercise progression to improve dynamic spinal stability. *Arch Phys Med Rehabil* 86: 216-223, 2005.

9. **Elphinston J and Hardman SL**. Effect of an integrated functional stability program on injury rates in an international netball squad. *J Sci Med Sport* 9: 169-176, 2006.

10. **Gentil P, Oliveira E and Bottaro M**. Time under tension and blood lactate response during four different resistance training methods. *J Physiol Anthropol* 25: 339-344, 2006.

11. **Hodges PW**. Core stability exercise in chronic low back pain. *Orthop Clin North Am* 34: 245-254, 2003.

12. **Hubley-Kozey CL and Vezina MJ**. Muscle activation during exercises to improve trunk stability in men with low back pain. *Arch Phys Med Rehabil* 83: 1100-1108, 2002.

13. **Hughes CJ, Hurd K, Jones A and Sprigle S**. Resistance properties of Thera-Band tubing during shoulder abduction exercise. *J Orthop Sports Phys Ther* 29: 413-420, 1999.

14. **Hughes CJ, Hurd K, Jones A and Sprigle S**. Resistance properties of Thera-Band tubing during shoulder abduction exercise. *J Orthop Sports Phys Ther* 29: 413-420, 1999.

15. **Kravitz L, Akalan C, Nowicki K and Kinzey SJ**. Prediction of 1 repetition maximum in high-school power lifters. *J Strength Cond Res* 17: 167-172, 2003.

16. **MacDougall JD, Tuxen D, Sale DG, Moroz JR and Sutton JR**. Arterial blood pressure response to heavy resistance exercise. *J Appl Physiol* 58: 785-790, 1985.

17. **MacDougall JD, Tuxen D, Sale DG, Moroz JR and Sutton JR**. Arterial blood pressure response to heavy resistance exercise. *J Appl Physiol* 58: 785-790, 1985.

18. **Narloch JA and Brandstater ME**. Influence of breathing technique on arterial blood pressure during heavy weight lifting. *Arch Phys Med Rehabil* 76: 457-462, 1995.

19. **Narloch JA and Brandstater ME**. Influence of breathing technique on arterial blood pressure during heavy weight lifting. *Arch Phys Med Rehabil* 76: 457-462, 1995.

20. **Page SJ, Gater DR and Bach YR**. Reconsidering the motor recovery plateau in stroke rehabilitation. *Arch Phys Med Rehabil* 85: 1377-1381, 2004.

21. **Palatini P, Mos L, Munari L, Valle F, Del Torre M, Rossi A, Varotto L, Macor F, Martina S, Pessina AC and .** Blood pressure changes during heavy-resistance exercise. *J Hypertens Suppl* 7: S72-S73, 1989.

22. **Pereira MI and Gomes PS**. Movement velocity in resistance training. *Sports Med* 33: 427-438, 2003.

23. **Reynolds JM, Gordon TJ and Robergs RA**. Prediction of one repetition maximum strength from multiple repetition maximum testing and anthropometry. *J Strength Cond Res* 20: 584-592, 2006.

24. **Reynolds JM, Gordon TJ and Robergs RA**. Prediction of one repetition maximum strength from multiple repetition maximum testing and anthropometry. *J Strength Cond Res* 20: 584-592, 2006.

25. **Stone M, Plisk S and Collins D**. Training principles: evaluation of modes and methods of resistance training--a coaching perspective. *Sports Biomech* 1: 79-103, 2002.

26. **Stone M, Plisk S and Collins D**. Training principles: evaluation of modes and methods of resistance training--a coaching perspective. *Sports Biomech* 1: 79-103, 2002.

27. **Tesch PA, Ekberg A, Lindquist DM and Trieschmann JT**. Muscle hypertrophy following 5-week resistance training using a non-gravity-dependent exercise system. *Acta Physiol Scand* 180: 89-98, 2004.

28. **Tesch PA, Ekberg A, Lindquist DM and Trieschmann JT**. Muscle hypertrophy following 5-week resistance training using a non-gravity-dependent exercise system. *Acta Physiol Scand* 180: 89-98, 2004.

29. **Wolfson L, Whipple R, Derby C, Judge J, King M, Amerman P, Schmidt J and Smyers D**. Balance and strength training in older adults: intervention gains and Tai Chi maintenance. *J Am Geriatr Soc* 44: 498-506, 1996.

Chapter 20

Functional Training Concepts

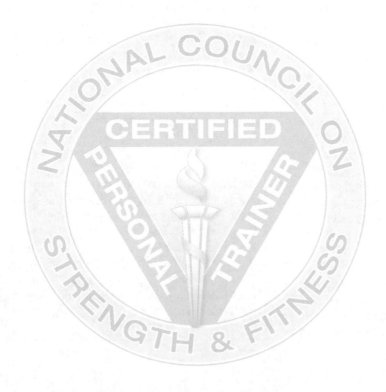

Introduction

It is often felt that the average personal training client requires improvements in endurance, strength, power, balance, speed, and coordination, but for what purpose? Earlier text suggested that all of these components of fitness are necessary to reduce the risk of functional decline, which leads to loss of independence with age. If this is, in fact, the ultimate goal of physical activity, then it makes more sense to train people to enhance their performance in everyday activities and those they enjoy participating in for recreation than to train them as weight lifters or body builders. This logic questions the traditional methods of training used in the normal gym setting. Is there a way to train people to improve in the aforementioned components that works better than the standard prescribed method? In sports training for improved performance the activities mirror totally, or in part, the sport-specific actions performed on the field. Therefore, it stands to reason that if improved human performance or function is the goal, the training should resemble wholly, or in part, the activities that are performed by the client everyday.

Defining Function

The term function is synonymous with purpose. So when function or "functionality" is applied to human movement, it suggests that the mechanical action of the body serves a specific purpose. Since normal body movements are proprioceptively integrated and multi-planar, the activities designed to make the body more functional should also meet the same description. Traditional resistance training employs movements that are isolated and often performed in a single plane of motion. These movements fail to duplicate the complex tasks that the body experiences during normal everyday activities. For instance, a person carrying a bag of groceries drops his or her house keys on the ground when attempting to unlock the front door of their house; the actions of holding the bag without spilling out the contents while bending and picking up the dropped keys cannot be modeled by a single plane resistance machine. Rather, the movement requires the neuromuscular system to account for concentric, eccentric, and isometric contractions with varying acceleration, deceleration, and stabilization (6). With the body constantly reacting to gravity, ground reaction forces, and momentum, it is important to realize that isolated or traditional resistance training does not effectively condition the central nervous system (CNS) to efficiently handle everyday movement patterns.

To accomplish better movement economy, activities should increase the requirements of the CNS, in conjunction with peripheral neural adjustments, to optimize neuromuscular control. Since a complex relationship exists between all segments of the musculoskeletal system and the central nervous system, the activities used in a **functional training** program should exploit the need for dynamic, multidimensional strength development (5). This new training paradigm, often called functional training, proposes the fundamental concept of training movements, instead of specific body parts. Functional training should enhance coordinated movements directed at a target activity. For this to be accomplished, the fitness professional must first understand what makes movement so complex.

~Quick Insight~

Proprioception

Proprioception is the unconscious perception of spatial orientation, movement, and muscular tension arising from stimuli within the body itself. The mind's awareness of the orientation of the body in space and the direction, extent, and rate of movement of the limbs depend, in part, upon information derived from sensory receptors in the joints, tendons, and muscles. Information from these receptors, called proprioceptors, is normally integrated with signals arising from vestibular receptors in the inner ear (which signal gravitational acceleration and changes in velocity of movements of the head), as well as from visual, auditory, and tactile receptors. Sensory information from certain proprioceptors, particularly those in muscles and tendons, need not reach consciousness; however, it can be used by the motor system as feedback to guide postural adjustments and control of well-practiced or semiautomatic movements, such as those involved in walking. A simple example of how the proprioception system works is when you place your hand in front of your face with your eyes closed. Though you can not visually see your hand, you mind is aware of its position in front of your face. This awareness exists because sensory organs in your muscles and tendons send signals to your brain, indicating the position and movement of the arm. When learning complicated movements, such as swinging a golf club, your body uses feedback from proprioceptors to tell the brain the exact position and angular velocity of the limbs, as well as tension in muscles of the trunk and lower extremities to maintain adequate balance and coordinate the movement, even though one is visually focused on the golf ball. For the beginner, these movements may initially feel awkward. However, after repeated drilling, the feedback from the proprioceptors aids the body in reinforcing the neuromuscular signals that control muscular contraction so that the coordinated movements can be performed without thinking.

Motor learning, from a conventional approach, involves the concept of sequential phases of learning - cognitive, associative, and autonomous. The fully developed concept suggests that attention requirements needed to perform a task are progressively reduced as motor development increases. This model contrasts with the theory that skill learning is actually a process of recall and recognition, in which motor programs are learned and stored in the nervous system. This theory implies that sensory input from physical environments is recorded as movements are performed and is then used to duplicate the neuromuscular activity when a similar physical environment or condition is experienced (10). Repeated movement patterns combined with external neuromuscular stimulus reinforce duplicable physiological responses, which enhance movement efficiency.

This theoretical discussion simply suggests that when a person performs something routinely they become proficient at it. The more proficient they become, the less focus or attention to the task is necessary to perform it gracefully. A task that was once challenging when first attempted becomes "second nature" because it requires such little attention to perform. Essentially, the body has effectively "learned" the movement. A circus clown is not born with the ability to juggle, but after doing it for a number of years, he or she becomes so proficient that he or she can juggle with different objects and engage in different movements at the same time to entertain a crowd. He or she spends little focus on the act of juggling, even though it is a very difficult task for most people. The same proficiency can be attained at any reasonable physical task, as long as it is properly instructed and adequately practiced.

Traditional Training vs. Functional Training

Traditional strength training requires a certain muscle group to produce force and move repeatedly in a single plane – as seen in a standard bicep curl or bench press. Repetitive single plane movement, under the application of load increases the specific neuromuscular action of that particular movement, explaining why the bench press weight can be increased over a training cycle. However, this simple movement pattern only improves the efficiency of the muscles used for the specific task. If the goal of the training is to bench press high amounts of weight then the training is appropriate. But what benefit does this training provide if the goal is improved function in life activities? How often does one find the need to lie on the floor and press a weighted bar off one's chest within an average day? The same question can be asked of an athlete: when are you going to need to duplicate a supine bench press in your sport? In most cases, when forward pressing occurs in sports, the load is applied asymmetrically; the body provides the stability, and the ground contact is maintained with varying stance positions. When forward pressing occurs in the average person's day, it is usually to push something into the back of an SUV or to move things back on a shelf. In both cases, the person is standing on the ground with varying amounts of hip flexion and without the back support of a bench for stability.

Movement is a complex, interdependent series of events that involves synergists, neutralizers, stabilizers, agonists and antagonists. Therefore, the training program should reflect the need to incorporate the muscles used for each of these responsibilities (5). This suggests that, instead of isolating muscles and movements during traditional weight training, integrating coordinated movement patterns better teaches the CNS to orchestrate acceleration, deceleration, and stability to accomplish a real life movement efficiently (8). By forcing a synchronicity between the neuromuscular system and the musculoskeletal system, the movements become more fluid and provide greater economy when the body encounters similar situations during sports, activity, and everyday life. Cases in point, which machines do you use to train for bowling, water skiing, or doing the laundry?

Training for human function is a relatively new training paradigm that offers alternatives to machine-dominated resistance training, using the traditional training principles because functional training integrates the need for additional physiological support mechanisms (4, 9). The focus shifts from training a single muscle or muscle group to training movements designed to target a specific activity or desired outcome. For instance, the seated dumbbell press and box step-ups are used routinely in traditional programs for shoulder and leg strength. Both are in a single plane of movement. Applying the functional concept, multi-planar movements and increasing stability can be created by performing a lateral box step-up with a single arm overhead dumbbell press. Combining activities and loading the body asymmetrically addresses numerous factors that challenge the body in ways the use of the traditional methods can not.

Employing functional based training allows the trainer to elicit physiological adaptations from varied environments and modified movements, as well as promotes an increased neural response from the activity. Ideally, the program activities are aimed at a carry-over response for enhanced performance and functionality in everyday activities. Performing a squat with a low to high medicine ball twist may produce a similar movement to picking up a laundry basket full of clothes and placing it on the dryer. Step-ups with an asymmetrical and laterally held medicine ball duplicate carrying a child in one arm while going up the stairs. It is all a matter of identifying the challenges of life or a select activity and duplicating the difficulties the activities present in an exercise routine.

In most cases, traditional strength training is combined with some added complexity. The different resistance modalities used in function-based training still require force production for increased muscular strength, but extend beyond the isolated contraction to cause proprioception and muscle recruitment from additional areas of the body. A good example would be a standing, single-leg chest press, using a cable machine for resistance. A movement such as this encourages total body muscle activity via a small base of support, kinetic transfer of energy through the tibia, trunk stabilization and asymmetrical force application, rather than just externally stabilized force production exerted by the **pectoralis major**, **anterior deltoids**, and triceps, as seen in a seated machine press. The forward press becomes increasingly challenging when the other difficult tasks are applied simultaneously.

The resistance applied to each movement can be as diverse as the movements themselves. As mentioned earlier, skill acquisition for new movements and less stable environments is often best applied using only body weight. New training techniques or previously mastered movements executed in an unfamiliar environment should be performed with the focus on proper movement technique rather than heavy resistance. The body must develop neuromuscular efficiency to balance and coordinate fluid movement before additional resistance can be applied safely and effectively. A natural continuum exists which requires proper progressions from the simple static maintenance of position to increased movement complexity under greater resistive loads. For example, before the single leg cable chest press can be introduced, the client must first become proficient at chest pressing with a cable and also be trained at standing on one leg. When the two acts are combined, the focus shifts from performing one task to performing two tasks simultaneously. If neither task has adequate efficiency, the movement technique is compromised.

The body uses its proprioceptors to control muscle contractions, which create the tension in the muscle and connected structures required to prevent undesirable action. For instance, standing on a single leg requires balance so that one does not fall over. Muscle contractions within the leg, hip, and trunk allow an erect posture to be maintained while standing on one foot.

These contractions are obviously different in specific tension development from those needed to stand on two feet. Whether sitting on a physioball or performing an asymmetrical press, each position requires proprioceptors to help stabilize the body. When a person first attempts to balance on one foot, the body often sways back and forth as the proprioceptors attempt to communicate the proper balance of muscle tension medially, laterally, anteriorly, and posteriorly. The faster the body commands harmonious tension, the more rapidly a person becomes balanced.

Stability in all three planes stems from trunk muscle activation. The responsibilities of the trunk musculature extend beyond the basic actions of trunk flexion, rotation, and the intra-abdominal pressure control associated with conventional abdominal training (5). This group of muscles finds additional responsibility once the movement switches from single plane activity to a multi-planar movement. Take the laundry example, for instance; bending over and rotating the spine to pick-up a basket of clothes that sits in lateral proximity to the body requires numerous trunk actions. First, the muscles must contract to rotate the trunk to the desired position to be able to grab the basket; next, the internal trunk musculature must stabilize the spine to transfer ground reaction force up through the kinetic chain to initiate the lift through the legs, and then counter rotate and extend the trunk while still maintaining spinal stability to exert prime mover force of the upper body to raise the basket up to the top of the dryer.

In a **closed kinetic chain**, the trunk muscles must act to stabilize activities in all three planes of movement. They function synergistically to eccentrically decelerate trunk extension and rotation, while combining with the lumbo-pelvic hip complex to produce dynamic force. Other force couples act to accelerate, decelerate, and counter force agents so that movements can be performed without undesired interference (10). The complex interrelationship of the trunk and hip enables synergistically accomplished movements in a controlled fashion, such as described in the example.

This fact is extremely relevant when additional force production is considered. Before extremity strength can be developed, it is necessary to understand how the body's musculoskeletal system is linked. Although squatting is basically leg and hip extension, the support mechanism of the trunk necessitates strong core musculature to stabilize the spine, allowing the resistance to be controlled by the prime movers. If the connecting bridge between peripheral movements is weak, then optimal strength cannot be developed because the middle will give way to the external stress. Simply put, "you are only as strong as your weakest link." Increased trunk stabilization properties allow for the transfer of energy from the ground to the active prime movers of the upper body. The bar-loaded back squat exemplifies the need for stability in the trunk to support the top loaded weight; if it does not, the body will cave into flexion during the lift and the leg pressing action cannot be effectively performed. The ability to apply hip extension to weights held on the shoulder requires a fused, isometrically contracted system, so when the hips and legs provide vertical acceleration force, the stable **axial skeleton** also accelerates at the same rate pushing the weight upward. This is true for all top-loaded exercises. A standing military press, for instance, often necessitates less resistance than the seated military press due to the trunk stabilization requirements. When seated, the back support and reduced lower and central body stabilization requirements allow for more resistance to be applied upward. In the standing version, ground reaction force is lost along the kinetic chain where the stabilizers are not efficient, so the potential force is lost before it can be transferred to the bar. Power athletes, body builders, and older adults alike can all benefit from improved stabilization properties within the body, particularly during closed-chain erect posture movements. The better the body can stabilize its motion segments, the better it can transfer force.

Key Terms

Functional training – Training targeted at enhancing coordinated movements specifically designed at improving function in activity necessary for everyday living.

Motor learning – A series of sequential phases (cognitive, associative, and autonomous) involved in learning to perform a movement task in response to a given stimulus.

Synergists – The name given to a muscle which assists in performing the same joint movement as the agonist.

Pectoralis major – The large muscle connecting the anterior aspect of the chest with the shoulder and upper arm.

Anterior deltoid – The muscle of the anterior part of the shoulder connecting from the anterior border of the clavicle to the lateral aspect of the humerus.

Closed kinetic chain – Energy transferred through the tibia from a fixed distal position.

Axial skeleton – The bones of the skeleton including the skull, spinal column, sternum and rib cage.

A strong core foundation is also essential for actions that require movement with simultaneous changes in the center of gravity or force shifts from one position to another. This is particularly true when the body is required to stabilize the center of gravity over the changing base of support. This situation can be illustrated by shifting a bag of groceries from one carrying arm to the other under a normal gait cycle or carrying a box up a flight of stairs. When a new center of gravity is established, the body must stabilize this shift or the movement will fail. This may mean dropping the object to prevent a fall, or in some cases, the body can completely lose stability and yield to gravity. The core musculature is central to activities performed for enhanced functionality.

Functional training under these parameters expands training philosophies beyond the traditional exercise approach. For the fitness professional, functional training integrated into a personal training regimen provides answers for many of the concerns facing today's clients. A lack of neuromuscular coordination results in compromised movement patterns and contributes to muscle imbalances which can lead to injury. In addition, and because normal movements are predominantly asymmetrical or one side dominant, using single plane muscle isolation activities to maximize strength does little to serve the physical training needs of most people (9). Fitness professionals need to recognize what activities will best elicit improvements in total health and functionality in their clients. Functional training works for all populations because the training enhances the performance of everyday actions and also expands the potential for improved performance in all activities.

Functional training provides a wide-ranging spectrum of exercise and movement options. Many new modalities have been developed to exploit the concept of movement with purpose. Physioballs, resistance bands and tubing, and specialized stability devices join the more traditional medicine ball and dumbbells as training equipment for movement enhancement. Each provides unique benefits in a well-planned training regimen. This is not to suggest that all other resistance tools have become obsolete but rather reflects the idea that a continuum exists between absolute scores of fitness and functional health for optimal quality of life. The graphs below represent the training responses from machine, free weight, and functional resistance modalities, respectively.

Training Responses

Functional vs Single Plane

Single plane stabilization

Functional training

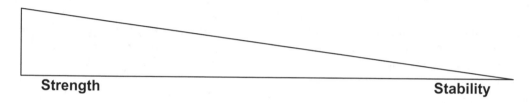

Strength / **Hypertrophy**

Coordination / **Stability**

The above diagram represents the training response focus between the two training paradigms. While single plane stabilization training maximizes single plane strength and hypertrophy, functional training, by design, is employed to enhance stabilization and multi-planar function.

Resistance Machines

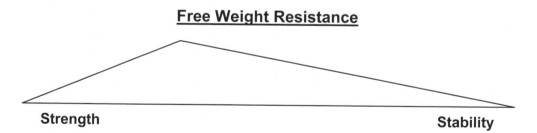

Strength

Stability

The above diagram demonstrates the relationship between stability and machine training. Machine movements are typically performed in a single plane of motion and require little to no respective joint stabilization to execute the movement pattern. This is due to the "fixed" plane of motion that accompanies most resistance training machines.

Free Weight Resistance

Strength

Stability

The above diagram demonstrates that there is a closer relationship between strength and stabilization when free weight resistance is used. This can be attributed to the increased neuromuscular control requirements of free weight training. However, typical free weight resistance training is generally performed in a single plane of motion, and once motor control has been accomplished the contribution from respective joint stabilizers diminishes.

Functional Resistance

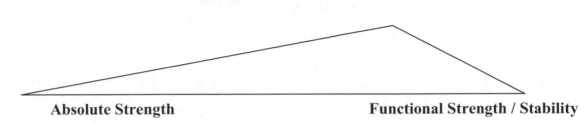

Absolute Strength   Functional Strength / Stability

The above diagram shows the different relationship between absolute strength and functional strength. This can best be exemplified by a power lifter and a lumberjack. The nature of the two physical tasks draws on separate components of functionality. While the power lifter may be able to lift a lot of weight a single time, he or she may not be able to optimally perform the daily physical requirements of a lumberjack, who must possess strength and endurance in multiple planes under asymmetrically loaded conditions.

Exercise Selection

Proprioception can be enhanced further using new movement patterns, changing sequences, adding less stable environments or postures, and even combining instability with asymmetrically resisted movements. Infinite movement combinations can be created from just a few categories. They include, but are not limited to, conventional resistance training movements, ballistic resistance training movements, stability training movements, multi-planar movements, and asymmetrical movements. Each holds merit as a single stress to the body but offers increasing benefits with categorical synergy when combined.

Exercise selection for function is based on the same factors as traditional resistance training; the only differences are the neuromuscular progressions (complexity of the movement) and a general understanding of two continuums: safety/effectiveness and stable-single plane/unstable-multi-planar. Almost any combination of categories can be used to transition from isolated to integrated training. The most important aspect of the programming is that the exercises be combined in the proper progression, accounting for proficiency and safety. As with any professionally developed exercise program, the modalities and techniques employed should be based on sensible evaluation criteria. It doesn't make sense to utilize activities just because they exist but rather to select exercises that reflect the desired response for an individual client. Ideally, the program components should have a high degree of carryover to the target activity or goal.

Exercise Variations

Traditional	Hybrid	Functional
Bench press	Bench press on ball	Bench push-up with feet on ball
Squat	Asymmetrically loaded squat	Lateral asymmetrical cable squat
Romanian deadlift	Single arm deadlift	Single arm/single leg deadlift
Seated shoulder press	Single arm standing press	Walking lunge w/SA shoulder press
Seated row	Standing single arm cable row	SA cable row with reverse lunge
Ab flexion	Ab flexion on ball	SL ab flexion on ball
Back extension	Back extension on ball	Single leg good morning w/MB
	SA=Single Arm SL=Single Leg	

Programming Considerations

The decision to incorporate functional exercises into a fitness training regimen requires forethought and design so that the activities complement the system of training with a focus on a goal-oriented response. Too often, exercise selection is based on convenience, or on "what's new," which does not lend itself well to the preset progressive design model. Programming decisions should first analyze what was found from a needs assessment. Secondly, the fitness professional should identify factors that may limit goal attainment or present obstacles for later improvements. Thirdly, the programming concept should be holistic in nature but goal-oriented by design. This means incorporating regular activities for each of the health-related components of fitness, while implementing a periodized approach to the goals of the client. This basic program model is further complicated when the decision for functional integration is introduced. Questions of: "When do I do it?", "How does it fit in?", and "Will it take away from tangible results?" often arise as fitness professionals are faced with limited time and a wide assortment of exercise modalities.

Functional training can easily be integrated into any program, as long as the fitness professional understands the function of the exercise and the demands it requires for proper performance. In many cases, the functional activity modifies a conventional movement, so rather than replace an existing exercise, it expands the range of effectiveness. As previously mentioned, once a client has mastered a particular movement, the activity can be advanced to provide more difficulty in completing it. This is not to suggest that the leg press can never be performed or traditional exercises aimed at hypertrophy are all replaced with unstable, multi-planar movements but rather that activities that incorporate a functional approach improve the performance of movements. Look at these common examples of how functionality can be put into practice by just modifying a few variables.

When programmed into an exercise session, functional-based activities can be integrated with other exercises. Program order should reflect the difficulty of the movement and consider the effects of fatigue on stabilization. In most cases, the traditional order of operations remains consistent. In general, larger muscle group exercises should precede smaller muscle group exercises, and less stable, more complex movements should precede simple, more stable ones. The following program is just one example of how functional activities can be added to a traditional program.

Traditional Program with Functional Activities	
Back squat	12, 10 ,10
Chest press on a physioball	3 x 12
Step-up with single arm overhead press	2 x 8 per side
Modified pull-up w/feet on stability disc	3 x10
Walking lunge with trunk rotation	3 x 6 per side
Front raise superset with rear delt band pull	2 x 15 each
Lateral asymmetrical squat walks up and back	3 x 20 feet
Closed chain single arm cable row	2 x 12
Tricep kickback with theraband	3 x 10
Single leg abdominal curl-up on ball	2 x 12
Bicep curl superset with calf raises	3 x 12
Opposite raise	3 x 12

The resistance used for each exercise will vary according to the neuromuscular demands of the stability and the complexity of the action. If strength and power are desired outcomes of the exercise, then the traditional formats, including intensity and set-repetition schemes should be used. On the other hand, if neuromuscular coordination and balance are the goal, more functional exercises should be emphasized. This allows a single exercise bout to address numerous variables as defined within the needs analysis. Essentially, the basic guide is logic. If it doesn't make sense, it should not be included. If the movement patterns become faulty, exchange the complexity for an easier movement, increase stability or reduce the resistance. Again, exercise proficiency is necessary before adding any new stress.

Increasing the Functionality of Common Exercises	
Standing cable torso twist	Cable torso twist in isometric lunge stance
Push-up on floor	Push-up with hands on physioball
Forward lunge	Forward lunge with diagonal MB chop
Bench press	Single arm alternating press on physioball
Back squat	Overhead squat on stability discs
High row	Modified pull up with feet on ball
Low row	Single leg/single arm band row
Leg curls	Supine leg curls w/feet on physioball
Side lateral raise	Single arm/single leg asymmetrical raise

Stability Considerations

A fitness professional can select a variety of tools when incorporating a stability component into a client's workout; however, the client must be able to perform the activity with proper mechanics in a stable environment prior to utilizing a destabilization modality. For example, a client must be able to properly execute a stationary lunge with proper proficiency before using a stability disk under one foot. The rule applies to all forms of stability activities. Begin with stable, single-plane movement and progress to unstable, multi-planar movements. Taking small steps in a progressive manner allows the body to adapt to the new training stimuli while maintaining the integrity of the movement.

Stability Progression

1. Standing cable press
2. Standing cable press one arm
3. Standing cable press one leg
4. Standing cable press one arm, one leg
5. Standing cable press on Bosu or balance disc
6. Standing cable press one arm on Bosu
7. Standing cable press one leg on Bosu
8. Standing cable press one arm one leg on Bosu

Multi-task or Multiplanar

Using the previous example, the press can also be performed in conjunction with any number of other exercises. For example, when combining the cable press with a forward lunge, the movement becomes more neuromuscularly challenging. To further add to complexity, the press can be done with one arm, causing asymmetrical loading while lunging. If more stability is required the lunge can be performed on a stability disc. Combining planes of movement can also be used to create more neuromuscular difficulty. Performing the lunge with high to low cable rotation employs the sagittal and transverse planes simultaneously. The combination of planar movements increases the proprioception and stability requirements throughout the body.

Example of Increasing Neuromuscular Difficulty

1. Walking forward lunge
2. Walking forward lunge with trunk rotation
3. Walking forward lunge with high to low alternating diagonal chop
4. Reverse lunge with trunk rotation
5. Reverse lunge with high to low alternating diagonal chop

Types of Resistance

Consistent with all forms of resistance training, the resistance used must meet the specific goals of the client and must also best match his or her abilities. General skill acquisition principles apply before progressing to different forms of resistance. The type of resistance used may make the exercise easier or more difficult, depending on the characteristics of the movement. Bands, balls, cables, dumbbells, and gravity all hold merit within a program but should be evaluated on a case-by-case basis. Bands offer increasing and decreasing resistance based on the lengthening-elastic properties and can be used in any direction, independent of gravity, to provide resistance. Cables provide the same variation of resistance angle, yet the resistance remains constant throughout the range of motion. Dumbbells and medicine balls use gravity and therefore, reduce lateral pull unless asymmetrically loaded. Even barbells and body bars can be used asymmetrically for greater resistance and stability requirements, which are increased due to the long length of the bars. The exercise selection and number of repetitions performed will often dictate the appropriateness of the resistance. Higher intensity lifts require stable movements; as stability decreases, resistance should decrease proportionately. There comes a point when an activity has reached its safety/effectiveness limitation and adding more resistance becomes undesirable. Making responsible program decisions is necessary to maintain safety while implementing exercise progressions.

Example of Increasing Training Resistance

1. Box step-up
2. Box step-up with two dumbbells
3. Box step-up with single dumbbell
4. Box step-up with asymmetrical medicine ball loaded on the shoulder
5. Box Step-up with medicine ball front pass

Range of Motion

The client's functional ROM and his or her ability to adhere to proper technique throughout the activity should determine the movement range of the exercise. The first rule of thumb is to lessen the resistance if the desired ROM is not attained. In some cases, the non-traditional movements identify flexibility limitations and muscle imbalances. If flexibility limits proper technique, the exercise should either be exchanged for a different movement or performed within the limited functional range. Flexibility is a factor of the range of motion attained during physical activity. Therefore, encouraging exercises in uncommon planes of movements may enhance ROM, particularly when complemented by a comprehensive flexibility program used in conjunction with the resistance training program.

Velocity

Velocity has particular relevance and application when using complex movements and ballistic activities. Throws can be performed in any number of ways and directions to incorporate a wide variety of force couples in the trunk and **appendicular musculature**. The intensity of the activity can be easily manipulated by adjusting the speed of movement or weight of the ball. The standing medicine ball chest pass, for instance, can be a relatively high intensity activity when requiring the user to produce maximum force and velocity, or it can be of relatively low intensity when only working on coordination and dynamic ROM. The speed of the movement should comply with the desired outcome and allow for proper movement execution. If the speed causes incorrect movement patterns, it should be reduced.

Sets and Reps

The number of sets and reps used in functional training will be client and goal specific. In some exercises, the client may have difficulty executing the movement, so repetitions should be designed around skill acquisition. As the client improves, total training volume and exercise intensity can be increased. The evaluation of exercise execution during multiple sets and the performance of higher repetition schemes will determine the time and the quantity of any subsequent increases in difficulty.

Equipment Considerations

Each piece of exercise equipment designed to enhance functionality works to move the body from stabilized single-plane training into less stable multi-plane environments. Therefore, the equipment selected should reflect this goal. The ideal piece of training equipment for functionally-based training combines resistance with a high proprioceptive demand. This can only be accomplished if receptors in the joints and muscles

---

Functional Training Program Recommendations (9)

- *Programming* – Use a holistic approach with sound training principles applied to goal attainment.

- *Focus* – Concentrate on the desired outcome with a balance of the safety/effectiveness continuum.

- *Progressions* – Analyze all physiological considerations before deciding on the direction and rate of progress. Use appropriate levels of training for each phase of training.

- *Skill acquisition* – Only utilize an external load after central nervous system proprioception feedback develops successful stabilizing patterns used for postural equilibrium. Act on system and joint stabilization.

- *Multiplanar* – As progress is made, attempt to engage all three planes simultaneously.

- *Move in 360 degrees* - Identify the role of gravity, momentum, and ground reaction forces and attempt to incorporate activities which exploit their benefits.

- *Velocity specific* – Once the movement becomes efficient, attempt to mimic the speed of the activity being trained for.

- *Activity specific* – Rehearse the activity within progressively different environments and conditions.

- *Balance* – Incorporate unstable environments to increase proprioception and develop improved functional strength.

- *Multijoint* – Follow the kinetic chain sequence of the movement to cause all joints to function synergistically.

- *Integrated exercise* – Combine muscle systems and movements for neuromuscular efficiency and fluid movement performance.

- *Diversify* – Make exercise selections based on outcome specific response; this may require a combination of traditional training, functional training, and general conditioning all in the same workout.

experience neuro-challenging stimuli, which generally suggests multi-planar instability. The neuromuscular control feedback develops movement efficiency, as muscles and nerves adjust to the demands and establish postural equilibrium. Stability requirements change based on the contact surface, direction of resistive force, asymmetrical loading, and tendency of an object to move. Other considerations for stability and neuromuscular control are variations in resistive tension and changes in the center of gravity of a moving object. Equipment that can present these challenges is ideal for functional training. Some common pieces of functional equipment include physioballs, foam rollers, cables, rubber bands and tubing, and a variety of medicine balls.

Key Terms

Appendicular musculature – The primary musculature of the arms and legs.

Examples of Functional Based Training Movements

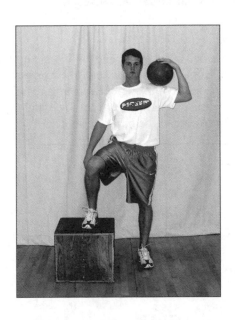
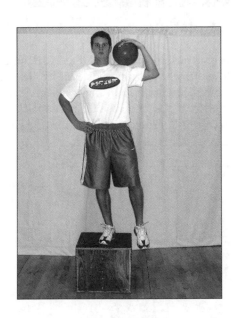

Asymmetrical Step-up

Start with one foot centered on the box, with the hip and knee flexed to approximately 90 degrees; the other leg will be located lateral to the box and under the hip. Hold a medicine ball or similarly weighted object over the outside shoulder. Step-up by extending and adducting the hip while extending the knee; the spine should remain in neutral position. Once the hip and knee are fully extended descend back to the start position. The back should remain flat during the entire movement. The speed of the movement will vary based on the objective of the exercise.

Examples of Functional Based Training Movements Continued

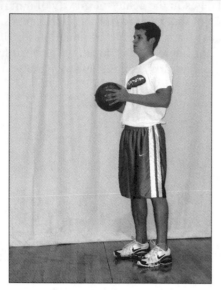 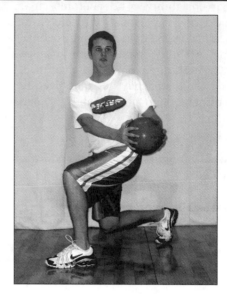

Lunge with Rotation

Start in an upright posture with feet under the hips holding a medicine ball at chest height with a neutral grip, arms flexed. Step forward into a lunge position by flexing the knee and hip. Simultaneously extend the arms and rotate the trunk moving the medicine ball in the transverse plane to a position outside the hip; the back should remain flat. Once full range of motion is reached counter rotate back to the start position while extending the front knee and hip. Once the start position has been reached repeat the movement to the same side or alternate to the opposite side.

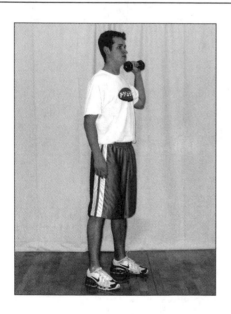 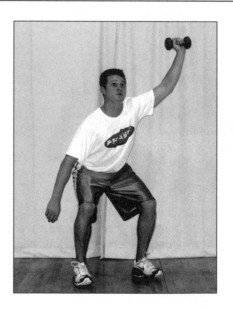

Overhead Asymmetrical Squat

Standing in an upright posture with feet at shoulder width, grasp a dumbbell in one hand and hold it just above the shoulder with a flexed arm position. Descend into a squat position by flexing the hips and knees while keeping the back straight. As the descent is initiated press the dumbbell over head by abducting the shoulder and fully extending the arm. The opposite arm should remain at the side of the body. Once a full squat position has been attained extend the knees and hips to return to the start position with the arm extended overhead. Bring the resistance back down to the initial position and repeat the movement. Latissimus dorsi flexibility is a factor in this movement which may cause the resistance to migrate into the sagittal plane.

Examples of Functional Based Training Movements Continued

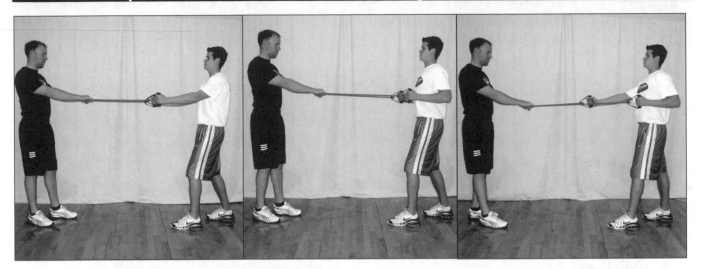

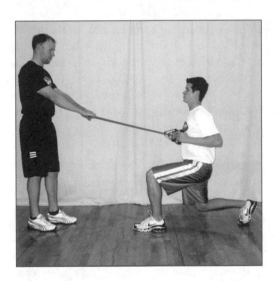
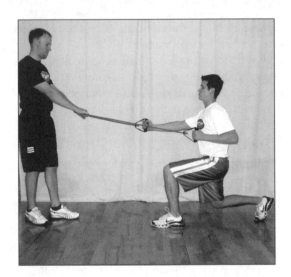

Band Row Sequence

Start in a split stance position holding the band handles with the arms extended and shoulders horizontally adducted at chest height. Initiate the movement by retracting the scapula and flexing the arms while horizontally abducting and extending the shoulder. The back should remain flat with the abdominals isometrically contracted. Return to the start position in a controlled manner moving through the same plane of motion. Once proficiency has been established the exercise can be advanced by alternating rows and asymmetrically loading the movement. To increase the complexity, the exercise can be performed while stepping backward into a reverse lunge position. The movement is initiated with a backward step. As the knees and hip flex the shoulders are horizontally abducted and extended while the scapula retracts and arms flex in a fluid manner. Once the full lunge and pull position have been reached the client returns to the start position and alternates sides. This movement can also be performed using the asymmetrical row for increased trunk activation.

Examples of Functional Based Training Movements Continued

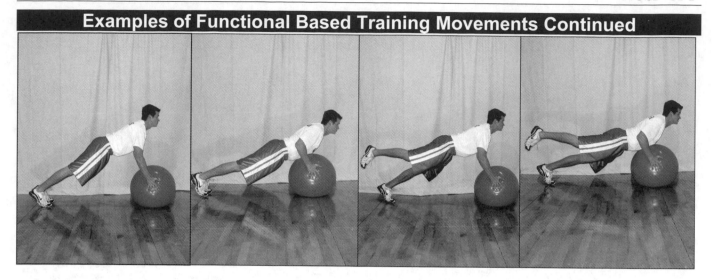

Physioball Push-up

Assume a straight body bridge position on the ball; feet on the floor with arms extended and hands in a neutral position. Descend to the ball by horizontally abducting and extending the shoulder while flexing the elbow. Lower the body to a point just above the ball in a controlled manner. Keeping the spine and hips in neutral position, press the body back to the start position stabilizing the ball to prevent any lateral movement. The feet should remain fixed throughout the movement. Once the arms are fully extended, but not locked, repeat the movement through the same plane of motion. The exercise can be made more difficult by aligning the feet close together or lifting one leg by extending the hip during the movement. The larger the ball, the easier the exercise is to perform. The trainer should spot the ball to prevent undesirable lateral movement.

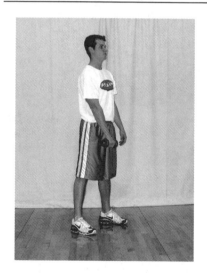
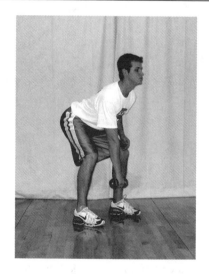
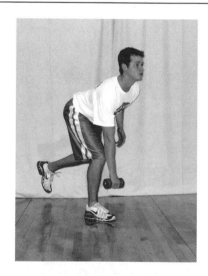

Asymmetrical Romanian Deadlift

Standing in an upright posture with feet located under the hips grasp a single dumbbell using a pronated grip. The arm should be extended with the resistance located just in front of the hip. Initiate the movement by flexing the hips while slightly flexing the knees. The back should remain flat as the resistance is reached downward toward the ground. Once full range of motion has been reached the hip, back, and knees should be extended maintaining a flat back position. The exercise can be made more difficult by performing the lift on one foot. A common error is to continue to flex the knees throughout the downward phase often due to tight hip extensors. In many cases hamstring flexibility limits the movement range.

Examples of Functional Based Training Movements Continued

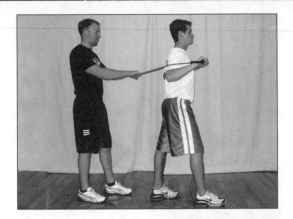 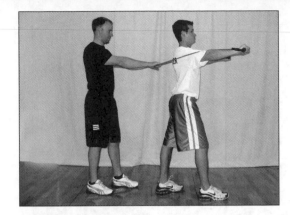

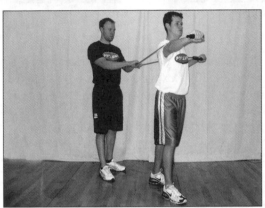

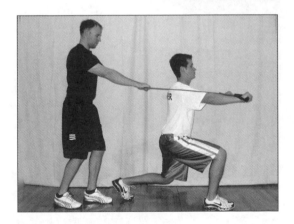 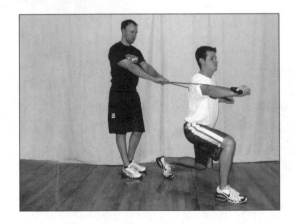

Band Press Sequence

Start in a split stance position holding the band handles with the arms flexed and shoulders horizontally abducted at chest height. Initiate the movement by pressing forward extending the arms while horizontally adducting the shoulder. The back should remain flat with the abdominals isometrically contracted. Return to the start position in a controlled manner moving through the same plane of movement. Once proficiency has been established the exercise can be advanced by alternating presses and asymmetrically loading the movement. To increase the complexity the exercise can be performed while stepping into a lunge position. The movement is initiated with a forward step. As the knees and hip flex the shoulders are horizontally adducted and arms extended in a fluid manner. Once the full lunge and press position have been reached the client returns to the start position and alternates sides. This movement can also be performed using the asymmetrical press for increased trunk activation.

Examples of Functional Based Training Movements Continued

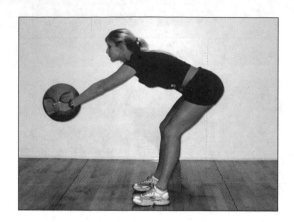 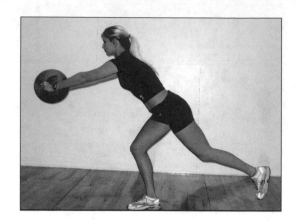

Medicine Ball Reach

Standing in an upright posture with feet approximately shoulder width apart, grasp a medicine ball using a neutral grip. Initiate the movement by flexing the hips and slightly flexing the knees. The shoulders will flex as the arms are reached forward. The back should remain flat throughout the entire movement. In most cases, hamstring flexibility will determine the degree of knee flexion and latissimus dorsi flexibility may limit the degree of attainable shoulder flexion. Once full functional range has been attained, return to the start position by extending the back, hips, and knees while maintaining the flat back position. The exercise can be varied by reaching in different directions. To increase stability the exercise can be performed on one leg and/or asymmetrically loaded. The back should not round during any phase of the activity.

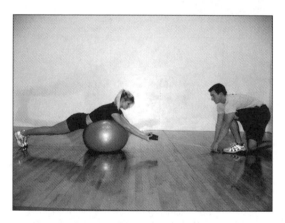 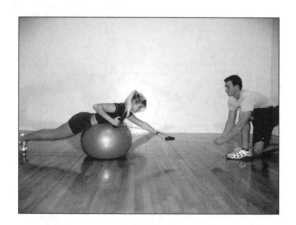

Alternating Prone Row

Lying in a prone position on the physioball with feet on the ground in a parallel position, flex both shoulders and extend the arms forward toward the line of the resistance. Grasp the handles of the bands or cable using a neutral grip. The body should be straight with the pelvis and spine in neutral position. Initiate the movement by extending the shoulder while flexing the arm. Pull the handle to a position in line with the chest as the shoulder is hyperextended. The body should remain in a stable straight position. Return the resistance to the start position in the same plane of motion while simultaneously contracting the latissimus dorsi and flexing the arm, pulling the opposite handle toward the body. The exercise will become more difficult by employing a single arm, loaded asymmetrically or by lifting one leg off the ground using hip extension during the pull phase.

Examples of Functional Based Training Movements Continued

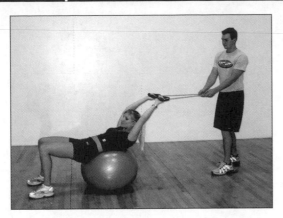 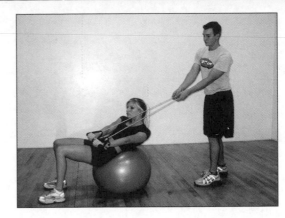

Physioball Lateral Pullovers

Lying in a supine position on the physioball establish a bridge position with the hips extended and knees flexed with feet flat on the floor. Reach the arms overhead by flexing the shoulder and extending the elbows. Grasp the handles with a pronated grip. Initiate the movement by extending the shoulders and flexing and rotating the trunk. Maintaining a straight arm position, pull the handles to a position lateral to the hip. Once full range of motion has been attained, return to the start position through the same plane of motion. At the start position perform the same movement to the other side of the body.

Chapter Twenty References

1. **Chaitow, L.** [Muscle Energy Techniques]. New York: Churchill Livingstone. 1997.
2. **Gambetta, V.** [Back to the Basics]. 1998. www.Gambetta.com/a97001p.html
3. **Gambetta, V and Gray, G.** [Following the Functional Path]. 1997. www.Gambetta.com/a97004p.html
4. **Gambetta, V.** [Force and function]. Training & Conditioning 9:5, 1999.
5. **Gambetta, V.** [Hard core training]. Training & Conditioning 9:4, 1999.
6. **Gambetta, V.** [Leap of strength]. Coaching Management. 8:3, 2000.
7. **Gambetta, V.** [Too Lose Too Much]. 2002. www.Gambetta.com/a97003p.html
8. **Gray, G and Gambetta.** Functional Balance. 2002. www.gambetta.com/a97002p.html
9. **Santanna, J.C.** Functional Training: Breaking the bonds of traditionalism. Video. 2000
10. **Seeley, R., Stephens, T.D., Tate, D.A.** [Anatomy and Physiology]. St. Louis: Mosby College Publishing. 1989

Chapter 21

Creating an Exercise Program

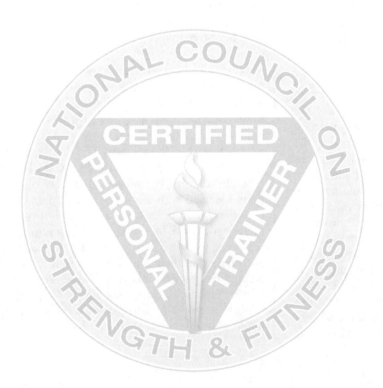

Introduction

The exercise prescription is technically defined as a premeditated, structured format of quantified stress, applied in appropriate dosages in a manner that stimulates adaptations in the physiological systems of the body. This suggests that each action defined by the exercise program has a specific purpose related to the intended outcome. To successfully create an exercise prescription, a personal trainer must identify the physiological needs of the client and determine the specific exercise components that will attend to them. This requires a multi-dimensional approach and a thorough review of all the factors involved (19).

Writing an effective exercise program is the most difficult task required of the personal trainer. Due to the number of health-related considerations, different personal goals, training aptitudes, and the limitations in contact time needed to address all the physiological issues, exercise programming for even the average personal training client can become somewhat complicated. Although programming may present different challenges for the personal trainer, the task can be managed effectively by using the proper approach.

In previous chapters, the needs analysis was addressed as a means to identify how to extract the relevant information from the findings of the health screening and behavior questionnaire, resting and physical evaluations, subjective reports, and observational data collection (18). Recording each finding provides the basis for the program decision making process. Identifying the needs of the client, ranking the needs, coming up with solutions, and integrating the solutions in a program matrix so that they adhere to the client's individual goals is how personal trainer programs are designed to individually cater to each client (28).

Prioritizing Needs

The easiest way to become proficient in program design is to 1) become knowledgeable enough to identify the important findings during a comprehensive screening and evaluation, 2) be able to correctly prioritize the defined needs, 3) know what activities and exercises address the problems, based on physiological adaptation response, and 4) be able to competently implement the exercise principles and program components in a manner specific to the goals (16). Thoroughly evaluating the findings that create the needs analysis often indicates broad categories of need. Early conclusions about what the program should entail can be refined to create a specific list of objectives. This list should further be refined to identify solutions that can be combined to provide the needed adaptation-based stress in the most efficient manner and within the reasonable capabilities of the client. Segmenting the exercise bout and using a weekly format will also aid in covering the relevant issues, while still maintaining a focus on client specific goals.

Most personal trainers find that the needs analysis identifies more relevant issues than are indicated by the initial goals defined by the client. The prevention of disease and age-limiting factors should be addressed with priority. Deficiencies in health-related fitness and musculoskeletal imbalances should also be ranked among the most important issues. In many cases, the actions used within the program can cover many benefits and address more than one area of concern simultaneously (11). For instance, aerobic exercise will aid in cardiorespiratory fitness, while also contributing to reductions in weight and blood pressure (22). Time management within the program becomes an important factor to ensure that the necessary issues and defined goals are attended to within the limited contact time a personal trainer has with a given client.

~Quick Insight~

The traditional approach to exercise programs uses the FITT principle. FITT represents F-frequency, I-intensity, T-time, and T-type. This principle suggests that all programming is based on frequency, duration, intensity, and mode of exercise. In personal training, the principle is somewhat limited, as the frequency is dictated by client finances and available time, and the duration has been standardized to reflect one hour of work. This leaves the options of intensity and mode to the discretion of the trainer. Due to the limited frequency and duration, most programming is forced to combine all of the aspects of a comprehensive program into a 120 to 180 minute time period per week.

Maximizing the exercise or contact time with a client is vital to goal attainment. Personal trainers should account for every minute of a workout session. In the early stages of an exercise program, the rest interval may necessitate complete recovery. After improved fitness status has been attained, different activities can be used during the rest interval to work on progressive skills. For instance, if a chest press is completed and a sixty-second rest period is used between sets, it may be an opportune time to work on stability, dynamic flexibility, or low level therapeutic back activities. If future progressions will require activities which require balance, a client could be acclimated to standing on a single foot, or practice stabilizing on a stability disc. These ideas ultimately save time. Personal trainers should always be looking for ways to promote improvements when any contact time is made available.

The following section covers three case studies intended to provide some ideas on how to program for multiple factors within the same workout session. Each workout is segmented, with specific emphasis based on the individual's presented needs analysis. Training in adaptation specific segments allows for more total body improvements than emphasizing a single adaptation response in each exercise session. A dose-response relationship is associated with physical adaptations (4). Therefore, the more often the stress can be applied, the faster the rate of improvement.

Case Study One

Mr. Thomson is a 51-year old High School principal. He is 5' 11" tall and weighs 224 lbs. He was previously sedentary and has hired a trainer based on his doctor's recommendation during a recent physical examination. In the initial meeting Mr. Thomson identified his personal goals as reducing body fat, reducing his blood pressure, and increasing his overall stamina. He has been cleared for exercise by his physician. During his initial screening and subsequent evaluation, the following information was collected.

Identified Need	Current Status	Solution
Resting Blood Pressure	140/87 mmHg	Aerobic exercise Behavior education
Resting Heart Rate	82 bpm	Aerobic exercise
Activity Status	Sedentary	Increase activity
Body Composition	23%	Negative caloric balance
Abdominal Girth	38 inches	Negative caloric balance Increase caloric expenditure
Cardiorespiratory Fitness	$37 \ ml \cdot kg^{-1} \cdot min^{-1}$	Aerobic activity
Upper Body Strength	Moderate deconditioning	Resistance training
Lower Body Strength	Mild deconditioning	Resistance training
Trunk Endurance	Poor	Increase strength and endurance
Flexibility	Poor ROM hamstrings, glutes, trunk rotators, hip flexors	Increase specific ROM
Additional	Intermittent low back pain	Muscle balance Pelvic stability

The initial needs analysis has provided general recommendations for activities that should be used within the exercise training bout. The solutions require refinement to identify the specific activities to be used in the exercise program. Due to the fact that Mr. Thomson will be able to train two days a week limits any particular emphasis within the program design but will provide enough stress application for health improvements.

Course of Action

Need	Solution
Aerobic Exercise	Steady state training 60-65% HRR
Behavior Education	Diet and lifestyle coaching
Increase Activity	Maximize daily activity
Negative Caloric Balance	300-400 kcal expenditure per session
Increase Caloric Expenditure	Daily task sheet
Resistance Training	Total body activities 50-70% 1RM
Increase Specific ROM	Static and dynamic ROM exercises

Refined Program Criteria

Cardiovascular Recommendation
- 60-65% HRR
- 15-20 minutes per exercise session

Diet and Lifestyle Coaching
- Reduce salt and increase potassium dietary intake
- Reduce total fat and simple carbohydrate intake
- Identify causes of stress
- Increase hydration

Caloric Expenditure Recommendation
- 300-400 kcal expenditure per session
- 150 kcal aerobic training
- 200 kcal resistance training

Daily Task Sheet
- Use stairs twice per day
- Walk dog for 15 minutes 3x/week
- Park away from the school

Total Body Resistance Training Activities

Trunk flexion	Ab-curl on ball, supine ankle reach
Trunk extension	Back extension, goodmorning, opposite raise
Trunk rotation	Seated diagonal chop, cable torso twist
Hip adduction	Lateral step up, lateral half squat, lateral cone shuffle
Hip extension	Body squat, modified deadlift, static lunge
Knee extension	Narrow stance ball squat, leg extension
Knee flexion	Supine leg curl, seated leg curl
Plantar flexion	Standing calf raise
Shoulder flexion	Standing front raise, kneeling MB front raise
Shoulder extension	Pullover, reverse grip pulldown
Shoulder horizontal flexion	Chest press, push-ups
Shoulder horizontal extension	Rear delt raise, 45 degree high row
Shoulder adduction	Lat pulldown, modified pull-up
Shoulder abduction	Dumbell press, side raise
Arm extension	Tricep pushdown, tricep extension
Arm flexion	Bicep curl, hammer curl

Flexibility Recommendation
- Static and dynamic ROM
- Static hamstring stretch
- Dynamic and static glute stretch
- Dynamic trunk rotation
- Dynamic hip flexor stretch

Following the refinement phase, the specific activities to address the need have been defined. The next step is to place them in a two-day program that is appropriate to the client's capabilities. For this individual, the program must emphasize caloric expenditure and provide time for aerobic activity, flexibility, and resistance training exercise. Reviewing the protocols used for resistance training in Chapter 18, it makes sense to employ some time-saving systems. Due to the fact that he is new to exercise, the sets, repetitions, intensity, and rest periods should be moderate in nature. Using higher repetition ranges will aid in movement proficiency and allow for work of a more continuous nature to meet caloric expenditure goals. The nervous system will not require significant stress for adaptations due to his current fitness status. An effort should be made to combine exercises whenever possible to save time and increase functional demands. It normally takes several sessions to ensure movement economy before adding any new level of complexity (3). The following program assumes the client has been adequately instructed and has gained appropriate levels of efficiency in performing the prescribed exercises.

Exercise Program Format

Day 1

Warm-up
5 minutes of biking

Day 2

Warm-up
5 minutes of walking

2 x 15 second

Dynamic hip flexor stretch
Dynamic trunk rotation

Dynamic glute stretch
Dynamic low back stretch

Resistance 1   2 x15 (40 seconds rest interval)
Body squat to overhead MB press
Lunge to side raise
Chest press
Back extension

Box step to MB press
Modified deadlift to front raise
Modified pull-up
Supine ankle touch

2 minute rest period

Resistance 2   2 x12 reps (Tri-set*); transitional rest; 2 min rest after each Tri-set
Lat pulldown
Ab-curl-up
Leg curl

Bench push-ups
Cable rotation
Lateral half squat

Resistance 3   2 x Circuit; 30 seconds; transitional rest; 2 min rest after each circuits
Seated diagonal chop
MB pullover
Good morning
Kneeling front raise
Bicep curl
Tricep push-down

Body squat
Rear delt raise
Opposite raise
Tricep extension
Calf raise
Hammer curl

Cardiovascular Component
15 min Biking w/ 3 min cool down

15 min incline walking w/3 min cool down

Range of Motion   2 x 15 second holds
Static hamstring stretch
Static low back stretch
Static lat stretch

Static hamstring stretch
Static glute stretch
Static hip flexor stretch

Total Duration of Work 46.5 minutes   Total Rest 13.5 minutes

Average MET intensity 4.5   Total calories: 366 kcal

*Tri-set = three exercises performed in a row

The program format allowed for the application of the appropriate stress within the desired period of time. Based on the current rest to work ratio, the client is able to accomplish more than 45 minutes of work and attain the intended caloric expenditure in the designated time allotment. In some cases, additional rest may be required to address individual exercise tolerance, but by varying the muscle groups used and employing reasonable intensity expectations, the desired amount of work can be accomplished. As the client adapts to the stress, intensities may increase, consistent with recommended progression rates, and rest intervals may be reduced or manipulated to reach the goal effect.

Many trainers do not utilize aerobic conditioning during the personal training workout, which may be a mistake. Aerobic exercise is necessary for improved health and the reduction of disease risk (26). Additionally, it adds to the total caloric expenditure (32). For this individual, it is certainly necessary to contribute to caloric expenditure, as he presents the pre-stages of hypertension and metabolic disease risk. As the client improves in aerobic capacity, interval training can be added to further the adaptation response.

Case Study Two

Miss Carter is a 25-year-old real estate agent. She is 5' 6" tall and weighs 135 lbs. She has been previously active and is an avid tennis player. She has hired a trainer to improve her tennis performance and is looking for overall conditioning. During the initial meeting, she identified her personal goals as improving her strength and speed on the court and would like to create better muscle tone throughout her body. During her initial screening and subsequent evaluation, the following information was collected.

Identified Need	Current Status	Solution
Resting Blood Pressure	116/68 mmHg	Maintain
Resting Heart Rate	65 bpm	Maintain
Activity Status	Active	Maintain
Body Composition	27%	Negative caloric balance
Waist Girth	27 inches	Negative caloric balance
Hip Girth	34 inches	Negative caloric balance
Cardiorespiratory Fitness VO$_2$max	43 ml $\cdot$ kg^{-1} $\cdot$ min^{-1}	Aerobic activity
Upper Body Strength	Moderate levels	Resistance training
Lower Body Strength	Moderate levels	Resistance training
Trunk Endurance	Good	
Flexibility	Bilateral difference in shoulder range ROM Mild hip flexor tightness	Increase specific ROM
Anerobic Power	Moderate	Increase power
Agility Test	Moderate	Increase lateral speed

The exercise prescription for Miss Carter places less emphasis on training for health purposes and emphasis more on enhancing fitness and movement capabilities. The exercise program will need to address power, strength, and performance endurance. The program should emphasize muscle balance due to the higher risk for injury associated with her sport activity, especially within the shoulder and elbow joints (17). The activities should address each body segment but focus on coordinated movements with particular consideration for the acceleration and deceleration requirements of her stop and go movements on the tennis court (12).

Course of Action

Need	Solution
Aerobic Training	70-80% HRR
Resistance Training	Total Body 65-80% 1RM
Flexibility Training	Shoulders, Hips
Body Composition	Caloric Expenditure
Sport Specific Training	Power, Agility

Refined Program Criteria

Cardiovascular Recommendation
- Weight bearing interval training
- 70-80% HRR

Total Body Resistance Training Activities

Trunk flexion	Weighted trunk flexion, knee rolls, reverse crunch
Trunk extension	Back extension on ball, goodmorning, cone reach
Trunk rotation	MB* side pass, incline MB twist, cable torso twist
Hip adduction	Lateral step-up, lateral lunge
Hip extension	Back squat, Romanian deadlift, single leg squat
Knee extension	Front MB squat, leg extension
Knee flexion	Supine curls on ball, supine leg curl
Plantar flexion	Standing calf raise, seated calf raise
Shoulder flexion	Standing front raise, kneeling MB front raise
Shoulder extension	Pullover, reverse grip pulldown
Shoulder horizontal flexion	Standing cable press, push-ups, flyes on ball
Shoulder horizontal extension	Rear delt raise, rear delt pulls
Shoulder adduction	Lat pulldown, mod pull-up, single arm pulldown
Shoulder abduction	Dumbell press, side raise, upright row
Arm extension	Tricep pushdown, tricep extension
Arm flexion	Bicep curl, hammer curl

* MB = medicine ball

Power Training
DB squat jumps
Box jumps
Low tuck jumps
Lateral box jumps
Lateral cone hops
Split squat jumps

Agility Training
Lateral shuttle
T-drill
Z-drill

Flexibility Recommendation
- Dynamic trunk stretch
- Dynamic and static hip flexor stretch
- Dynamic and static internal/external rotator
- Static pectoralis stretch
- Static lat stretch

Due to the sport specific nature of the training, energy system considerations will dictate the order of the program components so that fatigue does not negatively affect the activity performance (10). Recalling the recommended order of operations from Chapter 12, power and speed activities should be performed early in the session, followed by complex activities and those that utilize the most resistance (13; 14). In many cases, rate of perceived exertion can be used to adjust rest intervals for client-specific tolerance to the exercise volume and intensity (6).

Exercise Program Format

Day One

Warm-up
3 minute jump rope; 2 minute step-ups

Circuit: 15 reps each x 2

Dynamic internal rotator stretch
Dynamic trunk stretch
Empty can raises
Cone reach

Power	60-90 sec rest interval
Box jumps	3 x 8
Low knee tuck jumps	3 x 8
Medicine ball side passes	3 x 7 per side

Agility	30 sec rest interval
Lateral shuttle	6 x

Resistance 1	3 sets; 60 sec rest interval
Back squat	10, 8, 7
Standing cable press	12, 10, 8
Modified pull-up	3x number of reps to failure
Standing dumbbell press	3 x 8-10

Resistance 2   2 x 8-12 repetitions; 60 sec rest interval
Lateral step-up s/s* with back ext. on ball
Kneeling front raise s/s* with seated calf raise
Weighted trunk flexion s/s tricep pushdown

Cardiovascular Component
Aerobic Interval Biking
15 minutes 70-80% HRR
3 minute cooldown

Range of Motion	
Static hip flexor stretch	2 x 30 sec
Static lat stretch	2 x 30 sec

*S/S = Superset

Sport-specific training differs from general health and fitness training as the emphasis is on the performance components of fitness. During the early stages of the program, developmental strength and movement proficiency are very important to support the subsequent progressions. More strength is needed in performance activities due to the deceleration requirements of most sports. The pace of the workout bout should challenge the systems but not be so rigorous that movement technique becomes compromised. As motor patterns are reinforced, greater stability components can be added, consistent with the functional-based training paradigm.

Exercise Program Format

Day Two

Warm-up
5 minute Biking

Circuit: 15 reps each x 2; 30 sec rest interval

Dynamic external rotator stretch
Dynamic hip flexor stretch
Dynamic trunk rotation stretch
Back extension on ball

Power   60-90 seconds rest interval

Lateral box jumps   3 x 10 total jumps
Split squat jumps   3 x 6 per side
Lateral cone hops   3 x 8 per side

Agility   20 sec rest interval
T-drill   6 x

Resistance 1   60 sec rest
Romanian deadlift   12,10,8
Reverse grip pulldown   3 x 8-10
Upright row   2 x 12
Lateral lunge   3 x 8

Resistance 2   60 sec rest; 2 x 8-12
Single leg squat s/s* with cable torso twist
Lat pulldown s/s with tricep extension
Leg extension s/s hammer curl

Cardiovascular Component
Aerobic Interval Jogging
15 minutes 70-80% HRR
3 minute cooldown

Range of Motion
Static pectoralis stretch   2 x 30 sec
Static hip flexor stretch   2 x 30 sec

Total Duration of Work   43 minutes   Total Rest 17 minutes

Average MET intensity: 7.5   Total calories: 344 kcal

* s/s = superset

Case Study Three

Mr. Jones is a 67-year-old retired lawyer. He is 6' tall and weighs 208 lbs. He has been sedentary, but has decided to join the fitness center to occupy his time. Upon meeting Mr. Jones, he clearly has no particular goals, but would like to become more mobile, as he feels he has slowed down with advancing age. He required a medical referral, but has been cleared for exercise. During his initial screening and subsequent evaluation, the following information was collected.

Identified Need	Current Status	Solution
Resting Blood Pressure (medicated)	131/88 mmHg	Aerobic exercise Behavior education
Resting Heart Rate	78 bpm	Aerobic exercise
Activity Status	Sedentary	Increase activity
Body Composition	21%	Negative caloric balance
Abdominal Girth	36 inches	Negative caloric balance Increase caloric expenditure
Cardiorespiratory Fitness VO$_2$max	29 ml $\cdot$ kg^{-1} $\cdot$ min^{-1}	Aerobic activity
Upper Body Strength	Deconditioned	Resistance training
Lower Body Strength	Mod. deconditioning	Resistance training
Trunk Endurance	Poor	Resistance training
Flexibility	Poor ROM hamstrings, glutes, trunk rotators, hip flexors, back extensors trunk flexors, shoulder flexors	Increase specific ROM

Mr. Jones has notable limitations due to muscle imbalance and poor flexibility. Based on his overall deconditioning, he will only be able to train at low to moderate levels until his muscular and aerobic fitness improve (8). He requires physical activity aimed at movement range and functional applications (25). Conventional training can be utilized, but to more dramatically affect his performance, dynamic, closed-chain, compound movements are warranted (30).

Need	Solution
Aerobic Exercise	Steady-State Training 50-55% HRR
Behavior Education	Diet and lifestyle coaching
Increase Activity	Maximize daily movement through a full range of motion
Negative Caloric Balance	150-200 kcal expenditure per session
Increase Caloric Expenditure	Daily tasks sheet
Resistance Training	Total body compound activities 50-70% 1RM
Increase Specific ROM	Static and dynamic ROM

Refined Program Criteria

Cardiovascular Recommendation
- 50-55% HRR
- 10 minutes per exercise session

Diet and Lifestyle Coaching
- Reduce salt and increase potassium intake
- Reduce total fat and simple carbohydrate intake
- Identify causes of stress
- Increase hydration

Caloric Expenditure Recommendation
- 150-200 kcal expenditure per session
- 75 kcal aerobic training
- 75 kcal resistance training

Daily Task sheet
- Walk 10 minutes every day

Total Body Resistance Training Activities

Trunk flexion	Seated incline ab flexion, MB forward reach
Trunk extension	Standing floor reach, goodmorning, prone raise
Trunk rotation	Seated trunk rotation, standing rotation punch
Hip adduction	Lateral stepping, assisted lateral step-up
Hip extension	Body bench stands, MB deadlift, assisted lunge
Knee extension	Physioball squat, single leg extension
Knee flexion	Supine leg rolls, supine leg curl
Plantar flexion	Standing calf raise, seated calf raise
Shoulder flexion	Standing front raise, close grip band press
Shoulder extension	Pullover, incline band pullover
Shoulder horizontal flexion	Standing modified push-up, machine press
Shoulder horizontal extension	Seated rear delt band pulls, high row
Shoulder adduction	Lat pulldown, band rows
Shoulder abduction	Single arm band press, side raise
Arm extension	Tricep pushdown, tricep machine dips
Arm flexion	DB* bicep curl, hammer curl

Flexibility Recommendation
- Static hamstring stretch
- Static glute stretch
- Static trunk rotation
- Static hip flexor stretch
- Static low back
- Static shoulder stretch
- Static calf stretch

Movement Efficiency Recommendation
- Varied cone drills

*DB = dumbbell

Many of the exercises have been modified from their traditional forms to cater to the reduced physical capacity of Mr. Jones. Combining exercises whenever possible can help create more functional-based activities (29). The aerobic exercise component may be done in two segments to avoid leg fatigue unless otherwise tolerated by the client. Repetitions should be high due to lower intensity load assignments and the need for motor patterning and increased range of motion (9). The flexibility component is necessary to reduce the limitations associated with the client's current conditions and will make good use of the training time. Additionally, movement cone drills will allow for increased activity and encourage movements in different directions at controlled speeds to enhance gait stability.

Exercise Program Format

Day One

Warm–up
5 minutes walking on treadmill

Resistance 1   2 x 30 seconds activity or fatigue; 1 minute rest interval
MB bench stand to overhead press
Seated incline ab reach
Limited range MB deadlift
Modified push-ups
Calf raise

Cardiovascular Component
Exercise bike 5 minutes

Resistance 2   2 x 30 seconds activity or fatigue; 1 minute rest interval
Supine leg rolls
Band rows
Side raise
Lateral cone step
Tricep push down

Movement Efficiency Component   6 x 30 seconds rest interval
Cone movement drill

Cardiovascular Component
Walk on treadmill 5 minutes

Flexibility Component   2 x 20 second holds
Static hamstring stretch
Static glute stretch
Static trunk rotation
Static hip flexor stretch
Static low back
Static shoulder stretch
Static calf stretch

Exercise Program Format

Day Two

Warm–up
5 minutes walking on treadmill

Resistance 1   2 x 30 seconds activity or fatigue; 1 minute rest interval
Assisted lunge
MB forward reach w/flexion
Single leg extension
Band forward press
Seated calf raise

Cardiovascular Component
Exercise bike 5 minutes

Resistance 2   2 x 30 seconds activity or fatigue; 1 minute rest interval
Leg curls
Lat pulldown
MB front raise
Assisted lateral step-up
Tricep machine dips

Movement Efficiency Component
Cone movement drill   6 x 30 seconds rest interval

Cardiovascular Component
Walk on treadmill 5 minutes

Flexibility Component
Static hamstring stretch   2 x 20 second holds
Static glute stretch
Static trunk rotation
Static hip flexor stretch
Static low back
Static shoulder stretch
Static calf stretch

Total Duration of Work 32.5 minutes	Total Rest 27.5 minutes
Average MET intensity: 3	Total calories: 161 kcal

With program components for limited mobility, new exercisers often use modified versions of the traditional movements to allow for a building block approach, while reducing the deleterious effects from excess fatigue from the exercise (24). If overly aggressive movements are used early in the exercise bout, the total number of quality movements performed later may be limited. For example, performing abdominal flexion from the floor may be too demanding, and the deconditioned muscle may only allow for a limited number of proper repetitions. Moving Mr. Jones to a seated incline position provides for a mechanically advantaged start position but still activates the intended muscle group.

Progressions should focus on increased movement range and more complex actions. One of the goals of the early stages of this program is to stimulate activity in as many movements and muscle groups as is reasonably possible in a single exercise session (1). Total body flexibility should be encouraged in each workout to enhance ROM for later, progressively applied techniques.

Case Studies in Review

Each of the three case studies demonstrates the variety of training possibilities that exists in programming for diverse populations. Personal training clients may each require different methods and systems to best address the issues they present. Based on this fact, the employment of numerous program options is necessary to cater to the various client characteristics, which often results in a program as diverse as the clients themselves. Traditional approaches to personal training follow a modified body builder/strength program that is often ineffective at meeting the needs of most clients. Although 8-10 exercises performed using three sets of ten repetitions is a stress that will cause adaptations, it does not provide for the many individual needs of the average client.

Writing exercise prescriptions requires appropriate management of the needs assessment and the defined goals. Based on the three case studies, it should be evident that an individualized approach is necessary for long-term success. Testing results and evaluation criteria should be incorporated into the program and used to create the foundations of the prescribed stress (21). Using the test scores as baseline values, appropriate application of the exercise principles will help ensure each defined objective is met (31). Recalling the use of effective goal strategies, focusing on daily and weekly objectives is necessary to stay on track for short-term goal attainment. Keep the goals measurable and consistent with the tests and evaluation criteria used to assess training effectiveness. A recommended approach is to use movements and systems in the program that are similar or the same as those used in testing. This strategy will provide for quantified improvements that the clients can see, fostering a positive psychological impression as to their capabilities. When setting the goals, be conscious of time constraints and the dose-response gradient of physiological adaptations. The nervous system is quick to respond to stress, whereas the muscular and cardiovascular systems experience a slower adaptation process.

Effective use of exercise principles is another key consideration in the exercise prescription. The principle of specificity should be based on the physiological and biomechanical analysis, as well as the goals established for the client (5). The principle of specificity is necessary to ensure the proper energy pathways and movements are utilized to impose the appropriate demand. Progressive overload should be consistent with the physiological adaptation process (15). Early stages of the exercise experience warrant progressively applied overload that matches the individual's performance.

Neural efficiency often contributes to a rapid adaptation rate in the first 4 to 6 weeks, when adequate volume is used. During this preparation cycle, clients may experience improvements beyond the norm, and progressions can accelerate, necessitating supported adjustments. The emphasis should still be on skill acquisition and motor learning rather than resistance-based overload. Once the body reaches its initial adjustment response, shifting back to a progression rate of 2.5% per week is usually an appropriate progressive overload goal (2). More aggressive progressions usually lead to faulty movement patterns, incorrect performance via neuromuscular compensation and can potentially result in injury. Monitoring individual performance will best define the progression rate for each individual client. One key consideration is that the body adapts to stress based on its duration of exposure, intensity, and the frequency of application. Therefore, the number of times a client engages the program components will determine the rate of adaptation and subsequent progression. A client who participates at a frequency of 3x per week will progress at a proportionately faster rate than if he or she used a frequency of only 2x per week (20). Notable adaptations often require 7-12 exposures to the stress, but again, the nervous system is more expeditious in responding to exercise demands.

Individual considerations are the foundation of exercise programming in personal training. As mentioned earlier, each person presents a unique group of characteristics that shapes the exercise prescription. Exercise experience, physical limitations, exercise tolerance, genetic factors, and daily lifestyle factors all must be considered to shape the program in a manner that best caters to the individual client. This notion supports the need for a thorough evaluation of every client before designing a client-specific exercise regimen. Tweaking the traditional program concept to reflect the client-specific interests is often warranted for optimal results. Taking advantage of the multitude of variables presented under the auspices of physical activity helps to facilitate an effective program and positive experience for the client.

Modification Techniques

Almost every component of exercise can be modified in a way that refines the delivery of stress. Exercises, movements, environments, set-repetition schematics, intensities, speeds, stability, complexities, and a host of other variables can all be adjusted to fit the client's needs. The continuum that exists between ease of movement and movement difficulty allows for an immeasurable number of possible scenarios. The goal should be to identify the exact compilation of stresses that allows the client to experience ongoing improvements in health, fitness, and movement efficiency without being overtrained. This compilation of stress involves adding or reducing the actual training demand. This fine balance must be adjusted to prevent the demand from being too great where the client struggles or too little where the client does not progress due to lack of intensity. The decision to adjust the situation should be based on observation, experience, and logic.

Duration of Program Cycles

Exercise programs are aimed at eliciting an adaptation response. Once the degree of adaptation has been attained, the program must progress to create a new perceived stress in order for the next level of physiological improvement to occur. With regard to the priority of the adaptations, programs evolve from different emphases and foci, to new directions. The priority focus should continually address physiological need and goal attainment. Recalling the characteristics of effective goal setting, there is a designated time period in which efforts should concentrate on achieving short- and long-term goals. Programming activities and components, including the application of progressive overload and physiologically specific stress, should reflect the time period of the training cycle. In most cases, training cycles last 6, 8, 10, or 12 weeks in length (23). Utilizing a designated length of time allows for a premeditated and structured application of stress. Retesting the emphasized components at the end of the training cycle identifies the effectiveness of the programming and sets the values for the next training cycle.

When the needs list is extensive, the training cycles may employ specific emphasis in a building block approach and change at the beginning of each new cycle. For instance, the initial training cycle may be a 6-week program to emphasize motor learning, movement patterning, baseline endurance, and general conditioning in preparation for more challenging training protocols. The next training cycle may emphasize specific movement strength and more coordinated activities requiring 8 weeks of training to attain the necessary adaptation response. The actual training cycle length will be based on the client contact time, fitness status, training experience, and training aptitude. If a client does not comply with the initially programmed frequency, the training cycle may have to be lengthened to allow for adequate exposure to the exercise stress. Concentrating on specific goals, rather than taking a broad approach to address everything at one time increases the likelihood of timely goal attainment. This is not to suggest selecting only one or two issues and ignoring the rest of the needs list but

rather implies planned emphasis, based on a system of priority.

Program Tracking

Program components should be tracked on a daily basis to gauge the program's effectiveness and progress. Trainers should record each performance so that progressive overload is properly applied in each training bout. When adaptation to the exercise occurs, the body requires a new perceived stress to support continued improvements. Many exercisers use the same stress routinely, which explains why they spend so much time in the gym without experiencing any change to their physique or measured performance. Tracking is also valuable in identifying how effective each program component is at addressing its intended purpose. If certain areas of improvement are noticed, the

~Quick Insight~

Periodization Model

The periodization model is a programming method that plans for specific emphasis within a given training cycle, directed at focusing on specific goals (27). In a sense, this model partitions each cycle to highlight certain deficiencies or objectives. Ultimately, over the course of several individual cycles, all goals can be achieved. In most cases, an extensive program cycle of six or eight months is broken down into smaller cycles. It works on the same concept of goal-oriented behavior, which uses short-term goals to reach long-term goals. This is a relevant concept for client psychology, because short-term goal attainment reinforces efforts and contributes to motivation and compliance. Likewise, breaking the training into segments aids in effective tracking, and planned routine evaluations at the end of each cycle can identify effective and ineffective components of the program. This strategy will help prevent prolonged periods of programming errors by identifying them earlier and can help to distinguish areas that warrant modification.

In periodization, the concept is to accomplish one group of adaptations to support the next. The traditional periodization approach uses a preparation phase, endurance/hypertrophy phase, strength phase, and performance phase(7). Each phase reflects a progressive increase in complexity and intensity. In the sports model, the phases are characterized by ever-increasing sport-specific behavior. In personal training, the emphasis will be dictated by the client's overall goals, as well as identified needs. In both cases, the building block approach is used to gradually progress to more intensified focus on the program's ultimate purpose.

programmed activities are serving their intended role in those areas. If other areas are not showing signs of improvement, then the applied stress is incorrect on some level. Trainers should review the intensity, volume, rest interval used, and specificity of the stress to identify the problem. If tracking is not used, these errors may not be recognized until the end of the training cycle, which is an unnecessary waste of both time and effort. Identifying these obstacles early on allows for productive program adjustments. Likewise, if results are relatively slow, the stress should be analyzed to determine if it is adequate. In many cases, adaptations occur to the initial exercise stress and adjustments to new progressions are either overly aggressive or insufficient to stimulate the next level of physiological alterations.

Program tracking is also necessary from a liability standpoint. If a personal trainer finds him or herself involved in litigation, the program components are often reviewed for appropriateness. If the programming information is limited or non-existent, it becomes difficult to defend correct procedure because no tangible proof exists. Documenting and maintaining program records is a professional act that should be a standard of all personal training services. Additionally, using the programs to identify client improvements instills confidence in one's professional capabilities and can be used for motivation in the program. For example, clients who do not show improvements in body composition may want to give up or assume the personal trainer is not fully competent. Providing reinforcement through other adaptation improvements may be the justification needed to keep clients motivated and on track.

Chapter Twenty One References

1. American College of Sports Medicine Position Stand. The recommended quantity and quality of exercise for developing and maintaining cardiorespiratory and muscular fitness, and flexibility in healthy adults. *Med Sci Sports Exerc* 30: 975-991, 1998.

2. **Arnold P and Gentry M**. Strength training: what the team physician needs to know. *Curr Sports Med Rep* 4: 305-308, 2005.

3. **Bemben MG**. Age-related physiological alterations to muscles and joints and potential exercise interventions for their improvement. *J Okla State Med Assoc* 92: 13-20, 1999.

4. **Blair SN and Connelly JC**. How much physical activity should we do? The case for moderate amounts and intensities of physical activity. *Res Q Exerc Sport* 67: 193-205, 1996.

5. **Deschenes MR and Kraemer WJ**. Performance and physiologic adaptations to resistance training. *Am J Phys Med Rehabil* 81: S3-16, 2002.

6. **Dishman RK**. Prescribing exercise intensity for healthy adults using perceived exertion. *Med Sci Sports Exerc* 26: 1087-1094, 1994.

7. **Durell DL, Pujol TJ and Barnes JT**. A survey of the scientific data and training methods utilized by collegiate strength and conditioning coaches. *J Strength Cond Res* 17: 368-373, 2003.

8. **Feigenbaum MS and Pollock ML**. Prescription of resistance training for health and disease. *Med Sci Sports Exerc* 31: 38-45, 1999.

9. **Feigenbaum MS and Pollock ML**. Prescription of resistance training for health and disease. *Med Sci Sports Exerc* 31: 38-45, 1999.

10. **Konig D, Huonker M, Schmid A, Halle M, Berg A and Keul J**. Cardiovascular, metabolic, and hormonal parameters in professional tennis players. *Med Sci Sports Exerc* 33: 654-658, 2001.

11. **Kostka T**. [Resistance (strength) training in health promotion and rehabilitation]. *Pol Merkur Lekarski* 13: 520-523, 2002.

12. **Kraemer WJ, Hakkinen K, Triplett-Mcbride NT, Fry AC, Koziris LP, Ratamess NA, Bauer JE, Volek JS, McConnell T, Newton RU, Gordon SE, Cummings D, Hauth J, Pullo F, Lynch JM, Fleck SJ, Mazzetti SA and Knuttgen HG**. Physiological changes with periodized resistance training in women tennis players. *Med Sci Sports Exerc* 35: 157-168, 2003.

13. **Kraemer WJ and Newton RU**. Training for muscular power. *Phys Med Rehabil Clin N Am* 11: 341-68, vii, 2000.

14. **Kraemer WJ, Ratamess N, Fry AC, Triplett-McBride T, Koziris LP, Bauer JA, Lynch JM and Fleck SJ**. Influence of resistance training volume and periodization on physiological and performance adaptations in collegiate women tennis players. *Am J Sports Med* 28: 626-633, 2000.

15. **Kraemer WJ, Ratamess NA and French DN**. Resistance training for health and performance. *Curr Sports Med Rep* 1: 165-171, 2002.

16. **Malek MH, Nalbone DP, Berger DE and Coburn JW**. Importance of health science education for personal fitness trainers. *J Strength Cond Res* 16: 19-24, 2002.

17. **Mayer F, Axmann D, Horstmann T, Martini F, Fritz J and Dickhuth HH**. Reciprocal strength ratio in shoulder abduction/adduction in sports and daily living. *Med Sci Sports Exerc* 33: 1765-1769, 2001.

18. **Morrison CA**. Using the exercise test to create the exercise prescription. *Prim Care* 28: 137-158, 2001.

19. **Morrison CA**. Using the exercise test to create the exercise prescription. *Prim Care* 28: 137-158, 2001.

20. **Nakamura Y, Tanaka K, Yabushita N, Sakai T and Shigematsu R**. Effects of exercise frequency on functional fitness in older adult women. *Arch Gerontol Geriatr* 44: 163-173, 2007.

21. **Nied RJ and Franklin B**. Promoting and prescribing exercise for the elderly. *Am Fam Physician* 65: 419-426, 2002.

22. **Okura T, Nakata Y and Tanaka K**. Effects of exercise intensity on physical fitness and risk factors for coronary heart disease. *Obes Res* 11: 1131-1139, 2003.

23. **Rhea MR, Ball SD, Phillips WT and Burkett LN**. A comparison of linear and daily undulating periodized programs with equated volume and intensity for strength. *J Strength Cond Res* 16: 250-255, 2002.

24. **Singh MA**. Exercise to prevent and treat functional disability. *Clin Geriatr Med* 18: 431-vii, 2002.

25. **Singh MA**. Exercise to prevent and treat functional disability. *Clin Geriatr Med* 18: 431-vii, 2002.

26. **Stewart KJ, Bacher AC, Turner K, Lim JG, Hees PS, Shapiro EP, Tayback M and Ouyang P**. Exercise and risk factors associated with metabolic syndrome in older adults. *Am J Prev Med* 28: 9-18, 2005.

27. **Stone MH**. Muscle conditioning and muscle injuries. *Med Sci Sports Exerc* 22: 457-462, 1990.

28. **Topp R**. Development of an exercise program for older adults: pre-exercise testing, exercise prescription and program maintenance. *Nurse Pract* 16: 16-1, 25, 1991.

29. **Topp R, Mikesky A and Bawel K**. Developing a strength training program for older adults: planning, programming, and potential outcomes. *Rehabil Nurs* 19: 266-73, 297, 1994.

30. **Topp R, Mikesky A and Bawel K**. Developing a strength training program for older adults: planning, programming, and potential outcomes. *Rehabil Nurs* 19: 266-73, 297, 1994.

31. **Welsch MA, Pollock ML, Brechue WF and Graves JE**. Using the exercise test to develop the exercise prescription in health and disease. *Prim Care* 21: 589-609, 1994.

32. **You T, Murphy KM, Lyles MF, Demons JL, Lenchik L and Nicklas BJ**. Addition of aerobic exercise to dietary weight loss preferentially reduces abdominal adipocyte size. *Int J Obes (Lond)* 30: 1211-1216, 2006.

Chapter 22

Working with Special Populations

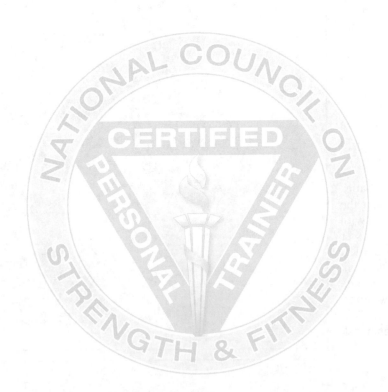

Exercise & Asthma

Asthma is a chronic inflammatory pulmonary disorder that is characterized by reversible obstruction of the airways. The disease is classified as a chronic obstructive pulmonary disorder caused by smooth muscle contraction and airway reactivity, leading to bronchospasms. The narrowing of the airway passages due to constriction is further worsened by the swelling of the windpipe lining and an increase in mucus produced along the tract, making it difficult to breathe. Major episodes of asthma can restrict breathing to a point that becomes life threatening. Over 5,000 Americans die each year from asthma, with the highest incidence among African-Americans (134). Of the nearly 17 million asthmatics in the United States, more than one third of them are under 18 years of age (21).

Asthma symptoms include shortness of breath, coughing, wheezing, and labored respiration. Asthma is induced by several mechanisms, including allergens, chemical irritants, smoke and pollutants, cold air, and exercise. **Exercise induced asthma (EIA)** occurs when the onset of symptoms is triggered by physical activity. EIA affects most asthmatics and is considered a significant barrier to activity participation and overall health in the young and old alike.

Asthma can be managed effectively via preventative strategies, medication, and regular exercise. Preventing the onset of asthma requires several environmental considerations. Avoiding poorly ventilated rooms, allergen exposure from dust, mold, animal dander, inhaling cold air or smoke, and avoiding rapid changes in exertion all reduce the incidence of asthma. Exercise has demonstrated significant improvements in the physical fitness measures of asthmatics. Many asthmatics avoid physical activity for fear of initiating an asthmatic episode, but exercise has been shown to reduce the occurrence of asthmatic conditions with routine participation and should be part of the overall management strategy (129).

Exercise should be introduced to asthmatics early on to reduce the psychosocial impact the disorder can have on children. Children with moderate or severe asthma present lower measures of aerobic capacity, lower left ventricular mass, and impaired systolic function, compared to healthy children of the same age (22). This may partially explain why they report participating in fewer physical activities. In addition, children with asthma have a higher risk for being overweight and experience higher levels of emotional difficulties compared to healthy children (89; 100; 159). Interview reports demonstrate that both children and their parents identify asthma as a barrier to the child's health (55; 90; 159).

Exercise can effectively prevent many of these condition-related problems. Therefore, strategies to promote exercise within this population should be explored to protect children from mental and physical health limitations. Children who exercise have shown the ability to achieve a level of exercise performance similar to that of healthy children when they participate in comparable levels of routine exercise (199). Studies comparing the two groups found improvements in maximal aerobic oxygen consumption and anaerobic threshold (121; 128; 199). Asthmatic children experience additional benefits of improved ventilatory capacity and decreased hyperapnea (83; 163; 198). When anaerobic activities were performed using 1 minute sprints, both mild and moderately asthmatic children demonstrated parity in exercise tolerance,

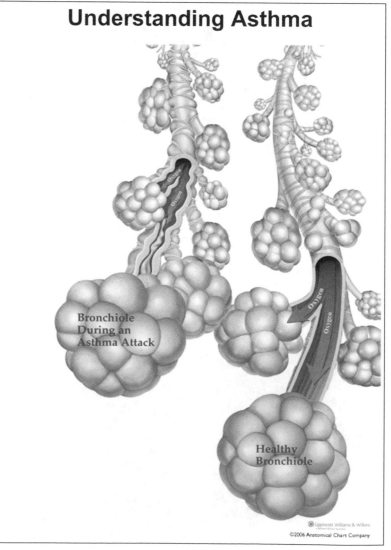

Understanding Asthma

Bronchiole During an Asthma Attack

Healthy Bronchiole

©2006 Anatomical Chart Company

compared to healthy children (18). Probably the most significant finding is that asthmatics experience reduced incidence of EIA with regular exercise participation and in many cases, EIA was not triggered during the participation (164). It is recommended that asthmatic children be encouraged to participate in both aerobic and anaerobic exercise activities to promote improvements in health and fitness.

Adults demonstrate similar improvements with routine exercise participation. Adults new to exercise also present deficiencies consistent with asthmatic children. Researchers attribute reduced physical condition states as a more prominent factor in limiting exercise performance rather than the obstruction of airflow (36). Adults are likely to experience the same mental barriers to exercise expressed by children. Fear of the onset of an asthmatic episode may be the greatest reason for avoiding exercise participation.

When adults engage in routine aerobic exercise, they experience a significantly higher level of oxygen consumption, lower blood lactate and heart rates at submaximal intensities, as well as significant improvement in 2-mile run times (70; 82). Additionally, routine exercise reduces occurrence and severity of EIA. When acute exercise measures are compared to healthy controls, asthmatics show consistent endocrine and metabolic response and similar **tidal volume** (the volume of air inhaled and exhaled with each breath), but demonstrate reduced breathing frequency (81; 119). Interestingly, asthmatics demonstrate only small increases in breathing rate but a better maintenance of tidal volume during aerobic exercise participation. The maintenance of tidal volume may compensate for airflow obstruction and therefore, allow for the successful participation in aerobic activities by asthmatics. Individuals with mild and moderate asthma can attain high measures of oxygen consumption and, with appropriate training and medications, can successfully participate in endurance sports at a competitive level (80; 180).

Even when the intensity is high (80-90% maxHR), trained asthmatics have a reduced occurrence of EIA. Following a 10-week

period of supervised, high-intensity training, adult asthmatics reported a reduced fear of experiencing breathlessness during exercise and less anxiety related to exercising at higher intensities. It was reported that asthma symptoms abated significantly during routine participation in aerobic exercise (69). Other studies have reported that regular submaximal exercise improved quality of life, exercise capacity, reduced need for medication, and reduced overall symptoms in adults and children alike (79; 160). When land and water-based exercise were compared, similar findings were noted (51). Aerobic exercise on land and in water resulted in reduced incidence of EIA during and after the training sessions, similar improvements in aerobic capacity, as well as reduced total symptoms (52). This suggests that multiple forms of exercise promote similar effects when the exercise intensity is consistent.

Physical fitness training programs can be designed to improve both anaerobic and aerobic fitness in asthmatic clients. Regular participation increases physical fitness measures and lowers ventilation during mild and moderate exercise, thereby lowering the incidence and likelihood of triggering an EIA event (78). Additionally, exercise exhibits a profound psychological effect on exercise confidence, perception of breathlessness, and reduced anxiety toward an EIA event. Although no change in lung function seems to occur in response to exercise, the corresponding benefits of routine physical activity provide significant improvements in overall health.

Personal trainers need to be familiar with the signs and symptoms of asthma, conditions and environments that induce or trigger the onset of symptoms, and

Asthma General Recommendations

- Evaluate the training environment for common asthma trigger factors including cold, dry air, presence of allergens, and poorly ventilated areas.
- Employ longer warm-up and cool down periods to acclimate the body to changing physiological conditions.
- Swimming, cycling, and walking are less likely to trigger an event than running, particularly outside.
- Sport participation that uses stop and go activities, such as tennis, volleyball, and basketball are less likely to trigger EIA, compared to longer, continuous, and more intense activities.
- High intensity exercise triggers EIA more often than moderate intensity exercise. It is recommended to use 60%-80% HRR when prescribing aerobic training.
- Encourage controlled nasal breathing whenever possible.
- Maintain appropriate medications on site, and have an emergency plan.

medications prescribed to manage the condition when working with asthmatic clients. Forms or documents used for pre-exercise screening should include items that identify clients with asthma and whether or not they use medication in the treatment of the disorder. Individuals who use medication to control asthma must be required to properly comply with recommendations for use before exercise or possess their prescribed inhaler when exercising, in the event EIA occurs. When implementing exercise strategies, personal trainers should use longer warm-ups, avoid rapid changes in intensity, and avoid activities that cause rapid respiration rates. Additionally, personal trainers should attempt to control environmental conditions to reduce the risk of an event.

Exercise & Diabetes

Diabetes is characterized by high blood glucose levels due to an impairment of sugar regulation within the body. Type I diabetes is an autoimmune disorder where the body produces antibodies against the Islet cells of the pancreas. This causes the destruction of beta cells and the consequent reduction or, more commonly, the cessation of insulin production. Type I diabetes is often referred to as Insulin Dependent Diabetes Mellitus due to the need to supply insulin via an external source, as the body cannot produce it. Type II diabetes is a more common form, characterized by insulin insensitivity and beta cell dysfunction in the later stages of the disease. Type II diabetes is caused by several mechanisms including genetic predispositions, obesity, sedentary lifestyle, and poor diet. In some cases, pregnant females develop the disease due to genetic predisposition, advanced maternal age, pre-diabetic condition before pregnancy exacerbated by the pregnancy, and obesity. Gestational diabetes (diabetes that occurs during pregnancy) will often subside following delivery but increases the risk for later development of Type II diabetes.

Physical activity plays a significant role in improving symptoms of diabetes (39). The positive role exercise plays in managing diabetes has been known for decades. During exercise, cellular uptake of glucose increases significantly, resulting in reduced circulating levels of glucose without the presence of high insulin concentrations. This insulin-like effect of active muscle tissue reduces the requirements for insulin in the regulation of glucose, thereby, improving blood glucose levels in diabetics.

Low cardiorespiratory fitness is a powerful and independent predictor of mortality in people with diabetes (32). Individuals with Type II

diabetes are often at the greatest risk due to the presence of compounding factors, including dyslipidemia, obesity, and hypertension. Aerobic training performed at an intensity of 50%-75% VO$_2$max for at least 30 minutes has been shown to improve cardiorespiratory function in diabetics (181; 202). In addition, participation in aerobic exercise demonstrates positive effects on visceral and subcutaneous adiposity, insulin response, and plasma triglyceride levels (201).

Resistance training yields similar, and in some cases more profound, effects than aerobic training on diabetes (30). With regard to acute response, resistance training exercise was effective in improving integrated glucose concentration. Compared to aerobic training, Type II diabetics who participated in 4 months of strength training significantly improved blood glucose levels and insulin resistance, reduced LDL and triglycerides, and increased HDL above diabetic subjects who performed aerobic training for the same period of time (31).

When aerobic and resistance activities were combined in an exercise circuit, positive adaptations on glucose control, insulin action, muscular strength, and exercise tolerance were observed. In a related review, circuit training had a significant effect on indices of glycemic control, cardiorespiratory fitness, muscular strength, and body composition (147). Following 8 weeks of circuit training, submaximal heart rate and blood pressure were reduced, skinfold and waist to hip measures significantly decreased, glycosylated hemoglobin (a measure of disease control) and fasting blood plasma glucose were reduced, while functional capacity, muscular strength, lean body mass, and glycemic control all increased significantly (132; 133). Based on these and other findings, it seems that both resistance

---

Benefits of Exercise on Diabetes

Improved insulin sensitivity

Improved glucose regulation

Improved blood lipid profile

Reduced visceral fat storage

Improved cardiovascular fitness

Improved muscle fitness

Prevents loss of muscle mass

Reduced risk for cardiovascular disease

Reduced risk for peripheral vascular disease

Reduced risk for heart attack and stroke

Increased quality of life

training and aerobic training are necessary components to an effective exercise program for those with diabetes either performed independently of each other or combined in a circuit training program (73; 179).

Although exercise is a staple for proper management of the disease, certain conditions may be exacerbated by exercise participation. Diabetics should have a thorough medical examination prior to initiating an exercise program so that a physician can rule out any possible factors that may lead to macro- or microvascular complications or injury. Within this screen, it is particularly important to analyze the disease effects upon the heart, kidneys, eyes, and nervous system. Additional screening criteria used to determine risk for injury include:

Age >35 years
Presence Type I Diabetes > 15 years
Presence of Type II Diabetes > 10 years
Presence of additional risk factors for heart disease
Presence of microvascular disease, including retinopathy and nephropathy
Peripheral vascular disease
Autonomic neuropathy

High risk diabetics require appropriate supervision and program modification to address the heightened risk for cardiovascular incidence and tissue damage associated with compromised vascular dynamics. The American Diabetic Association (ADA) provides guidelines and recommendations to aid in managing exercise programs for Type I and II diabetics. The differences between the classifications of the disease are also seen in the recommendations for safe participation. Due to the fact that Type I diabetics do not produce insulin, it must be injected, usually subcutaneously, to regulate glucose in the blood. Exercise has a profound effect on cellular uptake of glucose, and when insulin is injected prior to exercise, the combination of heightened cellular absorption can lead to dangerously low levels of blood glucose, a

conditioned known as hypoglycemia. This can cause light headedness, fainting, or, on rare occasions, diabetic coma. For this reason, Type I diabetics are required to monitor metabolic indices and plan insulin use around physical activity participation. Type I diabetics should not exercise within one hour of taking insulin, and insulin injection sites should not be at, or near, the location of the prime mover for the exercise.

Type I diabetics can compete at high performance levels with appropriate management of the disease (48). With prolonged and more intense exercise, carbohydrate regulation becomes more important. Planned pre-exercise meals and adequate carbohydrate availability during prolonged exercise are warranted to avoid hypoglycemia. Diabetics do not all respond the same way to exercise, and therefore, individual attention is necessary. Tracking the techniques that promote the best performance and glucose regulation response can aid in formulating the ideal management strategy. Record insulin injection time and dosage, food by ingestion time and quantity of carbohydrates, and intensity/duration measures to identify the specific outcomes.

Type II diabetics do not have the same concerns related to hypoglycemia from insulin injected but rather, must

General Recommendations for Type I Diabetics

- Maintain proper identification of the diabetic condition.
- Avoid exercise if fasting glucose levels are >250 mg/dl and ketosis is present.
- Use caution if fasting glucose levels are >300 mg/dl without ketones.
- Monitor blood glucose before and after exercise, and identify when adjustments to food or insulin are necessary (most diabetics possess a hand-held glucometer.
- Track glycemic response to exercise conditions for future preparations.
- Use carbohydrates to avoid hypoglycemic response.
- Keep fast-acting carbohydrate foods available during and after exercise.
- Pay close attention to signs of fatigue and metabolic shifts during exercise.
- Avoid high intensities with the introduction of new exercise activities.

General Recommendations for Type II Diabetics

- Maintain proper pre-exercise metabolic control.
- Consume adequate fluids.
- Perform regular physical activity most days of the week.
- Include client-appropriate aerobic and anaerobic activities.
- Focus on caloric expenditure and weight loss, with a minimum goal of 1,000 kcal per week from physical activity.
- Initiate exercise with appropriate acclimation periods.
- Work up to aerobic intensities of 60%-80% HRR.
- Modify exercise activities for microvascular complications.
- Comply with medication recommendations and monitor blood indices appropriately.

Exercise Considerations for Diagnosed Microvascular Complications

Retinopathy – (small vessel disease of the eyes) Avoid exercises that produce high blood pressure, and particularly high intensity, strenuous resistance training. Do not utilize activities that lower the head below the waist, such as yoga, or that may jar the head, such as plyometrics.

Nephropathy – (small vessel disease of the kidneys) Avoid moderate to heavy weightlifting, high intensity aerobic activity, and breath holding during exercise. Avoid any activity that notably raises blood pressure. Maintain adequate hydration.

Peripheral Neuropathy – (small vessel disease in nerves) Avoid exercise that causes pounding or repetitive stress to the feet. Select non-weight bearing exercises and ensure proper footwear is always worn during physical activity.

---

regulate carbohydrate intake and monitor blood glucose to avoid exercise related complications. Type II diabetics may present more difficulty with exercise management due to the fact that the disease is often accompanied by low levels of physical fitness, obesity, and additional cardiovascular risk factors. Higher risk Type II diabetics should be acclimated to exercise with similar precautions for those with cardiovascular risk, as well as specific considerations for the presence of microvascular complications. In addition, different medications for Type II diabetes exist and each has a unique action. Type II diabetic medications work by increasing insulin production (Sulfonylurea, Meglitinide, Nateglinide), sensitizing the body to circulating insulin present in the blood (Biguanide), helping insulin to work better in the muscle and fat cells (Thiazolidinedione), or acting to regulate carbohydrate digestion (Alpha-glucose Inhibitor). Due to the different mechanisms of action, physician recommended adjustments may need to be made before exercise participation, and clients need to comply strictly with medication instructions.

Exercise & Pregnancy

Physical activity, including structured exercise, has been shown to provide numerous and significant benefits for the health and fitness of the expecting mother (153). Pregnant females who engage in moderate exercise demonstrate improvements in cardiorespiratory fitness, reduced maternal weight gain, reduced musculoskeletal discomfort (including reduced incidence of low back pain during and following pregnancy), reduced postural compromise, decreased incidence and severity of varices (dilated veins due to valvular incompetence), thrombosis, delivery closer to term, fewer complications during delivery, and shorter delivery lengths (204). In addition, they have reduced risk for pregnancy-related disorders, improved glucose tolerance, improved psychological well-being, and quicker recovery from the stresses and strains of delivery.

Recommendations concerning exercise during pregnancy have gone through significant changes during the past three decades. Today, there is considerable support for the beneficial effects of moderate exercise during pregnancy, even in formerly inactive women (105; 145). It is now suggested that healthy pregnant women can engage in numerous types of physical activity, using gestational age-adapted exercise for safe and effective support of health for the mother and fetus. In most cases, it is recommended that pregnant women should practice exercise in a moderate, submaximal range based on individual criteria and physician approval.

Exercise has demonstrated a variety of effects on the pregnant woman, the developing fetus, and the placenta. The naturally occurring physiological adjustments related to pregnancy on the maternal cardiorespiratory system include increases in oxygen consumption, cardiac output, heart rate, stroke volume, and plasma volume (37; 72). These hormonally driven alterations improve aerobic capacity without the addition of any physical activity related adaptations.

In general, maternal resting oxygen consumption (VO_2) and cardiac output increase in the early stages of pregnancy. Heart rate becomes progressively elevated through gestation, with a concurrent increase in stroke volume until the third trimester, at which time it begins to decline until term. The decline is likely attributed to diminished venous return. Plasma volume increases earlier and to a greater magnitude than red cell volume, resulting in mild dilution of the blood, causing a decline in its oxygen-carrying capacity. This occurs despite increased red blood cell production, which warrants a compensatory increase in dietary iron intake. Pulmonary shifts cause tidal volume to increase with an unchanged rate of breathing, causing increased ventilation during pregnancy. However, **residual volume** (lung volume after maximum inspiration) is reduced, especially in the third trimester due to elevation of the diaphragm by the fetus. In addition, there is a gestation-proportionate increase in metabolism associated with increased mass.

When exercise is performed during pregnancy, exercise-induced cardiopulmonary changes are essentially the same or slightly exaggerated compared to non-pregnant females. Females maintain aerobic work capacity during pregnancy and may improve in exercise performance related to the hormonal effects on the cardiovascular system, depending on pre-training status. The typical training adaptations associated with exercise can also be found during pregnancy. The increase in oxygen reserve seen in early pregnancy is reduced later, related to the reductions in stroke volume as mentioned above, suggesting that maternal exercise may present a greater physiological stress in the third trimester (118). Relatively minor changes occur in the blood concentrations of O_2 and energy substrates during prolonged exhaustive exercise, demonstrating no loss in exercise performance due to metabolic alterations (68; 188). In addition, despite a temperature increase of 1 to 2 degrees C, there is little evidence for significant alteration in fetal metabolism, cardiovascular hemodynamics, or blood catecholamine concentrations (104; 115). The risk of neural tube defects due to exercise-induced hyperthermia that is suggested by animal studies is less likely in women, because of more effective mechanisms of heat dissipation in humans (5). These observations suggest that acute exercise normally does not represent a major distress for the fetus or mother.

Reduced Risk for Complications

Evidence-based guidelines indicate that participation in regular physical activity is an important component of a healthy pregnancy (7). In addition to promoting physical fitness, exercise may be beneficial in preventing or treating maternal-fetal diseases. Women who are the most physically active demonstrate the lowest prevalence of gestational diabetes (GDM), and preventing the occurrence of GDM using physical activity and proper diet may decrease the incidence of obesity and type II diabetes in both mother and offspring following birth (28). **Gestational diabetes mellitus (GDM)** is the most common medical complication of pregnancy (14; 207). Women with GDM are at elevated risk for numerous maternal health complications, and their infants are at elevated risk for death and morbidity (208).

Physically active women are also less likely to develop **pre-eclampsia** (the development of elevated blood pressure and protein in the urine after the 20th week of pregnancy) during pregnancy, compared to sedentary females (162; 197; 205). Pre-eclampsia occurs in 2-7% of all pregnancies and is a leading cause of maternal and fetal morbidity and mortality. Although not fully understood, it is proposed that pre-eclampsia is caused by abnormal placental development, predisposing maternal constitutional factors, oxidative stress, immune maladaptation, and genetic susceptibility. Exercise may reduce risk of developing pre-eclampsia via several mechanisms, including the stimulation of placental growth and vascularity, a reduction of oxidative stress, and exercise-induced reversal of maternal endothelial dysfunction (196; 206) . Whatever the actual mechanism that serves in prevention, physical activity seems to be an important part of reducing the risk for pre-eclampsia.

Maternal obesity associates with reproductive complications, including an increased risk of infertility and miscarriage (29). Exercise may be an optimal strategy when combined with proper diet to reduce the probability of obesity-related complications during pregnancy. Regular exercise following conception may prevent excessive gestational weight gain and reduce post-partum weight retention.

Fetal Considerations

Aerobic physical activity during pregnancy may be an important determinant of birth weight within the normal range. Studies suggest that aerobic exercise is strongly and inversely associated with fetal growth ratio. In cross comparisons, infants born to women with the highest levels of physical activity weighed an average 21 ounces less than infants born to sedentary women. It is suggested that women who engage in regular and appropriate physical activity throughout pregnancy have leaner babies than sedentary mothers (9; 34).

Although exercise results in an elevation of the fetal heart rate and breathing rate, training has not proved to be associated with increased risk of negative consequences (38). Other measures of fetal condition have equally demonstrated very little risk to the fetus during exercise participation at appropriate levels. The offspring of women who train during pregnancy manifest fewer signs of stress during delivery and are usually characterized by better general condition (e.g., higher Apgar scores) (35).

Contraindications to Exercise

- Pregnancy-induced hypertension.
- Premature rupture of membranes.
- Incompetent cervix.
- Persistent bleeding.
- Intrauterine growth retardation.
- Pre-term labor during prior or current pregnancy.
- Pre-existing cardiopulmonary diseases and pregnancy pathologies have to be considered as contraindications.

Training Considerations

The level of training that is defined as appropriate for a pregnant female is individual-specific and based on numerous physiological and genetic factors. To date, no upper level of intensity and training volume has been determined (20). However, moderate intensity aerobic exercise has been shown to be safe during pregnancy (187). A number of studies now indicate that for trained athletes, it may be possible to exercise at a higher level of physical activity than is currently recommended by the American College of Obstetricians and Gynecologists (4; 111). Although impairment of sufficient oxygen and substrate supply to the fetus has not been demonstrated with aerobic activity, it is usually recommended to perform exercise in a submaximal range.

One study analyzed the effects of high volume training versus moderate volume exercise on forty-two healthy females who had performed exercise regularly prior to conception (110). The athletes were split into one of two exercise groups and followed from gestational week 17 until 12 weeks postpartum while they performed standardized exercise programs. No complications were found in either the high volume or moderate volume groups. Researchers concluded that well-trained women can benefit substantially from training at high volumes during an uncomplicated pregnancy (33; 109).

The physiological adaptations to exercise during pregnancy appear to protect the fetus from potential harm, and the benefits of continued activity during pregnancy appear to outweigh any potential risks (139). All decisions about participation in physical activity during pregnancy should, however, be made by women in consultation with their medical advisers (19). Restriction of physical activity should be dictated by obstetric and medical indications. Health care providers should inform pregnant women of potential risks and individualize exercise prescription to reflect the safest level of participation.

In addition to aerobic exercise, other types of exercise have demonstrated positive outcomes with maternal participation during pregnancy. Studies of resistance training that incorporates moderate resistance and avoids maximal isometric contractions have shown no adverse outcomes for maternal exercises, while showing improvements in strength and flexibility (10; 127). Moderate resistance exercise may provide additional benefits for preventing back pain and muscle strain during pregnancy. It seems that women can participate in many fitness-related activities without consequence, provided that consideration is given to contraindications and warning signs (126).

General Recommendations

Although a wide range of physical activities seem to be safe for pregnant females, some considerations must be applied. The overall health of a woman, including obstetric and medical risks, should be evaluated before

Key Terms

Exercise induced asthma (EIA) - A medical condition characterized by shortness of breath induced by sustained aerobic exercise.

Tidal volume – The volume of air inspired or expired in a single breath during regular activity.

Gestational diabetes mellitus (GDM) – A form of diabetes affecting pregnant women with no specific cause.

Retinopathy – A non-inflammatory disease of the retina.

Nephropathy – A disease or abnormality of the kidney.

Peripheral Neuropathy – A small vessel disease or damage to the nerves predominantly in the arms and legs.

Residual volume – The volume of air remaining in the lungs after a maximal expiratory effort.

Pre-eclampsia – An abnormal state of pregnancy in which there are signs of elevated blood pressure, water retention, and protein excretion in the urine.

General Recommendations for Pregnancy

- Consult the primary health care provider prior to participating in exercise.
- Avoid motionless standing.
- Avoid exercise in the supine position following the 1st trimester.
- Avoid jumping or jarring activities.
- Avoid exercise in the heat.
- Maintain adequate hydration before, during, and following exercise.
- Ensure adequate caloric intake during pregnancy and lactation.
- Stop exercise upon fatigue, and never exercise to exhaustion.
- Weight-bearing exercise produces a greater decrease in oxygen reserve than non weight-bearing exercise; adjust intensity accordingly.
- Avoid contact sports.
- Beware of joint laxity during activity selection.
- Immediately report vaginal spotting or bleeding to primary physician.
- Avoid exercise during high risk pregnancies, including twins.

---

component of cardiopulmonary rehabilitation programs. Each type of cardiovascular disease has specific characteristics which determine the type and extent of activity that can safely be utilized. Participation levels and recommended guidelines will depend on the specific disease-related factors, such as the progressive stage of disease, degree of damage or symptoms, the current state of the individual, and the presence of other health-limiting factors. In most cases, individuals with disease can participate in physical activity, although the actual mode, intensity, and volume of participation will vary by the relative level of health risk.

prescribing an exercise program (6). Each activity should be reviewed individually for its potential risk, and women should discuss their intentions for physical activity with their primary health care provider. The physiologic and morphologic changes of pregnancy may interfere with the ability to engage safely in some forms of physical activity. Increases in body weight, the forward shift of the center of gravity, and ligamentous laxity experienced during pregnancy can increase the risk of injury (77). Contact sports, activities requiring significant balance or those that increase the risk of falling, and activities with a high potential for injury are not suitable during pregnancy.

To prevent pregnancy complications, such as pre-term labor or placental abruption, exercises with a risk of blunt abdominal trauma or forward fall are not recommended in the 2nd and 3rd trimester. Exercising in the supine position in late pregnancy has also raised concerns because supine cardiac output is decreased compared to cardiac output in the lateral position at rest. The reported 25% decrease in uterine blood flow during supine exercise in women late in gestation is caused by uterus obstruction upon the inferior vena cava experienced in the supine position (13).

Exercise & CVD

Exercise has become a universally accepted component for cardiac rehabilitation and therapy for heart disease. For more than 30 years, aerobic exercise has been an integral part of post-cardiac event rehabilitation and has been used as a key strategy in improving aerobic capacity, while reducing the risks associated with comorbities. Recently, resistance training, particularly performed in circuit format, has become a more popular

Hypertension

Hypertension is characterized by high blood pressure in the circulatory arteries. Blood pressure measures at, or above 140/90 mmHg, are considered hypertensive. The high circulatory pressure causes turbulent blood flow and excessive stress upon the inner lining of the blood vessels, resulting in damage referred to as endothelial lesions. The damage associated with high blood pressure leads to the formation of atherosclerotic plaque and the onset of coronary artery disease. In addition, high blood pressure can lead to kidney damage, stroke, and chronic heart failure.

It has been well documented that hypertension is present in epidemic proportion and is associated with a markedly increased risk of developing cardiovascular disorders (24; 200). For individuals with mild or moderate hypertension, all current treatment guidelines emphasize the role of nonpharmacological interventions, such as modifications to diet and participation in routine physical activity. A large number of studies have demonstrated that regular aerobic exercise reduces the incidence of hypertension and plays a significant role in managing the early stages of the disease (11; 56; 107). In addition to preventing hypertension, regular aerobic exercise has been found to lower blood pressure by an average 10 mmHg in both systolic and diastolic measures, while at the same time improving blood lipid profiles and insulin sensitivity (12; 57). It also improves endothelial function, platelet activation and inflammatory response (84). For individuals with stage 1 hypertension (140-159/90-99 mmHg), with no other coronary risk factors and no evidence of cardiovascular disease, exercise and dietary management are used as the initial treatment, generally lasting twelve months (116). Individuals with diabetes, cardiovascular disease, or with more marked elevations in blood pressure (>180/105 mm Hg) should add endurance exercise training to their treatment regimen only after initiating pharmacologic therapy. Endurance exercise training appears to elicit even greater reductions in blood pressure in medicated patients with hypertension (1).

Dynamic exercise of moderate intensity, 50-75% VO_2max, (e.g. brisk walking, cycling) for 40-60 minutes, 3-5 times per week, is preferable to vigorous exercise because it reduces acute blood pressure response to exercise and appears to be more effective in lowering blood pressure in general (154). Exercise training at somewhat lower intensities (40-70% VO2max) appears to lower blood pressure as much as exercise at higher intensities, which may be important in specific hypertensive populations with lower levels of cardiorespiratory fitness (156; 158). Due to the fact that physically active and fit individuals with hypertension have markedly lower rates of mortality than sedentary, unfit hypertensive individuals, aerobic exercise should be used to manage the disease while serving to improve cardiorespiratory fitness. When addressing program priorities in the exercise prescription among clients with hypertension, cardiorespiratory training should be emphasized because of the above mentioned improvements in reducing morbidity and mortality.

Aerobic activity used to treat hypertension does not have to be performed in single long duration bouts. Research has indicated that several ten minute sessions of brisk walking throughout the day provided the same benefits as 30 minutes of continuous walking at the same intensity (157). The relative intensity and cumulative total duration of work seem to be more important than the activity duration per session. This suggests that individuals with hypertension can manage the disease with planned, short bouts of exercise throughout the day, rather than being required to use a single, long duration workout session. Personal trainers can use this information to acclimate clients to routine exercise without the full commitment of a single, long-duration session.

Resistance training exercise does not provide the same benefits as aerobic training for the treatment of hypertension. Both high intensity aerobic training and resistance training exercise can cause dramatic increases in blood pressure. Although light-moderate resistance training performed using circuit training shows benefits, aerobic training must be a staple component of any exercise program used to manage hypertension (86).

CAD

Coronary artery disease (CAD) is the most common form of heart disease and accounts for the most disease-related deaths in the United States (161). It is characterized by the narrowing, hardening, and blockage of coronary vessels from the build-up of atherosclerotic plaque. It is commonly attributed to several factors, including obesity, physical inactivity, high blood pressure, poor lipid profile, and smoking. Based on these risk factors, a multi-factoral approach is necessary to reduce the risk of progressive atherosclerosis, which leads to coronary artery occlusion and heart attack.

Aerobic training and general increases in physical activity have been recommended as an integral part of prevention and treatment therapies. Exercise improves cardiovascular risk factors by reducing dyslipoproteinemia, sympathetic tone, insulin resistance, and inflammation, while enhancing **fibrinolysis**, normalizing endothelial function, and retarding **atherosclerosis** in the vessels (16; 50). Individuals with established CAD demonstrate improvements in symptoms of **angina** and congestive heart failure and experience attenuation of exercise-induced ischemia (94; 146; 174). Due to the strong evidence of the benefit of exercise in cardiovascular prevention and rehabilitation, it is recommended that exercise should be included in the multidimensional therapy of cardiovascular disease.

Regular aerobic exercise results in an increase in exercise capacity, improved circulatory function and lower myocardial oxygen demand, leading to cardiovascular benefits. It is recommended that individuals with heart disease who have been cleared

---

General Guidelines for Hypertension

- Aerobic exercise – accumulate 40-60 minutes using 50-80% HRR on most, if not all, days.
- Resistance training – use 12-15 repetitions, preferably in circuit format; avoid heavy resistance training and breath holding.
- Reduce salt intake.
- Adequate potassium intake (90 mmol per day).
- Reduce body weight if overweight.
- Limit or avoid alcohol.

for exercise gradually build up to 60 accumulated minutes of aerobic exercise most days, progressing to continuous exercise performed 3 or more times per week for 30 to 60 minutes (49). The initial goal of the exercise is to attain a work rate that results in the expenditure of 100 to 200 kcal per exercise session. Exercise at this level has been shown to reduce systolic blood pressure and heart rate at rest. While performing submaximal work, exercise can increase the level of physical work capacity, reduce the myocardial oxygen cost at rest and during performance of submaximal exercise, aid in the reduction of body fat with a concomitant increase in muscle mass, and reduce plasma triglyceride levels (85; 122). When combined with pharmacologic intervention and diet therapies, the benefits are more significant. Studies show that aerobic exercise, combined with cholesterol reducing agents such as statins, can lead to atherosclerotic plaque regression.

As an adjunct to endurance training, individuals with CAD can benefit from resistance training via improved muscle strength and endurance, increased metabolism and cardiovascular function, enhanced psychosocial well-being and quality of life, and concurrent reductions of cardiovascular risk factors (8; 203). Individuals with disease that present good cardiac performance capacity may include resistance training without any restraints as part of cardiac rehabilitation programs for CAD (168). However, based on the current data, resistance training is not recommended for all persons with heart disease (135). Individuals with CAD should be clinically screened and perform a symptom-limited maximal graded exercise test prior to engaging in resistance training. Individuals who have characteristics associated with an increased risk of cardiac event during exercise should avoid heavy resistance training. The level of appropriate participation is highly dependent on the individual's clinical status, cardiac stress tolerance, and the presence of comorbidities. Persons with myocardial ischemia and/or poor left ventricular function should not engage in resistance training, as the exercise may lead to cardiac wall motion disturbances and severe ventricular arrhythmias. Individuals who may safely engage in resistance exercise activities should

possess moderate-to-good left ventricular function, cardiac capacity greater than 5-6 METS, with no symptoms of angina pectoris or ST segment depression (a finding on EKG) (136). Given the complicated nature of these tests, inclusion of resistance training in the exercise prescription should be made by the client's physician and not the personal trainer.

The criteria for participation in resistive training are the same as those used for the more traditional cardiac and high risk exercise programs. Of primary concern is the risk of cardiovascular complications related to the dramatic rise in blood pressure associated with heavy resistance training. What must be considered is that the actual blood pressure response depends on a variety of controllable factors, including magnitude of the isometric component, the intensity of the movement, the amount of muscle mass involved, and the number of repetitions or duration of the load. Recent studies have demonstrated that when the resistance is limited to lower intensities, the blood pressure response is fairly

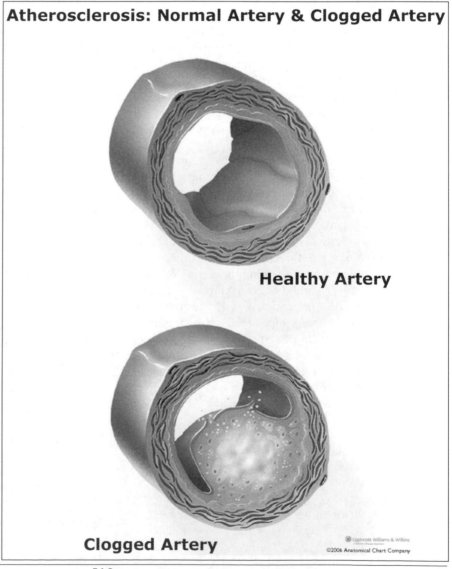

Atherosclerosis: Normal Artery & Clogged Artery

Healthy Artery

Clogged Artery

Lippincott Williams & Wilkins
©2006 Anatomical Chart Company

General Recommendations for CAD

- Aerobic exercise
- Accumulate up to 40-60 minutes of low intensity aerobic activity most days of the week. Increase to a frequency of 3-4 sessions per week, at an intensity of 40-75% HRR for 20-40 minutes.
- Use 10 minute warm-up and cool down periods
- Resistance training
- Introduce resistance training using closed-chain, body weight activities: 1 set, 15-20 repetitions. Circuits may include one exercise per muscle group to start and gradually progress at a client-appropriate pace.
- Cardiovascular measures should be monitored, and RPE should be used to gauge intensity.
- Medications should be accounted for and used in accordance with physician recommendations.
- Flexibility should be encouraged, utilizing proper breathing techniques.
- Avoid heavy resistance, isometric training, and breath holding during activities.

---

minimal. Intra-arterial blood pressure measurements in cardiac patients have demonstrated that, during low-intensity resistance training (40-60% maximum voluntary contraction) with 15-20 repetitions, only modest elevations in blood pressure occur (166; 191). The blood pressure response to low intensity weight training is similar to the values seen during moderate endurance training and can be safely utilized in medically cleared clients with CAD (137; 167; 190).

Resistance training activities may include any number of modalities consistent with standard strength training. Activities aimed at improved functional strength support activities of daily living and may enhance daily physical activity participation. Body weight exercises, free weights, elastic bands, and other resistive modalities may be used for exercise of major muscle groups in cardiopulmonary rehabilitation. Resistive training workloads should be determined by gradual acclimation to movement proficiency. Higher repetition schemes with light resistance encourage improved neuromuscular movement patterns and present minimal effect on the blood pressure response. The exercise prescription should be managed using heart rate, blood pressure, rate-pressure product, and rating of perceived exertion criteria to determine lifting loads and movements.

Circuit weight training is an ideal method for implementing strength training activities in cardiac-compromised clients. It has been reported to improve strength, lean body mass, self-efficacy, and may decrease risk factors for coronary artery disease (76; 189). This mode of exercise may allow clients to perform daily strength tasks safely, more efficiently, and with greater self-confidence. Circuit training has become an accepted component of exercise programs for populations with cardiac risk. Although reports are somewhat limited, studies have shown that high risk clients can attain increases in fitness similar to those seen in healthy populations (114). Furthermore, the hemodynamic responses to circuit weight training suggest that it is a clinically safe and acceptable form of exercise for most individuals with CAD (23).

Circuit training activities should be client specific and adapted to acceptable MET levels of work output. Cardiovascular measures should be monitored during the training, and adjustments should be made based on heart rate response and guided by RPE. Longer warm-ups prior to engagement and increased periods of transitional rest should be utilized based on rate of perceived exertion. Closed-chain body weight exercises are effective in enhancing fitness components that may transfer to daily life activities. Proper breathing techniques should be monitored to avoid breath holding, and isometric abdominal contractions should be avoided. In general, one exercise for each major muscle group can be used with approximately 15-20 repetitions. Programs should start out with single sets and may be moved to two sets per muscle group as a client improves in function and work capacity (172).

Congestive Heart Failure

Congestive heart failure (CHF) is caused by an enlargement of the left ventricle and central portion of the heart in response to CAD and the strain against vascular peripheral resistance. The hypertrophic adapatation alters the efficiency of the heart in mobilizing blood through the chambers and leads to a significant reduction in stroke volume, as well as reduced valvular function. The compromised cardiac output limits oxygen availability and decreases work capacity. Individuals with CHF demonstrate poor cardiovascular status and impaired exercise capacity due to both cardiac limitations and peripheral maladaptations of the skeletal musculature. The reduced work capacity often leads to significant peripheral muscle atrophy and functional decline.

According to researchers, individuals with congestive heart failure who participate in an aerobic exercise training program can improve their circulation, increase the pumping capacity of their hearts, and may positively affect heart enlargement (71; 103). Due to the related pathology and low levels of exercise tolerance, individuals with CHF have limited selection in the activities they can effectively participate in with adequate success. Walking and stationary cycling have both shown to be tolerable to individuals with CHF and lead to improvements in aerobic capacity (182). Initially, lower-intensity steady-state training should be used but can be exchanged for interval training as improvements in function are documented. Interval training has demonstrated a positive effect upon peripheral musculature, above that seen with steady-state training, without inducing greater cardiovascular stress. At present time, an optimal parameter for measuring intensity has not been established, but the intensity range of 40-80% peak oxygen consumption has been applied successfully (113; 141). A heart rate reserve of 60-80% may be used in conjunction with RPE to guide exercise intensity (142). RPE is generally a better measure of intensity than heart rate when gauging intensity, given that most clients with CHF are on medicines (B-Blockers and Ca^{++} channel blockers) that block the heart rate response. Due to the inability to sustain work for long periods of time, initial exercise should utilize 40-50% peak VO_2 with exercise duration lasting at least 3-5 min per session, performed several times daily (143). Progression order should emphasize duration before frequency, with intensity being the last stage of progression.

Peripheral muscular weakness is of significant concern with CHF clients (43). Recent scientific evidence suggests that the application of specific resistance exercise activities are safe and induce significant and important metabolic and functional adaptations in the peripheral skeletal muscles (102; 124; 192). These adaptations are valuable in addressing the issues of muscle weakness and atrophy facing the majority of CHF patients. Resistance training has been shown to improve exercise tolerance and peak oxygen consumption, stimulate changes in muscle composition and muscle hypertrophy, lead to alterations in skeletal muscle metabolism, and contribute to improvements in muscular strength and endurance, particularly when applied in combination with aerobic exercise (101; 123; 192).

Resistance training activities must be modified to cater to the specific limitations of individuals with CHF. The main focus of the exercise program is to effectively train the skeletal muscles without producing significant cardiovascular stress. Therefore, resistance training activities differ for clients with CHF compared to prescriptions for other cardiac impairments. Resistance training should emphasize small muscle groups, using short bouts of work and appropriate repetitions to avoid excessive stress on the cardiac muscle (144).

When performing dynamic strength exercises, the movements should be slow and controlled at intensity values of 50-60% of one repetition maximum. The number of repetitions can range between 15 and 20, or as tolerated, but work durations should not exceed 60 seconds (112; 192). Following the performance of the exercise, adequate recovery periods should be utilized. In general, a recovery period greater than twice the set duration is necessary. Individuals who present low cardiac reserve may be required to lift very limited loads, such as small free weights (2-6 lbs), or utilize elastic bands with 8-10 repetitions. Exercise machines may also be used effectively by clients with CHF (192). It is important to understand that CHF represents a wide spectrum of disability. Some CHF clients will tolerate close to normal training stress, whereas others may be severely limited. Since there exists such variability in this client population, it is very important that these clients get medical clearance and that the personal trainer adhere closely to physician recommendations.

Children & Exercise

Over the past few decades, the prevalence of overweight and obesity among children and adolescents in the United States has increased dramatically. The number of overweight children between ages 2 and 5 has more than doubled since the 1970s. In school-aged children, that number has almost tripled (26). Children and adolescents who are overweight have a high susceptibility to becoming obese as adults (46). In addition, the level of obesity found in adults is related to childhood weight (138).

General Recommendations for Congestive Heart Failure

- Short bouts of aerobic activity 40-50% peak oxygen capacity, performed several times per day for durations of at least 3-5 minutes per session.
- Resistance training, using smaller amounts of muscle mass with intensities of 50%-60% 1RM performed as tolerated, with longer rest intervals.
- Activities should use RPE and avoid excessive stress due to the limited work capacity.
- Progressions should mirror individual tolerance and work capacity.

Overweight children and adolescents are at risk for an increased number of health problems during their youth and into adulthood. Overweight and obese children experience an elevated risk for the development of risk factors associated with cardiovascular disease, including high blood pressure, high cholesterol, and Type II diabetes (117). In a population-based sample of 5 to 17-year-olds, almost 60% of overweight children had at least one CVD risk factor, while 25% of overweight children had two or more CVD risk factors (91). Less common health conditions associated with increased weight in children include asthma, hepatic steatosis (fatty degeneration of the liver), and **sleep apnea** (intermittent breathing cessation) (47). Additional consequences of childhood and adolescent overweight stem from psychosocial-related factors. Overweight children and adolescents are targets of early and systematic social discrimination (193). Overweight children report lower self-esteem than non-overweight children and may develop impaired social function, a condition which often persists into adulthood (194).

Exercise and routine physical activity can have a pronounced effect on the health and fitness of children and adolescents (149). Routine participation in exercise and sports-related activities can improve cardiovascular fitness, bone health, reduce susceptibility to weight gain, improve glucose tolerance, and reduce the risk of the early development of health problems (27; 148). Children can benefit from all types of activity, including strength training, flexibility, and aerobic conditioning.

Differences Between Children & Adults

Although children and adults experience similar benefits from aerobic and resistance training, physiological differences exist between these populations. The muscle characteristics of children are quantitatively and qualitatively different from those of adults. Performance differences between adults and children seem to be metabolically and hormonally mediated. Children are similar to adults in the ability to use the immediate anaerobic energy system. Children tolerate short, intense exercise similarly to adults but demonstrate a greater ability to

recover (63). This is likely due to lower peak power outputs, attributed to less muscle mass and lower stimulation of type II fibers. Additionally, faster phosphocreatine resynthesis, greater oxidative capacity, better acid-base regulation, faster readjustment of initial cardiorespiratory parameters, and higher removal of metabolic by-products in children could explain their faster recovery following high-intensity exercise.

When the glycolytic pathway is employed during exercise, children demonstrate a reduced performance capacity compared to adults (15). Children seem to maintain an immature glycolytic system in both storage and enzyme concentration until puberty (177). The reduced activity of phosphofructokinase-1 and lactate dehydrogenase enzymes (two key enzymatic reactions in glycolysis) likely limit the rate of glycolytic ATP generation in children. This assumption is supported by a lower production of muscle lactate relative to adults, suggesting less reliance on this energy system during the performance of work.

Upon comparisons of aerobic metabolism, children are better in terms of achieving steady-state heart rate during endurance activities (184). Children are well adapted to prolonged exercise of moderate intensity due to efficient utilization of lipids, as demonstrated by lower respiratory exchange ratio values during moderate

---

General Guidelines for Children

Aerobic Training

- Children can train at steady-state levels similar to adults.
- Avoid extended periods of activity.
- Children can perform short bouts (10 minutes) of intense aerobic exercise on an intermittent basis.
- Emphasize enjoyable activities that simulate play.
- Be cautious of overheating, and make sure children remain hydrated.

Resistance Training

- Higher repetition schemes are more effective for pre-pubescent children.
- Encourage motor learning and proper technique.
- In general, 2 sets are sufficient for improvements in strength and endurance.
- Multi-joint activities that develop motor skill are preferred over isolated training.
- It is not recommended that children lift loads greater than their 8 RM.
- Progressive overload should emphasize increased repetitions, rather than load.
- Pubescent adolescents can follow similar prescriptions as adults, but the emphasis should be on motor learning and efficient movement patterns.

Key Terms

Fibrinolysis – The process where a fibrin clot (blood clot), the product of coagulation, is broken down.

Atherosclerosis – The build up of plaque on the inside of blood vessels.

Angina – Chest pain or discomfort, often resulting from restricted blood flow to the heart.

Congestive heart failure (CHF) – A condition caused by the heart's inability to maintain adequate blood circulation in the peripheral tissues and the lungs, marked by a significant reduction in stroke volume, reduced valvular function, and shortness of breath.

Sleep apnea – A condition in which breathing is interrupted or even stops periodically during sleep.

Thermoregulation – The process of actively maintaining a constant internal body temperature regardless of the surrounding environment.

endurance exercise. Data indicate that children rely more on fat oxidation than adults, which is likely attributed to increased free fatty acid mobilization, greater glycerol release, and increases in growth hormone release in prepubescent children during exercise (165).

Differences between adults and children are also observed within the cardiovascular system. Children demonstrate higher heart rates with lower stroke volume and total cardiac output at a given submaximal work rate (183). Likewise, at maximal exercise intensities, heart rates are higher, while stroke volume and cardiac output remain lower in children compared to adults (185). Physiological differences, including heart size and blood volume likely account for the differences in stroke volume. Recovery heart rates occur at a faster rate in children compared to adults, which may be due to the greater reliance on lipid metabolism during steady-state exercise.

Thermoregulation in response to exposure to hot and cold environments differs between children and adults (96). Many physical and physiological changes occur during growth and maturation that can affect thermoregulation during resting and active states. In most cases, the physical and physiological differences between children and adults explain the different responses to thermal stress (170).

The primary physiological difference affecting the thermoregulation of heat between children and adults is related to the sweating mechanism. Children produce less sweat and have a lower sweating rate per gland, even though the heat-activated sweat glands are present in higher densities than in adults (95). The lower sweating rate per gland may be explained by the smaller sweat gland size, a lower sensitivity of the sweating mechanism to thermal stimuli, and possibly, a lower sweat gland metabolic capacity. Additional differences in thermoregulation between children and adults include metabolic, circulatory, and hormonal disparities (97). Adults have a much higher surface-area-to-mass ratio than children, allowing for greater heat loss to the environment, thereby placing less reliance on evaporative cooling. Likewise, children have a lower blood volume than adults, which may limit the internal transfer of heat to the body's surface for dry release (170). Children are also at a thremodynamic disadvantage when walking or running in heated environments due to higher metabolic costs of locomotion and greater cardiovascular strain from a lower cardiac output and less hemoglobin (40; 98). The increased physiological demand leads to more rapid increases in internal temperatures when exercising in the heat (99).

Program Considerations

Children can perform aerobic exercise using prescriptions that are similar to adults. With running, children experience a reduced heart rate, but training zones can be used to reflect appropriate intensity and pace. Cycling response is similar between children and adults, so no adjustment is required (186). The key to getting children active in aerobic-based training is to select activities that they enjoy. If the activity is not perceived as fun, it is not likely they will engage in it on a routine basis. Pushing children into structured exercise rather than activities that are perceived as play may turn them off to participation in the future. Children should pick their own activities and be encouraged to perform either intermittent, high-intensity work or moderate, steady-state paced training to take advantage of their physiologic differences.

Children can also benefit from routine resistance training activities. Previous research has shown that children can increase their muscular strength and muscular endurance as a result of regular participation in a progressive resistance training program (140; 195). Interestingly, higher repetition schemes (13-15 repetitions), using lighter resistance provide better results than lower repetition prescriptions (6-8 repetitions) using heavier loads, when performed two times per week with only single sets per exercise (59; 62). When high repetition training (13-15 repetitions) was compared to moderately-heavy resistance training

(6-8 repetitions), and contrast training (totaling 12-16 repetitions) similar results occurred (58; 61). Dramatic, and almost identical, improvements were found in the high repetition resistance and contrast training above the heavier resistance loads.

Children do not experience the same dramatic endocrine response as adults with heavy resistance training due to immature hormonal glands. Adaptations to strength training in children are neurally driven. Therefore, higher repetition activities cause greater motor enhancements when compared to low repetition training. Children should be encouraged to focus on motor efficiency rather than heavy resistance training for optimal improvements. Following puberty, adolescents can engage in repetition schemes that are similar to adults, but again, the emphasis should be on proper technique rather than maximal attainable loads. Children demonstrate significant adaptation response to routine strength training, even at limited volumes (64). One day of strength training on child-sized weight machines per week, using one set of 10-15 repetitions for 12 exercises, demonstrated limited gain in upper body strength, but a 14% improvement in lower body strength (60). When a second day of strength training was added per week, significant improvements were found in all measures. These findings support the concept that muscular strength can be improved during the childhood years with limited volume, and that a frequency of only twice per week is required for improvements in children participating in an introductory strength training program.

Exercise & the Elderly

Age-related losses in physiologic capacities contribute to the decline in physical function in the elderly population. Diminution in aerobic capacity, muscular fitness and power have significant implications for aging adults. A general lack of physical activity contributes to a 10%-30% loss of biological function between the ages of 40 and 65, with the most pronounced decline affecting the physically inactive (171; 178). Further decline may be related to the presence of disease, genetic and environmental factors, poor mental health, or pre-existing injuries, including chronic low back pain. Sedentary elderly, in particular have an elevated susceptibility to hypertension and coronary artery disease, the onset of metabolic disease often related to obesity, and limitations related to structural changes in the connective tissues (93).

Fifty percent of individuals between 65 and 74 years of age report at least one physical limitation, with 30% reporting significant limitations (25). It is suggested that 50% of individuals over 65 have hypertension, and at least 27% have been diagnosed with heart disease (150). In many cases, the limitations experienced by older adults are caused by a decrease in muscle mass and range of motion due to limited physical activity.

Sarcopenia signifies the age-related loss of muscle mass with consequential reductions in muscle strength and power (152). The loss of power and strength appear to be caused by both muscular and neural factors (130). Following age sixty, the decline becomes accelerated, leading to a pronounced loss of function. Although all older adults experience some level of decline, sedentary older adults experience the greatest reduction in muscle quantity and quality and physical performance (17). This situation is worsened by the steady decline in aerobic capacity. These factors contribute to a loss of quality of life and independence. Strength training increases muscle strength and muscular power in the elderly, thus counteracting part of the age-related loss (106). Improvements, however, depend on the initial strength of the elderly person. The benefit of strength training is greatest in frail elderly and the very old, although all older adults can benefit from strength training. Considering the growing segment of the elderly population, the focus on sarcopenia and measures to counteract it are becoming increasingly more important.

Benefits of Exercise

Independent older adults gain significant functional benefits from both aerobic and strength training activities (120). Aerobic exercise results in improvements in functional capacity and may reduce blood pressure and risk of developing type II diabetes in the elderly. Adaptations to routine aerobic exercise occur similarly between younger and older men and include increased cardiac output and oxygen extraction capabilities (75). The adaptations in older women, however, are almost exclusively related to improvements in oxygen extraction capabilities (173). Although comparisons between the young and the old identify differences in maximal oxygen extraction and cardiac output, older adults may improve their aerobic capacity by 10%-30% with routine aerobic exercise (155). The yearly decline in maximal heart rate accounts for the greatest reduction in cardiac output with age, while decline in oxygen extraction capabilities are likely attributed to the progressive loss of lean mass in the elderly.

Resistance exercise demonstrates the greatest capacity to arrest decline and substantially improve physical function in the elderly (131). It has been clearly demonstrated that skeletal muscle in older, untrained men and women will respond with significant strength gains, accompanied by considerable increases in muscle fiber size and capillary density (66). Maximal working capacity, VO₂max, and serum lipid profiles also benefit from high-intensity resistance training. Resistance training has been shown to significantly increase energy requirements, insulin sensitivity and yield positive effects on multiple risk factors for osteoporotic fractures in previously sedentary, post-menopausal women (92). Interestingly, overall physical activity seems to increase in those participating in exercise programs compared to sedentary controls (125). This may be related to increased physical confidence and a reduced concern for falling. In the frail elderly, strength training demonstrates such remarkable effects that it is recommended above aerobic training to maintain adequate function in performing daily tasks, such as getting out of bed and rising from a seated position (87; 151).

Consideration for Training

A combination of aerobic activity, strength training, and flexibility exercises, plus increased general daily activity have shown to enhance functional independence and improve quality of life in older adults. Aerobic activity can be prescribed in the same manner as it would be for healthy young adults but most often requires an acclimation phase in the lower end of the normal training zones (108). Deconditioned older adults can start by accumulating 30-40 minutes of aerobic exercise performed throughout the day before progressing to continuous, low end (50%-60% HRR)

steady-state training (3; 169). Healthy older adults should also begin at appropriate lower-end starting points before being progressed to higher exercise intensity.

Flexibility training should be encouraged for older adults, following adequate warm-up periods. Static stretching is beneficial when performed 2-3 days per week, using all the major muscle groups (45). Functional based activities, particularly those performed with a closed-chain through full ranges of movement, can also contribute to improved functional range (65). Encouraging tasks of daily activity using multi-planar movements can improve balance, movement efficiency, and dynamic range of motion. Older adults are particularly susceptible to limited range of motion in trunk extension, trunk rotation, shoulder flexion, and external humeral rotation due to postural adjustments common with age. Limitations should be identified, and dynamic movements and static stretching should be used to encourage improved range of motion in deficient areas.

Resistance training is an integral part of the exercise prescription for older adults. Heavy, moderate, and low intensity resistance training protocols have shown to be effective in improving muscular strength and size in older adults (42). This suggests that low-intensity resistance training can be beneficial for muscular fitness in individuals who cannot safely perform high-intensity exercise or where heavy resistance training is contraindicated (44).

General Guidelines for Older Adults

Resistance Training

- 2-3 times per week, using 8-10 exercises, 10-15 repetitions. Progressions can be similar to healthy, young adults.
- Encourage functional-based full range of motion activities, particularly loaded closed-chain movements.
- Include functional power activities, including hip flexion and extension.
- Healthy older adults can use heavy resistance training but should avoid breath holds and isometric contractions.

Aerobic Training

- Deconditioned older adults should accumulate 30-40 minutes in 10 minute sessions most days of the week using 50%-60% HRR.
- For healthy older adults 60%-80% HRR for 30-60 minutes is appropriate.

Flexibility

- Static stretching through pain free range should be performed 2-3 times per week, using 2-3 sets of 15-30 second holds.
- Encourage appropriate breathing techniques.
- Dynamic ROM – 2-3 sets, 10-15 repetitions.

Improvements in muscular strength and endurance can be attained with limited exercise volume, something to consider when initiating an exercise program for the elderly (2; 54; 175). Similar to children, training the major muscle groups once or twice per week, at moderate intensity, is sufficient for improvement (88; 176). Likewise, resistance training consisting of only single-set exercises provides adequate stress to significantly enhance muscle function and physical performance in new exercisers (74).

The aging neuromuscular system is highly responsive to resistance training. Therefore, following the initial adaptations to strength programs, older adults should be encouraged to participate in higher-volume work. In most cases, the elderly are most challenged by daily tasks that require the ability to generate short bursts of energy anaerobically. The performance of daily tasks, such as stair climbing or lifting an object, requires both muscle strength and power. Due to the fact that high levels of physical function are associated with elevated levels of anaerobic power in older adults, and that muscle power recedes at a faster rate than strength with age, it is necessary to emphasize power training in programs for the elderly where appropriate (53). Peak muscle power may be improved similarly using light, moderate, or heavy resistances, which allows for different options based on the capabilities of the client (67). Research suggests that using heavy loads during explosive resistance training may be the most effective strategy to achieve simultaneous improvements in muscle strength, power, and endurance in older adults

(41). It is important to realize that the high intensity is relative to the client's maximal values, which are often relatively low. Individual capacity will determine the most appropriate exercise prescription.

Exercise plays an important role in enhancing the quality of life of the older adult. Improved physiologic and psychological function helps to maintain personal independence and reduces the effects of aging. One of the largest obstacles to helping older adults is getting them to start participating in physical activities. Initially, many older persons have low physical confidence and fear they will become injured by engaging in physical activities. Older adults must be educated to the importance of physical activity, individually encouraged to participate, and appropriately supported during and after participation to ensure sustained involvement.

Chapter Twenty-Two References

1. Nonpharmacological interventions as an adjunct to the pharmacological treatment of hypertension: a statement by WHL. The World Hypertension League. *J Hum Hypertens* 7: 159-164, 1993.

2. The recommended quantity and quality of exercise for developing and maintaining cardiorespiratory and muscular fitness in healthy adults. Position stand of the American College of Sports Medicine. *Schweiz Z Sportmed* 41: 127-137, 1993.

3. American College of Sports Medicine Position Stand. The recommended quantity and quality of exercise for developing and maintaining cardiorespiratory and muscular fitness, and flexibility in healthy adults. *Med Sci Sports Exerc* 30: 975-991, 1998.

4. SMA statement the benefits and risks of exercise during pregnancy. Sport Medicine Australia. *J Sci Med Sport* 5: 11-19, 2002.

5. SMA statement the benefits and risks of exercise during pregnancy. Sport Medicine Australia. *J Sci Med Sport* 5: 11-19, 2002.

6. Exercise during pregnancy and the postpartum period. *Clin Obstet Gynecol* 46: 496-499, 2003.

7. Impact of physical activity during pregnancy and postpartum on chronic disease risk. *Med Sci Sports Exerc* 38: 989-1006, 2006.

8. **Ades PA, Savage PD, Brochu M, Tischler MD, Lee NM and Poehlman ET**. Resistance training increases total daily energy expenditure in disabled older women with coronary heart disease. *J Appl Physiol* 98: 1280-1285, 2005.

9. **Artal R**. Exercise and pregnancy. *Clin Sports Med* 11: 363-377, 1992.

10. **Avery ND, Stocking KD, Tranmer JE, Davies GA and Wolfe LA**. Fetal responses to maternal strength conditioning exercises in late gestation. *Can J Appl Physiol* 24: 362-376, 1999.

11. **Baster T and Baster-Brooks C**. Exercise and hypertension. *Aust Fam Physician* 34: 419-424, 2005.

12. **Baster T and Baster-Brooks C**. Exercise and hypertension. *Aust Fam Physician* 34: 419-424, 2005.

13. **Bell R and O'Neill M**. Exercise and pregnancy: a review. *Birth* 21: 85-95, 1994.

14. **Ben Haroush A, Yogev Y and Hod M**. Epidemiology of gestational diabetes mellitus and its association with Type 2 diabetes. *Diabet Med* 21: 103-113, 2004.

15. **Beneke R, Hutler M, Jung M and Leithauser RM**. Modeling the blood lactate kinetics at maximal short-term exercise conditions in children, adolescents, and adults. *J Appl Physiol* 99: 499-504, 2005.

16. **Bertoli A, Di Daniele N, Ceccobelli M, Ficara A, Girasoli C and De Lorenzo A**. Lipid profile, BMI, body fat distribution, and aerobic fitness in men with metabolic syndrome. *Acta Diabetol* 40 Suppl 1: S130-S133, 2003.

17. **Binder EF, Yarasheski KE, Steger-May K, Sinacore DR, Brown M, Schechtman KB and Holloszy JO**. Effects of progressive resistance training on body composition in frail older adults: results of a randomized, controlled trial. *J Gerontol A Biol Sci Med Sci* 60: 1425-1431, 2005.

18. **Boas SR, Danduran MJ and Saini SK**. Anaerobic exercise testing in children with asthma. *J Asthma* 35: 481-487, 1998.

19. **Brown W**. The benefits of physical activity during pregnancy. *J Sci Med Sport* 5: 37-45, 2002.

20. **Brown W**. The benefits of physical activity during pregnancy. *J Sci Med Sport* 5: 37-45, 2002.

21. **Burr ML**. Epidemiology of childhood asthma. *Allerg Immunol (Paris)* 23: 348-350, 1991.

22. **Burr ML**. Epidemiology of childhood asthma. *Allerg Immunol (Paris)* 23: 348-350, 1991.

23. **Butler RM, Palmer G and Rogers FJ**. Circuit weight training in early cardiac rehabilitation. *J Am Osteopath Assoc* 92: 77-89, 1992.

24. **Callow AD**. Cardiovascular disease 2005--the global picture. *Vascul Pharmacol* 45: 302-307, 2006.

25. **Campbell VA, Crews JE, Moriarty DG, Zack MM and Blackman DK**. Surveillance for sensory impairment, activity limitation, and health-related quality of life among older adults--United States, 1993-1997. *MMWR CDC Surveill Summ* 48: 131-156, 1999.

26. **Carrel AL and Bernhardt DT**. Exercise prescription for the prevention of obesity in adolescents. *Curr Sports Med Rep* 3: 330-336, 2004.

27. **Carrel AL, Clark RR, Peterson SE, Nemeth BA, Sullivan J and Allen DB**. Improvement of fitness, body composition, and insulin sensitivity in overweight children in a school-based exercise program: a randomized, controlled study. *Arch Pediatr Adolesc Med* 159: 963-968, 2005.

28. **Case J, Willoughby D, Haley-Zitlin V and Maybee P**. Preventing type 2 diabetes after gestational diabetes. *Diabetes Educ* 32: 877-886, 2006.

29. **Catalano PM**. Management of obesity in pregnancy. *Obstet Gynecol* 109: 419-433, 2007.

30. **Cauza E, Hanusch-Enserer U, Strasser B, Ludvik B, Metz-Schimmerl S, Pacini G, Wagner O, Georg P, Prager R, Kostner K, Dunky A and Haber P**. The relative benefits of endurance and strength training on the metabolic factors and muscle function of people with type 2 diabetes mellitus. *Arch Phys Med Rehabil* 86: 1527-1533, 2005.

31. **Cauza E, Hanusch-Enserer U, Strasser B, Ludvik B, Metz-Schimmerl S, Pacini G, Wagner O, Georg P, Prager R, Kostner K, Dunky A and Haber P**. The relative benefits of endurance and strength training on the metabolic factors and muscle function of people with type 2 diabetes mellitus. *Arch Phys Med Rehabil* 86: 1527-1533, 2005.

32. **Church TS, LaMonte MJ, Barlow CE and Blair SN**. Cardiorespiratory fitness and body mass index as predictors of cardiovascular disease mortality among men with diabetes. *Arch Intern Med* 165: 2114-2120, 2005.

33. **Clapp JF, III**. Oxygen consumption during treadmill exercise before, during, and after pregnancy. *Am J Obstet Gynecol* 161: 1458-1464, 1989.

34. **Clapp JF, III**. Exercise and fetal health. *J Dev Physiol* 15: 9-14, 1991.

35. **Clapp JF, III**. Exercise and fetal health. *J Dev Physiol* 15: 9-14, 1991.

36. **Clark CJ and Cochrane LM**. Physical activity and asthma. *Curr Opin Pulm Med* 5: 68-75, 1999.

37. **Cole PL and Sutton MS**. Normal cardiopulmonary adjustments to pregnancy: cardiovascular evaluation. *Cardiovasc Clin* 19: 37-56, 1989.

38. **Collings C and Curet LB**. Fetal heart rate response to maternal exercise. *Am J Obstet Gynecol* 151: 498-501, 1985.

39. **Constantini N, Harman-Boehm I and Dubnov G**. [Exercise prescription for diabetics: more than a general recommendation]. *Harefuah* 144: 717-23, 750, 2005.

40. **Davies CT**. Metabolic cost of exercise and physical performance in children with some observations on external loading. *Eur J Appl Physiol Occup Physiol* 45: 95-102, 1980.

41. **de Vos NJ, Singh NA, Ross DA, Stavrinos TM, Orr R and Fiatarone Singh MA**. Optimal load for increasing muscle power during explosive resistance training in older adults. *J Gerontol A Biol Sci Med Sci* 60: 638-647, 2005.

42. **de Vos NJ, Singh NA, Ross DA, Stavrinos TM, Orr R and Fiatarone Singh MA**. Optimal load for increasing muscle power during explosive resistance training in older adults. *J Gerontol A Biol Sci Med Sci* 60: 638-647, 2005.

43. **Delagardelle C, Feiereisen P, Autier P, Shita R, Krecke R and Beissel J**. Strength/endurance training versus endurance training in congestive heart failure. *Med Sci Sports Exerc* 34: 1868-1872, 2002.

44. **Delecluse C, Colman V, Roelants M, Verschueren S, Derave W, Ceux T, Eijnde BO, Seghers J, Pardaens K, Brumagne S, Goris M, Buekers M, Spaepen A, Swinnen S and Stijnen V**. Exercise programs for older men: mode and intensity to induce the highest possible health-related benefits. *Prev Med* 39: 823-833, 2004.

45. **DiBrezzo R, Shadden BB, Raybon BH and Powers M**. Exercise intervention designed to improve strength and dynamic balance among community-dwelling older adults. *J Aging Phys Act* 13: 198-209, 2005.

46. **Dietz WH**. Health consequences of obesity in youth: childhood predictors of adult disease. *Pediatrics* 101: 518-525, 1998.

47. **Dietz WH**. Health consequences of obesity in youth: childhood predictors of adult disease. *Pediatrics* 101: 518-525, 1998.

48. **Draznin MB and Patel DR**. Diabetes mellitus and sports. *Adolesc Med* 9: 457-65, v, 1998.

49. **Duncan GE, Perri MG, Anton SD, Limacher MC, Martin AD, Lowenthal DT, Arning E, Bottiglieri T and Stacpoole PW**. Effects of exercise on emerging and traditional cardiovascular risk factors. *Prev Med* 39: 894-902, 2004.

50. **Duncan GE, Perri MG, Anton SD, Limacher MC, Martin AD, Lowenthal DT, Arning E, Bottiglieri T and Stacpoole PW**. Effects of exercise on emerging and traditional cardiovascular risk factors. *Prev Med* 39: 894-902, 2004.

51. **Emtner M, Finne M and Stalenheim G**. High-intensity physical training in adults with asthma. A comparison between training on land and in water. *Scand J Rehabil Med* 30: 201-209, 1998.

52. **Emtner M, Finne M and Stalenheim G**. High-intensity physical training in adults with asthma. A comparison between training on land and in water. *Scand J Rehabil Med* 30: 201-209, 1998.

53. **Evans W**. Functional and metabolic consequences of sarcopenia. *J Nutr* 127: 998S-1003S, 1997.

54. **Evans WJ**. Exercise training guidelines for the elderly. *Med Sci Sports Exerc* 31: 12-17, 1999.

55. **Fabre OD, Caraballo PM, Gonzalez SS, Cabezas Gutierrez MJ, Arjona RR, Coutin MG, Aguilar FL and Rodriguez VR**. [Psychological factors contributing to asthma in asthmatic children and adolescents and their parents]. *Rev Alerg Mex* 52: 164-170, 2005.

56. **Fagard RH and Cornelissen VA**. Effect of exercise on blood pressure control in hypertensive patients. *Eur J Cardiovasc Prev Rehabil* 14: 12-17, 2007.

57. **Fagard RH and Cornelissen VA**. Effect of exercise on blood pressure control in hypertensive patients. *Eur J Cardiovasc Prev Rehabil* 14: 12-17, 2007.

58. **Faigenbaum AD, Loud RL, O'Connell J, Glover S, O'Connell J and Westcott WL**. Effects of different resistance training protocols on upper-body strength and endurance development in children. *J Strength Cond Res* 15: 459-465, 2001.

59. **Faigenbaum AD, Loud RL, O'Connell J, Glover S, O'Connell J and Westcott WL**. Effects of different resistance training protocols on upper-body strength and endurance development in children. *J Strength Cond Res* 15: 459-465, 2001.

60. **Faigenbaum AD, Milliken LA, Loud RL, Burak BT, Doherty CL and Westcott WL**. Comparison of 1 and 2 days per week of strength training in children. *Res Q Exerc Sport* 73: 416-424, 2002.

61. **Faigenbaum AD, Westcott WL, Loud RL and Long C**. The effects of different resistance training protocols on muscular strength and endurance development in children. *Pediatrics* 104: e5, 1999.

62. **Faigenbaum AD, Westcott WL, Loud RL and Long C**. The effects of different resistance training protocols on muscular strength and endurance development in children. *Pediatrics* 104: e5, 1999.

63. **Falk B and Dotan R**. Child-adult differences in the recovery from high-intensity exercise. *Exerc Sport Sci Rev* 34: 107-112, 2006.

64. **Falk B and Tenenbaum G**. The effectiveness of resistance training in children. A meta-analysis. *Sports Med* 22: 176-186, 1996.

65. **Fatouros IG, Kambas A, Katrabasas I, Leontsini D, Chatzinikolaou A, Jamurtas AZ, Douroudos I, Aggelousis N and Taxildaris K**. Resistance training and detraining effects on flexibility performance in the elderly are intensity-dependent. *J Strength Cond Res* 20: 634-642, 2006.

66. **Fatouros IG, Kambas A, Katrabasas I, Nikolaidis K, Chatzinikolaou A, Leontsini D and Taxildaris K**. Strength training and detraining effects on muscular strength, anaerobic power, and mobility of inactive older men are intensity dependent. *Br J Sports Med* 39: 776-780, 2005.

67. **Fielding RA, LeBrasseur NK, Cuoco A, Bean J, Mizer K and Fiatarone Singh MA**. High-velocity resistance training increases skeletal muscle peak power in older women. *J Am Geriatr Soc* 50: 655-662, 2002.

68. **Fierobe T, Pons JC, Edouard D, O'Donovan F and Papiernik E**. [Sports and pregnancy. A review of the literature]. *J Gynecol Obstet Biol Reprod (Paris)* 19: 375-381, 1990.

69. **Freeman W, Nute MG and Williams C**. The effect of endurance running training on asthmatic adults. *Br J Sports Med* 23: 115-122, 1989.

70. **Freeman W, Nute MG and Williams C**. The effect of endurance running training on asthmatic adults. *Br J Sports Med* 23: 115-122, 1989.

71. **Freimark D, Shechter M, Schwamenthal E, Tanne D, Elmaleh E, Shemesh Y, Motro M and Adler Y**. Improved exercise tolerance and cardiac function in severe chronic heart failure patients undergoing a supervised exercise program. *Int J Cardiol* 116: 309-314, 2007.

72. **Gaddi O, La Sala GB, Bruno G, Brandi L, Torelli MG, Dall'Asta D and Guiducci U**. [Cardiocirculatory adaptations during the initial phases of pregnancy. An echo-Doppler assessment]. *Minerva Cardioangiol* 37: 481-487, 1989.

73. **Gaesser GA**. Exercise for prevention and treatment of cardiovascular disease, type 2 diabetes, and metabolic syndrome. *Curr Diab Rep* 7: 14-19, 2007.

74. **Galvao DA and Taaffe DR**. Resistance exercise dosage in older adults: single- versus multiset effects on physical performance and body composition. *J Am Geriatr Soc* 53: 2090-2097, 2005.

75. **Giada F, Bertaglia E, De Piccoli B, Franceschi M, Sartori F, Raviele A and Pascotto P**. Cardiovascular adaptations to endurance training and detraining in young and older athletes. *Int J Cardiol* 65: 149-155, 1998.

76. **Goodman LS, McKenzie DC, Nath CR, Schamberger W, Taunton JE and Ammann WC**. Central adaptations in aerobic circuit versus walking/jogging trained cardiac patients. *Can J Appl Physiol* 20: 178-197, 1995.

77. **Hale RW and Milne L**. The elite athlete and exercise in pregnancy. *Semin Perinatol* 20: 277-284, 1996.

78. **Hallstrand TS, Bates PW and Schoene RB**. Aerobic conditioning in mild asthma decreases the hyperpnea of exercise and improves exercise and ventilatory capacity. *Chest* 118: 1460-1469, 2000.

79. **Hallstrand TS, Bates PW and Schoene RB**. Aerobic conditioning in mild asthma decreases the hyperpnea of exercise and improves exercise and ventilatory capacity. *Chest* 118: 1460-1469, 2000.

80. **Hallstrand TS, Bates PW and Schoene RB**. Aerobic conditioning in mild asthma decreases the hyperpnea of exercise and improves exercise and ventilatory capacity. *Chest* 118: 1460-1469, 2000.

81. **Hallstrand TS, Bates PW and Schoene RB**. Aerobic conditioning in mild asthma decreases the hyperpnea of exercise and improves exercise and ventilatory capacity. *Chest* 118: 1460-1469, 2000.

82. **Hallstrand TS, Bates PW and Schoene RB**. Aerobic conditioning in mild asthma decreases the hyperpnea of exercise and improves exercise and ventilatory capacity. *Chest* 118: 1460-1469, 2000.

83. **Hallstrand TS, Bates PW and Schoene RB**. Aerobic conditioning in mild asthma decreases the hyperpnea of exercise and improves exercise and ventilatory capacity. *Chest* 118: 1460-1469, 2000.

84. **Hambrecht R, Adams V, Erbs S, Linke A, Krankel N, Shu Y, Baither Y, Gielen S, Thiele H, Gummert JF, Mohr FW and Schuler G**. Regular physical activity improves endothelial function in patients with coronary artery disease by increasing phosphorylation of endothelial nitric oxide synthase. *Circulation* 107: 3152-3158, 2003.

85. **Hamer M**. The anti-hypertensive effects of exercise: integrating acute and chronic mechanisms. *Sports Med* 36: 109-116, 2006.

86. **Harris KA and Holly RG**. Physiological response to circuit weight training in borderline hypertensive subjects. *Med Sci Sports Exerc* 19: 246-252, 1987.

87. **Henderson NK, White CP and Eisman JA**. The roles of exercise and fall risk reduction in the prevention of osteoporosis. *Endocrinol Metab Clin North Am* 27: 369-387, 1998.

88. **Henwood TR and Taaffe DR**. Short-term resistance training and the older adult: the effect of varied programmes for the enhancement of muscle strength and functional performance. *Clin Physiol Funct Imaging* 26: 305-313, 2006.

89. **Hong SJ, Lee MS, Lee SY, Ahn KM, Oh JW, Kim KE, Lee JS and Lee HB**. High body mass index and dietary pattern are associated with childhood asthma. *Pediatr Pulmonol* 41: 1118-1124, 2006.

90. **Hong SJ, Lee MS, Lee SY, Ahn KM, Oh JW, Kim KE, Lee JS and Lee HB**. High body mass index and dietary pattern are associated with childhood asthma. *Pediatr Pulmonol* 41: 1118-1124, 2006.

91. **Horgan G**. Healthier lifestyles series: 1. Exercise for children. *J Fam Health Care* 15: 15-17, 2005.

92. **Hurley BF and Roth SM**. Strength training in the elderly: effects on risk factors for age-related diseases. *Sports Med* 30: 249-268, 2000.

93. **Hurley BF and Roth SM**. Strength training in the elderly: effects on risk factors for age-related diseases. *Sports Med* 30: 249-268, 2000.

94. **Immanuel S, Bororing SR and Dharma RS**. The effect of aerobic exercise on blood and plasma viscosity on cardiac health club participants. *Acta Med Indones* 38: 185-188, 2006.

95. **Inbar O, Morris N, Epstein Y and Gass G**. Comparison of thermoregulatory responses to exercise in dry heat among prepubertal boys, young adults and older males. *Exp Physiol* 89: 691-700, 2004.

96. **Inbar O, Morris N, Epstein Y and Gass G**. Comparison of thermoregulatory responses to exercise in dry heat among prepubertal boys, young adults and older males. *Exp Physiol* 89: 691-700, 2004.

97. **Inbar O, Morris N, Epstein Y and Gass G**. Comparison of thermoregulatory responses to exercise in dry heat among prepubertal boys, young adults and older males. *Exp Physiol* 89: 691-700, 2004.

98. **Inbar O, Morris N, Epstein Y and Gass G**. Comparison of thermoregulatory responses to exercise in dry heat among prepubertal boys, young adults and older males. *Exp Physiol* 89: 691-700, 2004.

99. **Inbar O, Morris N, Epstein Y and Gass G**. Comparison of thermoregulatory responses to exercise in dry heat among prepubertal boys, young adults and older males. *Exp Physiol* 89: 691-700, 2004.

100. **Jones SE, Merkle SL, Fulton JE, Wheeler LS and Mannino DM**. Relationship between asthma, overweight, and physical activity among U.S. high school students. *J Community Health* 31: 469-478, 2006.

101. **Jonsdottir S, Andersen KK, Sigurosson AF and Sigurosson SB**. The effect of physical training in chronic heart failure. *Eur J Heart Fail* 8: 97-101, 2006.

102. **Jonsdottir S, Andersen KK, Sigurosson AF and Sigurosson SB**. The effect of physical training in chronic heart failure. *Eur J Heart Fail* 8: 97-101, 2006.

103. **Jonsdottir S, Andersen KK, Sigurosson AF and Sigurosson SB**. The effect of physical training in chronic heart failure. *Eur J Heart Fail* 8: 97-101, 2006.

104. **Jovanovic L, Kessler A and Peterson CM**. Human maternal and fetal response to graded exercise. *J Appl Physiol* 58: 1719-1722, 1985.

105. **Kagan KO and Kuhn U**. [Sports and pregnancy]. *Herz* 29: 426-434, 2004.

106. **Kalapotharakos VI, Tokmakidis SP, Smilios I, Michalopoulos M, Gliatis J and Godolias G**. Resistance training in older women: effect on vertical jump and functional performance. *J Sports Med Phys Fitness* 45: 570-575, 2005.

107. **Karacabey K**. Effect of regular exercise on health and disease. *Neuro Endocrinol Lett* 26: 617-623, 2005.

108. **Karani R, McLaughlin MA and Cassel CK**. Exercise in the healthy older adult. *Am J Geriatr Cardiol* 10: 269-273, 2001.

109. **Kardel KR and Kase T**. Training in pregnant women: effects on fetal development and birth. *Am J Obstet Gynecol* 178: 280-286, 1998.

110. **Kardel KR and Kase T**. Training in pregnant women: effects on fetal development and birth. *Am J Obstet Gynecol* 178: 280-286, 1998.

111. **Kardel KR and Kase T**. Training in pregnant women: effects on fetal development and birth. *Am J Obstet Gynecol* 178: 280-286, 1998.

112. **Karlsdottir AE, Foster C, Porcari JP, Palmer-McLean K, White-Kube R and Backes RC**. Hemodynamic responses during aerobic and resistance exercise. *J Cardiopulm Rehabil* 22: 170-177, 2002.

113. **Karlsdottir AE, Foster C, Porcari JP, Palmer-McLean K, White-Kube R and Backes RC**. Hemodynamic responses during aerobic and resistance exercise. *J Cardiopulm Rehabil* 22: 170-177, 2002.

114. **Kelemen MH, Stewart KJ, Gillilan RE, Ewart CK, Valenti SA, Manley JD and Kelemen MD**. Circuit weight training in cardiac patients. *J Am Coll Cardiol* 7: 38-42, 1986.

115. **Kennelly MM, McCaffrey N, McLoughlin P, Lyons S and McKenna P**. Fetal heart rate response to strenuous maternal exercise: not a predictor of fetal distress. *Am J Obstet Gynecol* 187: 811-816, 2002.

116. **Ketelhut RG, Franz IW and Scholze J**. Regular exercise as an effective approach in antihypertensive therapy. *Med Sci Sports Exerc* 36: 4-8, 2004.

117. **Kjaer M, Andersen LB and Hansen IL**. [Physical activity--what minimal level is sufficient seen from health perspective?]. *Ugeskr Laeger* 162: 2164-2169, 2000.

118. **Koshino T**. [Management of regular exercise in pregnant women]. *J Nippon Med Sch* 70: 124-128, 2003.

119. **Kosmas EN, Milic-Emili J, Polychronaki A, Dimitroulis I, Retsou S, Gaga M, Koutsoukou A, Roussos C and Koulouris NG**. Exercise-induced flow limitation, dynamic hyperinflation and exercise capacity in patients with bronchial asthma. *Eur Respir J* 24: 378-384, 2004.

120. **Lanfranco F, Gianotti L, Giordano R, Pellegrino M, Maccario M and Arvat E**. Ageing, growth hormone and physical performance. *J Endocrinol Invest* 26: 861-872, 2003.

121. **Lecomte J**. [Asthma and exercise]. *Rev Med Brux* 23: A206-A210, 2002.

122. **Leon AS**. Physical activity levels and coronary heart disease. Analysis of epidemiologic and supporting studies. *Med Clin North Am* 69: 3-20, 1985.

123. **Levinger I, Bronks R, Cody DV, Linton I and Davie A**. The effect of resistance training on left ventricular function and structure of patients with chronic heart failure. *Int J Cardiol* 105: 159-163, 2005.

124. **Levinger I, Bronks R, Cody DV, Linton I and Davie A**. The effect of resistance training on left ventricular function and structure of patients with chronic heart failure. *Int J Cardiol* 105: 159-163, 2005.

125. **Liu-Ambrose T, Khan KM, Eng JJ, Lord SR and McKay HA**. Balance confidence improves with resistance or agility training. Increase is not correlated with objective changes in fall risk and physical abilities. *Gerontology* 50: 373-382, 2004.

126. **Lochmuller EM and Friese K**. [Pregnancy and sports]. *MMW Fortschr Med* 147: 28-9, 31, 2005.

127. **Lochmuller EM and Friese K**. [Pregnancy and sports]. *MMW Fortschr Med* 147: 28-9, 31, 2005.

128. **Lucas SR and Platts-Mills TA**. Physical activity and exercise in asthma: relevance to etiology and treatment. *J Allergy Clin Immunol* 115: 928-934, 2005.

129. **Lucas SR and Platts-Mills TA**. Physical activity and exercise in asthma: relevance to etiology and treatment. *J Allergy Clin Immunol* 115: 928-934, 2005.

130. **Macaluso A and De Vito G**. Muscle strength, power and adaptations to resistance training in older people. *Eur J Appl Physiol* 91: 450-472, 2004.

131. **Maeda S, Otsuki T, Iemitsu M, Kamioka M, Sugawara J, Kuno S, Ajisaka R and Tanaka H**. Effects of leg resistance training on arterial function in older men. *Br J Sports Med* 40: 867-869, 2006.

132. **Maiorana A, O'Driscoll G, Dembo L, Goodman C, Taylor R and Green D**. Exercise training, vascular function, and functional capacity in middle-aged subjects. *Med Sci Sports Exerc* 33: 2022-2028, 2001.

133. **Maiorana A, O'Driscoll G, Goodman C, Taylor R and Green D**. Combined aerobic and resistance exercise improves glycemic control and fitness in type 2 diabetes. *Diabetes Res Clin Pract* 56: 115-123, 2002.

134. **Malmstrom K, Kaila M, Kajosaari M, Syvanen P and Juntunen-Backman K**. Fatal asthma in finnish children and adolescents 1976-1998: Validity of death certificates and a clinical description. *Pediatr Pulmonol* 42: 210-215, 2007.

135. **McCartney N**. Role of resistance training in heart disease. *Med Sci Sports Exerc* 30: S396-S402, 1998.

136. **McCartney N**. Role of resistance training in heart disease. *Med Sci Sports Exerc* 30: S396-S402, 1998.

137. **McCartney N and McKelvie RS**. The role of resistance training in patients with cardiac disease. *J Cardiovasc Risk* 3: 160-166, 1996.

138. **McLean VA**. Overweight in children: definitions, measurements, confounding factors, and health consequences. *J Pediatr Nurs* 20: 201-202, 2005.

139. **McMurray RG, Mottola MF, Wolfe LA, Artal R, Millar L and Pivarnik JM**. Recent advances in

understanding maternal and fetal responses to exercise. *Med Sci Sports Exerc* 25: 1305-1321, 1993.

140. **Metcalf JA and Roberts SO**. Strength training and the immature athlete: an overview. *Pediatr Nurs* 19: 325-332, 1993.

141. **Meyer K**. Exercise training in heart failure: recommendations based on current research. *Med Sci Sports Exerc* 33: 525-531, 2001.

142. **Meyer K**. Exercise training in heart failure: recommendations based on current research. *Med Sci Sports Exerc* 33: 525-531, 2001.

143. **Meyer K**. Exercise training in heart failure: recommendations based on current research. *Med Sci Sports Exerc* 33: 525-531, 2001.

144. **Meyer K**. Resistance exercise in chronic heart failure-- landmark studies and implications for practice. *Clin Invest Med* 29: 166-169, 2006.

145. **Morris SN and Johnson NR**. Exercise during pregnancy: a critical appraisal of the literature. *J Reprod Med* 50: 181-188, 2005.

146. **Mosher PE, Ferguson MA and Arnold RO**. Lipid and lipoprotein changes in premenstrual women following step aerobic dance training. *Int J Sports Med* 26: 669-674, 2005.

147. **Mosher PE, Nash MS, Perry AC, LaPerriere AR and Goldberg RB**. Aerobic circuit exercise training: effect on adolescents with well-controlled insulin-dependent diabetes mellitus. *Arch Phys Med Rehabil* 79: 652-657, 1998.

148. **Nassis GP, Papantakou K, Skenderi K, Triandafillopoulou M, Kavouras SA, Yannakoulia M, Chrousos GP and Sidossis LS**. Aerobic exercise training improves insulin sensitivity without changes in body weight, body fat, adiponectin, and inflammatory markers in overweight and obese girls. *Metabolism* 54: 1472-1479, 2005.

149. **Nassis GP, Papantakou K, Skenderi K, Triandafillopoulou M, Kavouras SA, Yannakoulia M, Chrousos GP and Sidossis LS**. Aerobic exercise training improves insulin sensitivity without changes in body weight, body fat, adiponectin, and inflammatory markers in overweight and obese girls. *Metabolism* 54: 1472-1479, 2005.

150. **Oldridge NB, Stump TE, Nothwehr FK and Clark DO**. Prevalence and outcomes of comorbid metabolic and cardiovascular conditions in middle- and older-age adults. *J Clin Epidemiol* 54: 928-934, 2001.

151. **Orr R, de Vos NJ, Singh NA, Ross DA, Stavrinos TM and Fiatarone-Singh MA**. Power training improves balance in healthy older adults. *J Gerontol A Biol Sci Med Sci* 61: 78-85, 2006.

152. **Orr R, de Vos NJ, Singh NA, Ross DA, Stavrinos TM and Fiatarone-Singh MA**. Power training improves balance in healthy older adults. *J Gerontol A Biol Sci Med Sci* 61: 78-85, 2006.

153. **Paisley TS, Joy EA and Price RJ, Jr.** Exercise during pregnancy: a practical approach. *Curr Sports Med Rep* 2: 325-330, 2003.

154. **Papademetriou V and Kokkinos PF**. Exercise Training and Blood Pressure Control in Patients With Hypertension. *J Clin Hypertens (Greenwich)* 1: 95-105, 1999.

155. **Perini R, Fisher N, Veicsteinas A and Pendergast DR**. Aerobic training and cardiovascular responses at rest and during exercise in older men and women. *Med Sci Sports Exerc* 34: 700-708, 2002.

156. **Pescatello LS**. Exercise and hypertension: recent advances in exercise prescription. *Curr Hypertens Rep* 7: 281-286, 2005.

157. **Pescatello LS**. Exercise and hypertension: recent advances in exercise prescription. *Curr Hypertens Rep* 7: 281-286, 2005.

158. **Pescatello LS, Franklin BA, Fagard R, Farquhar WB, Kelley GA and Ray CA**. American College of Sports Medicine position stand. Exercise and hypertension. *Med Sci Sports Exerc* 36: 533-553, 2004.

159. **Reichenberg K and Broberg AG**. Emotional and behavioural problems in Swedish 7- to 9-year olds with asthma. *Chron Respir Dis* 1: 183-189, 2004.

160. **Robinson DM, Egglestone DM, Hill PM, Rea HH, Richards GN and Robinson SM**. Effects of a physical conditioning programme on asthmatic patients. *N Z Med J* 105: 253-256, 1992.

161. **Rosamond W, Flegal K, Friday G, Furie K, Go A, Greenlund K, Haase N, Ho M, Howard V, Kissela B, Kittner S, Lloyd-Jones D, McDermott M, Meigs J, Moy C, Nichol G, O'Donnell CJ, Roger V, Rumsfeld J, Sorlie P, Steinberger J, Thom T, Wasserthiel-Smoller S and Hong Y**. Heart disease and stroke statistics--2007 update: a report from the American Heart Association Statistics Committee and Stroke Statistics Subcommittee. *Circulation* 115: e69-171, 2007.

162. **Rudra CB, Williams MA, Lee IM, Miller RS and Sorensen TK**. Perceived exertion during prepregnancy physical activity and preeclampsia risk. *Med Sci Sports Exerc* 37: 1836-1841, 2005.

163. **Santuz P, Baraldi E, Filippone M and Zacchello F**. Exercise performance in children with asthma: is it different from that of healthy controls? *Eur Respir J* 10: 1254-1260, 1997.

164. **Santuz P, Baraldi E, Filippone M and Zacchello F**. Exercise performance in children with asthma: is it different from that of healthy controls? *Eur Respir J* 10: 1254-1260, 1997.

165. **Savage MP, Petratis MM, Thomson WH, Berg K, Smith JL and Sady SP**. Exercise training effects on serum lipids of prepubescent boys and adult men. *Med Sci Sports Exerc* 18: 197-204, 1986.

166. **Shaw BS and Shaw I**. Effect of resistance training on cardiorespiratory endurance and coronary artery disease risk. *Cardiovasc J S Afr* 16: 256-259, 2005.

167. **Shaw BS and Shaw I**. Effect of resistance training on cardiorespiratory endurance and coronary artery disease risk. *Cardiovasc J S Afr* 16: 256-259, 2005.

168. **Shaw BS and Shaw I**. Effect of resistance training on cardiorespiratory endurance and coronary artery disease risk. *Cardiovasc J S Afr* 16: 256-259, 2005.

169. **Shephard RJ**. Management of exercise in the elderly. *Can J Appl Sport Sci* 9: 109-120, 1984.

170. **Shibasaki M, Inoue Y, Kondo N and Iwata A**. Thermoregulatory responses of prepubertal boys and young men during moderate exercise. *Eur J Appl Physiol Occup Physiol* 75: 212-218, 1997.

171. **Simonsick EM, Lafferty ME, Phillips CL, Mendes de Leon CF, Kasl SV, Seeman TE, Fillenbaum G, Hebert P and Lemke JH**. Risk due to inactivity in physically capable older adults. *Am J Public Health* 83: 1443-1450, 1993.

172. **Sparling PB, Cantwell JD, Dolan CM and Niederman RK**. Strength training in a cardiac rehabilitation program: a six-month follow-up. *Arch Phys Med Rehabil* 71: 148-152, 1990.

173. **Spina RJ, Ogawa T, Kohrt WM, Martin WH, III, Holloszy JO and Ehsani AA**. Differences in cardiovascular adaptations to endurance exercise training between older men and women. *J Appl Physiol* 75: 849-855, 1993.

174. **Swain DP and Franklin BA**. Comparison of cardioprotective benefits of vigorous versus moderate intensity aerobic exercise. *Am J Cardiol* 97: 141-147, 2006.

175. **Taaffe DR**. Sarcopenia--exercise as a treatment strategy. *Aust Fam Physician* 35: 130-134, 2006.

176. **Taaffe DR**. Sarcopenia--exercise as a treatment strategy. *Aust Fam Physician* 35: 130-134, 2006.

177. **Tanaka H and Shindo M**. Running velocity at blood lactate threshold of boys aged 6-15 years compared with untrained and trained young males. *Int J Sports Med* 6: 90-94, 1985.

178. **Taylor AH, Cable NT, Faulkner G, Hillsdon M, Narici M and Van Der Bij AK**. Physical activity and older adults: a review of health benefits and the effectiveness of interventions. *J Sports Sci* 22: 703-725, 2004.

179. **Thomas DE, Elliott EJ and Naughton GA**. Exercise for type 2 diabetes mellitus. *Cochrane Database Syst Rev* 3: CD002968, 2006.

180. **Todaro A**. [Physical activities and sports in asthmatic patients]. *Minerva Med* 74: 1349-1356, 1983.

181. **Tokmakidis SP, Zois CE, Volaklis KA, Kotsa K and Touvra AM**. The effects of a combined strength and aerobic exercise program on glucose control and insulin action in women with type 2 diabetes. *Eur J Appl Physiol* 92: 437-442, 2004.

182. **Toman J, Spinarova L, Kara T, Soucek M, Zatloukal B and Lukas Z**. [Physical training in patients with chronic heart failure: functional fitness and the role of the periphery]. *Vnitr Lek* 47: 74-80, 2001.

183. **Turley KR**. Cardiovascular responses to exercise in children. *Sports Med* 24: 241-257, 1997.

184. **Turley KR**. Cardiovascular responses to exercise in children. *Sports Med* 24: 241-257, 1997.

185. **Turley KR**. Cardiovascular responses to exercise in children. *Sports Med* 24: 241-257, 1997.

186. **Turley KR and Wilmore JH**. Cardiovascular responses to treadmill and cycle ergometer exercise in children and adults. *J Appl Physiol* 83: 948-957, 1997.

187. **Uzendoski AM, Latin RW, Berg KE and Moshier S**. Physiological responses to aerobic exercise during pregnancy and post-partum. *J Sports Med Phys Fitness* 30: 77-82, 1990.

188. **van Doorn MB, Lotgering FK, Struijk PC, Pool J and Wallenburg HC**. Maternal and fetal cardiovascular responses to strenuous bicycle exercise. *Am J Obstet Gynecol* 166: 854-859, 1992.

189. **Verrill D, Shoup E, McElveen G, Witt K and Bergey D**. Resistive exercise training in cardiac patients. Recommendations. *Sports Med* 13: 171-193, 1992.

190. **Verrill D, Shoup E, McElveen G, Witt K and Bergey D**. Resistive exercise training in cardiac patients. Recommendations. *Sports Med* 13: 171-193, 1992.

191. **Vincent KR, Vincent HK, Braith RW, Bhatnagar V and Lowenthal DT**. Strength training and hemodynamic responses to exercise. *Am J Geriatr Cardiol* 12: 97-106, 2003.

192. **Volaklis KA and Tokmakidis SP**. Resistance exercise training in patients with heart failure. *Sports Med* 35: 1085-1103, 2005.

193. **Wadden TA and Stunkard AJ**. Social and psychological consequences of obesity. *Ann Intern Med* 103: 1062-1067, 1985.

194. **Wadden TA and Stunkard AJ**. Social and psychological consequences of obesity. *Ann Intern Med* 103: 1062-1067, 1985.

195. **Webb DR**. Strength training in children and adolescents. *Pediatr Clin North Am* 37: 1187-1210, 1990.

196. **Weissgerber TL, Wolfe LA and Davies GA**. The role of regular physical activity in preeclampsia prevention. *Med Sci Sports Exerc* 36: 2024-2031, 2004.

197. **Weissgerber TL, Wolfe LA and Davies GA**. The role of regular physical activity in preeclampsia prevention. *Med Sci Sports Exerc* 36: 2024-2031, 2004.

198. **Welsh L, Kemp JG and Roberts RG**. Effects of physical conditioning on children and adolescents with asthma. *Sports Med* 35: 127-141, 2005.

199. **Welsh L, Kemp JG and Roberts RG**. Effects of physical conditioning on children and adolescents with asthma. *Sports Med* 35: 127-141, 2005.

200. **Whelton SP, Chin A, Xin X and He J**. Effect of aerobic exercise on blood pressure: a meta-analysis of randomized, controlled trials. *Ann Intern Med* 136: 493-503, 2002.

201. **Wilmore JH, Green JS, Stanforth PR, Gagnon J, Rankinen T, Leon AS, Rao DC, Skinner JS and Bouchard C**. Relationship of changes in maximal and submaximal aerobic fitness to changes in cardiovascular disease and non-insulin-dependent diabetes mellitus risk factors with endurance training: the HERITAGE Family Study. *Metabolism* 50: 1255-1263, 2001.

202. **Wilmore JH, Green JS, Stanforth PR, Gagnon J, Rankinen T, Leon AS, Rao DC, Skinner JS and Bouchard C**. Relationship of changes in maximal and submaximal aerobic fitness to changes in cardiovascular disease and non-insulin-dependent diabetes mellitus risk factors with endurance training: the HERITAGE Family Study. *Metabolism* 50: 1255-1263, 2001.

203. **Winett RA and Carpinelli RN**. Potential health-related benefits of resistance training. *Prev Med* 33: 503-513, 2001.

204. **Wolfe LA, Hall P, Webb KA, Goodman L, Monga M and McGrath MJ**. Prescription of aerobic exercise during pregnancy. *Sports Med* 8: 273-301, 1989.

205. **Yeo S and Davidge ST**. Possible beneficial effect of exercise, by reducing oxidative stress, on the incidence of preeclampsia. *J Womens Health Gend Based Med* 10: 983-989, 2001.

206. **Yeo S and Davidge ST**. Possible beneficial effect of exercise, by reducing oxidative stress, on the incidence of preeclampsia. *J Womens Health Gend Based Med* 10: 983-989, 2001.

207. **Zhang C, Solomon CG, Manson JE and Hu FB**. A prospective study of pregravid physical activity and sedentary behaviors in relation to the risk for gestational diabetes mellitus. *Arch Intern Med* 166: 543-548, 2006.

208. **Zhang C, Solomon CG, Manson JE and Hu FB**. A prospective study of pregravid physical activity and sedentary behaviors in relation to the risk for gestational diabetes mellitus. *Arch Intern Med* 166: 543-548, 2006.

Chapter 23

Ethics & Professional Behavior

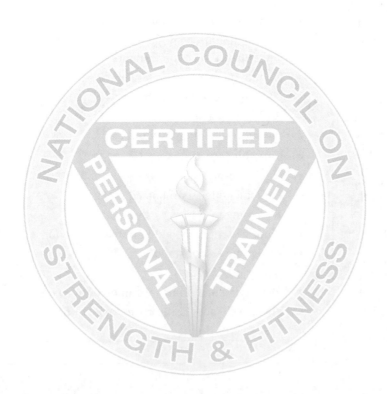

What Makes a Professional

The personal trainer profession is evolving into a recognized and respected part of the allied health care system of support. An important part of the ongoing development of the industry is the advancement of professional competencies and the elevation of standards of practice (21). Establishing the highest level of professionalism within the industry will ensure growth and future opportunity within the field. Professionalism starts with the desire to achieve greatness within one's chosen field of practice (7). Striving to reach the highest level of the profession is a personal attribute that leads to success (4). This suggests that to perform optimally within a profession, one must identify the qualities that are possessed and exemplified by the most successful and respected practitioners.

Professionalism is defined as the conduct, aims, or qualities that characterize or mark a profession or a professional person. It is not just attained from the desire to achieve in one's chosen field but also originates from performance of routine actions, compliance with industry standards, and management of external perceptions (20). Importantly, external perception is often the measure that consumers use for judgment of professionalism. Perception is commonly defined by outward appearance, ability to communicate, pursuit of inquiry to remain updated within the field, and conveying confidence. For many people, appearance is the first measure of professionalism (12). It suggests that the attention to detail and the level of seriousness one takes in appearance is similar to the considerations made for other components of the job. Proper grooming and appropriate attire conveys self-respect and an interest in how one is perceived. Presentation comprises a significant portion of impression. Therefore, personal trainers should routinely make a conscious effort to look professional.

The ability to communicate is often considered an extension of social intelligence. Successful professionals maintain the ability to instill confidence in their knowledge and abilities upon others by way of physical and verbal communication. Communication skills are valuable when working with people, as they are not only used to pass information but also convey emotions. Physical and verbal communications can express care, support, empathy, interest, and enthusiasm (13). All of these features are considered central to effective personal trainer services. Professional communication should be clear, accurate, and relevant. In some cases, it is challenging to state the facts rather than to simply say what wants to be heard. Thus, employing proper judgment and tact are part of being a good communicator.

Inquiry is a characteristic that is often attributed to successful personal trainer practice. Inquiry suggests the continued pursuit of knowledge and professional development. Complacency in the professional environments negatively impacts effectiveness. Due to the extensiveness of new information, research, and protocols that are emerging within the fitness industry, knowing everything is impossible. New information is presented everyday and practices are regularly evolving to include new techniques. However, interest in improving one's knowledge and competency is necessary to remain current in such a dynamic profession.

Confidence is a quality that people look for in a professional. Although less tangible, confidence can be observed. Confidence stems from a compilation of attributes, including self-assurance, belief in one's abilities and knowledge, self-efficacy, and experience. When someone does not have confidence in a particular environment, others perceive a deficiency or compromise in one's abilities. This is not to suggest that something is wrong with the person but rather that others place trust in those individuals who possess confidence in themselves and their ability to perform effectively.

Common Professional Behaviors

- Being punctual and schedule conscious.
- Responding in a timely manner to email, phone messages, and outstanding commitments.
- Communicating accurately and clearly.
- Upholding commitments.
- Premeditating action.
- Performing routine follow-up.
- Providing prompt feedback.
- Documenting operations.
- Implementing an organized system.
- Accessing resources.
- Thinking critically and in unbiased fashion.
- Accepting responsibility.
- Being task driven.
- Identifying and improving upon deficiencies.
- Proactively addressing issues and conflict.

The measure of professionalism encompasses more than personal characteristics and presentation, as it is also based on actions, principles, and an individual's decision making process. Professional actions are those that demonstrate effectiveness in one's job, convey aptitude and competency, and identify a practitioner as skilled, diligent, and resourceful (22). When a person acts in a professional manner, he or she exemplifies the traits expected of the model practitioner. Regardless of the profession, effective people present similarities within their daily routines and professional behaviors.

Professional Principles

Professional principles support actions and decisions and enable a practitioner to develop the appropriate behaviors pertaining to the chosen career. Each profession has a slightly different application of professional principles determined by governing bodies, employer requirements, and consumer expectations and demands. Professional principles provide the framework for conformity to an industry standard. They are used to adapt the proper behavior and attitude toward the job tasks which are relevant to the values of the profession and enable the developing professional to identify the competencies required in order to become an effective contributor to the profession.

Interpersonal Relations & Communication

The basic principle of communication defines the manner in which interpersonal skills are applied to maintain good relations within the work environment. They include use of professional language when speaking with clients and colleagues and the process of proper dissemination and articulation of information.

Professional Compliance

The principle of compliance suggests making decisions based on established norms within the profession. Providing evidence-based information and practice and acting in a manner appropriate to defined standards and guidelines falls under the principle of professional compliance.

Professional Judgment & Autonomy

Also based on preconceived values, this principle guides the decision-making process to protect the stakeholders of the profession, including those who receive professional services. Autonomy suggests self-governance in accordance with the highest expectations of the governing body. This principle supports professional accountability.

Professional Ethics

The principle of ethics holds those acting in a professional role to make an ethical covenant with society to exercise judgment in the best interest of all others. It encompasses all the principles and standards that underlie one's responsibilities and conduct in a particular field of expertise (profession). It requires practitioners to act in a fiduciary role to fulfill the highest ideals and core values of both the profession and discipline.

Self Discipline

This principle reflects the structured approach to the management of professional activity as it places expectations on premeditated and conscience-driven work ethics. Self discipline entails both restraint and diligence.

The principles of a profession embody the professional standards by which practitioners perform their trade (11). The personal trainer is held to a standardized code of conduct that, at a minimum, ensures safe and professional practice. Professional standards allow for critical evaluation and the accountability of the practitioner to all stakeholders of the profession. Most professional standards incorporate clearly articulated requirements and specific guidelines as to how to practice correctly. These requirements and guidelines are developed in accordance with evidence-based criteria, social responsibility, and uniformly accepted norms within a profession (8).

Professional Standards

Professional standards distill expectations of what constitutes sound and proper practices by identifying fundamental ethical considerations, while addressing more specific acts of professional conduct. Secondarily, they may serve as a basis for judging the merit of a formal complaint pertaining to violations of professional and ethical standards. Defined standards provide guidance for professional behaviors, activities, and decision-making process and serve as a framework for self-evaluation (10). They outline the benchmark as defined by peers within the profession and should be used as the foundation by which a professional practice is built. In addition, professional standards are as evolving as the profession they serve and provide ongoing contributions to the integrity and ultimately the respect of the profession.

Every day fitness professionals are required to make decisions regarding different aspects of their job responsibilities. In some cases, the decisions are rudimentary and imply minimal consequences, while other decisions may have serious repercussions if not

---

Common Standards of the Personal Trainer Profession

1. Validly assessed and documented attainment of the minimal competency standards.
2. Proper representation of one's academic achievement, skills, and abilities.
3. Practicing within the defined scope of the profession.
4. Commitment to continued learning and the maintenance of professional competency.
5. Protection of the privacy of clients by not disclosing information to third parties, unless required by law.
6. Maintaining appropriate files, and documenting all professional activity.
7. Providing proper screening and evaluation, acquiring proper medical clearance when required.
8. The referral of clients to the appropriate health care practitioners, as needed.
9. Establishing and delivering the highest quality services.
10. Implementing strategies and management services in accordance with evidence-based criteria.
11. Avoiding conflict of interest, improper dissemination of information, and false representation on any level.
12. Calling attention to unethical, illegal, and unsafe behaviors by other professionals.

---

made with prudent deliberation. The ability to make the right decision in a situation is based on several factors that stem from the aforementioned composite of what makes a quality professional. Professional decision making is actually a formatted cognitive process, which uses analytical and critical thinking to determine the ideal conclusion for a situation, conflict, or problem (14).

Professional decision making requires one to evaluate a problem, gather information, develop alternative solutions, weigh each alternative objectively, and select the best choice based on the facts presented. Essentially, the decision making process leads to the selection of a course of action among the alternatives. Decision making is a process of reasoning based on known and potential factors and assumptions. Structured rational decision making is an important part of all science-based professions. This identifies why adequate competency is necessary. One must apply one's knowledge in a given area when making informed decisions. As one's level of expertise increases, intuitive decision making may replace a more structured approach because the professional is better able to recognize a set of indicators from experience in similar situations (6). Expertise suggests the ability to define a course of action without weighing all the alternatives, secondary to accrued knowledge and experience.

The Professional Decision-Making Process

1) Identify the problem – Is it a goal, challenge, or opportunity?

2) Gather information – Collect facts and data; differentiate opinion and assumptions; consider professional boundaries; identify the stakeholders.

3) Develop alternatives – Establish criteria, consider all the aspects, and look at precedence.

4) Weigh the alternatives - Identify the advantages and disadvantages, benefits and consequences of each option.

5) Select the best course of action – Rank by appropriateness, suitability, and benefit vs. consequence relationship.

6) Implement the solution – Premeditate a plan, properly communicate; adapt to the situation or individual.

7) Monitor the effect – Analyze the process or the result, could anything be improved upon?

8) Analyze the outcome – Learn from your actions.

9) Record your findings – Use for future decision-making.

Following this process will help to create the best solution for the problems presented in professional situations. As one gains experience, the rapidity of the process and implementation of pre-learned actions to common problems creates an increased level of professional proficiency and expertise. Experts are those who have dealt with many situations, deliberated upon all of the alternatives and learned from the outcomes. This suggests that the decision-making process is a combination of both on-the-job learning, as well as more traditional knowledge attainment. This explains why inquiry is a fundamental component of effective professionalism.

The decision-making process calls on many aspects of cognitive function. One inherent component that is always applied within a professional decision is one's ethics. Personal ethics and professional ethics may differ, but they are linked by a single foundation. Ethics is defined as the enterprise of disciplined reflection on moral intuitions and moral choices, or, more simply put, a system of moral principles within each person (19). Professional ethics are the moral principles defined within a profession, which determine acceptable practices, including actions, communications, and behaviors. In most cases, governing organizations will define ethical conduct based on peer determined criteria which are intended to protect the primary stakeholders of the profession. Ethics help to formulate the standards of practice and therefore, are often categorized into specific components of the profession. In personal training, professional ethics include the following:

> Representation of Expertise
> Professional Client Relationship
> Aspiration of the Profession
> Professional Competence
> Conflicts of Interest
> Societal Responsibilities

Representation of Expertise

Personal trainers are expected to be honest and trustworthy. This includes factually representing one's academic background and degrees, validly measured knowledge, and experience. It has been suggested that nearly one-third of the resumes presented for American jobs are not accurate representations of the individual or have been falsified in some manner (16). Professional ethics suggest being truthful in all forms of communication. A common occurrence within the fitness industry that weighs on the ethics of representation is the assignment of a credential or distinction without valid assessment of one's competency. Taking a weekend course that provides a

certification does not represent the attainment of expertise. Often, the distinction of "specialist" or "certified" is used to make the education course more marketable, but unless the credential is backed by a validly-constructed, psychometrically-analyzed, and proctored examination, the document is simply a certificate of completion for a continued education course. The course may provide some valuable information on a subject, but it is inappropriate to represent oneself as an expert from a weeklong or weekend course. It is appropriate to market oneself as having taken educational course work in that particular area within the discipline.

Professional Client Relationship

Within the professional role, the personal trainer makes an ethical covenant with all stakeholders of the profession to act in the best interest of all others. This suggests placing the welfare of others central to all considerations within the professional domain. The client/professional relationship, in particular, has an ethical basis and is built on confidentiality, trust, and honesty (17). This requires the establishment of boundaries. Boundaries are the limits that allow for safe connection between individuals. With defined boundaries, appropriate levels of human intimacy and the maintenance of trust are possible. Unclear boundaries can lead to inappropriateness within the relationship. The professional is in a position of power because the expectation of trust rests on the assumption that the professional will operate in the context of the best interest of the client. Boundary violations occur when the power of trust is misused. If, at anytime, ethics may be compromised by the dynamics of the client/professional relationship, the personal trainer has the responsibility to withdraw from providing professional services.

Aspiration of the Profession

In addition to the responsibility a personal trainer has to the client, he or she also has responsibilities to the profession. The ethics of aspiration represent one's effort to attain a level of aptitude consistent with the defined professional standards and to represent the profession based on the ideals and core values of the discipline. Compliance with the professional standards and code of conduct is an ethical responsibility of all personal trainers. When the members of a profession strive to reach a higher standard, the entire profession reaches a new benchmark, leading to advancement. Performing at a sub-par level by not complying with accepted standards is unethical with regard to personal responsibility to the profession.

Professional Competence

Professional aspiration is consistent with the ethical responsibility of a personal trainer to remain current in the skills and knowledge of the profession. Personal trainers owe it to the stakeholders of the profession to attain appropriate competency and to maintain the defined acceptable level throughout one's career. Individuals who possess professional credentials are mandated by the governing body to earn continued education credits to maintain their certified or licensed status. With regard to considerations for professional ethics, personal trainers should identify their deficiencies and focus their efforts on improving their competency within those areas. Taking coursework that provides new challenges and leads to improved skill and comprehension is the ethical path, whereas collecting continued education credits in other manners, such as through professional contacts, or falsification of professional activities in any way, constitutes unethical practice (1).

Conflicts of Interest

It is the personal trainer's ethical responsibility to avoid conflicts of interest. A conflict of interest is defined by an influence that compromises the objectivity in one's professional decision making, based on self interest (18). When acting in a professional role, personal trainers have a duty to serve the stakeholders of the profession above serving self interest. Conflicts of interest interfere with objective professional judgment and may lead to concessions that are not in the best interest of others (3). Potential conflicts of interest may arise from commercial promotions of fitness or health related products and services which may generate bias unrelated to product merit, creating, or appearing to create, an inappropriate, undue influence. The trainer should be aware of this potential conflict of interest and offer fitness advice that is as accurate, balanced, complete, and devoid of bias. When the trainer receives anything of substantial value, including royalties, from companies in the healthcare industry, such as a manufacturer of supplements and fitness devices, this fact should be disclosed to clients and colleagues.

Societal Responsibilities

Responsibility to society is also of ethical concern to the personal trainer profession. Personal trainers should support and participate in those health programs, practices, and activities that contribute positively and in a meaningful and effective way to the welfare of individual clients, the health and fitness community, or the public good. Personal trainers who provide expert testimony in courts of law recognize their duty to testify truthfully. The trainer should not testify concerning matters about which he or she is not knowledgeable.

The trainer should be prepared to have testimony given in any judicial proceeding subjected to peer review by an institution or professional organization to which he or she belongs. It is unethical for a trainer to accept compensation that is contingent upon the outcome of litigation.

Risk Management

Ethics, standards, and guidelines are established to provide the framework for professional practices. In addition to accounting for the homogenous delivery of service, the peer-defined minimal acceptable standards are used as a guide for risk management, particularly as they pertain to litigation (5). The protection of the stakeholders is the primary objective of health and fitness professionals. This is accomplished through the anticipation, recognition, and control of risk in occupational environments. Similar to decision making, consideration for the existence of risk and how to manage it requires a structured process. The comprehensive framework for risk assessment and management includes several stages of analysis. It is simply a process of reviewing historical precedence related to the outcome of different strategies, looking at the probability of incidence, analyzing the factors that contribute to risk, and identifying control mechanisms that affect the probability of occurrence (15).

The first step to risk management is to be aware of possible risk factors and areas where they commonly exist. There are generally three categories of risk with which a personal trainer must contend. They include participant risk, environment risk, and professional risk (2). Within these categories exists internal and external risk factors. External risks are sources of risk that a trainer has no direct control over but may be able to predict. This may have to do with changes in business dynamics, such as the reduction in training hours over the holiday season, or be related to the risk of your client getting hit by an object dropped by a third party in the weight room. Although there exists no direct control over the risk, analyzing the situation and predicting the possibility of a circumstance arising allows one to better reduce the risk of the negative event occurring by being proactive. Internal risks are those over which a personal trainer has a level of control. The effect or level of control over the risk is based on all the activities incurred in a risk management program.

Participant Risk

Participant risk is of significant concern because, of the three categories of risk, it is most commonly linked with direct liability and legal action. Injury is inherent to physical activity and, therefore, risk for an injury occurring exists on a daily basis. Personal trainers must contend with this risk by implementing appropriate risk management behaviors. Screening participants, using client appropriate protocols, maintaining safe work environments, and instructing proper technique all contribute positively to this goal.

Environmental Risks

Environmental risks are those that affect your business. Changes in the business environment can lead to financial shifts; for instance, poor economy may reduce consumer spending and those who once had expendable income for personal training may not be able to afford the service. A hurricane or long period of inclement weather, a car accident, or an injury may all be forms of environmental risks that can adversely affect a personal trainer's ability to successfully participate in his or her trade. The degree of risk and the ratio of external to internal risk factors can be analyzed to determine what actions can be used to reduce the effect of any issues arising from environment risk.

Professional Risks

Professional risks are those that directly relate to one's professional activity. Every employee has a risk of being fired for one reason or another, but by performing at a high standard, the risk is well-managed and may never become an issue. Professional risks may come from employers, competition in a business environment, or changes within the profession. Forgetting to renew one's personal trainer or CPR certification may increase professional risk by removing the mechanisms which protect against a particular risk. Likewise, not maintaining professional liability coverage may increase susceptibility to a negative outcome.

Each area of risk presents different and unique situations that must be managed. In some cases, the risk is related to an independent and relatively rare circumstance and therefore, may not require ongoing effort to manage. In other cases, the risk may be experienced everyday, requiring a structured and consistent action or behavior as a staple to one's daily professional activities. When risk management planning occurs, the goal is to identify, prevent, and minimize problems. Assessing each situation will help identify any and all risks, as well as the level of risk and related circumstances that increase the prevalence of a particular risk so that a management plan to adequately address each possible problem is created. This process serves as an internal audit of one's business activities and commonly leads to dramatic improvements in the overall delivery of service, more efficient use of resources, better business management, and an improved grasp on one's professional career or business.

The six steps of risk management should be applied to each facet of one's professional career. In doing so, the actual extent of risk that exists becomes quantified. Many personal trainers do not realize the potential risks they experience everyday because they are not aware the risk exists and do not fully understand the magnitude of the risk and the associated consequences. The more educated a person becomes as a professional and about the environment he or she works in, the more the risks become evident. Professional governing bodies are most often comprised of individuals with high levels of expertise in the field of practice. Part of that expertise lies in understanding the dynamics of the profession and the risks associated with practicing within the trade. Standards and protocols are formed by peer committees as a way of helping the profession contend with risk by implementing standardized practices. Personal trainers should become proficient in the standards of conduct and practice, as well as the skill-set protocols defined by the profession as necessary for delivery of safe and effective professional activities.

In the context of the personal training profession, numerous strategies can reduce risk and aid in effective delivery of services. For most situations, there are clearly defined best approaches that have been developed from a historic perspective but have strong relevance in today's personal training environments. Other situations may require a level of resourcefulness and research to find an effective management strategy used by other professions for similar situations (9). The following recommendations will aid in the development of a comprehensive risk management plan and are in compliance with the minimum expectations of the professional personal trainer.

The Six Steps of Risk Management

1. Identifying risk.
2. Measuring its extent or the magnitude of the risk, and its associated level of consequence.
3. Formulating strategies to prevent or limit the risk.
4. Evaluating each strategy and comparing the benefit summary.
5. Selecting and implementing the strategy.
6. Continuously monitoring the effort and updating the plan as new risk is defined and new resources become available.

Scope of Practice

Although no licensure exists in personal training, the scope of practice has been defined to acknowledge acceptable and unacceptable activities based on credentialed qualifications and education. A personal trainer's emphasis is on improving health and physical fitness while acting to prevent disease, premature aging, and the onset of health problems. Personal trainers are not able to diagnose medical problems or serve the role of any other defined health care provider, including physical therapists, athletic trainers, registered dietitians, and rehabilitation therapists. Acting outside the scope of the profession is unethical and in many cases illegal.

Standard Protocols

Personal trainers must become proficient in the standardized protocols and guidelines used by the profession. These standards and guidelines have been established for safe and effective practice in the best interest of the client. Foregoing a standardized approach is within the rights of a professional when justified by adequate evidence. However, anytime activities fall outside the norm, the risk for negative consequences increases. The actual risk and extent of the consequences should be evaluated before making a professional decision.

Emergency/Safety Procedures

Personal trainers owe their clients a duty of care. This duty is often what is called into question during litigation. To satisfy their legal requirements, personal trainers must comply with established safety protocols and implement the necessary safety and emergency procedures, as warranted by a given situation. Although the highest degree of safety should be the goal, personal trainers are held responsible to an acceptable level as defined by what a sensible person would do in the same situation. Taking the time to ensure a client's safety and defining emergency procedures in the event of a serious situation contributes greatly to reducing risk for liability.

Documentation

In any health-related profession, documentation is required and necessary for effective delivery of services. Documenting test outcomes, tracking program activities, and maintaining client files are all requisite acts of the personal trainer. This allows for optimal use of the data as criteria for program decision making. If an incident occurs that requires evidence to the nature of the professional activities, personal trainers must present their documentation during a legal preceding. Improperly documenting activities, or not documenting

at all, will dramatically increase related risk. Some common documents used by personal trainers to manage risk and effectively deliver services include informed consent, screening forms, screening notes and findings, program documents and tracking records, accident reporting forms, emergency plans, and equipment safety check forms. Documents should be maintained for one year past the statute of limitations of the state where the services were rendered.

Program Implementation

It is expected that personal trainers comply with standard operational procedures to initiate client participation in an exercise program. This includes following the guidelines for screening, program decision making, physical evaluation, and program activity management. The everyday activities supervised by personal trainers should be performed with the highest regard for client safety. This includes instruction, supervision, and spotting, as well as implementing components such as warm-up and cool down protocols. Taking short cuts or not focusing on the job at hand may lead to increased risk.

Liability Coverage

Personal trainers should maintain an appropriate amount of personal liability insurance in the event that a lawsuit is filed and the verdict is not favorable. A general rule of thumb is to maintain enough coverage that one's professional practice will not be disabled due to a temporary loss of coverage related to aggregate limits. Validly credentialed professionals can purchase $2 million of coverage for about $200 per year.

Although the utopian situation in any profession is never to experience any negative consequences associated with one's job, inevitably some risk factors will create a situation that must be managed. When risk management evolves into situational management, the goal should be to minimize the effects of the problem. Taking the right steps during and immediately following an occurrence will aid in diffusing the problem or limiting the extent of the damage. Personal trainers should establish a plan to deal with each situation that has a high probability of occurring or which will have the greatest impact on a professional career.

When things go wrong, the following recommendations may assist in several different types of situations.

Caution
Take a cautious approach in the face of uncertainty. Waiting for more information or a better emotional state

will help with rational decision making. Jumping quickly to act may be a poor decision.

Communicate

Maintain open channels of communication and communicate effectively with all parties involved. Always be as respectful and genuine as possible and emphasize listening.

Follow-up

Follow-up on each aspect of the situation and with all parties involved. People are likely to react far more passively if they feel their interests are attended to.

Document

Document the situation as soon as possible to maintain the integrity of the facts; use witnesses whenever possible.

Evaluate

Evaluate the potential extent of the damage and identify controls that may limit the overall magnitude of damage.

The Best Risk Management Plans:

1. Are structured by comprehensive and sound principles, which provide the integral framework of the plan.

2. Consider the problem and the risk within the full context of the situation, using a broad perspective. This is done by acknowledging, incorporating, and balancing the multi-dimensions of risk.

3. Ensure the highest degree of reliability for all components of the risk management process so accuracy is validated, as assumption itself is a risk.

4. Commit to routine implementation of strategies and the ongoing process of tracking outcomes.

5. Change with the identification of new facts and resources.

Chapter Twenty-Three References

1. **Barnette M**. Credentialing, accountability, & ethics. Keys to home care PPS. *Caring* 20: 26-30, 2001.

2. **Bloche MG**. The invention of health law. *Calif Law Rev* 91: 247-322, 2003.

3. **Coulehan J, Williams PC, McCrary SV and Belling C**. The best lack all conviction: biomedical ethics, professionalism, and social responsibility. *Camb Q Healthc Ethics* 12: 21-38, 2003.

4. **Cruess RL**. Teaching professionalism: theory, principles, and practices. *Clin Orthop Relat Res* 449: 177-185, 2006.

5. **Feld AD and Walta D**. Malpractice, tort reform, and you: an introduction to risk management. *Am J Gastroenterol* 99: 192-193, 2004.

6. **Gagliardi J**. Management responsibility enables success. *Biomed Instrum Technol* 40: 222-224, 2006.

7. **Gauss JW**. Integrity is integral to career success. *Healthc Financ Manage* 54: 89, 2000.

8. **Hall KD**. Student development and ownership of ethical and professional standards. *Sci Eng Ethics* 10: 383-387, 2004.

9. **Heckman FD and Zaremski MJ**. The business plan to manage high-damage liability lawsuits. *Physician Exec* 20: 10-13, 1994.

10. **Keffer JH**. Guidelines and algorithms: perceptions of why and when they are successful and how to improve them. *Clin Chem* 47: 1563-1572, 2001.

11. **Keffer JH**. Guidelines and algorithms: perceptions of why and when they are successful and how to improve them. *Clin Chem* 47: 1563-1572, 2001.

12. **Livingston J**. Dressing for success: professionalism in appearance. *J Hosp Admit Manage* 13: 11, 1987.

13. **Lopopolo RB, Schafer DS and Nosse LJ**. Leadership, administration, management, and professionalism (LAMP) in physical therapy: a Delphi study. *Phys Ther* 84: 137-150, 2004.

14. **Oliphant CA**. Professionalism: key to success in time of crisis. *Hosp Manage Commun* 6: 2-4, 1982.

15. **Olver J, Jr. and West DJ, Jr.** Practice compliance programs: reducing therapeutic misadventures and adverse outcomes. *J Med Pract Manage* 15: 187-193, 2000.

16. **Sachs L**. Verifying a job applicant's factual credentials. *J Med Pract Manage* 17: 196-199, 2002.

17. **Schick IC and Guo L**. Ethics committees identify success factors: a national survey. *HEC Forum* 13: 344-360, 2001.

18. **Schick IC and Guo L**. Ethics committees identify success factors: a national survey. *HEC Forum* 13: 344-360, 2001.

19. **Summers JW**. Doing good and doing well: ethics, professionalism, and success. *Hosp Health Serv Adm* 29: 84-100, 1984.

20. **Surdyk PM, Lynch DC and Leach DC**. Professionalism: identifying current themes. *Curr Opin Anaesthesiol* 16: 597-602, 2003.

21. **Surdyk PM, Lynch DC and Leach DC**. Professionalism: identifying current themes. *Curr Opin Anaesthesiol* 16: 597-602, 2003.

22. **Urusmambetov S**. [High professionalism--a pledge of success]. *Med Sestra* 47: 22-24, 1988.

INDEX

*NOTE – **Bold** numbers indicate pages where "key term" definitions can be found in the text.